SECOND EDITION

ADVANCED ASSESSMENT

Interpreting Findings and Formulating Differential Diagnoses

SECOND EDITION

ADVANCED ASSESSMENT

Interpreting Findings and Formulating Differential Diagnoses

Mary Jo Goolsby, EdD, MSN, ANP-C, CAE, FAANP
Director of Research and Education
American Academy of Nurse Practitioners
Austin, Texas

Laurie Grubbs, PhD, MSN, ANP-C
Professor
Florida State University
College of Nursing
Tallahassee, Florida

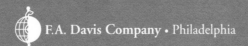
F.A. Davis Company • Philadelphia

F. A. Davis Company
1915 Arch Street
Philadelphia, PA 19103
www.fadavis.com

Printed in the United States of America

Last digit indicates print number: 10 9 8 7 6 5 4

Publisher: Joanne Patzek DaCunha, RN, MSN
Director of Content Development: Darlene D. Pedersen
Project Editor: Christina C. Burns
Design Manager: Carolyn O'Brien

As new scientific information becomes available through basic and clinical research, recommended treatments and drug therapies undergo changes. The author(s) and publisher have done everything possible to make this book accurate, up to date, and in accord with accepted standards at the time of publication. The author(s), editors, and publisher are not responsible for errors or omissions or for consequences from application of the book, and make no warranty, expressed or implied, in regard to the contents of the book. Any practice described in this book should be applied by the reader in accordance with professional standards of care used in regard to the unique circumstances that may apply in each situation. The reader is advised always to check product information (package inserts) for changes and new information regarding dose and contraindications before administering any drug. Caution is especially urged when using new or infrequently ordered drugs.

Library of Congress Cataloging-in-Publication Data

Advanced assessment: interpreting findings and formulating differential diagnoses / [edited by] Mary Jo Goolsby, Laurie Grubbs. —2nd ed.
    p. ; cm.
Includes bibliographical references and index.
ISBN-13: 978-0-8036-2172-5
ISBN-10: 0-8036-2172-8
1. Diagnosis, Differential. 2. Nursing assessment. 3. Nurse practitioners.
I. Goolsby, Mary Jo. II. Grubbs, Laurie, 1951–
[DNLM: 1. Nursing Assessment—methods. 2. Diagnosis, Differential.
3. Nurse Practitioners. WY 100.4]
RC71.5.A345 2011
616.07'5—dc22

2011002267

Preface

The idea for this book evolved over several years while teaching an advanced health assessment course designed primarily for nurse practitioner (NP) students. Although many health assessment texts have been available, they have lacked an essential component—the information needed to arrive at a reasonably narrow differential diagnosis of a patient who presents with one of the almost endless possible complaints. The response to the first edition of this text supported our idea. We hope that this edition, with the updates and new content, will continue to be helpful to advanced practice students, new practitioners, and experienced practitioners faced with new presentations.

As NPs increasingly become the providers of choice for individuals seeking primary and specialty care, the need for expertise in the assessment and diagnostic processes remains essential. In spite of the growth in available technology and diagnostic studies, performing assessment skills correctly, obtaining valid data, and interpreting the findings accurately are necessary for the safe, high-quality, and cost-effective practice for which NPs are known.

Even once these skills are accomplished, accurate diagnosis remains a difficult aspect of practice. However, it was our experience that students and practicing clinicians rarely referred to their health assessment book after completing their assessment course. Instead, they tended to turn to clinical management texts, which focus on what to do once the diagnosis is known. This supported our belief that although assessment texts cover common findings for a limited range of disorders, most are not perceived as helpful in guiding the diagnostic process. Novice practitioners often spend much energy and time narrowing their differential diagnosis when they have no clear guidance that is driven by the patient and/or complaint. For this reason, our aim has been to develop a text that serves as a guide in the assessment and diagnostic process, is broad in content, and is suitable for use in varied settings.

Advanced Assessment: Interpreting Findings and Formulating Differential Diagnoses is designed to serve as a textbook during advanced health assessment course work and as a quick reference for practicing clinicians. Studying the text will help students to develop proficiency in performing assessment and interpreting findings and to recognize the range of conditions that can be indicated by specific findings. For practicing clinicians, the text will be an aide to guide the assessment and the narrowing of differential diagnosis.

The book consists of three parts. Part I provides a summary discussion of assessment and some matters related to clinical decision-making. In addition to discussing the behaviors involved in arriving at a definitive diagnosis, the chapter discusses some pitfalls that clinicians often experience and the types of evidence-based resources that are available to assist in the diagnostic process.

A new feature of this edition is the chapter on conducting a genetic assessment. This component of health assessment has great potential, with recent advances in the information and technology related to genetics and genomics. It is critical that clinicians be able to address the potential of hereditary diseases and genetic variations that may affect their patients. This new chapter is placed in Part I as, like clinical decision-making, genetic assessment is relevant to the content of all subsequent chapters.

Part II serves as the core of the book and addresses assessment and diagnosis using a system and body region approach. Each chapter in this part begins with an overview of the comprehensive history and physical examination of a specific system, as well as a discussion of common diagnostic studies. The remainder of the chapter is then categorized by chief complaints commonly associated with that system. For each complaint, there is a description of the focused assessment relative to that complaint, followed by a list of the conditions that should be considered in the differential diagnosis, along with the symptoms, signs, and/or diagnostic findings that would support each condition.

Part II of this edition includes a more extensive color atlas than was included in the original version. Previously limited to the skin assessment chapter, the expanded color atlas includes color photographs for several chapters. New figures have been added to select chapters, to better depict examination techniques or expected findings. Descriptive captions have been added to support photographs and figures within the body of the text and the color atlas. Additional complaints and conditions have been included in several differential diagnosis sections.

Finally, Part III addresses the assessment and diagnosis of specific populations: those at either extreme of age (young and old) and pregnant women. This part has also been updated and is designed to include a heavy emphasis on the assessments that allow clinicians to evaluate the special needs of individuals in these populations, such as growth and development in children and functionality in older patients.

To aid the reader, we have tried to follow a consistent format in the presentation of content so that information can be readily located. This format is admittedly grounded on the sequence we have found successful as we presented this content to our students. However, we have a great appreciation for the expertise of the contributors in this edited work, and some of the content they recommended could not consistently fit our "formula." We hope that the organization of this text is helpful to all readers.

Acknowledgments

We express our sincere appreciation for the support and assistance provided by so many in the development of this book. Their contributions have made the work much richer.

Particular mention goes to all at F. A. Davis for their enthusiasm, support, and patience during the process. Most specifically, we acknowledge the invaluable assistance of Joanne DaCunha, our publisher. Joanne's continued belief in the concept and in our ability to develop the content was a vital factor in our work and she was always available to guide us throughout the process. We also want to express our gratitude to Christina C. Burns, our project editor, for coordinating so many tasks and pushing us to ensure as much consistency as possible between chapters.

We are immensely grateful to the contributors of this edition, who shared their expertise and knowledge to enhance the content. They were a pleasure to work with. We appreciate the contributions to this second edition by those who provided content to the first edition: Saundra Turner, Randolph Rasch, Karen Koozer-Olson, Diane Mueller, and Phillip Rupp. In addition to the contributors, we also want to thank the many reviewers of the first edition for their timely and thoughtful feedback.

Personal Acknowledgments From Laurie Grubbs

Most of all, I would like to thank my friend and coauthor, Mary Jo, for providing the impetus to write this book—an often talked about aspiration that became a reality; and to F. A. Davis for their enthusiasm, support, and patience during the process.

I would like to thank my children, Jennifer and Ashley, for their support and for being themselves—intelligent, talented, beautiful daughters.

Personal Acknowledgments From Mary Jo Goolsby

I must also express thanks to my dear friend and colleague, Laurie. Throughout the majority of my time in academia, I had the pleasure and honor of being "tied at the hip" with Laurie, from whom I learned so much.

Above all else, I thank my husband, H. G. Goolsby. Without his constant support and encouragement, this work would not have been possible.

Contributors

SARA F. BARBER, MSN, ARNP
Professional Park Pediatrics
Tallahassee, Florida

DEBORAH BLACKWELL, PHD, RNC, WHCNP
Dean, Carolinas College of Health Sciences—
School of Nursing and Mercy School of Nursing
Charlotte, North Carolina

JAMES BLACKWELL, MS, APRN, BC
Nurse Practitioner, Department of Internal
Medicine Carolinas HealthCare System
Charlotte, North Carolina

VALERIE A HART, EdD, APRN, CS
Associate Professor of Nursing, College of
Nursing and Health Professions
University of Southern Maine
Private Practice Portland, Maine

PATRICIA HENTZ, EdD, CS, PMH/NP-BC
Associate Professor, College of Nursing and
Health Professions University of Southern Maine
Portland, Maine

CHARON A. PIERSON, PhD, RN, GNP, BC,
FAANP
Assistant Professor, Department of Geriatric
Medicine
University of Hawaii, John A. Burns School
of Medicine
Editor-in-Chief, *Journal of the American
Academy of Nurse Practitioners*
Honolulu, Hawaii

SUSANNE QUALLICH, APRN, BC, NP-C, CUNP
Nurse Practitioner, Division of Andrology
and Microsurgery
Michigan Urology Center
University of Michigan Health System
Ann Arbor, Michigan

QUANNETTA T. EDWARDS, PhD, RN,
FNP-BC, WHNP-BC, FAANP
Associate Professor, College of Health &
Human Development Graduate Nursing,
Department of Nursing, Cal State University,
Fullerton, CA
Western University of Health Sciences,
Pomona, CA

ANN MARADIEGUE, PhD, RN, FNP-BC,
FAANP
Assistant Professor, College of Health &
Human Services, School of Nursing
George Mason University
Fairfax, Virginia

DIANE SEIBERT, PhD, RN, ANP, WHNP-BC,
FAANP
*Assistant Associate Professor, Program
Director Family Nurse Practitioner
Program,*
Graduate School of Nursing
Uniformed Services University
Bethesda, Maryland

SUSANNE HAVEL, MSN, RN, CPNP, APNG
Lieutenant Colonel, United States Air Force
Nurse Corps
Little Rock Air Force Base, Arkansas

MICHELLE LAJINESS, APRN, BC
Nurse Practitioner, Department of
Urology
Beaumont Hospital
Royal Oak, Michigan

Reviewers

xi

Table of Contents

The Art of Assessment and Clinical Decision-Making

Chapter 1

ASSESSMENT AND CLINICAL DECISION-MAKING: AN OVERVIEW

Mary Jo Goolsby & Laurie Grubbs

Clinical decision-making is often fraught with uncertainties. However, expert diagnosticians are able to maintain a degree of suspicion throughout the assessment process, to consider a range of potential explanations, and then to generate and narrow their differential diagnosis on the basis of their previous experience, familiarity with the evidence related to various diagnoses, and understanding of their individual patient. Through the process, clinicians perform assessment techniques involving both the history and physical examination in an effective and reliable manner and then select appropriate diagnostic studies to support their assessment.

History

Among the assessment techniques essential to valid diagnosis is performing a fact-finding history. To obtain adequate history, providers must be well organized, attentive to the patient's verbal and nonverbal language, and able to accurately interpret the patient's responses to questions. Rather than reading into the patient's statements, they clarify any areas of uncertainty. The expert history, like the expert physical examination, is informed by the knowledge of a wide range of conditions, their physiologic bases, and their associated signs and symptoms.

The ability to draw out descriptions of the patient's symptoms and experiences is important because only the patient can tell his or her story. To assist the patient in describing a complaint, a skillful interviewer knows how to ask salient and focused questions to draw out necessary information without straying, i.e. avoiding a shotgun approach, with lack of focus. The provider should know, based on the chief complaint and any preceding information, what other questions are essential to the history. It is important to determine why the symptom brought the patient to the office—that is, the significance of this symptom to the patient—which may uncover the patient's anxiety and the basis for his or her concern. It may also help to determine severity in a stoic patient who may underestimate or underreport symptoms.

Throughout the history, it is important to recognize that patients may forget details, so probing questions may be necessary. Patients sometimes have trouble finding the precise words to describe their complaint. However, good descriptors are necessary to isolate the cause, source, and location of symptoms. Often, patients must be encouraged to use common language and terminology. For instance, encourage the patient to describe the problem just as he or she would describe it to a relative or neighbor.

The history should include specific components (summarized in Table 1.1) to ensure that the problem is comprehensively evaluated. The questions to include in each component of the history are described in detail in subsequent chapters.

Table 1.1

Components of History

Component	Purpose
Chief complaint	To determine the reason patient seeks care. Important to consider using the patient's terminology. Provides "title" for the encounter.
History of present illness	To provide a thorough description of the chief complaint and current problem. Suggested format: **P-Q-R-S-T.**
• **P:** precipitating and palliative factors	To identify factors that make symptom worse and/or better; any previous self-treatment or prescribed treatment, and response.
• **Q:** quality and quantity descriptors	To identify patient's rating of symptom (e.g., pain on a 1–10 scale) and descriptors (e.g., numbness, burning, stabbing).
• **R:** region and radiation	To identify the exact location of the symptom and any area of radiation.
• **S:** severity and associated symptoms	To identify the symptom's severity (e.g., how bad at its worst) and any associated symptoms (e.g., presence or absence of nausea and vomiting associated with chest pain).
• **T:** timing and temporal descriptions	To identify when complaint was first noticed; how it has changed/progressed since onset (e.g., remained the same or worsened/improved); whether onset was acute or chronic; whether it has been constant, intermittent, or recurrent.
Past medical history	To identify past diagnoses, surgeries, hospitalizations, injuries, allergies, immunizations, current medications.
Habits	To describe any use of tobacco, alcohol, drugs and to identify patterns of sleep, exercise, etc.

(Continued)

Table 1.1	

Components of History—cont'd

Component	Purpose
Sociocultural	To identify occupational and recreational activities and experiences, living environment, financial status/support as related to health care needs, travel, lifestyle, etc.
Family history	To identify potential sources of hereditary diseases; a genogram is helpful; the minimum includes first-degree relatives (parents, siblings, children), although second and third orders are helpful.
Review of systems	To review a list of possible symptoms that the patient may have noted in each of the body systems.

Physical Examination

The expert diagnostician must also be able to perform a physical assessment accurately. Extensive, repetitive practice; exposure to a range of normal variants and abnormal findings; and keen observation skills are required to develop physical examination proficiency. Each component of the physical examination must be performed correctly to ensure that findings are as valid and reliable as possible. While performing the physical examination, the examiner must be able to

- differentiate between normal and abnormal findings.
- recall knowledge of a range of conditions, including their associated signs and symptoms.
- recognize how certain conditions affect the response to other conditions in ways that are not entirely predictable.
- distinguish the relevance of varied abnormal findings.

The aspects of physical examination are summarized in the following chapters using a systems approach. Each chapter also reviews the relevant examination for varied complaints. Along with obtaining an accurate history and performing a physical examination, it is crucial that the clinician consider the patient's vital signs, and general appearance and condition when making clinical decisions.

Diagnostic Studies

The history and physical assessment help to guide the selection of diagnostic studies. Diagnostic studies should be considered if a patient's diagnosis remains in doubt following the history and physical. They often help establish the severity of the diagnosed condition or rule out conditions included in the early differential diagnosis. Just as the history should be relevant and focused, the selection of diagnostic studies should be judicious and directed toward specific conditions under consideration. The clinician should select the study (or studies) with the highest degree of sensitivity and specificity for the target condition while also considering cost-effectiveness, safety, and degree of invasiveness. Selection of diagnostics requires a range of knowledge specific to various studies as well as the ability to interpret the study's results.

Resources are available to assist clinicians in the selection of diagnostic studies. For example, the American College of Radiology's Appropriateness Criteria Web pages provide guidelines on selecting imaging studies (see http://acsearch.acr.org). A number of texts review variables relative to the selection of laboratory studies. Subsequent chapters identify specific studies that should be considered for varied complaints, depending on the conditions included in the differential diagnosis.

Diagnostic Statistics

In the selection and interpretation of assessment techniques and diagnostic studies, providers must understand and apply some basic statistical concepts, including the tests' sensitivity and specificity, the pretest probability, and the likelihood ratio. These characteristics are based on population studies involving the various tests, and they provide a general appreciation of how helpful a diagnostic study will be in arriving at a definitive diagnosis. Each concept is briefly described in Table 1.2; detailed discussions of these and other diagnostic statistics can be found in numerous reference texts.

Bayes's theorem is frequently cited as the standard for basing a clinical decision on available evidence. The Bayesian process involves using knowledge of the pretest probability and the likelihood ratio to determine the probability that a particular condition exists. Given knowledge of the pretest probability and a particular test's associated likelihood ratio, providers can estimate posttest probability of a condition based on a population of patients with the same characteristics. Posttest probability is the product of the pretest probability and the likelihood ratio. Nomograms are available to assist in applying the theorem to clinical reasoning. Of course, the process becomes increasingly more complex as multiple signs, symptoms, and diagnostic results are incorporated.

Reliable and valid basic statistics needed for evidence-based clinical reasoning are not always readily available. When available, they may not provide a valid representation of the situation at hand. Sources for the statistics include textbooks, primary reports of research, and published meta-analyses. Another source of statistics, the one that has been most widely used and available for application to the reasoning process, is the recall or estimation based on a provider's experience, although these are rarely accurate. Over the past decade, the availability of evidence on which to base clinical reasoning is improving, and there is an increasing expectation that clinical reasoning be based on scientific evidence. Evidence-based statistics are also increasingly being used to develop resources to facilitate clinical decision-making.

Table 1.2

Clinical Statistics

Statistic	Description
Sensitivity	The percentage of individuals with the target condition who would have an abnormal, or positive, result. Because a high sensitivity indicates that a greater percentage of persons with the given condition will have an abnormal result, a test with a high sensitivity can be used to rule out the condition for those who do not have an abnormal result. For example, if redness of the conjunctiva is 100% sensitive for bacterial conjunctivitis, then conjunctivitis could be ruled out in a patient who did not have redness on examination. However, the presence of redness could indicate several conditions, including bacterial conjunctivitis, viral conjunctivitis, corneal abrasion, or allergies.
Specificity	The percentage of healthy individuals who would have a normal result. The greater the specificity, the greater the percentage of individuals who will have negative, or normal, results if they do not have the target condition. If a test has a high level of specificity so that a significant percentage of healthy individuals are expected to have a negative result, then a positive result would be used to "rule in" the condition. For example, if a rapid strep screen test is 98% specific for streptococcal pharyngitis and the person has a positive result, then he or she has "strep throat." However, if that patient has a negative result, there is a 2% chance that that patient's result is falsely negative, so the condition cannot be entirely ruled out.
Pretest probability	Based on evidence from a population with specific findings, this probability specifies the prevalence of the condition in that population, or the probability that the patient has the condition on the basis of those findings.
Likelihood ratio	This is the probability that a positive test result will be associated with a person who has the target condition and a negative result will be associated with a healthy person. A likelihood ratio above 1.0 indicates that a positive result is associated with the disease; a likelihood ratio less than 1.0 indicates that a negative result is associated with an absence of the disease. Likelihood ratios that approximate 1.0 provide weak evidence for a test's ability to identify individuals with or without a condition. Likelihood ratios above 1.0 or below 0.1 provide stronger evidence relative to the test's predictive value. The ratio is used to determine the degree to which a test result will increase or decrease (from the pretest probability) the likelihood that an individual has a condition.

Clinical Decision-Making Resources

Clinical decision-making begins when the patient first voices the reason for seeking care. Expert clinicians immediately compare their patients' complaints with the "catalog" of knowledge that they have stored about a range of clinical conditions and then determine the direction of their initial history and symptom analysis. It is crucial that the provider not jump to conclusions or be biased by one particular finding; information is continually processed to inform decisions that guide further data collection and to begin to detect patterns in the data.

Depending on the amount of experience in assessing other patients with the presenting complaint, a diagnostician uses varied systems through which information is processed and decisions are made. Through experience, it is possible to see clusters or patterns in complaints and findings and compare against what is known of the potential common and urgent explanations for the findings. Experience and knowledge also provide specifics regarding the statistics associated with the various diagnostic options. However, experience is not always adequate to support accurate clinical decision-making, and memory is not perfect. To assist in clinical decision-making, a number of evidence-based resources have been developed to assist the clinician. Resources such as algorithms and clinical practice guidelines assist in clinical reasoning when properly applied.

Algorithms are formulas or procedures for problem solving and include both decision trees and clinical prediction rules. Decision trees provide a graphic depiction of the decision-making process, showing the pathway based on findings at various steps in the process. A decision tree begins with a chief complaint or physical finding and then leads the diagnostician through a series of decision nodes. Each decision node or decision point provides a question or statement regarding the presence or absence of some clinical finding. The response to each of these decision points determines the next step. An example of a decision tree is provided in Figure 13.5, which illustrates a decision-making process for amenorrhea. These devices are helpful in identifying a logical sequence for the decisions involved in narrowing the differential diagnosis and also provide cues to recommended questions and/or tests that should be answered through the diagnostic process. A decision tree should be accompanied by a description of the strength of the evidence on which it has been developed as well as a description of the settings and/or patient population to which it relates.

Clinical decision (or prediction) rules provide another support for clinical reasoning. Clinical decision rules are evidence-based resources, which provide probabilistic statements regarding the likelihood that a condition exists if certain variables are met with regard to the prognosis of patients with specific findings. Decision rules use mathematical models and are specific to certain situations, settings, and/or patient characteristics. They are used to express the diagnostic statistics described earlier. The number of decision, or predictive, rules is growing, and select examples are included in this text. For instance, the Ottawa ankle and foot rules are described in the discussion of musculoskeletal pain in Chapter 14. The Gail model, a well-established rule relevant to screening for breast cancer, is discussed in Chapter 9. Many of the rules involve complex mathematical calculations, but others are simple. In addition to discussions of tools, this text provides several sources of electronic "calculators" based on rules. Box 1.1 includes a limited list of sites with clinical prediction calculators. These resources should be accompanied by information describing the methods by which the rule was validated.

Clinical practice guidelines have also been developed for the assessment and diagnosis of various conditions. They are typically developed by national advisory panels of clinical experts who base the guidelines on the best available evidence. An easily accessible source of evidence-based guidelines is the National Guideline Clearinghouse, which provides summaries of individual guidelines as well as syntheses and comparisons on topics if multiple guidelines are available. Like decision trees and diagnostic rules, guidelines should be accompanied by a description of their supporting evidence and the situations in which they should be applied.

These resources are not without limitations, and it is essential that they be applied in the situations for which they were intended. In applying these tools to clinical situations, it is essential that the diagnostician determine the population in which the tool was developed, ensure the tool is applicable to the case at hand, and have accurate data to consider in the tool's application. For instance, a clinical prediction rule based on a population of young adult college students is not valid if applied to an elderly patient. The provider must also recognize that these resources are intended to assist in the interpretation of a range of clinical evidence relevant to a particular problem, but they are not intended to take the place of clinical judgment, which rests with the provider.

Box 1.1

Online Sources of Medical Calculators

Emergency Medicine on the Web
www.ncemi.org
Essential Evidence Plus
www.essentialevidenceplus.com
Med Students: Online Clinical Calculators
www.medstudents.com.br/calculat/index2.htm
Medical Algorithms Project
www.medal.org
National Center for Emergency Medicine Informatics
www.med.emory.edu/EMAC/curriculum/informatics.html
National Institutes of Health
www.nih.gov

Note: Sites active as of March 7, 2011. Other subscription-based sites are also available.

The Diagnostic Process

As data is collected through the history and physical examination, providers tailor their approach to subsequent data collection. They begin to detect patterns that guide the development of a differential diagnosis that is based on an understanding of probability and prognosis. This means that conditions considered are those that most commonly cause the perceived cluster of data (probability) as well as conditions that may be less common but would require urgent detection and action (prognosis).

Several adages are frequently used when teaching health assessment to encourage novice diagnosticians to always consider clinical explanations that are most likely to explain a patient's situation. For instance, students often hear, "Common diseases occur commonly." Most clinicians learn to use the term "zebra" to refer to less likely (and more rare) explanations for a presentation, using the adage "When you hear hooves in Central Park, don't look for zebras." Both adages direct novices to consider the most likely explanation for a set of findings. This text describes common conditions that should be considered in the differential diagnosis of common complaints as well as some of the less common possibilities. With the emergence of conditions, zebras may well be responsible for findings, and providers must always maintain some level of suspicion for these less common explanations.

Even though it is appropriate that conditions with high probabilities be considered in the differential diagnosis, it is also vital in the diagnostic process to consider conditions that put the patient at highest risk. To do otherwise places the patient in jeopardy of life-threatening or disabling complications. These life-threatening situations are often referred to as "red flags," which are clues signaling a high likelihood of an urgent situation requiring immediate identification and management. This text includes red flags for the various systems to promote their recognition in clinical practice.

Finally, as Chapter 2 on genetic assessment describes, some patients are at higher risk than others for certain conditions. The ability to identify genetic patterns is becoming increasingly important as we learn more about the role genetics play in many diseases.

As the potential list of conditions in the differential diagnosis develops, the provider determines what, if any, diagnostic studies are warranted to confirm or rule out specific diagnoses. A knowledge of the tests' specificity and sensitivity is helpful in the selection process. The diagnostician then combines the knowledge gained through the history and physical assessment with the findings from any diagnostic studies to assess the probability for the conditions remaining in the differential diagnosis.

Times arise when a definitive diagnosis is not identified, yet urgent explanations have been ruled out. In situations of this kind, options include moving forward with further diagnostic measures, including further history, physical examination, diagnostic studies, and/or referral or consultation. Another option involves waiting briefly before further diagnostic studies are performed in order to see whether or not the condition declares itself. In this case, serial assessments should be scheduled over a period of days or weeks in order to arrive at a diagnosis. An important factor involved in the decision to wait is the patient's ability and willingness to return for follow-up at the specified intervals. In situations, such as emergency department or urgent care center visits, the clinician has no long-term relationship with the patient, and the likelihood of the patient returning for follow-up is greatly decreased. A plan should be in place to complete the assessment and diagnosis, and the patient should be informed of and should verbalize his or her understanding of the plan as well as what symptoms would warrant reconsideration. Missed diagnosis and delayed diagnosis are among the most common causes of malpractice complaints, particularly the failure to diagnose myocardial infarctions and breast cancer.

Although not always to the patient's advantage, patient expectations often play a part in clinical decision-making. Some patients are less willing to wait; others are less willing to be treated. This can be the cause for errors, and clinicians should be aware that they should try to accommodate patients' wishes without putting them at risk.

Box 1.2 includes a list of common diagnostic errors. Although the list is far from exhaustive, avoidance of these errors will improve clinical decision-making.

Box 1.2

Common Diagnostic Errors

- Jumping to conclusion, being biased by an early finding (e.g., something in the patient's past medical history or recheck from a previous visit).
- Accepting previous diagnosis/explanation without exploring other possible explanations (e.g., diagnosis of chronic bronchitis as explanation of chronic cough in patient on ACE inhibitor).
- Using a shotgun approach to assessment without adequate focus.
- Focusing solely on the most obvious or likely explanation.
- Relying solely on memory, which limits the diagnostician's knowledge and options to only what is memorized or recalled.
- Using the wrong rule, decision tree, or other resource to guide analysis or using the correct device incorrectly.
- Performing skills improperly.
- Misinterpreting or using wrong data.
- Allowing the patient to make diagnosis (e.g., "I had sinusitis last year, and the symptoms are exactly the same").
- Allowing other health care professionals to lead the diagnosis in the wrong direction.
- Accepting the "horses" without contemplating the "zebras"; contemplating zebras without adequately pursuing the possibility of a more common condition.

Common Diagnostic Errors—cont'd

- Accommodating patient wishes against clinician judgment.
- Ignoring basic findings, such as vital signs.
- Failing to consider medical conditions as the source of "psychiatric" symptoms and psychiatric conditions as the source of "medical" symptoms.

Summary

The content of this book is directed toward assisting clinicians to adequately assess presenting complaints and then to consider reasonable explanations for the complaint and findings. For each complaint, a summary of the relevant history and physical assessment is provided, along with a list of conditions that should be considered in the differential diagnosis. The lists of conditions are not exhaustive. However, by noting the possibility of those included, clinicians will consider various potential etiologies and, by weighing the likelihood of these options, begin to develop critical-thinking skills necessary for clinical decision-making. Very brief descriptions of the possible findings for each of the conditions are listed to help guide the reader in recognizing definitive clusters of signs and symptoms.

Above all, practice and experience provide the skills necessary for accurate diagnosis. These skills are supported by life-long learning through which clinicians maintain an awareness of the highest level of evidence relative to assessment and diagnosis.

SUGGESTED READINGS

Ebell, M.H. (2001). *Evidence-Based Diagnosis: A Handbook of Clinical Prediction Rules.* New York: Springer.

Elstein, A.S., & Schwarz, A. (2002). Evidence base of clinical diagnosis: Clinical problem solving and diagnostic decision making: Selective review of the cognitive literature. *BMJ,* 324: 729–732.

Guyatt, G., & Ronnei, D. (Ed.). (2008). *Users' Guides to the Medical Literature: A Manual for Evidence-Based Clinical Practice, Second Edition.* Chicago: AMA Press.

Saint, S., Drazen, J., & Solomon, C. (2006). *The New England Journal of Medicine Clinical Problem Solving.* Waltham, MA: Massachusetts Medical Society.

Chapter 2

AN OVERVIEW OF GENETIC ASSESSMENT

Quannetta T. Edwards, PhD, RN, FNP-BC, WHNP-BC, FAANP •
Ann Maradiegue, PhD, RN, FNP-BC, FAANP •
Diane Seibert, PhD, RN, ANP, WHNP-BC, FAANP •
Susanne Havel, MSN, RN, CPNP, Advanced Practice Nurse in Genetics
(APNG)

In April 2003, researchers heading up the Human Genome Project (HGP) announced that they had sequenced all 3 billion base pairs in the human genome, which is the complete set of DNA in the body. The HGP's goal was to provide researchers with the tools they needed to identify the genetic factors in human disease, paving the way for novel diagnostic, treatment, and prevention options (National Institutes of Health [NIH], 2008). Advances in genetic and genomic information and technology make it necessary to reconsider the way primary health care is delivered. *Genetics* is the study of single genes and their effects on the body; *genomics* is the functions and interactions of all the genes in the genome (Guttmacher & Collins, 2002). See Table 2.1.

In the early 1960s, Dr. Victor A. McKusick initiated development of Mendelian Inheritance in Man (MIM), a catalog of mendelian traits and disorders. An online version, Online Mendelian Inheritance in Man (OMIM), was created in 1985 by the National Library of Medicine and the William H. Welch Medical Library at Johns Hopkins University and, in 1995, was developed for the Internet by the National Center for Biotechnology Information: www.ncbi.nlm.nih.gov/omim. Currently, OMIM features over 18,750 entries of hereditary conditions containing autosomal dominant, autosomal recessive, X-linked, Y-linked, and mitochondrial inheritance, and more are added every year. Genetic variations not only are associated with rare diseases or hereditary disorders affecting infancy or childhood but also contribute to common chronic diseases such as cancer, Alzheimer's disease, mental health, human immunodeficiency virus infection, tuberculosis, and heart disease as well as hereditary disorders manifesting in adulthood (Guttmacher & Collins, 2002). All healthcare providers (HCPs), including nurse practitioners (NPs), must understand

Table 2.1

Selected Definitions Used in Genetics and Genomics

Genetic/Genomic Terms	Definition
Affected	Individual who manifests the disorder
Consanguinity[a]	Related in descent by a common ancestor
De novo mutations	A new, spontaneous mutation (noninherited)
Expressivity (variable)[b]	The range of clinical features observed in individuals with a particular disorder. Variable expressivity applies to disorders following all patterns of inheritance
Genes	The functional and physical unit of heredity passed from parent to offspring. It is estimated that each cell of the human body contains 30,000 genes[c]
Genetics[c]	The study of heredity, the process by which parents pass genes to their children; the study of single genes and their effects. A person's appearance (height, hair color, skin color, and eye color) is determined by genes. Other characteristics, such as mental abilities, natural talents, and susceptibility to develop certain diseases, are also affected by heredity
Genome[a]	All the DNA contained in an organism or a cell, which includes both the chromosomes within the nucleus and the DNA in mitochondria
Genomics[d]	The study of not only single genes but the functions and interactions of all the genes in the genome
Mutation[a]	A permanent structural alteration in DNA. In most cases, DNA changes either have no effect or cause harm, but occasionally a mutation can improve an organism's chance of surviving and passing the beneficial change on to its descendants
Pedigree	A graphic illustration of a family health history using standardized symbols.[e] The simplified diagram of a family's genealogy shows family members' relationships to each other and how a particular trait or disease has been inherited[f]
Penetrance[b]	The proportion of individuals with a mutation causing a particular disorder who exhibit clinical symptoms of that disorder
Phenotype[a]	Observable traits or characteristics
Proband[b]	The affected individual through whom a family with a genetic disorder is ascertained

[a]Nussbaum et al., 2007; [b]GeneTests, 2004; [c]U.S. National Library of Medicine, 2008; [d]Guttmacher & Collins, 2002; [e]Bennet et al., 1995; [f]National Human Genome Research Institute, 2008b.

genetics and genomics well enough to be aware of and appreciate the wide variety of diseases and genetic conditions that might be encountered in primary care as well as other health-care settings. The ability to assess and recognize the potential for hereditary disease and other conditions affected by genetic variations is critical for implementation of primary and secondary prevention, diagnostic and management of care strategies, appropriate early-intensified surveillance, and referral consultation when needed.

A critical first step in genetic assessment is the use of a family history. Family history is considered the first "genetic screen" (Berry & Shooner, 2004) and is rapidly becoming a critical component of care because it reflects shared genetic susceptibilities, shared environment, and common behaviors (Yoon, Scheuner, & Khoury, 2003). The value of the family history must not be underestimated. A comprehensive family history provides for (a) early diagnosis; (b) identification of family members at risk; (c) risk assessment for potential disease; (d) preventive strategies through increased surveillance, life-style changes, and prophylactic measures to include chemoprevention and surgery when indicated; (e) individualized treatment strategies; and (f) referral and clinical decision-making for testing and management of care when appropriate. A comprehensive family history assessment is essential in identifying individuals and family members for hereditary conditions as well as diagnosing and identifying at-risk individuals and family members for numerous medical conditions. Essential nursing core competencies and curricula guidelines in genetics and genomics were established by the Consensus Panel on Nursing Genetics/Genomic and published by the American Nurses Association (ANA) as a means to prepare the nursing workforce to deliver competent genetic- and genomic-focused care (Consensus Panel on Genetic/Genomic Nursing Competencies [CPGGNC], 2006). Examples of application of genetic and genomic nursing assessment noted in these guidelines include the following:

- Demonstrating an understanding of the relationship of genetics and genomics to health, prevention, screening, diagnostics, prognostics, selection of treatment, and monitoring of treatment effectiveness.
- Demonstrating the ability to elicit a minimum of three-generation family health history information.
- Constructing a pedigree from collected family history information using standardized symbols and terminology.
- Collecting personal, health, and developmental histories that include genetic, environmental, and genomic influences and risks.
- Conducting comprehensive health and physical assessments that incorporate knowledge about genetic, environmental, and genomic influences and risk factors.
- Assessing client's knowledge, perceptions, and responses to genetic/genomic information.
- Developing a plan of care that incorporates genetic and genomic assessment information. (CPGGNC, 2006)

The National Coalition of Health Professionals Education in Genetics (NCHPEG), established in 1996 by the American Medical Association, the National Human Genome Research Institute, and the ANA, has established genetic core competencies for all health-care professionals, and family history is a critical element in those competencies. According to the NCHPEG core competencies, all health-care professionals should, at a minimum, (1) examine one's competence of practice on a regular basis, identifying areas of strength and areas where professional development related to genetics and genomics would be beneficial; (2) understand that health-related genetic information can have important social and psychological implications for individuals and families; and (3) know how and when to make a referral to a genetics professional (NCHPEG, 2007). Also, NCHPEG notes specific genetics skills for all health-care professionals that include the following:

- Gathering genetic family history, including a minimum of a three-generation history.
- Identifying and referring clients who might benefit from genetic services or consultation with other professionals for management of issues related to genetic diagnosis.
- Explaining the reasons for and benefits of genetic services.
- Using information technology to obtain credible, current information about genetics.
- Assuring that the informed-consent process for genetic testing includes appropriate information about the potential risks, benefits, and limitations of the test in question. (NCHPEG, 2007)

Online resources for the CPGGNC and NCHPEG guidelines are listed in Table 2.2.

Table 2.2

Selected Genetic and Genomic Online Resources

Resource	Purpose	Web Site
National Coalition of Health Professionals Education in Genetics (NCHPEG)	Prepare health professionals in genomics	www.nchpeg.org
Essentials for Nursing Competencies and Curricula Guidelines in Genetics/Genomics	Guidelines for nursing in genetics and genomics	www.genome.gov/Pages/Careers/HealthProfessionalEducation/geneticscompetency.pdf
Online Mendelian Inheritance in Man disorders (OMIM)	Database of a catalog of genes, genetic traits, and genetic disorders	www.ncbi.nlm.nih.gov/omim

Continued

Table 2.2

Selected Genetic and Genomic Online Resources—cont'd

Resource	Purpose	Web Site
GeneTests	Medical genetics resource: expert author disease review, international directory of genetic testing laboratories, internal directory of genetic and prenatal diagnosis laboratories, educational materials, genetic tools	www.genetests.org
Genetics Home Reference (U.S. National Library of Medicine, National Institutes of Health)	Guide to understanding genetic conditions	http://ghr.nlm.nih.gov
National Genome Research Institute, National Institutes of Health	Information on research, grants, education, health policy, ethics, careers and training; glossary of genetic terms	www.genome.gov
National Cancer Institute	Cancer genetics overview Physician Data Query (PDQ) for health-care professionals	www.cancer.gov/cancertopics/pdq/genetics/overview/HealthProfessional/page2
Centers for Disease Control and Prevention, National Office of Public Health Genomics	Genomics in public health research, policy, and practice; resources and training tools	www.cdc.gov/genomics/translation/competencies

Web sites current as of March 2011 and subject to change. Listing does not constitute an endorsement.

Genetic Assessment—The Family History

Family history is the key to an accurate genetic assessment. Several tools are available to assist in collecting a family history (Table 2.3), and regardless of which tool is used, *a minimum of three generations*, including information from both the maternal and paternal lineage, should be obtained. Whenever possible, this information should be recorded in the form of a *pedigree*, which is a visual diagram of the family history illustrating how traits cluster in families and move through generations (American Medical Association [AMA], 2004). Pedigrees are cost-effective tools for genetic diagnosis and risk assessment, but they must be recorded using standardized symbols so that interpretation is consistent across HCPs and practices. Pedigrees help HCPs make medical diagnoses, establish patterns of inheritance, identify at-risk family members, distinguish genetic

Table 2.3

Resources for Family History Tools, Genetic Referral Consultation, Genetic Education for Nursing, and Risk Assessment Models

Resources	Web Sites
Family History Resources	
American Medical Association: family history tools and links to resources: prenatal genetic screening questionnaire, pediatric clinical genetics questionnaire, adult family history form	www.ama-assn.org/ama/pub/category/2380.html
Centers for Disease Control and Prevention, National Office of Public Health Genetics: family history resources and tools	www.cdc.gov/genomics/famhistory/famhist.htm
U.S. Department of Health and Human Services, U.S. Surgeon General's Family History Initiative: patient-completed pedigree drawing software	www.hhs.gov/familyhistory
March of Dimes: pregnancy and newborn, birth defects and genetics, preconception counseling and checklist	www.marchofdimes.com/Pregnancy/trying_healthhistory.html www.marchofdimes.com/Baby/birthdefects_chromosomal.html www.marchofdimes.com/your_family_health_historypreconceptionprenatal.pdf
Genetic data management and pedigree construction software: Progeny; McIntosh software; Cyrillic	www.progenygenetics.com www.pedigree-draw.com/index.html www.cyrillicsoftware.com
Genetic Referral Consultation Resources	
National Cancer Institute, Physician Data Query Cancer Information Summaries	http://www.cancer.gov/cancertopics/pdq/cancerdatabase#summaries
Selected Genetic Resources for Nursing	
International Society of Nurses in Genetics	www.isong.org
Cincinnati Children's Hospital: genetics education program for nurses	www.cincinnatichildrens.org/ed/clinical/gpnf/default.htm
Risk Assessment Tools	
U.S. Department of Health and Human Service, National Institute of Health, National Heart, Lung and Blood Institute's health assessment tools: body mass index; 10-year heart attack risk calculator; Framingham Heart Study, and genetic data	www.nhlbi.nih.gov/health/index.htm#tools www.nhlbi.nih.gov/about/framingham/index.html
National Cancer Institute Breast Cancer Risk Assessment Model (Gail Model)	www.cancer.gov/bcrisktool

Web sites current as of March 2011 and subject to change. Listing does not constitute an endorsement.

from other risk factors, and make care and surveillance management decisions (Bennett, 1999).

Starting the Pedigree for Genetic Assessment

The following guidelines are intended to help HCPs construct an accurate family history:

1. *Use standardized pedigree symbols and nomenclature* such as those recommended by the Pedigree Standardization Task Force (Bennett et al., 1995) (Table 2.4). The use of standard pedigree symbols helps avoid misinterpretation of the pedigree data. Standardized pedigree symbols provide a consistent means of recording and interpreting family history; increases uniformity of medical information; and enhances quality control in clinical genetics, medicine, genetic education, and research. In addition, the pedigree enables visualization of important issues relevant to the health history, such as social and biological factors, consanguinity, reproductive factors, births, and deaths. A consanguineous family is one in which two mating individuals are related by descent to the same common ancestor (Nussbaum, McInnes, & Willard, 2007). Consanguinity increases the risk for hereditary disorders due to autosomal recessive inheritance like sickle cell, cystic fibrosis, and Tay-Sachs disease (Bennett, 1999).

2. *Always document the date the history was collected and who recorded the history.* Remember that family history is dynamic and ever changing. Assessing the family history at the initial visit and updating it on subsequent patient/client visits are important in assuring an accurate family assessment. Always add the new date to any subsequent addition to the pedigree and record the name of the historian if the history is not given by the patient.

3. *Begin the pedigree with the individual whose history is being assessed.* The person whose history is being assessed may be the *consultand* or *proband,* and he or she should be identified with an arrow on the pedigree (Figs. 2.1, 2.2, and 2.3). A consultand is an individual presenting for genetic counseling or testing (GeneTests, 2004; Nussbaum et al., 2007). This is the patient or client whose family history is being constructed using a pedigree and who may be seeking advice or consultation. The consultand can be healthy or can have a medical condition (see Fig. 2.3) (Bennett, 1999). A proband is an *affected* individual who has symptoms of a particular condition. This person might be the first person to be clinically identified, sometimes called the *index* case, in a given family (GeneTests, 2006; Nussbaum et al., 2007). The proband may be the affected individual who caused the consultand to seek advice, or the individual seeking advice can be both the proband and the consultand. Start the family history with the consultand, and *always* identify the consultand with an arrow symbol on the pedigree. Use an arrow with a designated *P* (for proband) to denote whether the patient is the proband or

Table 2.4

Examples of Commonly Used Standardized Pedigree Symbols and Nomenclature

Nomenclature	Symbol	Comment	Nomenclature	Symbol	Comment
INDIVIDUALS: Male	□	Unaffected	Male affected	▣	Use a "key" or legend to define condition
Female	○	Unaffected	Female affected	◉	
Gender unknown	◇	Unaffected	Gender unknown, affected	◈	
Multiple siblings unaffected put appropriate gender symbol & number inside	3 / ⑤	3 unaffected males / 5 unaffected females	Multiple individuals, gender unknown	◇4	4 unaffected members, gender unknown
Deceased individual (draw line through gender)	⧅ d. age 45	Deceased male	Deceased individual female	⊘ d. age 89	
Consultand: [Use appropriate gender]	↗□ / ↗○	Consultand (male) / Consultand (female)	Proband	↗○ P / ↗□ P	Proband (female) / Proband (male)
Pregnancy: Include gestational age below or last menstrual period (LMP)	P 38 weeks / ⓟ LMP 1/1/2008	Use 'P' inside appropriate gender symbol if known	Pregnancy	◇P 12 weeks	Pregnancy, gender unknown
Spontaneous abortion (SAB) (use "triangle" and write in gender below if known)	△ Female / △ Male	Use smaller symbol than standard	Termination of unaffected pregnancy	△	Termination of affected pregnancy
Stillbirth	⧅	⊘	Stillborn gender unknown	◈	
Include gestational age	SB 29 weeks	SB 32 weeks		SB 33 weeks	
RELATIONSHIPS: Married (insert male on left)	□——○		Divorced	□—//—○	
Consanguinuity Use double lines	□——○ =		Horizontal line = relationship line / Vertical line = Descent	□——○ / □ e.g., married with 1 son	
Parents with children and siblings (e.g., 3 children: 1 son and 2 daughters)	□——○ / □ ○ ○		Couple with no children by choice / Line with 1 bar / Female with infertility / Vertical line with 2 bars	□——○	
Adoption - brackets Solid descent line "adopted out"; broke adopted out	[□] : [□]		Twins boys; Monozygotic (with bar); Dizygotic (no bar)	/△\ / /△\ □ □	

Reference: Bennett, Steinhaus, Uhrich, O'Sullivan, Resta et al. (1994). This table is not intended to be exhaustive; refer to reference for more inclusive symbols.

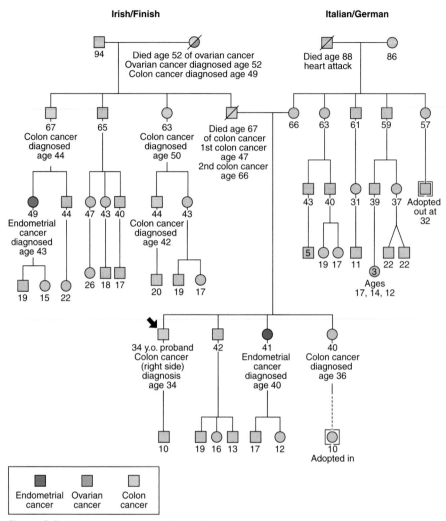

Figure 2.1 Four-generation pedigree (fictitious) depicting an autosomal dominant inheritance pattern of Lynch's syndrome (hereditary nonpolyposis colon cancer) on the paternal lineage.

is both the consultand and proband (see Figs. 2.1 and 2.2) (Bennett et al., 1995, Pritchard & Korf, 2008).

4. *Assessment of family history data.* To be complete, the pedigree should include the client/patient, siblings, children, parents, aunts/uncles, nieces/nephews, and grandparents so that a family history of at least three generations from both the maternal and paternal lineage is obtained. Assessment should include the following data elements:

   a. *Ethnic background or ancestry of each grandparent.* Some disorders have a higher incidence among certain populations. For example, sickle cell disease, an autosomal recessive hereditary condition, is

Ancestry: Ashkenazi Jewish

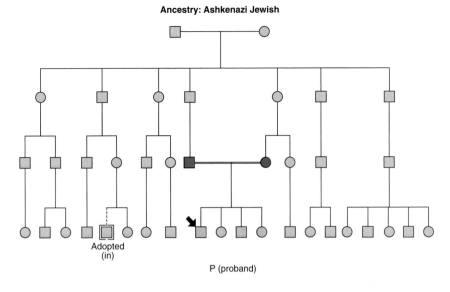

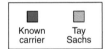

Figure 2.2 Four-generation pedigree (fictitious) with autosomal recessive inheritance pattern of Tay-Sachs disease in family of Ashkenazi ancestry with a consanguineous relationship.

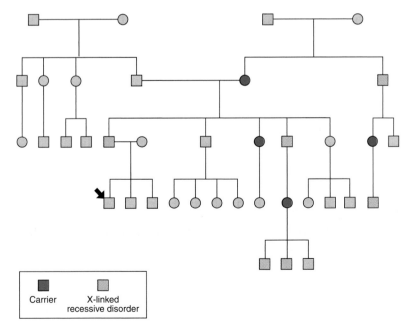

Figure 2.3 Five-generation pedigree (fictitious) of X-linked recessive pattern of inheritance, maternal lineage, with consultand noted by arrow.

found more frequently among individuals of African descent, and Tay-Sachs is more common among Ashkenazi Jewish individuals.

b. *Age of each family member* if known; use the symbol "?" if age is unknown, or denote the approximate age (e.g., age ~50s; ~60s, etc.). Recording birth year of family members rather than age can be more reliable when reviewing the pedigree at later dates. If approximate age is unknown, record approximate year of birth (e.g., birth year ~1952).

c. *Relevant medical information, including age of diagnosis* (e.g., maternal aunt, age 40, diagnosed with breast cancer at age 37; maternal cousin, age 38, diagnosed with ovarian cancer, age 37); and pertinent surgical history, including age and reason for surgery (e.g., mother with hysterectomy for fibroids, age 52) (Edwards et al., 2007).

d. *Age and cause of death of each family member* (e.g., father died at age 38 of massive heart attack; sister, age 40, died of motor vehicle accident).

e. *Consanguinity*, if present in the family history, using two horizontal lines to establish the relationship between the male and female partners (see Fig. 2.1).

f. *Adoption* (adopted in or out of the family using appropriate standardized pedigree symbol [e.g., brackets]), as noted in Figures 2.1 and 2.2.

g. *History of infertility, pregnancy complications* including gestational age, miscarriage, stillbirth, pregnancy termination, or ectopic pregnancy (e.g., proband with a history of three spontaneous abortions at 8 weeks' gestation).

h. *History of mental retardation or severe learning problems, mental illness, or depression* (Bennett, 1999; Spahis, 2002).

Drawing a legend to depict significant medical conditions provides a quick visualization of medical conditions and how they cluster within the family (see Figs. 2.1 and 2.2). Once the pedigree is completed, assess it for medical conditions that may show patterns of Mendelian inheritance due to single-gene alterations or medical conditions due to chromosomal or multifactorial inheritance.

■ Pedigree Interpretation

The human body contains 46 chromosomes: 22 pairs (44 chromosomes) known as *autosomes* and 1 pair (2 chromosomes: X and Y) known as *sex chromosomes*. A female has no Y chromosome but normally has two copies of X, while males normally have one X and one Y sex chromosome. While the sex chromosomes are different depending on gender, both males and females have exactly the same 22 pairs of autosomes (except in chromosomal abnormalities). The basic unit of heredity, consisting of a segment of DNA arranged in a linear manner along a chromosome, is known as a *gene* (GeneTests, 2004). Each gene has a specific location on a specific chromosome known as the *gene locus*. The genes located on the chromosomes form a specific protein or segment of protein leading to a particular characteristic or body function (GeneTests, 2004). The human genome contains approximately 30,000 genes, which make approximately 100,000 unique proteins (National Human Genome Research Institute [NHGRI], 2003).

Single-Gene Disorders

Single-gene disorders are a result of an alteration in the gene or a permanent heritable change in the sequence or arrangement of genomic DNA, commonly called a mutation (Nussbaum et al., 2007). A single-gene mutation may occur on the autosome, on the X or Y sex chromosome, or in the mitochondria. Single-gene disorders have a unique pattern of inheritance that can be identified in a family pedigree. Because the mutations are inherited in a predictable pattern, they are often classified as dominant or recessive or as autosomal or X-linked (Nussbaum et al., 2007).

Autosomal Dominant Inheritance

Autosomal dominant (AD) inheritance is a result of a gene mutation in one of the 22 autosomes. In AD disorders, gene mutations are transmitted from either the father or the mother, and each offspring has a 50% chance of inheriting the mutation. Unless the mutation originates spontaneously during conception (called a de novo mutation; see Table 2.1), individuals with an AD disorder have one parent (either a mother or father) who also has the mutation. Pedigrees associated with AD disorders typically reveal multiple affected family members with the disease or syndrome. When analyzing the pedigree for AD conditions, it is common to see a "vertical" pattern denoting several generations of affected members. Figure 2.1 denotes a four-generation pedigree with multiple affected family members on the paternal lineage with colon cancer. Note that each of the four generations has at least one member with colon cancer. The presence or absence of affected members in a given family with an AD condition depends on the family structure, such as familial size, gender concentrations (e.g., lots of men but few females), early age of death from other causes (e.g., accidents), and features of the disease (age of onset at which the gene typically expresses symptoms or clinical features). Not all genetic disorders are observed at birth. For example, women with a *BRCA* mutation that predisposes to hereditary breast and ovarian cancer are not born with breast or ovarian cancer but are at risk for developing these cancers in adulthood. Gender may also influence the presence of affected members in a family with a genetic mutation. For instance, in a limited family structure with few women over age 50, paternal inheritance of a *BRCA* mutation may be missed or the probability of a familial *BRCA* mutation underestimated (Edwards et al., 2007; Weitzel et al., 2007). Table 2.5 lists characteristics of AD disorders.

Autosomal Recessive Inheritance

In autosomal recessive (AR) disorders, the offspring inherits the condition by receiving one copy of the gene mutation from each of the parents. *Autosomal recessive disorders must be inherited through both parents* (Nussbaum et al., 2007). Individuals who have an AR disorder have two mutated genes, one on each locus of the chromosome. Parents of an affected person are called *carriers* because each carries one copy of a mutation on one chromosome and a normal gene on the other chromosome. Carriers typically are not affected by the disease because one gene usually produces enough normal protein to

Table 2.5

Definition and Characteristics of Single-Gene Patterns of Inheritance

Terms	Definition	Characteristics
Autosomal dominant (AD)	A gene on one of the autosomes that may be expressed even if only one copy is present	Fifty percent chance of parental transmission; males and females affected; phenotype is observed in multiple or every generation with each affected person having an affected parent (vertical transmission on pedigree). NOTE: Exceptions may be de novo variable expressivity, penetrance,[b] family structure, early onset of deaths; gender-related conditions (e.g., breast and ovarian cancer syndromes) may not be observed in families of limited size or with small number of females or males.
Autosomal recessive (AR)	A genetic disorder that appears only in a patient who received two copies of a gene mutation, one from each parent.[a] Two genetic mutations on the autosomes.	50% chance of the offspring inheriting one gene mutation carrier; 25% chance of inheriting disease/phenotype; horizontal transmission on the pedigree proband may have affected siblings but not parents (carriers), offspring, or other relatives. Males and females affected equally.[b]
X-linked[a] dominant	Genetic mutations located on the X chromosome requires only one copy for phenotype or disease in male or females	Disorders are rare; most are lethal in pregnancy with male fetus;[b] no male-to-male transmission; no carrier state—affected males transmit to affected daughters only.[c]
X-linked recessive	Genetic mutation located on the X chromosome requires both X chromosomes to be affected in females; males with affected gene will have the disorder	Males are affected, females are typically unaffected carriers. Rare but possible for females to be affected if they inherit two X mutations (one from each parent). Affected fathers: 100% of daughters are carriers, and no affected sons (only sons inherit Y chromosome); no male-to-male transmission.[b] Carrier mother: 50% of daughters are carriers, and 50% of sons affected.
Mitochondrial DNA (mtDNA)	Mutations located in the mitochondria inherited by the mother	Mitochondria present in egg only (not in sperm), so all offspring (male and female) inherit mutations. Daughters pass mutation to all offspring;[b] sons do not pass mutation.

[a]National Human Genome Research Institute, 2008b; [b]Nussbaum et al., 2007; [c]Lashley, 2005.

sustain cellular function. Because AR disorders affect the autosomes rather than the sex chromosomes, the disease can manifest in either males or females who receive two copies of the mutated genes. The offspring of two parents who both are carriers of an AR condition has a 50% chance of receiving one copy of a mutation and will be a carrier (like the parents); a 25% chance of receiving two copies of the mutation (one from each parent) and having the AR disorder; and a 25% chance of receiving two normal genes. It is important that parents understand that if they both carry a mutation, the risk to each of their offspring (each pregnancy) is an independent event: 25% disease free, 25% affected, and 50% carrier. In pedigrees with an AR inheritance pattern, *males and females will be equally affected* because the gene mutation is on the autosome. In addition, the pedigree will have a "horizontal" presentation (many unaffected generations followed by an affected generation). If more than one family member is affected by an AR disorder, the pedigree will usually show disease in the proband and his or her siblings, *not* in the parents (who are carriers) or other relatives, as noted in Figure 2.2 (Nussbaum et al., 2007). Consanguineous families are at increased risk for AR disorders because they share many genes (including rare ones), so it is important to denote consanguinity on the pedigree (see Fig. 2.2). Ancestry of origin and ethnicity are also important because some ethnic groups have a higher incidence of AR disorders (Table 2.6; see Fig. 2.2). AR disorders are most commonly

Table 2.6			

Examples of Genetic Conditions Commonly Seen Among Racial/Ethnic Groups or by Ancestry of Origin

Genetic Condition Pattern of Inheritance	Race/Ethnicity Ancestry of Origin	Estimated Prevalence	Carrier Frequency (Recessive Disorders)
Sickle cell anemia (AR)	African Americans	1/600	1/12
Tay-Sachs disease (AR)	Ashkenazi Jewish American non-Jewish	1/3,600 1/360,000	1/30 1/300
Cystic fibrosis (AR)	Caucasians African Americans Asian Americans	1/2,500 1/15,000 1/32,100	1/25 1/65[a] 1/90[a]
Alpha-thalassemia (AR)	Southeast Asians and Chinese	1/2,500	1/25
Beta-thalassemia (AR)	Mediterranean (Greeks, Italians)	1/3,600	1/30
Gaucher's disease (AR)	Ashkenazi Jewish	1/25,000	1/15
Hemochromatosis (AR)	Caucasians	1/400	1/10

AR = autosomal recessive.
[a]Statistics obtained from March of Dimes Pregnancy and Newborn Health Education Center (2008).
Table adapted from Pritchard & Korf, 2008.

seen in newborns, infancy, or early childhood and frequently involve disorders of inborn errors of metabolism affecting known enzymes and metabolism (Bennett, 1999).

X-Linked Disorders

The X and Y chromosomes determine gender. Females have two X chromosomes, and males have an X and Y chromosome. An estimated 1,100 genes are thought to be located on the X chromosome, and 40% of them are known to be associated with disease (Nussbaum et al., 2007). X-linked diseases may be dominant (mutation required on only one X chromosome) or recessive (both X chromosomes must carry the mutation).

X-Linked Dominant Inheritance

Only one X chromosome mutation is required for X-linked dominant disorders to occur, and fortunately, these disorders are extremely rare. Everyone born with an X-link dominant disorder will be affected with the disease. Transmission of the disorder to the next generation varies by gender, however. A woman will transmit the mutation to 50% of all her offspring (male or female), while a man will transmit the mutation to 100% of his daughters (they receive his X chromosome) and none of his sons (they receive his Y chromosome). The pedigree of a family with an X-linked dominant disorder would reveal *all the daughters and none of the sons affected with the disorder if the father has an X-linked disorder.* It is rare to see an X-linked dominant disorder in men, because these disorders *are often lethal in males* during the prenatal period, and as a result, one striking feature of an X-linked dominant disorder is a relative absence of male family members (Bennett, 1999; Nussbaum et al., 2007). Females with one copy of an X-linked dominant mutation survive because they have a second, healthy X chromosome capable of producing normal protein. Pedigrees of a family with an X-linked dominant disorder will be markedly different depending on which parent carries the mutation, but they follow the general rule for dominant pedigrees, demonstrating a vertical pattern of inheritance. A pedigree may also be helpful in ruling out an X-linked dominant disorder. If a father is affected with a suspected X-linked genetic disorder, but the pedigree shows unaffected daughters or affected sons, the inheritance pattern does not conform to an X-linked pattern. The mutation must therefore be on an autosome and not a sex chromosome (Nussbaum et al., 2007). One example of an X-linked dominant disorder is incontinentia pigmenti, an extremely rare disorder affecting the skin, hair, teeth, nails, eyes, and central nervous system (Scheuerle & Ursini, 2010).

X-linked Recessive Inheritance

Some X-linked disorders are recessive, which means that in a woman, both X chromosomes must have the mutation if she is to be affected. If only one X chromosome carries the mutation and the other is normal, she will be a carrier and typically will be unaffected. Because males have only one copy of the X chromosome, they will be affected if their X chromosome carries the mutation. Because of the rarity of X-linked recessive disorders, it is unusual for a female to have two affected X chromosomes unless her father had an X-linked disorder and her mother was either a carrier or also affected with the disorder. Thus, *X-linked recessive disorders occur typically in males.* There is no male-to-male transmission because the father with an X-linked disorder can transmit the Y chromosome only to his male offspring. *All daughters of affected fathers with an X-linked recessive disorder will be carriers.* Female carriers have a 50% chance of transmitting the gene mutation to their sons, who will all be affected (see Fig. 2.3). One example of an X-linked recessive disorder is hemophilia A, and additional disorders are listed in Table 2.7.

Table 2.7

Examples of Single-Gene Disorders With Associated Pattern of Inheritance, Estimated Prevalence, and Clinical Characteristics

Pattern of Inheritance and Genetic Conditions *Autosomal Dominant*	Estimated Prevalence	Clinical Characteristics
Polycystic kidney disease[a]	1/300 to 1/1,000	Progressive renal failure characterized by bilateral renal cysts; cysts in other organs (e.g., hepatic, pancreatic, ovarian, splenic); mitral valve prolapse; intracranial saccular aneurysms; hypertension
Marfan's syndrome[b]	1/5,000 to 1/10,000	Systemic disorder of connective tissue with a high degree of clinical variability. Cardinal manifestations involve the ocular, skeletal, and cardiovascular systems
Familial hypercholesterolemia[c]	1/200 to 1/1,000	Hypercholesterolemia; atherosclerosis
Autosomal Recessive		
Hemochromatosis[d]	1/200 to 1/400 (Caucasians) 1/7,000 (rare in African Americans)	Inappropriately high absorption of iron by the gastrointestinal mucosa, resulting in excessive storage of iron, particularly in the liver, skin, pancreas, heart, joints, and testes
X-Linked Recessive		
Fragile X[c]	16–25/100,000 males	Moderate mental retardation (males); mild mental retardation in females, most with behavioral abnormalities
Duchenne muscular dystrophy[c]	1/3,500 males	Progressive myopathy leading to muscle degeneration and weakness

Continued

Table 2.7		

Examples of Single-Gene Disorders With Associated Pattern of Inheritance, Estimated Prevalence, and Clinical Characteristics—cont'd

Pattern of Inheritance and Genetic Conditions *Mitochondria (mtDNA)*	Estimated Prevalence	Clinical Characteristics
Leber hereditary optic neuropathy[e]	Varies throughout the world; 1/8,500 (Northeast England) with mutation and 1/31,000 with visual loss; 1/39,000 (Netherlands); similar in other Caucasian populations	Bilateral, painless, subacute visual failure; minor neurologic abnormalities

[a]Harris & Torres, 2009; [b]Dietz, 2009; [c]Nussbaum et al., 2007; [d]Kowdley, Tait, Bennett, & Motulsky, 2006; [e]Yu-Wai-Man & Chinnery, 2008.

Chromosomal Disorders

In addition to single-gene mutations, entire chromosomes or large sections of chromosomes can be affected, resulting in disease. Abnormalities of any of the chromosomes (autosomes and/or sex chromosomes) can be a consequence of numerical or structural problems. There can be too few (less than 46) or too many (more than 46) chromosomes. An individual with an abnormal number of chromosomes has a condition called *aneuploidy*, which is frequently associated with mental or physical problems or both (Nussbaum et al., 2007). The normal structural appearance of the chromosome may also be altered because of deletions, duplications, inversions, translocations, rearrangements, insertions, or other changes of segments of the chromosomes. These structural alterations can result in positional changes of the gene leading to nonfunctional genes, excessive or inadequate protein production, or the development of cancer (Lashley, 2005). Chromosomal disorders have also been associated with mental retardation; failure to thrive; developmental delay; low birth weight; infertility; and histories of frequent spontaneous abortions, stillbirths, or neonatal births. Approximately 50% of spontaneous abortion have chromosomal abnormalities (Lashley, 2005; Nussbaum et al., 2007). An estimated 1 in 160 newborns have a chromosomal abnormality (Nussbaum et al., 2007). For instance, a newborn with trisomy 21 (Down's syndrome) has an extra chromosome 21 and therefore has a total of 47 chromosomes instead of the usual 46. A complete family history includes inquiring about prior pregnancy outcomes such as spontaneous abortions, stillbirths, and neonatal deaths. In addition, maternal age is important because Down's syndrome and other trisomies have been associated with advanced maternal age (older than 35 years at time of delivery). Although most aneuploidy conditions involve autosomes (particularly chromosomes 21, 13, and 18), sex chromosomes may also be duplicated or omitted, resulting in disorders like Turner's and Klinefelter's syndromes. Chromosomal alterations affecting the sex chromosomes may not be apparent until later in life. Individuals with Klinefelter's syndrome have too many sex chromosomes (47 XXY) and may appear normal until adolescence when signs of hypogonadism become apparent. Individuals with Turner's syndrome (45 X) are missing a sex chromosome and may be identified at birth (clinical features of webbed neck and lymphedema of hands and feet) or later because of primary amenorrhea (Nussbaum et al., 2007).

Mitochondrial DNA (mtDNA) Inheritance

Mitochondria are found in every cell in the body, and they have a critical function in producing energy. They have a unique ring of DNA that can carry mutations very similar to the single mutations discussed previously. Because mitochondrial mutations involve oxidative phosphorylation and metabolic energy, mitochondrial abnormalities often involve the central nervous and musculoskeletal systems, but they can also be multisystem (Lashley, 2005; Nussbaum et al., 2007). Mitochondrial inherited disorders have a distinct *maternal inheritance* because, at conception, the sperm contribute only the nuclear content (chromosomes) while the ovum provide mitochondria and all the other cellular structures (Nussbaum et al., 2007). Fathers therefore cannot transmit a mitochondrial condition to their offspring. The pedigree of a family with an mtDNA disorder is unique in that *all offspring (regardless of gender) of an affected female will have disease, and none of the offspring from an affected male will have disease* (see Table 2.5). Because mutations may be present in all mtDNA (homoplasmy) or in some (heteroplasmy), the risk and severity of mtDNA diseases often varies widely among family members. One example of an mtDNA disorder is Leber hereditary optic neuropathy (see Table 2.7).

Special Consideration in Genetic Assessment

■ Preconception/Prenatal Counseling

A comprehensive personal and family history is an integral part of preconception counseling and care. Assessing the family history with a minimum of a three-generation pedigree can help to identify hereditary conditions so that appropriate information, education, genetic testing, and referral for genetic counseling can be implemented (Edwards et al., 2004). Some individuals or couples have unique identifiable risks that should be discussed prior to conception whenever possible. For example, women who will be older than 35 years at delivery (advanced maternal age) are at increased risk for aneuploidy, and certain racial/ethnic groups are at higher risks for specific genetic conditions (see Table 2.6). During a preconception visit, prior adverse pregnancy outcomes such as congenital birth defects, pregnancy loss, or fetal death can be explored and may offer important information about future reproductive risks or may be an indicator of chromosomal abnormalities. Table 2.3 contains online resources for preconception and prenatal assessment.

■ Hereditary Cancer Syndromes

A cancer diagnosis in one or more family members is commonly found when a minimum of a three-generation pedigree is collected. While the majority of cancers are sporadic or multifactorial due to a combination of genetic and environmental factors, approximately 5% to 10% of all cancers are due to a single-gene mutation (Garber & Offit, 2005). Family history is a key tool in the early recognition of individuals at increased risk for cancer due to a hereditary cancer syndrome. This early identification provides an opportunity to offer genetic counseling, discuss genetic testing if available, and develop a management of care strategy. One example of the use of hereditary cancer syndrome screening is screening at-risk women for a *BRCA* mutation. Women with a *BRCA* mutation are at a high risk for developing breast and ovarian cancers (Ford et al., 1998; Garber & Offit, 2005; Nussbaum et al., 2007). Appropriate measures for women diagnosed with a *BRCA* mutation might include enhanced surveillance, possible chemoprevention, or optional surgery to reduce their risk for developing the disease. In 2005, the United States Preventive Service Task Force (USPSTF) issued guidelines for genetic risk assessment and *BRCA* mutation testing to determine susceptibility for breast and ovarian cancer (USPSTF, 2005).

Most hereditary cancer syndromes like that of *BRCA* mutations are autosomal dominant, and it is not uncommon to find multiple family members with a specific cancer, an unusual presentation of a disease (a male with breast cancer), and/or early age of onset in the family pedigree. These genetic red flags are associated with an inherited predisposition to the disease (see Red Flag box). Some hereditary cancer syndromes are associated with several different cancers or other clinical characteristics. For example, in Figure 2.1 (fictitious family), the four-generation pedigree reveals many relatives in the paternal lineage with early age–onset colon, endometrial, and ovarian cancers, red flags for the AD condition Lynch's syndrome (also known as hereditary nonpolyposis colorectal cancer [HNPCC]).

RED Flag ◄ Example of Family History Red Flags

Hereditary Cancer Syndromes
- Early-age onset (e.g., breast cancer at age 45 or younger; colon cancer at age 45–50 or younger)
- Occurrence of cancer in the less-often affected sex (e.g., male breast cancer)
- Multiple family members with cancer, especially if age of onset is earlier than usual

---

RED Flag ◀ Example of Family History Red Flags—cont'd

- AD pattern of inheritance
- Known hereditary cancer gene mutation in the family (e.g., *BRCA* mutation)
- Family member with multiple primary cancers
- Clustering of syndromes associated with a hereditary cancer (e.g., breast and ovarian cancer; colon cancer and endometrial cancer)
- Two or more unusual cancers in the same person or close relative

Medical Disorders
- Heart disease before age 40 to 50 years
- Dementia before age 60
- Hearing loss before age 50 to 60
- Venous thromboembolism before age 50
- Three or more pregnancy losses
- Several family members with the same condition
- Multisystem or bilateral occurrences (e.g., deafness and nephritis suggestive of Alport's syndrome)

Family GENES mnemonic
- **G** Group of congenital anomalies
- **E** Extreme or exceptional presentation of common conditions (e.g., multiple primary cancers seen with hereditary cancer syndromes such as *BRCA* mutation)
- **N** Neurological delays or degeneration (e.g., early age–onset Alzheimer or dementia)
- **E** Extreme or exceptional pathology (e.g., medullary thyroid cancer; multiple adenomatous polyps in familial adenomatous polyposis)
- **S** Surprising laboratory values (e.g., familial hypercholesterolemia, cholesterol greater than 500)

Adapted from American Medical Association, 2004; GeneTests, 2006; Lashley, 2005; Nussbaum et al., 2007.
Family GENE mnemonic taken from Whelan, et al., 2004.

Analyzing and Interpreting Family History Findings

Once completed, the family history must be evaluated for patterns of inheritance that may indicate a genetic disorder. Key points to look for include the presence of consanguinity, male-to-male transmission or female-to-male transmission, whether males and females are affected in equal numbers or if only males are affected, all of which can aid in distinguishing autosomal from X-linked disorders. Pedigree can sometimes be difficult to evaluate, and errors in interpretation can occur for many reasons. It is important, there-fore, that all HCPs take as careful, thorough, and detailed a family history as possible. Even if an accurate family history is obtained, other difficulties can arise in interpreting the pedigree. Several common problems include the following:

1. A new or de novo mutation. The proband is the first person to have the disease. New mutations are a frequent cause of dominant and X-linked diseases (Nussbaum et al., 2007). For example, over 80% of children born with achondroplasia, an AD disorder, have a de novo mutation and are born to parents of normal stature (Francomano, 2006).

2. Nonpaternity. The person identified as the father on the pedigree is not the biological father.

3. The family is very small (limited in structure) or is limited by gender. This is particularly important when assessing for gender-associated conditions. For example, if a *BRCA* mutation occurs in the paternal lineage with mostly male members, a vertical pattern of the disease may not be noted on the pedigree. The sole family member, a female daughter with newly diagnosed breast cancer at age 35, might be the red flag that is indicative of a *BRCA* mutation that she inherited from the paternal lineage.

4. The person providing the history is not aware of all the details of the family history, has inaccurate information ("ovarian cancer" was actually "cervical cancer"), or is deliberately withholding information (perhaps from fear of discrimination).

5. Early death of a family member from other causes (e.g., in a war or an accident) limits the family structure, particularly when there are genetic diseases that express symptoms in adulthood.

6. Disorders inherited from an individual who does not typically express the disorder. For example, color blindness, an X-linked recessive disor-der, is not usually seen in women because they are typically carriers and unaffected. It is difficult to assess for color blindness patterns in a family with many females but few males or in families in which males died early of other causes or never mentioned having any visual prob-lems. In these situations, color blindness can appear to be a new con-dition, when in fact it may have been present in the family for many generations.

7. Some disorders have a range of expression from mild to severe. For example, patients with neurofibromatosis (NF1), an AD disorder of the nervous system, may manifest with many forms of the disease (variable expressivity). The diagnosis may be further complicated by the variability in symptoms. For instance, some patients with NF1 may have mild symptoms like café-au-lait spots or axillary or skin freckling, while others may have life-threatening spinal cord tumors or malignancy (Nussbaum et al., 2007).

8. Some gene mutations are more penetrant than others. In mutations of varying penetrance, some individuals will have the gene mutation but will never develop disease (GeneTests, 2004). Some genetic disorders are not 100% penetrant. For example, a woman with a *BRCA* mutation is at a 50% to 85% life-time risk of developing breast cancer and a 35% to 50% life-time risk of developing ovarian cancer (Ford et al., 1998). While these risks are higher than the population risk, carrying a *BRCA* mutation does not confer a 100% risk for disease. Reduced penetrance may be attributed to a combination of genetic, lifestyle, and environmental factors.

While pedigree interpretation may be at times difficult, assessing the family history for red flags is very important because it can lead to early recognition of hereditary disorder (see Red Flag box).

■ Questionable Medical History

Critical family medical information may be missing that could be important in determining whether a family member is at risk for a genetic condition. If a hereditary condition is being considered but family medical information is unclear or unknown, requesting medical records and pathology or autopsy reports may be warranted. For instance, the cause of early death (age 35) of a patient's mother might be unknown. The death certificate or an autopsy report, however, may reveal that the cause of death thought to be a stomach problem was actually metastatic ovarian cancer diagnosed at age 34. Coupling this information with the family history reveals a red flag for a hereditary cancer syndrome, leading to the patient's (consultand's) genetic referral, testing, and diagnosis of a *BRCA* mutation.

Importance of Physical Examination

A physical examination should be conducted on all patients suspect for a genetic condition or who, based on family history, may be at risk for a medical problem. Physical examination should be focused on the characteristics of the disease and the system(s) needed to aid in diagnosing or excluding the genetic condition. Special attention to height and weight, head circumference, and physical development to include hearing, vision, motor skills, language, linguistic, behavior, and social skills are important components when assessing for genetic disorders in infants and children (Pritchard & Korf, 2008). Assessing for dysmorphic features may enable identification of certain syndromes or genetic or chromosomal disorders (Lashley, 2005; Pritchard & Korf, 2008). For example, epicanthal folds, up-slanted palpebral fissures, single transverse palmar crease, and a low nasal bridge are clinical features of Down's syndrome. Enlarged head circumference, tongue and skin lesions, and/or thyroid nodules may suggest Cowden's syndrome if hereditary breast cancer syndrome is suspected. Individuals with Cowden's syndrome, a rare AD disease caused by a mutation in the *PTEN* gene, are at high risk for benign and malignant tumors of the breast, thyroid, and endometrium as well as other benign disorders such as multiple hamartomatous polyps and fibrocystic breast disease (Eng, 2009). Clinical signs suggestive of Cowden's syndrome often include macrocephaly (occipital frontal circumference 97th percentile or greater), facial trichilemmomas, acral keratoses, papillomatous papules, palmoplantar keratoses, cobblestone-like pattern of oral mucosa especially the buccal and gingival mucosae, and/or a multinodular thyroid (Kovich & Cohen, 2004; Zbuk et al., 2006). In another physical finding, assessment of the skin with noted lesions of café-au-lait spots, axillary freckling, or neurofibromas might meet the diagnostic criteria suggestive of NF1, formerly known as von Recklinghausen's disease (Lashley, 2005). Examples of selected single-gene disorders and hereditary cancer syndromes by body systems are listed in Tables 2.8 and 2.9.

Table 2.8

Examples of Selected Genetic Single-Gene Disorders by Body Systems

System	Medical Condition and (Frequency)	Inheritance Pattern	Characteristics
Skin	Neurofibromatosis type 1: *NF1* mutation (1/3,000–1/5,000)	AD; 80% de novo	Variable expression: skin café-au-lait spots; axial or inguinal freckling; neurofibromas; Lisch nodules on retina; optic gliomas; malignant tumors of peripheral nerve sheath[a]
Ear	Deafness: *GJB2* mutation (1/500–1/1,000 neonates)	AD and AR	Congenital hearing impairment or deafness (nonsyndromic); congenital in AR; progressive childhood in AD[b]
Respiratory	α_1-antitrypsin deficiency: α1AT (1/5,000 Caucasians) (2% carriers)	AR	Increased risk of chronic obstructive lung disease, emphysema, and liver cirrhosis[b]
Cardiovascular	Familial hypercholesterolemia: low-density lipoprotein receptor mutation (1/500 Caucasians)	AD	Hypercholesterolemia; atherosclerosis; xanthomas; Arcus corneae[b]
	Long QT syndrome: cardiac ion channel gene mutation (~1/5,000–1/7,000)	AD	Tachyarrhythmias; syncope episodes; QT prolongation; sudden death[b]

ASSESSMENT FINDINGS

Vesicles

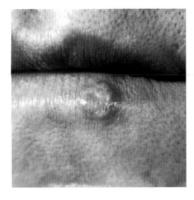

Plate 1 Herpes Simplex Herpes simplex is a virus that causes painful vesicular lesions on the skin and mucosal surfaces. Shown here are grouped vesicles on an erythematous base on the skin. (Courtesy of CDC and Dr. Herrmann, 1964)

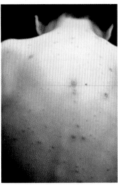

Plate 2 Varicella Hallmark skin eruptions of the acute viral disease known as chickenpox. Typical lesions are generalized papules, vesicles, and crusted lesions in various stages. (Courtesy of CDC, 1995)

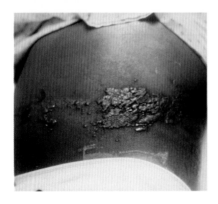

Plate 3 Herpes Zoster (Shingles) Reactivation of the varicella (chickenpox) virus leads to inflammation of a few peripheral nerves causing, as shown here, a dermatomal distribution of erythematous papules, vesicles, and eroded vesicles in various stages. (Courtesy of CDC, 1995)

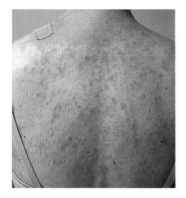

Plate 4 Contact Dermatitis In response to skin contact with allergens or irritating substances, erythematous papulovesicular lesions in distribution of causative agent can occur. (Reprinted with permission by Margaret Bobonich, DNP, DCNP, FNP-C)

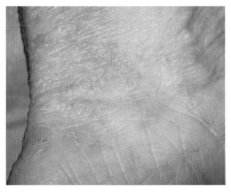

Plate 5 Scabies Skin manifestations of the highly contagious infections of the mite *Sarcoptes scabiei* show erythematous papules in a burrows pattern, rarely some vesicles, and excoriations from scratching because of extreme itching. (Barankin & Friemann, 2006; Image courtesy of Loretta Fioroillo, MD.)

Bullae (Large Blisters)

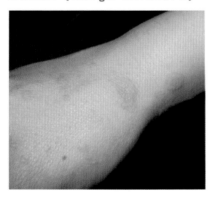

Plate 6 Erythema Multiforme The rash shown here often is caused by an immune response to drugs or an infection, such as herpes simplex virus. It presents with a target lesion with three rings and a vesicular or dusky center. (Barankin & Friemann, 2006)

PUSTULES

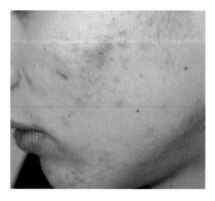

Plate 7 Acne Vulgaris An inflammatory skin condition of the sebaceous follicles exhibiting inflammatory papules, pustules, and nodules. (Barankin & Friemann, 2006)

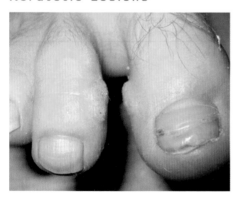

Plate 8 Bacterial Folliculitis Infection of the hair follicles caused most commonly by *S. aureus, Pseudomonas,* or *Pityrosporum folliculitis.* It is identified by pustules and papules in a distribution of hair follicles. (Barankin & Friemann, 2006)

Keratotic Lesions

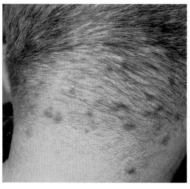

Plate 9 Warts Firm, hyperkeratotic, skin-colored lesions caused by infection from the human papilloma virus. Warts are most commonly found on the hands but can occur anywhere. (Barankin & Friemann, 2006)

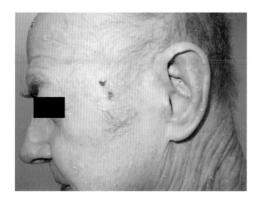

Plate 10 Actinic Keratoses Rough, scaly lesions on skin surfaces exposed to the sun. These are the most common precancerous lesions. (Barankin & Friemann, 2006)

Raised, Skin-Colored Lesions

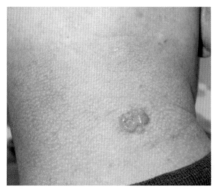

Plate 11 Basal Cell Carcinoma Pearly, raised border with central induration, often with telangiectasia that defines the most common human cancer. The malignancy is associated with exposure to sun or other ultraviolet light. (Barankin & Friemann, 2006)

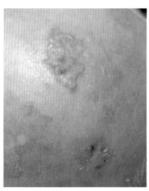

Plate 12 Squamous Cell Carcinoma Nonhealing, usually slow-growing lesions, often with scaly surface, that appear on skin exposed to sunlight and ultraviolet light. Second most common form of human cancer after basal cell carcinoma. (Barankin & Friemann, 2006)

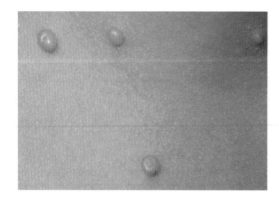

Plate 13 Molluscum Contagiosum Small, umbilicated, flesh-colored, and dome-shaped lesions caused by infection with poxvirus. The contagious infection occurs mainly in children and immunocompromised patients. (Barankin & Friemann, 2006)

White Lesions

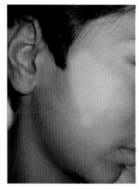

Plate 14 Pityriasis Alba Hypopigmented patches with fine, scaly surface that are commonly seen on the face in children. (Barankin & Friemann, 2006)

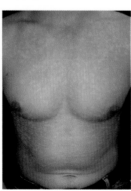

Plate 15 Tinea Versicolor Macules and patches ranging from hypopigmentation to various colors, with fine, scaly surface caused by infection with the fungus *Malassezia furfur.* (Barankin & Friemann, 2006)

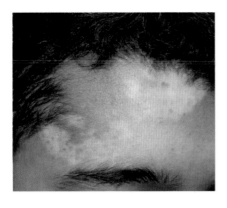

Plate 16 Vitiligo Hypopigmented/white, well-defined patches caused by localized loss of melanocytes. (Barankin & Friemann, 2006)

Brown Lesions

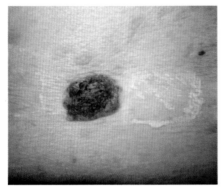

Plate 17 Seborrheic Keratosis Papules of varying size and pigmentation with roughened surface and adhesive appearance, commonly seen in older adults. These are benign tumors, and the cause is not known. (Barankin & Friemann, 2006)

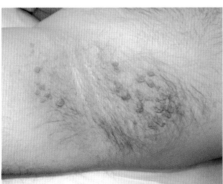

Plate 18 Acanthosis Nigricans Hyperpigmented plaques with velvety surface, typically on neck, axillae, or groin. This may be associated with endocrine disorders and obesity and with the use of certain drugs. It runs in families and can be seen with some malignancies. (Barankin & Friemann, 2006)

7

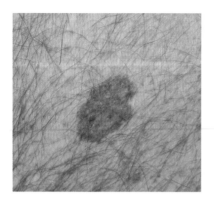

Plate 19 Melanoma A potentially aggressive form of skin cancer of the melanocytes characterized by asymmetric lesions with irregular borders, variegated coloring, and/or diameter greater than 6 mm, resulting from exposure to sun and ultraviolet light. (Barankin & Friemann, 2006)

Inflammatory Or Red Lesions

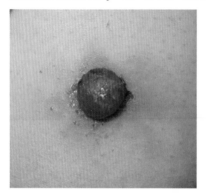

Plate 20 Pyogenic Granulomas Firm, red, isolated papule that may ulcerate and crust. This is a benign tumor often referred to as "proud flesh." (Barankin & Friemann, 2006)

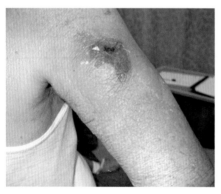

Plate 21 Cellulitis Erythematous and edematous warm area of tenderness caused by a bacterial infection, most commonly *Streptococcus pyogenes* or *Staphylococcus aureus.* (Barankin & Friemann, 2006)

8

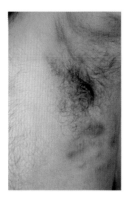

Plate 22 Hidradenitis Suppurativa Pustules, nodules, abscesses, and/or sinus tracks in area of hair follicles caused by inflammation of the sweat glands. Often associated with obesity, diabetes, and smoking. (Barankin & Friemann, 2006)

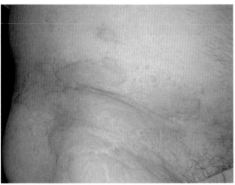

Plate 23 Urticaria An allergic reaction that causes extremely itchy erythematous, edematous papules, and/or plaques in varied distributions. (Barankin & Friemann, 2006)

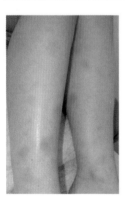

Plate 24 Erythema Nodosum Inflammation of the subcutaneous fat (panniculitis) that causes a dull erythematous and tender nodule, frequently on anterior lower leg. (Barankin & Friemann, 2006)

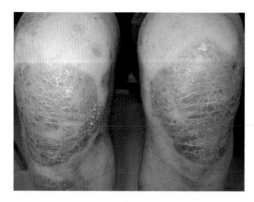

Plate 25 Psoriasis A chronic skin disorder of unknown etiology that causes erythematous and scaly, silvery plaques over an erythematous base, frequently found on extensor surfaces. Many variations are possible. (Barankin & Friemann, 2006)

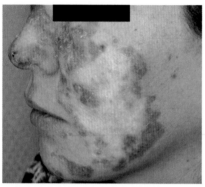

Plate 26 Lupus Erythematosus A chronic autoimmune disease of connective tissue that causes a characteristic "butterfly rash" on the face presenting as a fixed erythematous rash that occurs on the cheeks but not in the nasolabial folds. (Courtesy of the CDC)

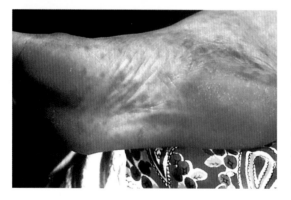

Plate 27 Secondary Syphilis Characteristic nontender maculopapular lesions that commonly appear on the soles of the feet or palm of the hand and occur up to several months after infection with the spirochete *Treponema pallidum* if the condition is untreated. (Courtesy of CDC and Susan Lindsley, 1977)

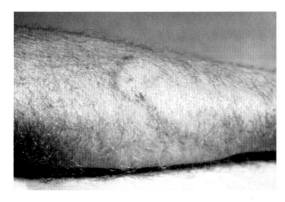

Plate 28 Tinea Corporis
Annular lesion with raised, erythematous, scaly border and central clearing that occurs after infestation of the fungus *Trichophyton, Microsporum,* or *Epidermophyton.* (Courtesy of the CDC, 1975)

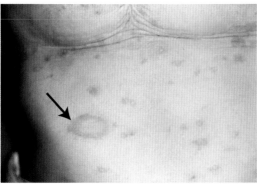

Plate 29 Pityriasis Rosea A mild, acute inflammatory condition with a characteristic early rash that is a large macular herald patch and is followed by ovoid, fawn-colored, scaly lesions with a "Christmas tree" pattern, or diagonal, orientation. Occurs most commonly in the spring and fall. (Courtesy of the CDC, 1975)

Eczematous Lesions with Excoriations

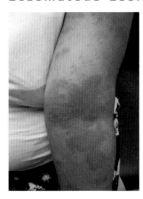

Plate 30 Atopic Dermatitis A chronic condition often seen in families that presents with erythematous, scaly patches and plaques, often along the flexor surfaces, as in this flare affecting the antecubital area. (Reprinted with permission by Margaret Bobonich, DNP, DCNP, FNP-C)

11

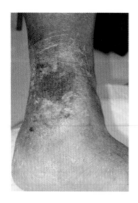

Plate 31 Stasis Dermatitis Erythematous, scaly patches on lower leg, associated with edema, varicosities, and/or hyperpigmentation associated with impaired blood return from the legs. (Barankin & Friemann, 2006)

Variations In Skin Color

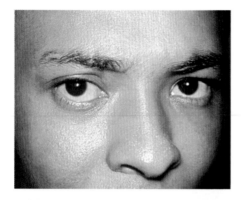

Plate 32 Jaundice Yellow staining of skin and sclera associated with elevated bilirubin. (Courtesy of CDC and Dr. Thomas F. Sellers/ Emory University, 1963)

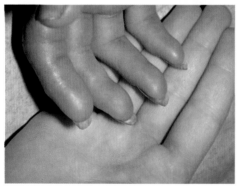

Plate 33 Cyanosis Blue to purple tinge associated with hypoxemia. (Dillon, 2007)

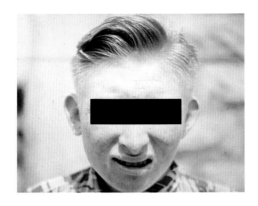

Plate 34 Albinism Inherited condition with little or no pigmentation in skin, hair, eyes. (Dillon, 2007)

Exterior Eye Abnormalities

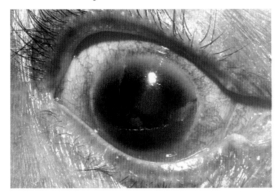

Plate 35 Ciliary Flush A condition in which conjunctival vessels are most dilated around the corneal edge. (Reprinted with permission from Dr. Julia Haller, Ophthalmologist in Chief. Permission granted by Michael D. Allen, Esquire, at Wills Eye Institute)

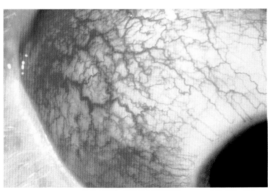

Plate 36 Episcleritis Inflammation of the subconjunctival layer of the sclera characterized by localized, sectoral conjunctival vessels dilated peripherally. (Reprinted with permission from Dr. Julia Haller, Ophthalmologist in Chief. Permission granted by Michael D. Allen, Esquire, at Wills Eye Institute)

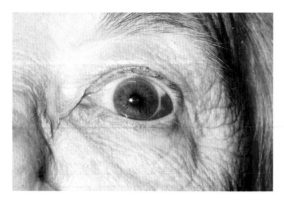

Plate 37 Subconjunctival Hemorrhage **Hemorrhage** beneath the conjunctiva usually caused by injury. (Reprinted with permission from Dr. Julia Haller, Ophthalmologist in Chief. Permission granted by Michael D. Allen, Esquire, at Wills Eye Institute)

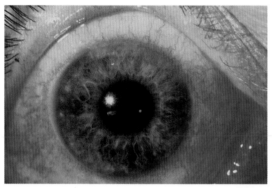

Plate 38 Conjunctivitis Inflammation of the conjunctiva that is most commonly caused by viral, gonococcal, and chlamydial organisms. Presentation is generalized vessel injection with dilation greatest peripherally. (Reprinted with permission from Dr. Julia Haller, Ophthalmologist in Chief. Permission granted by Michael D. Allen, Esquire, at Wills Eye Institute)

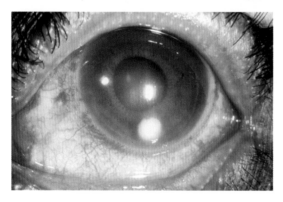

Plate 39 Corneal Ulceration Well-circumscribed ulcer following fluorescein staining. Not always visible to the naked eye. (Reprinted with permission from Dr. Julia Haller, Ophthalmologist in Chief. Permission granted by Michael D. Allen, Esquire, at Wills Eye Institute)

14

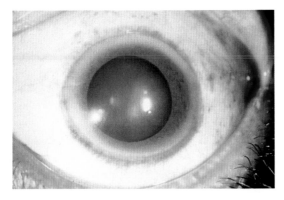

Plate 40 Corneal Arcus White or gray ring at corneal margin seen in older adults and caused by fat deposits in the cornea or hyaline degeneration. (Reprinted with permission from Dr. Julia Haller, Ophthalmologist in Chief. Permission granted by Michael D. Allen, Esquire, at Wills Eye Institute)

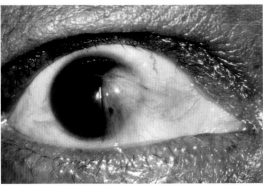

Plate 41 Pterygium Wedge-shaped, raised conjunctival growth, usually extending from nasal side. May be related to chronic irritation. (Reprinted with permission from Dr. Julia Haller, Ophthalmologist in Chief. Permission granted by Michael D. Allen, Esquire, at Wills Eye Institute)

Ophthalmoscopic Findings

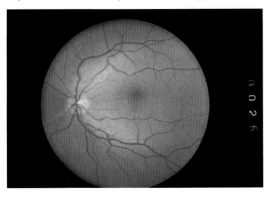

Plate 42 Normal Fundus Well-defined disk; paired arteries and veins; bright red arteries; arteriovenous (AV) ratio 2:3; no nicking, exudates, hemorrhages. (Reprinted with permission from Dr. Julia Haller, Ophthalmologist in Chief. Permission granted by Michael D. Allen, Esquire, at Wills Eye Institute)

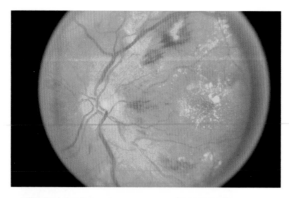

Plate 43 Diabetic Retinopathy Soft and hard exudates, dot and blot hemorrhages. (Reprinted with permission from Dr. Julia Haller, Ophthalmologist in Chief. Permission granted by Michael D. Allen, Esquire, at Wills Eye Institute)

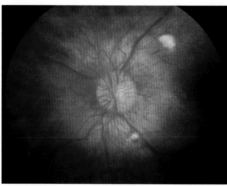

Plate 44 Diabetic Proliferative Retinopathy Extensive microvascular changes with exudates and other background changes that occur in advanced-stage diabetes when abnormal new blood vessels and scar tissue form on the surface of the retina. (Courtesy of National Eye Institute, National Institutes of Health)

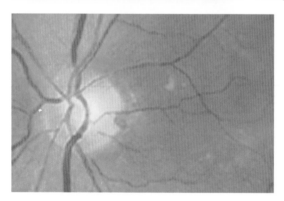

Plate 45 Hypertensive Changes Narrowing arteries, increased light reflex, crossing changes, and exudates commonly seen with long-term hypertension. (Reprinted with permission from Dr. Julia Haller, Ophthalmologist in Chief. Permission granted by Michael D. Allen, Esquire, at Wills Eye Institute)

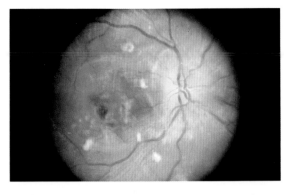

Plate 46 Malignant Hypertension Blurred disk margins, papilledema, narrowed arteries, crossing changes, and exudates seen in malignant hypertension. (Reprinted with permission from Dr. Julia Haller, Ophthalmologist in Chief. Permission granted by Michael D. Allen, Esquire, at Wills Eye Institute)

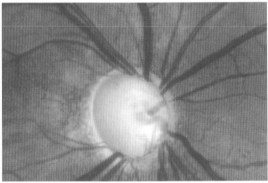

Plate 47 Glaucomatous Optic Nerve Increased cup-and-disk ratio is a common finding when visualizing the optic nerve in a patient with glaucoma. (Reprinted with permission from Dr. Julia Haller, Ophthalmologist in Chief. Permission granted by Michael D. Allen, Esquire, at Wills Eye Institute)

EAR INSPECTION

Otoscopic Findings

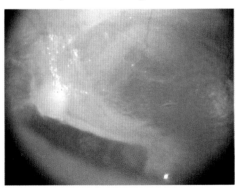

Plate 48 Normal Tympanic Membrane Bony landmarks are visible through translucent membrane (tympanic membrane) in the ear with intact light reflex. (Permission from Kevin Kavanaugh, MD of Cumberland Otolaryngology Consultants)

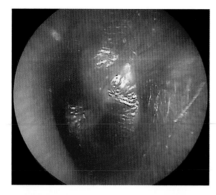

Plate 49 Acute Otitis Media Reddened and opaque tympanic membrane with distorted light reflex is a usual otoscopic finding with middle ear infection. (Permission from Kevin Kavanaugh, MD of Cumberland Otolaryngology Consultants)

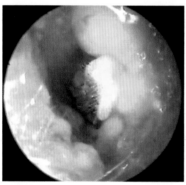

Plate 50 Otitis Externa Inflammatory swelling of canal, often with exudates seen in infection of the external ear canal. Shown is otomycosis.
(Permission from Kevin Kavanaugh, MD of Cumberland Otolaryngology Consultants.)

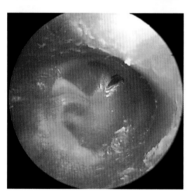

Plate 51 Acute Otitis Media With Perforation Perforation may stem from increased pressure associated with infection, physical trauma, or barotraumas. (Permission from Kevin Kavanaugh, MD of Cumberland Otolaryngology Consultants)

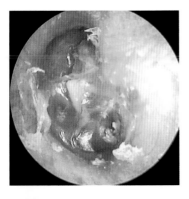

Plate 52 Cholesteatoma Cystlike sac of keratin debris, which may erode ossicles. (Permission from Kevin Kavanaugh, MD of Cumberland Otolaryngology Consultants)

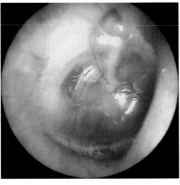

Plate 53 Otitis Media With Effusion Fluid level is visible through retracted membrane, and a distorted light reflex occurs when middle ear infection produces exudates. (Permission from Kevin Kavanaugh, MD of Cumberland Otolaryngology Consultants)

MOUTH INSPECTION

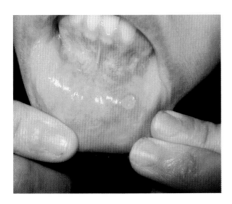

Plate 54 Aphthous Ulcer Painful, open, well-circumscribed lesion on mucous membranes. (Barankin & Friemann, 2006)

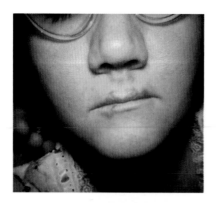

Plate 55 Herpes Simplex Herpes simplex is a virus that causes painful vesicular lesions on the skin and mucosal surfaces. Shown here are individual or clustered vesicles, eroding to ulcers and crusted lesions on the lips. (Courtesy of CDC and Dr. Sellars/Emory University, 1963)

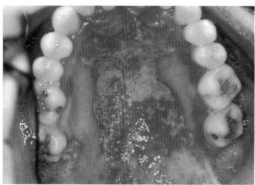

Plate 56 Candidiasis A fungal infection caused by *Candida,* especially *Candida albicans,* that causes an erythematous mucosa often with white patches. Shown here is an infection of the roof of the mouth; this commonly is seen on the tongue as well. (Permission and photo from Dr. Levine)

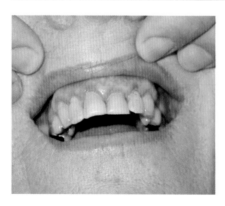

Plate 57 Oral Lichen Planus A chronic autoimmune inflammatory condition affecting the lining of the mouth, usually resulting in characteristic lacy white striations, papules, and patches. (Barankin & Friemann, 2006)

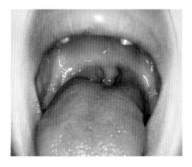

Plate 58 Tonsillitis Moderate redness of oropharynx, 3+ tonsils caused by group A streptococcus. (Courtesy of CDC, 1975)

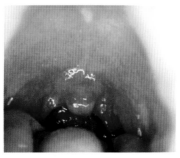

Plate 59 Tonsillitis Redness of the soft palate and tonsillitis caused by group A streptococcus bacteria. (Courtesy of CDC, 1975)

NAIL INSPECTION

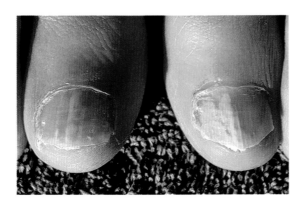

Plate 60 Onychomycosis Associated with dermatophyte infection of the nail plate, the nail may be yellowed, thickened, and separate (onycholysis). (Courtesy of CDC/Dr. Ewing Jr., 1997)

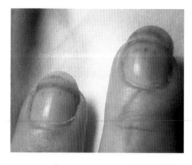

Plate 61 Splinter Hemorrhages Narrowed, reddish streaks beneath the nail, which can be nonspecific or related to either bacterial endocarditis or trauma. (Courtesy of CDC/Dr. Thomas Sellers/Emory University, 1963)

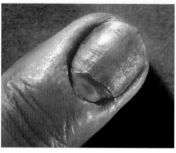

Plate 62 Candidiasis of Fingernail Candidiasis can cause nails to be cracked and deformed with surrounding erythema. (Courtesy of CDC and Sherry Brinkman, 1963)

HEAD INSPECTION

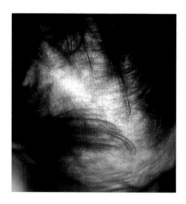

Plate 63 Alopecia Alopecia due to secondary syphilis. (Courtesy of CDC, 1971)

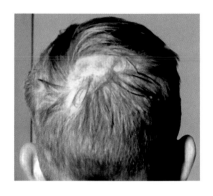

Plate 64 Tinea Capitis Dermatophyte infection causing hair loss with skin changes. (Courtesy of CDC, 1959)

REFERENCES

Barankin, B., & Friemann, A. (2006). *Derm Notes: Clinical Dermatology Pocket Guide.* Philadelphia: F.A. Davis.

Centers for Disease Control and Prevention (CDC). http://www.cdc.gov.

Dillon, P.M. (2007). *Nursing Health Assessment: A Critical Thinking, Case Study Approach,* 2nd ed. Philadelphia: F.A. Davis.

National Eye Institute, National Institutes of Health. Photos, images, and videos. http://www.nei.nih.gov/photo/keword.asp?narrow=Photo&match=all (accessed March 21, 2011).

Table 2.8

Examples of Selected Genetic Single-Gene Disorders by Body Systems—cont'd

System	Medical Condition and (Frequency)	Inheritance Pattern	Characteristics
Genitourinary	Polycystic kidney disease: *PKD1* and *PKD2* mutations (1/300–1/1,000)	AD	Progressive renal failure;[b] see Table 2.7
Musculoskeletal	Huntington's disease: *HD* mutation (3–7/100,000 Western Europeans)	AD	Progressive movement, cognitive and psychiatric abnormalities[b]
Neurological	Alzheimer's disease: *PSEN1, PSEN2, APP* genes (varies)	Multifactorial or AD	Middle to late adulthood age of dementia (40s to early 60s; mean age 45)[b]

AD = autosomal dominant; AR = autosomal recessive.
[a]Pritchard & Korf, 2008; [b]Nussbaum et al., 2007.

Table 2.9

Selected Hereditary Cancer Syndromes by Body Systems

Body System	Genetic Condition (Gene Mutation)	Inheritance Pattern	Characteristics/Associated Cancer
Skin	Malignant melanoma *(CDKN2A [p16]; CDK4)*	AD	Earlier than usual age of onset (median age ~36 years); increased pancreatic cancer risk *(CDKN2A)*[a]
Eye	Retinoblastoma *(RB1* mutation)	AD	Bilateral disease usually presents the first year of life; unilateral ~24–30 months; rare neoplasm of retina; strabismus; visual deterioration; other neoplasms (e.g., osteosarcomas, soft tissue sarcomas, melanomas)[b]
Breast[a,c]	Hereditary breast and ovarian *(BRCA* mutation)	AD	High-risk breast and ovarian cancer; multiple primary tumors; increased risk of other cancers (e.g., prostate, pancreatic)

Continued

Table 2.9

Selected Hereditary Cancer Syndromes by Body Systems—cont'd

Body System	Genetic Condition (Gene Mutation)	Inheritance Pattern	Characteristics/Associated Cancer
Breast	Li-Fraumeni syndrome (*p53* mutation)	AD	Osteo and soft tissue sarcomas; leukemia, brain, and adrenocortical cancer
	Cowden's disease (*PTEN* mutation)	AD	Associated cancers: thyroid (especially follicular), endometrial
	Peutz-Jeghers syndrome (*STK11LKB1* mutation)	AD	Associated cancer: gastrointestinal, ovarian, lung
	Ataxia telangiectasia (*ATM* mutation) (heterozygous carriers)	AR	Progressive cerebellar ataxia (homozygous)
	CHEK2	AD	Possibly colorectal cancer
Gastrointestinal (colon cancers)	Lynch's syndrome (hereditary non-polyposis colon cancer [HNPCC]) (*MLH1, MSH2, MSH6, PMS2* mutation)	AD	Extracolonic cancer: ovary, endometrium, stomach, small bowel, bile duct, urinary tract (sebaceous skin tumors, keratoacanthomas with Muir-Torre syndrome, an HNPCC variant), brain tumors (e.g., glioblastomas, Turcot's syndrome, HNPCC variant)[a,d]
	Familial adenoma-tous polyposis (FAP) (*APC* mutation)	AD	Colorectal adenomatous polyps greater than 100 (~10–100 in attenuated FAP); Turcot's syndrome: colon cancer and central nervous system tumors (e.g., medulloblastoma); Gardner's syndrome: adenomatous polyps, soft tissue tumors, osteomas, congenital hypertrophy of the retinal pigment epithelium[b]
Genitourinary	von Hippel-Lindau syndrome (*VHL* mutation)	AD	Clear cell renal cell carcinoma (CCRCC); multiple tumor types with great variability (e.g., retinal angiomas, cerebellar and

Table 2.9			

Selected Hereditary Cancer Syndromes by Body Systems—cont'd

Body System	Genetic Condition (Gene Mutation)	Inheritance Pattern	Characteristics/Associated Cancer
			spinal cord hemangioblastoma, pheochromocytoma, pancreatic cysts, islet cell/neuroendocrine tumors); endolymphatic sac tumor (inner ear); 70% of patients with CCRCC have the VHL mutation[a]
Neurological	Ataxia telangiectasia (*ATM* mutation)	AR	Progressive cerebellar ataxia; facial and conjunctiva telangiectasia; infant may appear normal at birth, symptoms occurring usually by 1–4 years; most wheelchair bound by adolescence; humoral and cellular immune dysfunction; associated cancer: lymphoreticular malignancies (e.g., lymphosarcoma, leukemias), breast cancer, melanoma[a,e]
Endocrine	Multiple endocrine neoplasia (MEN) type 2 (*RET* mutation)	AD	MEN type 2A: medullary thyroid cancer (MTC), hyperparathyroidism, and pheochromocytoma; MEN type 2B: MTC pheochromocytoma **No hyperparathyroidism** Marfanoid appearance[a,e]

AD = autosomal dominant; AR = autosomal recessive.
[a]Offit et al., 2004; [b]Nussbaum et al., 2007; [c]Edwards et al., 2007; [d]Maradiegue et al., 2008; [e]Lashley, 2007.
Note: Only selected hereditary cancer syndromes are presented; table is not all inclusive.

Additional Medical and Social History

Assessment of the social, environmental, occupational, and medication history is important when caring for any patient, including those with genetic conditions. Individuals living with an X-linked recessive disorder known as glucose-6-phospate dehydrogenase (G6PD) deficiency, for example, may be impacted by numerous external factors such as drugs, viral and bacterial infections, toxins, and metabolic acidosis (Nussbaum et al., 2007). For some individuals with G6PD, acute hemolytic anemia can occur when taking certain medications such as antimalarial primaquine, NSAIDS, aspirin, quinine, nitrofurans, and sulfonamides. Also, some people with G6PD may be sensitive to certain chemicals, such as mothballs, and must avoid eating fava beans (Nussbaum et al., 2007). Many environmental factors, such as trauma, surgery, malignant disease, immobility, oral contraceptives, and advanced age, increase the risk for deep vein thrombosis (DVT). The risk for DVT is further enhanced in some patients with a mutation in the factor V Leiden gene.

Clinical Decision-Making and Differential Diagnoses

When the family history is suspect for a hereditary condition, patients should be informed about genetic counseling resources and referred when necessary. Genetic counseling visits include the collection and validation of the family and medical history, a further assessment of genetic risk, genetic education and testing options, management and screening recommendations if indicated, discussion of insurance and employment issues, posttest genetic test results disclosure and interpretation, treatments and options, and the implications of the results for the individual and family members as well as anticipatory guidance and support (Lashley, 2005; Resta et al., 2006). Genetic services should be provided by genetic experts or a team of professionals that often includes physicians, geneticists, genetic counselors, and advanced practice nurses in genetics. Referral to a physician specialist may also be warranted for patients who require immediate medical consultation (e.g., a new obstetrical case with an abnormal genetic test finding). Several online resources are available to assist in locating genetic counseling services (see Table 2.3).

Ethical, Legal, and Social Implications

On May 21, 2008, President George W. Bush signed the *Genetic Information Nondiscrimination Act* (GINA) that protects Americans against discrimination based on their genetic information when it comes to health insurance and employment, paving the way for patient-personalized genetic medicine without fear of discrimination (NHGRI, 2008a). Keeping with the ethical principles of beneficence, nonmaleficence, patient respect, autonomy, and fairness will ensure that HCPs provide patient privacy and confidentiality of information throughout assessment of personal and family history and when referring patients for genetic consultation and testing if indicated and agreed upon by the patient. Major ethical issues in genetics include (a) genetic testing (e.g., risks, benefits, informed consent, who to screen, when, and what age), (b) privacy of the genetic information and duty and permission to warn other family members, (c) misuse of genetic information by insurers, and (d) the potential stigmatization that may occur with genetic testing and results (Nussbaum et al., 2007). These issues are complex and can result in psychological distress, change in family dynamics, false security, or stigmatization in some patients (Offit et al., 2004). Genetic consultation and referral to genetic counselors or HCPs with specialized genetic training should be provided to all patients suspect for a hereditary condition so that appropriate ethical, legal, and social implications can also be addressed.

Genetic Health Assessment: Putting It All Together

Time constraints are often the biggest barrier for HCPs to obtaining an in-depth three-generation family history. Asking the patient to complete a family history worksheet prior to the appointment saves time in the visit while offering the patient an opportunity to contribute to the collection of an accurate family history. Reviewing the family information can also help establish family rapport while verifying medical conditions in individual family members. Several family history collection tools are available to assist in gathering this important information. Some of the well-established tools include the U.S. Surgeon General's Initiative and the American Medical Association tools (see Table 2.3).

HCPs, including NPs, can achieve and maintain genetic core competency established by NCHPEG and the ANA through continuing education in medical genetics and genomics. They should also continuously compare their personal competence in genetics against NCHPEG's core competencies and identify areas of strength as well as areas where professional development in genetics and genomics would be beneficial. Continuing education can assist HCPs to better use and interpret medical family histories while reducing barriers to family history assessment in primary care practice (CPGNC, 2006; NCHPEG, 2007). The rapid pace of genetic and genomic knowledge and technology require that all health-care professionals keep abreast of advances in human genetics in order to integrate current and new genetic and genomic information into clinical practice. HCPs will find the translation of genetic and genomic research into practice playing an increasingly important role in patient care.

One area of genetic health care where advances are perhaps most striking is in genetic testing. Genetic tests now play an important role in diagnosing, monitoring, and treating many diseases. As new genetic tests emerge, all primary care providers will be expected to have a level of comfort and competence in genetics, and interpreting genetic test results will soon become routine in primary care (Suther & Goodson, 2003). Today's consumers also have access to a considerable amount of genetics information on the Internet, and HCPs must understand the content so that they can help patients fully understand the implications of genetic information as it applies to their particular situation. Finally, most common medical conditions, such as diabetes, coronary heart disease, and Alzheimer's disease, as well as the majority of cancers, are multifactorial, resulting from the interaction of both genetics and the environment. Family history has long been an important tool in identifying people at risk for early onset of coronary heart disease (Scheuner et al., 2006). Prevention of many multifactorial diseases requires that HCPs conduct risk assessment based on patient and family history in order to implement strategies to reduce disease. Resources for genetic and genomic continuing education, risk assessment tools, and family history and pedigree resources are listed in Tables 2.2 and 2.3 to assist HCPs in the process of integrating genetics into their practice.

REFERENCES

American Medical Association (AMA). (2004). "Family Medical History in Disease Prevention." www.ama-assn.org/ama1/pub/upload/mm/464/family_history02.pdf (accessed May 27, 2008).

Bennett, R.L. (1999). *The Practical Guide to the Genetic Family History.* New York: Wiley.

Bennett, R.L., Steinhaus, K.A., Uhrich, S.B., O'Sullivan, C.K., Resta, R.G., Lochner-Doyle, D., et al. (1995). Recommendation for standardized human pedigree nomenclature. *American Journal of Human Genetics, 56,* 745–752.

Berry, T.A., & Shooner, K.A. (2004). Family history: the first genetic screen. *Nurse Practitioner, 29*(11), 18, 23–25.

Consensus Panel on Genetic/Genomic Nursing Competencies (CPGNC). (2006). *Essential Nursing Competencies and Curricula Guidelines for Genetics and Genomics.* Silver Spring, MD: American Nurses Association.

Dietz, H.C. (2009). "Marfan Syndrome." In *GeneReviews* at GeneTests: Medical Genetics Information Resource (database online). Copyright University of Washington, Seattle, 1997–2011. Available at http://www.genetests.org (accessed March 7, 2011).

Edwards, Q.T., Seibert, D., Maradiegue, A., MacDonald, D., Jasperson, K., Lowstuter, K., et al. (2007). Breast cancer and the family tree. *Advance for Nurse Practitioners, 15*(5), 34–41.

Edwards, Q.T., Seibert, D., Macri, C., Covington, C., & Tilghman, J. (2004). Assessing ethnicity in preconception counseling: genetics—what nurse practitioners need to know. *Journal of the American Academy of Nurse Practitioners, 16*(11), 472–480.

Eng, C. (2009). "PTEN Hamartoma Tumor Syndrome (PHTS)." In *GeneReviews* at GeneTests: Medical Genetics Information Resource (database online). Copyright University of Washington, Seattle, 1997–2011. Available at http://www.genetests.org (accessed March 7, 2011).

Ford, D., Easton, D.F., Stratton, M., Narod, S., Goldgar, D., Devilee, P., et al. (1998). Genetic heterogeneity and penetrance analysis of the BRCA1 and BRCA2 genes in breast cancer families. *American Journal of Human Genetics, 62*(3), 676–689.

Francomano, C.A. (2006). "Achondroplasia." In *GeneReviews* at GeneTests: Medical Genetics Information Resource (database online). Copyright University of Washington, Seattle, 1997–2011. Available at http://www.genetests.org (accessed March 7, 2011).

Garber, J.E., & Offit, K. (2005). Hereditary cancer predisposition syndrome. *Journal Clinical Oncology, 23*(2), 276–292.

GeneTests: Medical Genetics Information Resource (database online). (2004). "Illustrated Glossary." University of Washington, Seattle, 1993–2008. www.ncbi.nlm.nih.gov/books/NBK5191 (accessed March 7, 2011).

GeneTests: Medical Genetics Information Resource (database online). (2006). "Genetic Tools." University of Washington, Seattle, 1993–2008. www.ncbi.nlm.nih.gov/books/NBK1335 (accessed March 7, 2011).

Guttmacher, A.E., & Collins, F.S. (2002). Genomic medicine—a primer. *New England Journal of Medicine, 347*(19), 1512–1520.

Harris, P.C., & Torres, V.E. (2009). "Polycystic Kidney Disease, Autosomal Dominant." In *GeneReviews* at GeneTests: Medical Genetics Information Resource (database online). Copyright University of Washington, Seattle, 1997–2011. Available at http://www.genetests.org (accessed March 7, 2011).

Kovich, O., & Cohen, D. (2004). Cowden's syndrome. *Dermatology Online Journal, 10*(3), http://dermatology.cdlib.org/103/NYU/case_presentations/102103n3.html (accessed March 7, 2011).

Kowdley, K.V., Tait, J.F., & Bennett, R.L. (2006). "HFE-Associated Hereditary Hemochromatosis." In *GeneReviews* at GeneTests: Medical Genetics Information Resource (database online). Copyright University of Washington, Seattle, 1997–2011. Available at http://www.genetests.org (accessed March 7, 2011).

Lashley, F.R. (2005). *Clinical Genetics in Nursing Practice*, 3rd ed. New York: Springer.

Maradiegue, A., Jasperson, K., Edwards, Q.T., Lowstuter, K., & Weitzel, J. (2008). Scoping the family history: assessment of Lynch syndrome (hereditary non-polyposis colorectal cancer) in primary care settings—a primer for nurse practitioners. *Journal American Academy of Nurse Practitioners, 20*(2), 76–84.

March of Dimes, Pregnancy and Newborn Health Education Center. (2008). "Carrier Screening for Cystic Fibrosis (CF)." www.marchofdimes.com/Pregnancy/prenatalcare_cysticfibrosis.html (accessed March 7, 2011).

National Coalition of Health Professional Education in Genetics (NCHPEG). (2007). "Core Competencies in Genetics for Health Professionals," www.nchpeg.org (accessed March 7, 2011).

National Human Genome Research Institute (NHGRI), National Institutes of Health. (2003). "The Human Genome Project Completion: Frequently Asked Questions." www.genome.gov/11006943 (accessed March 7, 2011).

National Human Genome Research Institute, National Institutes of Health. (2008a). "Genetic Information Nondiscrimination Act: 2007–2008." www.genome.gov/24519851 (accessed March 7, 2011).

National Human Genome Research Institute (NHGRI), National Institutes of Health. (2008b). "Talking Glossary of Genetic Terms." www.genome.gov/glossary/index.cfm? (accessed March 7, 2011).

National Institutes of Health. (2008). "Human Genome Project: Fact Sheet." http://www.genome.gov/18016863 (accessed March 7, 2011).

Nussbaum, R.J., McInnes, R.R., & Willard, H.F. (2007). *Thompson & Thompson Genetics in Medicine*, 7th ed. Philadelphia: Saunders.

Offit, K., Garber, J., Grady, M., Greene, M.H., Gruber, S., Peshkin, B., et al. (2004). *ASCO Curriculum: Cancer Genetics & Cancer Predisposition Testing*, 2nd ed. Alexandria, VA: American Society of Clinical Oncology.

Pritchard, D.J., & Korf, B.R. (2008). *Medical Genetics at a Glance*, 2nd ed. Malden, MA: Blackwell.

Resta, R., Biesecker, B.B., Bennett, R.L., Blum, S., Hahn, S.E., Strecker, M.N., et al. (2006). A new definition of genetic counseling: National Society of Genetic Counselor's Task Force report. *Journal of Genetic Counseling, 15*(2), 77–83.

Scheuner, M.T., Whitworth, W.C., Henraya-McGruder, H., Yoon, P.W., & Khoury, M.J. (2006). Familial risk assessment for early-onset coronary heart disease. *Genetics in Medicine, 8*(8), 525–531.

Scheuerle, A., & Ursini, M.V. (2010). "Incontinentia Pigmenti." In *GeneReviews* at GeneTests: Medical Genetics Information Resource (database online). Copyright University of Washington, Seattle, 1997–2011. Available at http://www.genetests.org (accessed March 7, 2011).

Spahis, J. (2002). Human genetics: constructing a family pedigree. *American Journal of Nursing, 102*(7), 44–50.

Suther, S., & Goodson, P. (2003). Barriers to the provision of genetic services by primary care physicians: a systematic review of the literature. *Genetics in Medicine, 5*(2), 70–76.

U.S. Department of Energy Office of Science, Office of Biological & Environmental Research, Human Genome Project. (2007). "Genome Glossary." www.ornl.gov/sci/techresources/ Human_Genome/glossary (accessed March 7, 2011).

U.S. National Library of Medicine. (2008). "Genetics Home Reference (Glossary)." http://ghr .nlm.nih.gov/glossary=genetics (accessed March 7, 2011).

U.S. Preventive Service Task Force (USPSTF). (2005). "Genetic Risk Assessment and *BRCA* Mutation Testing for Breast and Ovarian Cancer Susceptibility." www.ahrq.gov/clinic/ uspstf/uspsbrgen.htm (accessed March 7, 2011).

Weitzel, J.N., Lagos, V.I., Cullinane, C.A., Gambol, P.J., Culver, J.O., et al. (2007). Limited family structure and *BRCA* mutation status in single cases of breast cancer. *Journal of the American Medical Association, 297*(23), 2587–2595.

Whelan, A.J., Ball, S., Best, L., Best, R.G., Echiverri, S.C., Ganschow, P., et al. (2004). Genetic red flags: clues to thinking genetically in primary care practice. *Primary Care, 31*, 497–508.

Yoon, P., Scheuner, M., & Khoury, M. (2003). Research priorities for evaluating family history in the prevention of common chronic disease. *American Journal of Preventive Medicine, 24*(2), 128–135.

Yu-Wai-Man, P., & Chinnery, P.F. (2008). "Leber Hereditary Optic Neuropathy." In *GeneReviews* at GeneTests: Medical Genetics Information Resource (database online). Copyright University of Washington, Seattle, 1997–2011. Available at http://www.genetests .org (accessed March 7, 2011).

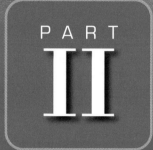

PART

II

Advanced Assessment and Differential Diagnosis by Body Regions and Systems

Chapter 3

SKIN

Mary Jo Goolsby

The skin is the largest of all organs. In addition to the obvious protective functions, the skin helps regulate body heat and moisture, and it is a major sensory organ. Even though many skin disorders are self-limiting, almost any skin condition can be extremely distressing for an individual. Not only is a large portion of the skin clearly visible, so that all can see any abnormality, but the skin is also an extremely sensitive organ, and its disorders invoke a wide range of symptoms, including pruritus, pain, burning, and stinging. However, in addition to minor, self-limited conditions, the skin serves as a barometer for overall health because it often exhibits changes occurring in response to serious systemic problems. Moreover, some dermatologically specific conditions, such as skin cancer, present significant risks to a patient's health.

Because the skin is such a large organ and exhibits changes in response to so many elements in the internal and external environments, the list of skin disorders is extensive. This chapter is organized to provide information to assist providers in making a definitive diagnosis for most common conditions. Information is provided on these common conditions and on some less-common mimics to assist the reader in applying the content in a practical manner.

History

■ General Integumentary History

When a patient presents with a skin-related complaint, there is an inclination to immediately examine the skin, as the lesion or change is often readily observable. However, it is crucial to obtain a history before proceeding to the examination in order to understand the background of the problem. A thorough symptom analysis is essential and should include details regarding the onset and progression of the skin change; anything the patient believes may trigger, exacerbate, or relieve the problem; how it has changed since first noticed; and all associated symptoms, such as itching, malaise, and so on. When a patient has a skin complaint, it is important to include a wide range of other integumentary symptoms in the review of systems. For instance, ask about the following: dryness, pruritus, sores, rashes, lumps, unusual odor or perspiration, changes in warts or moles, lesions that do not heal, or areas of chronic irritation. Establish whether the patient has noticed any changes in the skin's coloration or texture. Determine what the patient believes caused or contributed to the problem, any self-treatment and the response, and any distress caused by the complaint.

■ Past Medical History

The past medical history should include details on any previous dermatologic illnesses. Ask about infectious diseases associated with skin changes, such as chickenpox, measles, impetigo, pityriasis rosea, and others. Identify chronic skin problems, such as acne vulgaris or rosacea, psoriasis, and eczema. Ask about prior diagnoses of skin cancer. Determine the history of any previous skin treatments, biopsies, or procedures, as well as general surgical history. Because disorders in other systems frequently affect the skin, ask about the history of cardiovascular, respiratory, hepatic, immunologic, and endocrine disorders. Identify any recent exposures to others who have been ill and/or who have had obvious skin problems that might have been contracted. Many medications affect the skin, and a list of all prescribed and over-the-counter agents should be obtained, including herbal and nutritional supplements. The medication box below includes a nonexhaustive list of medications with potential adverse skin effects. Finally, ask the patient how he or she generally tolerates exposure to the elements, such as heat, cold, and sun, to determine whether environmental exposure is responsible for or may contribute to the patient's complaint.

MEDICATIONS AFFECTING SKIN

Classification	Agent	Possible Adverse Effects
Adrenocorticosteroids	Methylpred-nisolone, prednisone, corticotropin (adrenocorticotropic hormone [ACTH])	Urticaria, atrophy/thinning, acne, facial erythema, allergic dermatitis, petechiae, ecchymoses
Anticonvulsants	Carbamazepine, lamotrigine	Pruritic rash, toxic epidermal necrolysis, Stevens-Johnson syndrome
	Valproate	Alopecia
	Phenytoin sodium	Morbilliform (measleslike) rash, excessive hair growth
	Ethosuximide	Urticaria, pruritic and erythematous rashes

(cont. on page 46)

(cont. from page 45) MEDICATIONS AFFECTING SKIN

Classification	Agent	Possible Adverse Effects
Antimalarial	Chloroquine phosphate	Pruritis, pigmentary changes, lichen planus–like eruptions
Antineoplastic	Neomycin sulfate	Hypoesthesia, hyperesthesia, urticaria, erythematous swelling, hyperpigmentation, patchy hyperkeratosis, alopecia
	Busulfan	Cheilosis, melanoderma, urticaria, dry skin, alopecia, anhidrosis
	Cyclophosphamide	Pigmentary changes (skin/nails), alopecia
Barbiturates	Pentobarbital sodium, phenobarbital	Urticaria, varied rashes
Cephalosporins	Variety	Rash, pruritus, urticaria, erythema multiforme
Gold salts	Auranofin, gold sodium thiomalate	Rash, pruritus, photosensitivity, urticaria
NSAIDs	Variety	Rash, pruritus, erythema multiforme, Stevens-Johnson syndrome, photosensitivity
Oral antidiabetics	Variety	Photosensitivity, varied eruptions
Penicillins	Variety	Urticaria, erythema, maculopapular rash, pruritus
Phenothiazines	Chlorpromazine hydrochloride, thioridazine hydrochloride, trifluoperazine hydrochloride	Urticaria, pruritus, dermatoses, photosensitivity, erythema, eczema, exfoliative dermatitis

(cont. from page 46) **MEDICATIONS AFFECTING SKIN**		
Classification	Agent	Possible Adverse Effects
Sulfonamides	Cotrimoxazole, sulfamethoxazole, sulfasalazine, sulfisoxazole	Rash, pruritus, erythema nodosum, erythema multiforme, Stevens-Johnson syndrome, exfoliative dermatitis, photosensitivity
Tetracyclines	Demeclocycline hydrochloride, doxycycline hydrate, tetracycline hydrochloride	Photosensitivity
Miscellaneous	Allopurinal	Pruritis, maculopapular rash, exfoliative dermatitis, urticaria, erythematous dermatitis
	Captopril	Maculopapular rash, pruritus, erythema
	Oral contraceptives	Chloasma/melasma, rash, urticaria, erythema
	Thiazide diuretics	Photosensitivity
	Lithium	Acne
	Warfarin	Skin necrosis

Adapted with permission from Dillon, P. (2003). *Nursing Health Assessment: A Critical Thinking, Case Studies Approach.* Philadelphia: F.A. Davis, pp 147–148.

▪ Family History

The family history should include the occurrence of such skin diseases as eczema, psoriasis, and skin cancer, as well as other disorders commonly associated with skin problems, such as cardiovascular, respiratory, hepatic, immunologic, and endocrine disorders.

▪ Habits

Investigate habits related to skin, hair, and nail care. Identify any chemicals used in grooming, as well as potential exposures encountered through work and recreational activities. Identify occupational, daily living, and recreational activities that could be responsible for lesions resulting from friction, infestations, environmental extremes (heat, cold, sun), and other variables. Dietary history is helpful for identifying the potential sources of atopic reactions.

Physical Examination

■ Order of the Examination

As the history is obtained, a general survey is performed to determine the patient's general status. Notice the posture, body habitus, obvious respiratory status, and whether the patient is guarding or protecting any area of the skin. The general survey should provide an indication of the patient's overall skin condition, including color, visible lesions, moisture, and perspiration.

The progression for the skin examination can be completed in a systematic head-to-toe fashion or by region as other systems are being examined and are uncovered. Regardless of the sequence or system chosen, the examination of the skin consists of both inspection and palpation. During the general examination of the skin, compare side to side for symmetry of color, texture, temperature, and so on. Then look more closely at specific areas. Good lighting is essential. In many situations, additional equipment, such as a magnifier, measuring device, flashlight or transilluminator, and Wood's (ultraviolet) lamp, are helpful. Privacy is an important consideration because any area being examined must be completely bared. Keep in mind the structures underlying the skin and the amount of exposure a particular area is likely to receive to explain any particular "wear-and-tear" patterns, scars, calluses, stains, and/or bruises. For instance, an eczematous rash on the area of the nipple and/or areola should always trigger consideration of Paget's disease, a malignant breast condition.

Basic considerations for each section of skin inspected and palpated include the skin's color, temperature, moisture, texture, turgor, and any lesions.

Color

Color is highly variable among individuals of all racial and ethnic backgrounds. Color variation is even found among an individual's own various body regions, depending on several factors, including general exposure to the elements. For instance, coloring is typically darker in exposed areas, and calluses may be slightly darkened or have a yellow hue. Some patients develop a vascular flush over their face, neck, chest, and extremity flexor surfaces when they are exposed to warm environments or emotional disturbances.

Changes in color can also indicate a systemic disorder. For instance, cyanosis, which may indicate pulmonary or heart disease, a hemoglobin abnormality, or merely that the patient is cold, is observed for in the nail beds, lips, and oral mucosa. Jaundice indicates an elevation in bilirubin and often is evident in the sclera and mucous membranes before it is obvious in the skin. Pallor can indicate decreased circulation to an area or a decrease in hemoglobin. Like cyanosis, pallor is frequently first noticed in the face, conjunctiva, oral mucosa, and/or nail beds. Redness of the skin may indicate a generalized problem associated with a fever or localized problems, such as sunburn, infection, or allergic response. Table 3.1 lists several alterations in coloring associated with specific conditions.

Table 3.1	

Pigmentary Variations Associated With Systemic Conditions

Pigmentary Change	Associated Conditions
Bronze	Addison's disease (adrenal insufficiency)
	Hemochromatosis
Tan	Chloasma (pregnancy)
	Lupus
	Scleroderma
	Ichthyosis
	Sprue
	Tinea versicolor
Yellow	Uremia
	Jaundice, hepatic diseases
	Carotenemia
Dusky blue	Arsenic poisoning
	Cyanosis
Red	Polycythemia
Pallor	Anemia
	Vitiligo
	Albinism

Temperature

As each area is observed for visible changes, palpation helps to further explore the findings. Skin temperature is best assessed by the dorsal aspects of the hand and fingers. Situations that increase skin temperature include increased blood flow to the skin or underlying structures; thermal or chemical burns; local infections; and generalized, systemic infections and fever. Decreased skin temperature may result from atherosclerosis and shock.

Moisture

The moisture of the skin varies among body parts and with changes in the environmental temperature, activity level, or body temperature. Skin is typically drier during winter months and moister in warm months. Dehydration, myxedema, and chronic nephritis can all cause dry skin. Older patients tend to have drier skin than younger patients.

Texture

Skin texture is an important variable. Coarseness may be a sign of chronic or acute irritation as well as hypothyroidism. Extremely fine or smooth texture may indicate hyperthyroidism.

Turgor

Finally, skin turgor and elasticity are indications of several variables, including hydration and age. The skin should feel resilient, move easily, and return to place quickly after a fold is lifted. The skin overlying the forehead or dorsal hand is more likely to provide a false impression of tenting or decreased elasticity; therefore, turgor should be tested by gently pinching a fold of skin over the abdomen, forearm, or sternum. Some disorders, such as scleroderma, are associated with increased skin turgor.

■ Assessing Skin Lesions

All lesions must be assessed in detail for size, shape, configuration, color, and texture. There should be a determination of whether the lesion is elevated, depressed, or pedunculated. The color, odor, amount, and consistency of any exudate should be determined. If multiple lesions are present, consider their pattern, location, and distribution. All of theses variables, along with information obtained during the history and findings related to other systems, are important to making an accurate diagnosis. Specialized techniques such as magnification, diascopy, skin scrapings, and the use of Wood's lamp are helpful in assessing skin lesions.

Differential Diagnosis of Common Chief Complaints

Note: The color plate section includes photographs of many of the conditions described in this section.

■ Vesicles (Blisters)

Vesicles (blisters) are small, fluid-filled lesions. They may erupt at a site that initially appears inflamed, with a macule or papule. A wide range of conditions can cause vesicles, including infectious and atopic disorders as well as trauma. The history is very helpful in narrowing the differential diagnosis.

HERPES SIMPLEX (PLATE 1)

Herpes simplex is a viral infection that involves the skin and mucous membranes. It is transmitted via direct contact between a susceptible person and one who is shedding the herpes simplex virus (HSV). The infection can cause significant systemic symptoms. Orolabial lesions are typically caused by HSV-1 and genital lesions by HSV-2, although the prevalence of HSV-1 genital lesions is increasing.

Signs and Symptoms

The client may have a history of recurrent lesions in the same location. The skin lesions consist of multiple vesicles, which cluster and are usually preceded by an area of tender erythema. The vesicles erode, forming ulcerations. The lesions can occur anywhere on the body, although common sites include perioral and perigenital regions. Herpetic whitlow, a herpetic lesion on the finger, is usually a result of self-contamination of an infected patient to a skin break on the finger. The primary herpes simplex episode can be more severe, with a more painful lesion and greater likelihood of systemic symptoms such as malaise, aches, fever, and lymphadenopathy. Recurrent episodes may be more mild in nature. Regardless, herpes simplex is often associated with lymphadenopathy.

Diagnostic Studies

Diagnostic studies are typically not warranted or ordered. Definitive diagnosis can be made by viral culture of the lesion and Tzanck smear. The Tzanck smear does not differentiate between herpes simplex and varicella-zoster. There is a point-of-care test that is specific to HSV-2.

VARICELLA (PLATE 2)

The varicella-zoster virus causes chickenpox, which is considered a common childhood disease. Owing to the recent introduction of chickenpox vaccine, the incidence of chickenpox/varicella is decreasing.

Signs and Symptoms

The onset of the condition often is evident only when the characteristic skin lesions appear, although some patients describe a brief prodromal period of malaise and fever. The prodromal period is more common in adults with the disease than in children. The skin lesions appear first randomly scattered on the trunk and then extend to the extremities. Lesions may also appear on the mucosal surfaces. Similar to other herpes lesions, the lesions progress from an area of redness to form a vesicle, then become pustular, and finally ulcerate. The vesicles look like a dewdrop on a rose petal. New vesicles continue to appear while older lesions ulcerate and crust over, so that there is a range of lesion types at a given time. The lesions are intensely pruritic. The systemic symptoms may become severe, and complications include pneumonia, encephalitis, and death.

Diagnostic Studies

Diagnostic studies usually are not indicated but may be beneficial for atypical presentations or immunosuppressed patients.

HERPES ZOSTER (SHINGLES) (PLATE 3)

Herpes zoster is caused by the varicella-zoster virus. Patients who have circulating antibodies to the virus, usually adults, develop zoster with later exposure.

Signs and Symptoms

The skin lesions associated with herpes zoster are usually preceded by a period of regional neuralgia and discomfort as well as a period of malaise. Skin lesions appear as reddened macules, which later develop as clusters of vesicles and then ulcerate, crusting over. The distribution lies along a dermatome and is typically unilateral. There are many variations of the condition, depending on the affected dermatome. The healing of the lesions is frequently followed by development of postherpetic neuralgia. There is lymphadenopathy in the region of the skin lesions. In patients who are immunocompromised, the condition may be disseminated.

Diagnostic Studies

A Tzanck smear taken from the base of a vesicle is positive.

TINEA PEDIS

Tinea pedis is caused by a number of dermatophytes. The fungi invade the skin, and the infection is limited to the keratin layer.

Signs and Symptoms

There is often complaint of pruritus over scaling areas and pain at any developing fissures. The condition usually involves the interdigital areas, causing maceration, inflammation, and fissures. However, the plantar areas of the feet are prone to developing painful blisters in response to the infection. The vesicles often erode, and the patient is then prone to secondary infection.

Diagnostic Studies

None are needed. Scrapings will reveal hyphae.

CONTACT DERMATITIS (PLATE 4)

Contact dermatitis is an inflammatory response to contact with some chemical or other agent. The range of potential contactants is immense and includes agents used in grooming, recreation, and occupation as well as medications.

Signs and Symptoms

The affected area is usually intensely pruritic. The history helps in identifying the offending agent. The dermatitis appears within days following the contact or exposure. The first exposure usually results in a delayed response, whereas reactions to subsequent exposures develop more rapidly, commonly within 1 to 2 days. The distribution and configuration of skin lesions is determined by the exposure. The lesions can range in appearance; they emerge as reddened papules, which form vesicles and later erode and encrust. Any area of skin can be affected. As lesions erupt, the skin is at risk for developing secondary infection.

Diagnostic Studies

None are needed. A patch test will be positive.

DYSHIDROSIS

The cause of dyshidrosis is not clear. Although often associated with excessive sweating of the hands and feet, this is unlikely the direct cause. Instead, there is possibly an atopic contribution to the condition.

Signs and Symptoms

Dyshidrosis affects the hands and feet. Lesions often appear first along the lateral aspects of the digits and later involve the palms and/or soles. In very mild cases, there may be only a recurrent scaling or peeling of affected areas. However, the condition usually involves the appearance of small vesicles that itch and burn. With time, the vesicles open and crust. If secondary infection is present, the area will become inflamed. The distribution is usually symmetrical and there are often recurrences.

Diagnostic Studies

None are needed but may be done to rule out tinea pedis.

SCABIES (PLATE 5)

The mite *Sarcoptes scabiei* is responsible for this condition. Individuals are infected through direct contact. After the mites mate on the skin surface, the females burrow beneath the skin and the infected person develops a delayed sensitivity reaction to the mite, larvae, and fecal material.

Signs and Symptoms

The patient complains of intense pruritus, often worst at night. There is frequently a history of similar symptoms in other family members or contacts. The lesions appear as small red papules, which often form vesicles, erode, and crust. The distribution depends on the area of infestation. The hands, finger webs, wrists, axillae, and pubic areas are commonly involved. There can be secondary lesions related to the person's scratching the pruritic primary site. The lesions' configuration is typically linear, as the larvae burrow beneath the skin. Lesions become painful and reddened if secondary infection is present.

Diagnostic Studies

There is generally no reason to perform diagnostic tests, as the diagnosis is made on the basis of history and physical examination. However, skin scraping from a burrow viewed microscopically will often reveal the mite, egg, and/or fecal packet.

DERMATITIS HERPETIFORMIS

Dermatitis herpetiformis is an autoimmune skin disorder associated with a number of other conditions, including celiac disease, diabetes, rheumatoid arthritis, and lupus.

Signs and Symptoms

Pruritus, burning, or stinging at the site often preceeds the development of skin lesions. The lesions consist of clustered vesicles on a reddened base. The lesions have a herpetiform configuration, and the distribution is symmetrical. The extensor surfaces of the knees and elbows are often affected, as well as the posterior scalp, neck, back, and thighs. The condition is chronic. The oral mucosa is rarely involved, and the palms and soles are not affected.

Diagnostic Studies

Biopsy will demonstrate characteristic findings.

■ Bullae (Large Blisters)

Bullae are the fluid-filled lesions that are greater than 1 cm in diameter. They can be caused by thermal trauma as well as by infectious or atopic disorders.

ERYTHEMA MULTIFORME (PLATE 6)

Erythema multiforme is usually a self-limited skin condition that results from exposure to a medication or infection. This condition occurs in varying grades and is commonly classified as erythema multiforme minor, erythema multiforme major, and Stevens-Johnson syndrome. Erythema multiforme minor is caused by the herpes virus. Erythema multiforme major usually occurs in association with herpes or mycoplasma infection or in response to medications, although a range of infections are implicated. Stevens-Johnson syndrome is usually associated with medications.

Signs and Symptoms

The patient with erythema multiforme often provides the history of having recently taken a drug that caused the disorder or the history of another condition such as an autoimmune disorder, malignancy, or infection. The lesions are nonraised, reddened macules and/or plaques. They may have a "target" appearance, with a deep red outer rim and center, separated by a pale area. The lesions may progress to form vesicles and/or bullae that lie over the reddened base and form crusts as they erode. Although the lesions are generalized, they are usually most prominent over the limbs. The mouth, trunk, and soles of the feet are frequently involved.

Diagnostic Studies

Erythema multiforme may be associated with decreased white blood count and red blood cells and increased erythrocyte sedimentation rate (ESR) and increased blood urea nitrogen/creatinine in severe cases. In severe cases of Stevens-Johnson syndrome, the patient may be at risk for septicemia, particularly if immunocompromised, and therefore may require hospitalization for isolation.

CONTACT DERMATITIS

See p. 52.

BULLOUS IMPETIGO

Bullous impetigo is caused by *Staphylococcus aureus* and is less common than the nonbullous form. Although it can occur at any age, it is most common in children younger than 6 years old.

Signs and Symptoms

The patient or parent may recall being exposed to another person with similar lesions. The bullae progress rapidly, have a thin surface that bursts easily, and subsequently erode. A honey-colored crust is characteristic of impetigo, and smaller lesions may develop near the first. If the crust is removed, a reddened base is visible. Lesions can occur anywhere. There is no associated lymphadenopathy.

Diagnostic Studies

None are needed. Culture may be performed.

■ Pustules

Pustules are lesions that are filled with purulent fluid. The cause is typically infectious.

ACNE VULGARIS (PLATE 7)

Acne vulgaris affects most people at some time during their life. The multifactorial condition affects the sebaceous follicles.

Signs and Symptoms

The lesions may be tender. The areas most frequently involved include the face and the upper trunk. Patients with moderate acne commonly exhibit a range of lesions, including pustules. Other lesions include comedones, papules, and nodules.

Diagnostic Studies

None are needed.

ACNE ROSACEA

Although there are many theories regarding the cause of acne rosacea, including hair follicle mites and *Helicobacter pylori,* the cause is not clear. It is a condition affecting adults, with varying degrees of sebaceous hyperplasia.

Signs and Symptoms

The history includes facial flushing, which becomes more permanent over time. There is often some degree of facial edema. The central third of the face is most often involved. The lesions vary and include erythema, telangiectasia, and hyperplastic sebaceous glands. Rhinophyma tends to develop later in the condition and is more prevalent in middle-aged men.

Inflammatory papules and/or pustules are often present on the face, neck, and upper trunk.

Diagnostic Studies

None are needed.

BACTERIAL FOLLICULITIS (PLATE 8)

Folliculitis is an inflammation of the hair follicles and is typically associated with staphylococci. Other microorganisms and causes include pseudomonas (associated with hot tubs), Candida, tinea barbae, and herpes.

Signs and Symptoms

The patient complains of reddened areas of swelling often associated with a mild pruritic discomfort. Folliculitis lesions often develop as red papules that progress to form pustules. When the lesions erode, crusting occurs. Scarring often develops as the lesions heal. The site of previously healed lesions often have a keloid scar or atrophic scar with no hair growth. Lesions are located in the areas with greater hair growth, including the face, scalp, neck, upper trunk, axillae, and inguinal areas.

Diagnostic Studies

None are generally needed, although a Gram stain and/or culture may be performed.

■ Keratotic Lesions

Keratotic lesions are rough and generally raised. As the name implies, they contain a high amount of keratin.

WARTS (PLATE 9)

Warts are harmless skin tumors caused by the human papilloma virus.

Signs and Symptoms

Warts are raised lesions with no significant pigmentation, often paler than surrounding skin. The surface is irregular and may be stippled. If the surface is scraped or pared, minute bleeding points appear. The most common sites include the hands and feet, face, and genitalia. Lesions often occur in clusters.

Diagnostic Studies

None are needed. However, biopsy will reveal characteristic features.

ACTINIC KERATOSES (PLATE 10)

Actinic keratoses, also called solar keratoses, are premalignant lesions that appear in sun-exposed areas of skin. They typically are found in individuals with fair skin and who have a history of developing sunburns without tanning.

Signs and Symptoms

Typical sites include the face and hands, although any area of chronic sun exposure is at risk. The margins are irregular, as is the surface, which has slight scale and can be removed to reveal bleeding. The lesions vary in color and may be hypo- or hyperpigmented.

Diagnostic Studies

Biopsy will reveal features characteristic of this premalignant lesion.

CORNS AND CALLUSES

A callus is an area of skin thickening at a site exposed to repetitive force and wear and tear. With time, a callus may develop a central area of dead cells, which is the "corn."

Signs and Symptoms

Although calluses are generally painless, corns do become painful. Calluses have rather indistinct borders, yet corns have very distinct borders. The coloring varies. The sites include area exposed to wear-and-tear pressures, often against bony prominences, such as on the hands and feet. Unlike warts, these lesions will not reveal pinpoint black dots and bleeding if pared or scraped.

Diagnostic Studies

None are needed.

■ Raised, Skin-Colored Lesions

BASAL CELL CARCINOMA (PLATE 11)

Basal cell carcinoma is the most common form of human malignancy and involves sun-exposed skin. This malignancy is generally very slow growing. However, it can become quite destructive and invasive if not diagnosed and treated in a timely manner.

Signs and Symptoms

The typical complaint is of a nonhealing sore located on the face, ear, or other sun-exposed area. The patient may complain that the lesion is nonhealing because of repeated trauma. The history often includes previous incidences of basal cell or other skin cancers. Although the lesions can vary, the typical lesion has a waxy/pearly appearance with a central indentation. The surface often reveals telangiectasia. Over time, the central area erodes and becomes crusty. The border of the lesion typically has a "rolled" appearance. However, basal cell carcinoma appears in several variants and can be flat, hyperpigmented, and/or have very indistinct margins.

Diagnostic Studies

The diagnosis is made by biopsy.

SQUAMOUS CELL CARCINOMA (PLATE 12)

Squamous cell carcinoma is second in prevalence only to basal cell carcinoma and also involves sun-exposed areas of skin. These carcinomas are more rapidly growing and can become invasive over time.

Signs and Symptoms

The patient complains of a nonhealing lesion that is growing in size. The lesion is often tender. There is frequently also a history of a lesion consistent with actinic keratosis that progressed into the offending lesion. The appearance of squamous cell carcinoma varies. The lesion may have a warty appearance, a pink-colored plaque, a nodule, or a papule with eroded surface. The size is usually between 0.5 and 1.5 cm in diameter, although it can be much larger.

Diagnostic Studies

Diagnosis is made by biopsy.

EPIDERMAL INCLUSION CYST

Also called *epidermoid cysts*, these are formed of epidermal hyperplasia. The cause is unknown. Some epidermal inclusion cysts develop malignancy.

Signs and Symptoms

The patient complains of a cystic lesion that produces cheesy discharge with foul odor. The lesion is sometimes tender or painful. The lesion is nodular, round and firm, and subcutaneous; thus, it is flesh colored. The most common sites include the face, scalp, neck, upper trunk, and extremities. However, epidermoid cysts can involve the oral mucosa, breasts, and perineum.

Diagnostic Studies

Usually none are necessary. However, the contents can be cultured, and the lesion can be biopsied.

MOLLUSCUM CONTAGIOSUM (PLATE 13)

Molluscum contagiosum is a skin lesion caused by the DNA poxvirus. It affects persons of all ages.

Signs and Symptoms

On occasion, patients present with the complaint of burning or pruritus at the site of the lesion, although they are usually asymptomatic. The lesion has a smooth surface with exception of a central indentation. Although the lesion is skin-colored or pink, the area immediately surrounding the lesion may be red. If the surface over the center of the lesion is broken, pressure may express keratotic material. The skin over trunk and extremities is most often the site, although it can affect oral mucosa and the inguinal area.

Diagnostic Studies

Studies are not generally necessary because diagnosis is based on physical examination findings. Biopsy will reveal characteristic features.

XANTHOMAS

Xanthomas are reflective of lipid metabolism and are caused by accumulations of lipid-laden macrophages in the skin.

Signs and Symptoms

There may be a family history of similar lesions and/or a history of hyperlipidemia or heart, thyroid, or liver disorders. The lesion is asymptomatic. The color ranges from flesh to yellow. The distribution includes the area surrounding the eyes, including the eyelids, and the extensor areas of the elbows, knees, and elbows.

Diagnostic Studies

None are warranted specific to the skin lesion. Lipid studies will reveal elevations.

■ White Lesions

PITYRIASIS ALBA (PLATE 14)

The cause of pityriasis alba is unknown. It is very common in children and young adults.

Signs and Symptoms

There are usually no symptoms associated with the lesions, although patients complain of mild pruritus on occasion. There is commonly a family history of atopic diseases, such as asthma and eczema. Occurrence often has a seasonal pattern. The lesions consist of areas of hypopigmentation, usually covered with a very fine scale. The hypopigmented area is poorly defined and often dry. Over time, the dryness and/or scaling resolves to leave a smooth area of hypopigmentation. The lesions sometimes arise from an initial area of mild erythema. Common sites include the face and arms.

Diagnostic Studies

None are warranted.

TINEA VERSICOLOR (PLATE 15)

Caused by *Malassezia furfur* (formerly named *Pityrosporum orbiculare*), a yeast-like organism, tinea versicolor is not contagious.

Signs and Symptoms

Tinea versicolor, also know as *pityriasis versicolor*, consists of scaly patches of hyper- or hypopigmented skin. Although the color can range from paler than the surrounding skin to dark brown, an individual's multiple lesions are similar in color. Size ranges widely. The margins are well discriminated. Itching is often present. It usually occurs in the warm months and in adolescents and young adults.

Diagnostic Studies

Skin scrapings with potassium hydroxide solution reveal hyphae and spores.

MILIA

Milia occur in infants and are similar to epidermal inclusion cysts.

Signs and Symptoms

Milia consist of 1- to 2-mm pearl-colored lesions scattered over a newborn infant's face. They may involve the oral mucosa over the palate (Epstein's pearls).

Diagnostic Studies

None are warranted.

VITILIGO (PLATE 16)

Vitiligo is a progressive loss of pigmentation. The average age of onset is 20 years. The exact cause is unknown, although there appears to be a genetic component.

Signs and Symptoms

The patient often describes a history of the progressive development of small, multiple areas of depigmentation that, over time, become larger and confluent. The lesions are well demarcated. There is no overlying scale or vesicle development. Any area of skin can be involved. The hair in the affected area may also lose pigmentation. There is a higher incidence of vitiligo in patients with autoimmune disorders, particularly those affecting the endocrine system, including hypothyroidism, diabetes mellitus, and Addison's disease.

Diagnostic Studies

None are warranted except to rule out other causes of hypopigmented lesions. Thyroid studies and/or blood glucose should be considered.

■ Brown Lesions

FRECKLES

Freckles are usually benign lesions found in most individuals. They are responsive to sun exposure, usually becoming more evident in response to sun.

Signs and Symptoms

Freckles are asymptomatic, tan to brown macules ranging from 1 to 5 mm in diameter. The color is consistent on an individual.

NEVI

Melanocytic nevi are extremely common and have genetic predetermination for the number, distribution, and coloring among individuals. Nevi reflect "nests" of melanocytes with hyperpigmentation.

Signs and Symptoms

The lesions are less than 1 cm in diameter and are evenly pigmented. The margins are well demarcated, and the shape is round. The patient reports that the nevus has existed for a long period without change. The distribution is random.

Diagnostic Studies

None are necessary. Biopsy can be performed to rule out malignancy.

SEBORRHEIC KERATOSIS (PLATE 17)

Seborrheic keratoses are common, benign skin changes found in older adults. The cause is unknown, although they do appear most commonly on sun-exposed areas.

Signs and Symptoms

Seborrheic keratoses are usually asymptomatic. If the keratoses are subjected to frequent trauma, by location and exposure, patients may complain of itching, tenderness, or irritation at their site. Seborrheic keratoses appear as flat, light tan lesions that evolve to become raised and have keratotic surfaces, often with increased pigmentation. The mature lesion has a "stuck-on" appearance, and the keratotic cover can be scraped off. Although they can occur anywhere, the most common sites include the trunk, face, and arms.

Diagnostic Studies

None are warranted.

ACANTHOSIS NIGRICANS (PLATE 18)

Acathosis nigricans is associated with insulin resistance. It is most prevalent in individuals who are obese and in blacks and hispanics. Onset is usually in youth. More rarely, acanthosis nigricans with adult onset is associated with an underlying malignancy.

Signs and Symptoms

There is a history of progressively growing hyperpigmented areas that may be associated with pruritis. The lesions have a velvety surface and are often located in the skin of the axilla, neck, and groin. In malignant acanthosis nigricans, the lesions develop more rapidly, often involve the mouth, and are assocated with different forms of cancer.

Diagnostic Studies

The patient should be evaluated for diabetes. With late onset and/or rapid progression of lesions, patient should be evaluated for potential malignancy.

MELANOMA (PLATE 19)

Malignant melanomas are responsible for most skin cancer–related deaths each year. Most arise in sites without prior hyperpigmentation, but some arise from previously pigmented sites. The risk is increased among fair-skinned persons with extensive sun exposure, persons with a family history of melanoma, and persons who have had previous changes in moles.

Signs and Symptoms

There is usually a history of a changing mole or other area of hyperpigmentation. The lesion is usually greater than 0.5 cm in diameter and has notched or irregular edges, irregular pigmentation, and asymmetry of shape. Like other skin disorders, there are variations in appearance, and there should be a high suspicion for melanoma in any changing pigmented skin lesion.

Diagnostic Studies

Diagnosis is made by biopsy of the lesion.

CAFÉ AU LAIT

Café-au-lait spots are caused by increased melanin content and are associated with neurofibromatosis. The lesions vary in appearance and size, with color ranging from tan to brown.

Signs and Symptoms

There frequently is a history of a variety of developmental and congenital conditions. The lesions are asymptomatic. They range in size from millimeters to over 10 cm and are usually flat macules or patches. Although the color varies, most are coffee colored. Physical findings include signs of accompanying conditions, such as neurofibromatosis or Fanconi anemia.

Diagnostic Studies

Biopsy reveals specific characteristics.

GIANT HAIRY PIGMENTED NEVUS

Hairy pigmented lesions are congenital and vary in size. Those classified as "giant" are over 20 cm in diameter in adults and adolescents. In infants and children, giant lesions cover at least 5% of the body surface area. The lesions have a high likelihood of becoming malignant.

Signs and Symptoms

The lesions are typically round or oval in shape and have an irregular surface, with coarse hairs in approximately 50% of cases. They are usual single lesions, and the color ranges from light to dark brown. The coloring may be speckled.

Diagnostic Studies

Biopsy reveals specific features.

■ Inflammatory or Red Lesions

CHERRY HEMANGIOMAS

Cherry hemangiomas, or angiomas, arise from dilated venules. They are more common with advancing age. The cause is unknown, and they are not inflammatory lesions.

Signs and Symptoms

The patient may describe onset after age 30, with number and size increasing over time. The lesions are asymptomatic. The color is typically bright red, though they may be darker, including purple to black in coloring. They do not blanch.

Diagnostic Studies

None are warranted.

PYOGENIC GRANULOMAS (PLATE 20)

Pyogenic granulomas are benign lesions that stem from vascular proliferation. These hemangiomas often occur after a minor skin injury but also occur spontaneously. While the cause is not known, they are not caused by infection, as the name would imply.

Signs and Symptoms

The 1- to 10-mm lesion initially appears as a bright-red papule, which consists of capillaries and collagen and quickly evolves over a period of a few weeks to become a duller shade of red with a roughened and friable surface. They open and bleed with mild trauma. The lesions may become pale, flesh-colored, and chronic, but they rarely resolve spontaneously. It is important to diagnose them early so they can be treated at a more manageable stage.

Diagnostic Studies

Biopsy will reveal specific histopathologic findings, if performed.

FURUNCLES

Furuncles are also commonly called "boils." These lesions are staphylococcal infections of hair follicles or sebaceous glands. Multiple or clustered furuncles are called carbuncles.

Signs and Symptoms

Patients complain of pain, redness, and swelling at the affected site. The lesion may ooze pus. The most common sites are the axillae and groin. The patient's temperature may be elevated, and there is often lymphadenopathy. The size of lesion varies. There is significant tenderness.

Diagnostic Studies

None are generally indicated. Cultures can be performed.

CELLULITIS (PLATE 21)

Cellulitis is an infection of the skin and subcutaneous tissue. The causative organism varies, although staphylococcal and streptococcal infections are common. Superficial cellulitis, erysipelas, is associated with streptococcal infections.

Signs and Symptoms

The patient often describes a skin injury preceding the onset of redness, swelling, and pain at the site. The affected area is tender, swollen, reddened, and warm. There is regional lymphadenopathy. When streptococcal infection is involved, bullae may form on the surface.

Diagnostic Studies

Typically none are indicated unless the condition is severe; if so, complete blood count (CBC) and cultures may be warranted.

HIDRADENITIS SUPPURATIVA (PLATE 22)

Hidradenitis suppurativa involves occlusions of hair follicles. The site is commonly the axillae or groin. The cause or trigger of the occlusion is unknown.

Signs and Symptoms

The patient complains of pain at the site of swelling and redness. The lesions range from papules to nodules and are red, warm, and tender. Usually, multiple lesions are present. The lesions often become infected, drain, and/or may form abscesses. Lymphadenopathy is absent. Without treatment, the lesions can become chronic with prolonged drainage and/or scarring.

Diagnostic Studies

None are usually indicated, but CBC and blood chemistries and blood glucose may be ordered to assess contributing factors.

URTICARIA (PLATE 23)

Urticaria, also commonly called "hives," involves a histamine-mediated response that can be either acute or chronic. A wide range of situations are associated with hives, including a variety of infections, foods, and medications.

Signs and Symptoms

The patient may be able to identify a potential trigger based on experience. The complaint may include a recurrence of the pink or red wheals. The lesions are usually very pruritic and, depending on the severity, may cause localized pain and/or burning. The lesions are nonblanching and vary in size. There are often lesions of various stages, as they emerge from pink to red and then gradually fade before disappearing. New lesions appear as others resolve. The lesions are palpable, with a nonpalpable area of peripheral erythema. There may be associated signs of anaphylaxis and/or angioedema. Dermographism is frequently positive.

Diagnostic Studies

Diagnostic studies, performed based on the basis of recurrence and/or severity, include skin tests for allergen identification, CBC, and other studies specific to presentation.

ERYTHEMA NODOSUM (PLATE 24)

Erythema nodosum is not well understood but is believed to be an antigen-related reaction. The condition can be acute and isolated or chronic. Erythema nodosum is associated with the use of certain medications (sulfa drugs and oral contraceptives), chronic conditions (sarcoidosis), streptococcal infections, and pregnancy.

Signs and Symptoms

The patient may have experienced a period of arthralgia and malaise preceding the development of the skin lesion. The lesion is usually isolated, although multiple sites are possible. The lesion emerges as a firm, tender, reddened nodule, usually along the anterior aspect of the leg, although other sites can be involved. Over a period of up to 2 weeks, the lesion fades in color and the degree of firmness decreases.

Diagnostic Studies

The ESR is often elevated. Chest x-ray may reveal findings consistent with sarcoidosis or another chronic condition (performed only after pregnancy is excluded).

PSORIASIS (PLATE 25)

Psoriasis is a chronic condition that affects the skin and is associated with arthritis. There is a genetic predisposition.

Signs and Symptoms

The patient often provides the history of recurrent and/or chronic skin changes that most frequently involve the extensor surfaces of extremities and scalp, although other regions are frequently involved. The lesions are described often as itchy, although this is highly variable. There may be associated concurrent arthralgia. The typical psoriasis lesion has a well-demarcated border with a silvery colored scale overlying an area of obvious erythema. If the scale is removed, the erythemic base reveals minute bleeding points. The shape of most lesions is oval, and several often coalesce to form one larger lesion. Patients frequently exhibit nail pitting and oncholysis.

Diagnostic Studies

Diagnosis is typically made on physical findings. However, biopsy will reveal specific histopathologic features.

LUPUS ERYTHEMATOSUS (PLATE 26)

Lupus is described in more detail in Chapter 14, on the musculoskeletal system. However, this chronic connective tissue disorder does have specific dermatological findings.

Signs and Symptoms

The patient will have a range of symptoms relevant to the diagnosis, depending on the affected organs. There is often coexisting arthralgia and malaise. The rash is macular and erythematous. It is described as a "butterfly rash" because the distribution resembles a butterfly's wings overlying the forehead and cheeks. Other skin manifestations include discoid plaques, generalized photosensitivity, and lesions of erythema nodosum.

Diagnostic Studies

See Chapter 14, pp. 420–421.

LICHEN PLANUS

Lichen planus is believed to be a cell-mediated response. The highest incidence occurs in the winter months.

Signs and Symptoms

The lesions emerge initially on the extremities and then become generalized over a period of days to weeks. They persist for months and may involve the skin overlying all body parts. The lesions are red papules of 1 cm or greater in diameter. They can occur individually or in clusters. The presence and severity of pruritus is variable.

Diagnostic Studies

If performed, specific histopathologic features are identified.

SECONDARY SYPHILIS (PLATE 27)

Secondary syphilis is commonly called the "great imitator" because the associated skin lesions can have a variety of presentations and appearances. The condition is caused by infection with *Treponema pallidum*. The onset of the rash associated with secondary syphilis occurs weeks to months following the primary lesion.

Signs and Symptoms

The patient may provide the history of a more generalized rash developing 2 or more weeks following the primary lesion, which may still be evident. The primary lesion is usually an isolated, single red lesion, which ultimately ulcerates, forming a nontender chancre. There may be a period of malaise preceding the eruption of secondary lesions. These lesions vary in appearance and distribution, but the typical finding is of red maculopapular lesions smaller than 1 cm in diameter. Any portion of skin can be involved, including the scalp, mucous membranes, perineum, and the soles and palms. There is generalized lymphadenopathy. Depending on the involvement of other organs, there may be findings consistent with meningitis, hepatitis, iritis, and arthritis.

Diagnostic Studies

The diagnosis is confirmed by positive serology.

TINEA CORPORIS (PLATE 28)

Tinea corporis is caused by a dermatophyte infection. Depending on the site of the lesion, the condition is referred to differently: tinea capitis (scalp), tinea cruris (groin), and so on. The disorder is commonly called "ringworm."

Signs and Symptoms

The patient may recall exposure to another individual with similar lesions or an activity such as gardening or handling animals through which they were exposed to the dermatophyte. The lesion is pruritic. It begins as a small, annular, erythemic, and scaling lesion that develops a central area of clearing as it grows in diameter. The edge may develop vesicles, is typically scaling, and remains palpable and reddened, so that it presents as a ring.

Diagnostic Studies

The diagnosis is typically evident by the appearance of the lesion and the patient's history. However, skin scraping will reveal the hyphae.

PITYRIASIS ROSEA (PLATE 29)

Pityriasis rosea is believed to be caused by a virus. It is most common in the spring and autumn.

Signs and Symptoms

The patient is usually asymptomatic, although some complain of a prodromal period of malaise preceding the emergence of the rash. The rash is often pruritic. The first sign is typically a "herald patch," which is a 2- to 10-cm annular pink patch that, similar to tinea, has an area of central clearing with a fine scale. The herald patch is most commonly located on the trunk. The herald patch is followed several days later by a more diffuse set of smaller pink, salmon, or fawn-colored lesions, which, at 0.5 to 1.5 cm, are much smaller than the herald patch. The distribution of the smaller lesions is described as "Christmas tree distribution" because the lesions have a slightly diagonal axis and are distributed along the skin tension lines.

Diagnostic Studies

The diagnosis is made on history and physical findings. Skin scraping will differentiate the condition from tinea by the absence of hyphae.

■ Eczematous Lesions With Excoriations

ATOPIC DERMATITIS (PLATE 30)

Atopic dermatitis, commonly called eczema, is an atopic condition. The term *eczematous dermatitis* encompasses a broad set of conditions that include atopic dermatitis, contact dermatitis, and others. Atopic dermatitis, however, is differentiated by often having onset in infancy or early childhood and by its association with other atopic diseases, including asthma and rhinitis/hayfever.

Signs and Symptoms

The patient presents with complaint of recurrent, itchy skin rash. The most common sites involve the flexor surfaces of extremities, neck, and face, although the condition is certainly not limited to these areas. There may be a personal or family history of other atopic conditions. The lesions are erythematous, exudative eruptions that can be intensely pruritic. They often progress to form areas of lichenification, which may become chronic. The sites are prone to secondary infections.

Diagnostic Studies

The diagnosis is typically based on history and physical findings. However, eosinophilia and/or immunoglobulin E (IgE) elevations are present on laboratory testing.

DYSHIDROSIS

See p. 53.

STASIS DERMATITIS (PLATE 31)

Statis dermatitis is a condition affecting the skin in areas with venous insufficiency. It affects the lower extremities.

Signs and Symptoms

There is typically a gradual emergence of patches of erythemic scaling, associated with pruritus. Edema is often present. The most frequent site is the medial ankle. Over time, the lesions enlarge and become eczematous, so that they weep and/or form crusting. If the site heals, there is a residual area of discoloration caused by leaking of hemosiderin into the tissues.

Diagnostic Studies

Deep venous thrombosis may be revealed through Doppler studies. Biopsy reveals characteristic features.

SEBORRHEIC DERMATITIS

The cause of seborrheic dermatitis is believed to be immunologic. It is more common in males than females.

Signs and Symptoms

The patient typically presents with complaints of itching and/or burning associated with scaling lesions on the hairy parts of body, such as scalp, central face, and presternal areas. The lesion consists of a greasy scale lying over an erythematous patch. The problem is recurrent. It can become eczematous, allowing for secondary infection.

Diagnostic Studies

None are necessary; diagnosis is made on the basis of distribution and appearance of lesion and the history.

CONTACT DERMATITIS

See p. 52.

SUGGESTED READINGS

Bickley, L.S., & Szilagyi, P.G. (2004). *Bates' Guide to Physical Examination and History Taking.* Philadelphia: Lippincott, Williams, and Wilkins.

Dillon, P. (2003). *Nursing Health Assessment: A Critical Thinking, Case Studies Approach.* Philadelphia: F.A. Davis.

Goldsmith, L.A., Lazarus, G.S., & Tharp, M.D. (1997). *Adult and Pediatric Dermatology: A Color Guide to Diagnosis and Treatment.* Philadelphia: F.A. Davis.

Swartz, M.H. (2005). *Textbook of Physical Diagnosis: History and Examination.* Philadelphia: Saunders.

Chapter 4

HEAD, FACE, AND NECK

Laurie Grubbs

In the United States, malignancies of the head and neck are responsible for 2% to 5% of cancers. People with a history of tobacco and ethyl alcohol abuse are particularly susceptible. Other systemic diseases, such as thyroid, kidney, neurological, heart, skin, and autoimmune diseases, may manifest themselves as alterations in the appearance of the neck and face and may be detectable upon physical examination. This chapter focuses on causes of head, jaw, and facial pain; facial swelling; facial numbness; neck pain or neck mass; and dysphagia. Owing to the complexity of the head and neck examination, subsequent chapters pertain to the eye (Chapter 5) and the ear, nose, mouth, and throat (Chapter 6).

History

■ General Head, Face, and Neck History

The origins of head, face, and neck disorders vary. A history of acute trauma or injury to the head may require x-ray, computed tomographic (CT), or magnetic resonance imaging (MRI) technologies, depending on the location and extent of the injury. Chronic headaches need investigation, and CT scanning or referral to a neurologist may be warranted. A complaint of syncope or dizziness suggests the possibility of decreased cerebral blood flow. A complaint of enlarged lymph nodes or masses, in the absence of infection, suggests the possibility of a malignant process. Any changes in taste, dysphagia, frequent sore throats, mouth sores that do not heal, hoarseness, or voice changes may indicate oral or throat cancer. Ask about tobacco and alcohol use or abuse because those are significant risk factors for malignancies of the head and neck. Ask about dental disease and dental hygiene practices. A complaint of swelling or fullness in the neck may be related to thyroid disease. A psychosocial and mental health history should be done, especially for complaints of chronic pain, to determine any relation to stress, anxiety, or other mental health problems. More specific histories should be undertaken according to the chief complaint.

■ Past Medical History

A history of disorders of the head, face, and neck should be thoroughly reviewed. Past head trauma should be thoroughly investigated. Reports of past syncopal episodes, transient ischemic attacks (TIAs), or cerebrovascular accidents (CVAs) are red flags, and patients with such histories should be referred. A history of malignancies of the head, face, or neck raises a high index of suspicion for recurrence. Past radiation administered to the head and neck may cause long-term side effects, such as mouth sores, dysphagia, dry mouth, excessive salivation, or hoarseness. Past radiation to the thyroid may cause secondary malignancies.

■ Family History

A positive family history of cerebrovascular disease, thyroid disease, or migraine creates some increased risk in family members depending on the age and general health of the patient. Malignancies of any kind should be reviewed. A family history of smoking raises the risk of secondhand smoke exposure in the patient.

■ Habits

As previously mentioned, alcohol and tobacco use are significant risk factors for malignancies of the head and neck. Environmental exposures may also cause malignancies, and a thorough occupational and social history should be obtained.

Physical Examination

The physical examination includes inspection of the face for symmetry, sensation (cranial nerves [CNs] V and VII), color, lesions, edema, or masses. Palpate the head and neck for tenderness, paying particular attention to the sinuses, temporal areas, temporomandibular joints (TMJs), and lymph nodes. The mouth, ears, eyes, and nose (covering all the CNs) are included. See Chapters 5 and 6, and see chief complaints in this chapter for more detail.

Differential Diagnosis of Chief Complaints

■ Headache

See Chapter 15, pp. 456–467.

■ Jaw Pain and Facial Pain

Jaw pain or facial pain is often a manifestation of a problem in another area of the head and neck, such as ear infection, dental disease, sinusitis, or in an unrelated system, as is the case with angina.

History

A logical place to start is with a history of any disorders of the jaw, mouth, ear, or nose. You should inquire about psychosocial problems because bruxism and TMJ are often associated with increased stress. Recent trauma is a red flag and should alert you to a possible facial or mandibular fracture. A history of smoking could indicate a neoplasm of the mouth and its associated structures or of the neck. Characteristics of the pain are important—nerve pain is qualitatively different from the pain of soft-tissue, musculoskeletal, or cardiac origin. Nerve pain is usually described as burning or tingling. Pain of cardiac origin is more likely to occur with activity. Inquire about the timing of the pain because pain associated with TMJ syndrome or bruxism may be worse in the morning; pain with trigeminal neuralgia is usually paroxysmal. Pain in the frontal or maxillary area is often caused by sinus congestion or infection, and a history of allergies or a recent upper respiratory infection assists in identifying sinusitis as the cause.

Physical Examination

It is important to examine the entire head and neck, paying particular attention to the jaw, ears, mouth, sinuses, and lymph system. Be sure to include CNs V and VII, which govern jaw clench, facial sensation, and facial movement. If other systems are suspected, such as cardiac or musculoskeletal, those systems should be thoroughly examined.

TEMPOROMANDIBULAR JOINT (TMJ) SYNDROME

TMJ syndrome is a common syndrome with several causes, the most common being a psychosomatic response to stress. Such stress responses may be jaw clenching or bruxism, resulting in fatigue or spasm of the masticatory muscles and, in turn, TMJ pain. Other causes include malocclusion, dental disease, disease of the TMJ tissues, and poorly fitting dentures, or more serious conditions such as congenital anomalies, fractures and dislocations, intra-articular disk disease, arthritis, ankylosis, and neoplasias. The pain can be severe and debilitating and can interfere with daily activities, particularly eating.

Signs and Symptoms

The signs and symptoms range from mild aching to severe, sharp pain in and around the TMJs. Typically, there is pain with movement of the joint, particularly with chewing, and a clicking sound may be heard on movement. Although often present in TMJ syndrome, jaw clicking is not pathognomonic because many people who have jaw clicking are asymptomatic. There is tenderness of the masticatory muscles. The pain is often referred to the ear, causing tinnitus and hearing difficulties.

Diagnostic Studies

Clinical findings are most helpful for ruling in TMJ syndrome, but x-rays or MRI of the TMJ can assist in ruling out degenerative arthritis or possible neoplastic causes. Generally, treatment is supportive, and a referral to a dentist or maxillofacial specialist is recommended.

TRIGEMINAL NEURALGIA

The jaw pain associated with this condition is caused by inflammation, degeneration, or pressure on the trigeminal nerve, CN V.

Signs and Symptoms

The pain of trigeminal neuralgia is usually sharp and paroxysmal, lasting from seconds to minutes, but with recurrent paroxysms that may continue for hours. Bouts of neuralgia are recurrent and may be triggered by movement, but they may subside for weeks and months without an exacerbation. Because there are three branches to this nerve (ophthalmic, maxillary, and mandibular), the pain radiates from the angle of the jaw to one or more of the three places innervated: the forehead and eye area; the cheek and nose area; or the tongue, lower lip, and jaw area (Fig. 4.1).

Diagnostic Studies

The history is most helpful in the diagnosis of trigeminal neuralgia because no clinical or pathologic signs are present. Sensory changes or abnormalities in the

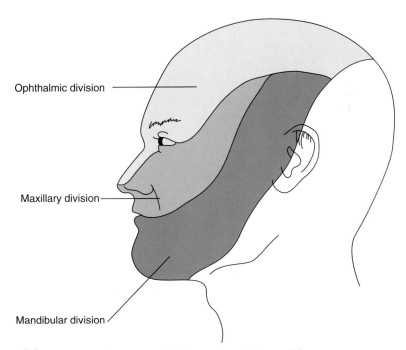

Figure 4.1 Branches of the trigeminal nerve (cranial nerve V). (From Swartz, M. *Textbook of Physical Diagnosis*, 3rd ed. Philadelphia: W.B. Saunders, 1998, p. 509. Reprinted with permission.)

function of CN V suggest a more serious cause, such as a neoplasm, brainstem lesion, cerebrovascular insult, multiple sclerosis, Sjögren's syndrome, rheumatoid arthritis, or migraine, although there are generally other defining symptoms with the systemic diseases.

ANGINA

The pain from myocardial ischemia can often be referred to the neck and jaw areas, and these can occasionally be the only areas of pain. The examiner should retain an index of suspicion for angina being the cause of jaw pain in order to elicit a proper history and physical.

Signs and Symptoms

A thorough history should lead the examiner in the right direction. Middle-age males with a history of cardiovascular disease in themselves or family members should raise the index of suspicion. The red flag complaints that should alert the examiner to the possibility of a cardiac origin are accompanying chest pain, pain with exertion, dyspnea, nausea, or diaphoresis.

Diagnostic Studies

The diagnosis can be made with electrocardiogram if it is obtained while the patient is having pain or with a graded exercise test (GXT).

DENTAL PAIN

The most common causes of dental-related jaw pain are the eruption of wisdom teeth and tooth decay or abscess, particularly in the molars. Wisdom teeth generally erupt in the late teens or early 20s, so they should be part of the differential diagnosis in patients of that age. In patients with obviously poor dental hygiene, decay should be included in the differential diagnosis at any age. Several other periodontal diseases can cause jaw pain, and these are more prevalent with aging and poor dental hygiene. Osteonecrosis of the jaw seen almost exclusively in cancer patients can also cause dental pain.

Signs and Symptoms

Jaw pain that is constant and throbbing in nature is typical when dental decay or abscess is the cause. The pain can be quite severe and requires analgesics and, if infection is present, antibiotics, until dental referral can be made. With the eruption of wisdom teeth, the pain is milder and generally not constant.

Diagnostic Studies

Diagnosis can be made with dental examination. Decay and abscess are obvious with a simple oral examination, whereas other forms of dental disease require in-depth dental evaluation. In any case, dental referral is necessary.

BRUXISM

Bruxism is the clenching or grinding of teeth during sleep. The most common causes are malocclusion or tension and stress.

Signs and Symptoms

Over the long term, bruxism can cause the teeth to wear down, erode, and loosen. Patients are usually not aware of the problem because it occurs during sleep, but they may experience TMJ pain.

Diagnostic Studies

The diagnosis is usually made via the report of family members or through a routine dental examination. Occlusal guards for the teeth are helpful to prevent dental injury. Fixing the underlying cause is most helpful.

PAROTITIS

There are two types of parotid infection—suppurative (usually caused by *Staphylococcus aureus*) and epidemic, more commonly called mumps (caused by a paramyxovirus). In developed countries, mumps is rarely seen because children are immunized against it within the first 2 years of life. Patients with Sjögren's syndrome are also predisposed to inflammation of the salivary glands (Fig. 4.2)—parotid or submandibular—termed *sialadenitis*.

Signs and Symptoms

In bacterial parotitis, the symptoms include fever, chills, rapid onset of pain, and swelling, usually in the preauricular area of the jaw. The gland is firm on palpation, with tenderness and erythema overlying the gland. Symptoms are similar to those of mumps, with both glands usually being affected.

Diagnostic Studies

Clinical signs and symptoms most often make the diagnosis of infectious parotitis. The examiner should attempt to express pus from Stensen's duct, which helps to make the diagnosis of infection. The pus will most often show gram-positive cocci. Treatment includes antibiotic therapy and massage of the gland to promote drainage. Surgery is rarely necessary in infectious parotitis.

SALIVARY GLAND TUMORS

The majority of these tumors occur in the parotid gland, and over 80% are benign. Those occurring in the submandibular gland are more likely to be malignant (about 50%).

Signs and Symptoms

Salivary gland tumors are often painless and may go unnoticed for months. If malignancy is present, the facial nerve is often affected.

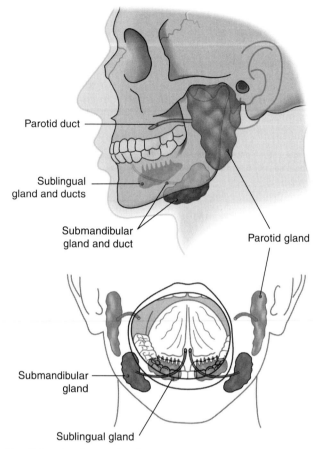

Figure 4.2 Parotid and salivary glands. (From Dillon, P.M. *Nursing Health Assessment: A Critical Thinking, Case Studies Approach.* Philadelphia: FA Davis, 2003, p. 199. Reprinted with permission.)

Diagnostic Studies

MRI or a CT scan is recommended once a mass is found. Fine-needle aspiration (FNA) is necessary for diagnosis and treatment. Surgical excision is necessary, and radiation is warranted for large tumors.

SALIVARY DUCT STONE (SIALOLITHIASIS)

The submandibular glands are affected more often than the parotid. Often these patients have a history of recurrent sialadenitis, and the stones are composed of calcium phosphate as a result of the pH of the saliva.

Signs and Symptoms

Anything that causes the affected salivary gland to be stimulated, usually related to eating, will elicit pain. Swelling also may be apparent over the affected gland.

Diagnostic Studies

Clinical diagnosis is made by inspection and palpation. The stones are expressed by manipulation or excision.

TRAUMA

A history of trauma to the jaw alerts the examiner to the need for x-ray to evaluate the presence of a fracture or dislocation of the mandible. Fist fighting, boxing, and other sources of trauma, such as motor vehicle accidents, are the most common causes.

Signs and Symptoms

Pain over a TMJ and difficulty with opening and closing the jaw are the hallmark symptoms.

Diagnostic Studies

The definitive diagnosis is made by x-ray.

SINUSITIS

An infection in the sinuses can cause referred pain to the jaw, especially if the middle ear is also involved and/or there is preauricular, tonsillar, or mandibular lymphadenopathy. Sinusitis is covered in Chapter 6, pp. 143–144.

■ Facial Swelling

Facial swelling is most often due to an allergic reaction, but systemic diseases can also be associated with facial swelling, as is the case with hypothyroidism, Cushing's disease, or hepatic disease.

History

Inquire about environmental allergies to plants, animals, or chemicals. A medication history is particularly important because facial swelling can be a sign of a medication allergy or a side effect of certain medications, particularly steroids. Ask about a history of thyroid disorders, which can be a cause of myxedematous facies. Ask the patient about any history of adrenal or renal disease, which can cause generalized edema and facial swelling. Inquire about any recent fever, although facial swelling related to infection is usually accompanied by redness and increased skin temperature, which will be evident on physical examination.

Physical Examination

The physical examination is straightforward in determining whether the swelling is localized, which may be caused by a problem or infection in the underlying tissues, or generalized, which suggests an allergic reaction or systemic disease. Look for redness, skin changes, tenderness, and lymphadenopathy, which indicate infection.

ANGIOEDEMA

Angioedema is basically anaphylaxis that is restricted to the skin and is generally benign and self-limiting. The causes are numerous and include insect stings; atopic conditions; food allergies (typically nuts, eggs, shellfish, fruit, sulfites); drug allergies; allergy desensitization injections; a reaction to blood products; a response to exercise, cold, or pressure; heredity; and vasculitis.

Signs and Symptoms

The edema is often accompanied by urticaria, which presents as wheals and is usually seen around the mouth, nose, eyes, mucous membranes, and hands and feet. It can be accompanied by a systemic reaction; therefore, the patient should be watched and questioned about any dyspnea or shortness of breath. Angioedema is usually self-limiting and lasts 1 to 7 days but can be a chronic, recurring condition depending on the cause.

Diagnostic Studies

The diagnosis is usually made by history. Allergy testing may give information if the cause is related to food or drug allergies.

CELLULITIS

Cellulitis is an acute inflammation of cellular or connective tissue, usually confined to the skin and subcutaneous tissue, but it may extend beyond to deeper tissues (see Chapter 3, pp. 63–64). Group A β-hemolytic streptococcus is the most common organism responsible for superficial cellulitis. It can occur from a wound or bite or as a complication of infections of the eyes, ears, mouth, or nose.

Signs and Symptoms

The symptoms include redness, warmth, edema, leukocyte infiltration, tenderness, and regional lymphadenopathy. The skin may have a thick, orange peel appearance, and the borders are usually indistinct. Systemic symptoms such as fever, tachycardia, and headache may be present. Tissue necrosis and suppuration may ensue.

Diagnostic Studies

The diagnosis can be made solely by history and physical examination, but wound or tissue cultures will help to identify the causative organism. Cellulitis in the head and face should be treated promptly and can usually be accomplished with outpatient antimicrobials.

CUSHING'S DISEASE

See "Fatigue" in Chapter 16, pp. 491–492.

LONG-TERM USE OF STEROIDS

A cushingoid look can occur in patients who take long-term steroids for chronic diseases, including respiratory, hematologic, and autoimmune.

Signs and Symptoms

The typical symptoms are those of Cushing's disease, with a rounded "moon face" appearance and truncal obesity.

Diagnostic Studies

In the case of steroid use, the diagnosis is made by history.

MYXEDEMA

Myxedema is related to hypothyroidism. See "Neck Fullness, Mass, or Pain" in this chapter, pp. 81–85.

NEPHROTIC SYNDROME

See "Fatigue" in Chapter 16, pp. 478–485.

■ Facial Numbness and Weakness

Numbness, tingling, or hypersensitivity in the face should be taken seriously because the causative conditions can be grave neurological diseases. Bell's palsy is the most common cause of facial neuropathy; rarely, infectious and inflammatory diseases such as HIV, Lyme disease, and sarcoidosis may present with facial numbness.

History

Inquire about the presence of other neurological symptoms, such as weakness, unsteadiness, hemiparesis, disequilibrium, diplopia or other visual changes, which are possible indications of either CVA or multiple sclerosis. Bell's palsy can occur at any age and is often a sequela of a viral illness. Multiple sclerosis occurs more in the young adult population, whereas CVA occurs more in the older population, especially in those with hypertension or diabetes. A thorough family history may disclose a predisposition to CVA, hypertension, diabetes, and other neurological diseases. Twin studies show a genetic susceptibility for multiple sclerosis.

Physical Examination

The physical examination should include testing facial sensation on each side of the face (CN V) as well as movement by having the patient perform various facial expressions (CN VII). Symptoms are almost always unilateral. Diagnostic imaging can be helpful to rule in CVA or MS.

BELL'S PALSY

Bell's palsy is a unilateral paralysis of the face. The etiology is uncertain, but the paralysis is thought to be due to an inflammation of CN VII, secondary to a viral infection, a large percentage being herpes simplex virus.

Signs and Symptoms

The onset of Bell's palsy is sudden, and the symptoms are unilateral. The affected side of the face droops with asymmetrical facial movement; there is pain in or around the ear, excessive lacrimation and salivation, and inability to close the eye. The result may be partial or complete paralysis. No sensory loss is demonstrable. The affected eye must be kept moist and patched to avoid excessive dryness.

Diagnostic Studies

The diagnosis is made by physical examination. There are no diagnostic tests for initial diagnosis, but an electromyogram can be helpful to determine the extent of the nerve damage. Recovery from partial paralysis occurs in 2 to 6 months; complete recovery from total paralysis varies from 20% to 90%. Corticosteroids and antivirals may hasten recovery.

MULTIPLE SCLEROSIS

Multiple sclerosis is a progressive disease of the central nervous system, resulting in a variety of neurological symptoms affecting the motor, sensory, mental, and central and autonomic nervous systems. See Chapter 15, pp. 475–476.

Signs and Symptoms

The onset is insidious and may go undiagnosed for months or years. Unilateral facial paresthesia or pain is seen occasionally early in the disease process, although most of the symptoms involve the eye.

Diagnostic Studies

A good history—especially one that describes remissions and exacerbations of the symptoms—can raise an index of suspicion. Computed tomography, MRI, lumbar puncture, and evoked potentials are all part of the diagnostic workup.

CEREBROVASCULAR ACCIDENT

Although it would be unusual for facial numbness to be the presenting complaint for stroke, it should be considered in the differential diagnosis. Age and medical history are very helpful in raising the index of suspicion for CVA. A thorough physical examination and diagnostic imaging are definitive. See Chapter 15, p. 455.

■ Scalp and Face Pruritis

History

It is unusual for pruritus in the head and neck to indicate anything except a skin condition/disease or infestation. If the patient is a school-age child, pediculosis is an obvious choice, and the child's friends and school administrators should be questioned about recent outbreaks. You should ask about sun exposure and blistering sunburns. A history of other skin cancers in the patient or family is important to determine.

Physical Examination

The physical examination includes careful inspection of the head and scalp for nits or actual lice. Nits are fixed to the hair shaft and are grayish-white in appearance. Unlike the flakiness of seborrhea, nits cannot be easily dislodged. The skin of the head and face should be inspected for lesions, color changes, new or changing moles, crusting, scaling, ulceration, or bleeding, which might be indicative of cancer or psoriasis. Chapter 3 further discusses dermatologic problems causing pruritis, and Chapter 18 addresses pediatric dermatologic problems.

■ Neck Fullness, Mass, or Pain

History

Start with a thorough history, including a medical history for cancer or exposure to environmental toxins. Ask about frequent infections; allergies; chronic ear, nose, and throat problems; and surgeries. Ask about living arrangements because close quarters, such as classrooms and college dormitories, can predispose the patient to a variety of infections. Ask about sexual practices. Inquire about family history, especially thyroid disease.

Symptoms vary depending on the underlying cause. In thyroid disease, patients may describe a feeling of having something in their throat. The complaint is more likely to be of fullness rather than of pain or dysphagia. The history should inquire about signs and symptoms of hyperthyroidism or hypothyroidism, such as weight loss or gain, nervousness or fatigue, diarrhea or constipation, intolerance to heat or cold, insomnia or lethargy, menstrual irregularities, and skin or hair changes. Laboratory studies and thyroid scanning can diagnose most problems.

Lymphadenopathy has numerous causes but can generally be categorized as infection or malignancy. Infection often presents with fever, sore throat, runny nose, cough, and malaise. A history of an upper respiratory infection is common.

Symptoms of malignancies are more likely to be fatigue, weakness, anorexia, weight loss, fever, night sweats, bleeding, and easy bruisability. A history of tobacco and/or alcohol abuse may be present in neoplasms of the head and neck.

Physical Examination

The physical examination includes palpation of the thyroid for enlargement, asymmetry, or nodules. Inspect the skin and hair for moistness or dryness. Look for periorbital edema, which may be present in hypothyroidism. Check the vital signs for hypertension or hypotension, tachycardia or bradycardia, and fever or subnormal temperature. Notice any tremor. Check the deep tendon reflexes (DTRs) for hyperreflexia or hyporeflexia. Abnormalities in any of these areas indicate the need for further thyroid studies, including thyroid-stimulating hormone (TSH), T_3, T_4, and possibly a thyroid scan.

A complete examination of the mouth, throat, nose, ears, and eyes should be performed as you look for infection. Palpate for lymphadenopathy in other areas of the body, which might be present in malignancies. Laboratory studies for a complete blood count (CBC) might be warranted to check for leukocytosis or leukopenia. A positive "mono spot" gives a definitive diagnosis of mononucleosis. If it is suspected, palpate for splenomegaly. A chest x-ray may be necessary to look for mediastinal lymphadenopathy, indicating Hodgkin's disease or other malignancy. Depending on sexual practices, a *Neisseria gonorrhoeae* (GC) or *Chlamydia trachomatis* culture of the throat or blood studies for rapid plasma reagin (RPR) or human immunodeficiency virus (HIV) may be necessary.

GOITER

A deficiency in thyroid hormone can result from thyroid failure, likely autoimmune in etiology (primary hypothyroidism), or failure of the hypothalamic-pituitary axis (secondary hypothyroidism). Goiter, an enlargement of the thyroid gland, may be associated with hypothyroidism or hyperthyroidism, but patients with goiter also may be euthyroid, a condition termed *nontoxic goiter.*

HYPOTHYROIDISM

The numerous causes of hypothyroidism include Hashimoto's thyroiditis; iodine deficiency; genetic thyroid enzyme defects; iodine deficiency; medications (amiodarone, iodine-containing contrast media, lithium, methimazole, phenylbutazone, sulfonamides, aminoglutethimide, interferon-α); thyroid cancer; and infiltrative disorders, such as sarcoidosis, amyloidosis, scleroderma, cystinosis, and hemochromatosis. Thyroid diseases in general are more common in women.

Signs and Symptoms

The severity of symptoms ranges from unrecognized states found only by TSH screening to striking myxedema. Symptoms include fatigue, cold intolerance, constipation, weight gain, depression, menorrhagia, hoarseness, dry skin and hair, cool skin with slow capillary refill, paresthesias of the hands and feet, bradycardia, delayed DTRs, periorbital edema, anemia, and hyponatremia. The thyroid may be of normal size or enlarged and nodular, depending on the cause. In rare and extreme cases, myxedematous coma may ensue, with severe hypothermia, hypoventilation, hyponatremia, hypoxia, hypercapnia, hypotension, and seizures.

Diagnostic Studies

Diagnosis is made by measurement of TSH, T_4, and radioiodine uptake. Because it is a feedback system, the TSH is elevated and the T_4 and radioiodine uptake are low. A thyroid ultrasound is helpful for determining the size and differentiation of nodules.

HYPERTHYROIDISM

Graves' disease is the most common cause of hyperthyroidism except in patients over 55, in whom multinodular goiter is a more common etiology. Onset of this condition can occur at any age, but it is most common between the ages of 20 and 40 years. Often patients have a family history of Graves' disease or other autoimmune thyroid diseases, such as Hashimoto's disease. See Box 4.1 for predisposing factors for hyperthyroidism.

Signs and Symptoms

Clinical manifestations include diffuse goiter, nervousness, irritability, tremor, heat intolerance, weakness, tachycardia, palpitations, widened pulse pressure, increased sweating, weight loss, insomnia, frequent bowel movements, menstrual irregularities, exophthalmos, and infiltrative dermopathy. Patients older than 50 years often present with cardiac symptoms, such as hypertension, atrial fibrillation, or heart failure.

Diagnostic Studies

A decreased TSH and elevated free T_4 and T_3 will generally make the diagnosis. Also consider the erythrocyte sedimentation rate, which can be elevated in Graves' disease; the CBC, to rule out anemia or an elevated white blood cell count; and the metabolic profile, with special attention to calcium, glucose, and potassium, to rule out pheochromocytoma or adrenal disease. Thyroid autoantibodies are elevated in Graves' disease and Hashimoto's thyroiditis. Radioactive iodine (RAI) imaging should be performed to look for increased uptake and the presence of hot or cold nodules. FNA is recommended. Most can be managed medically or with RAI ablation.

EUTHYROID GOITER

Simple, endemic, nontoxic diffuse and nontoxic nodular goiter indicate an enlargement of the thyroid gland with diminished thyroid hormone production but without clinical thyroid disease. Euthyroid goiter is the most common type of goiter and commonly occurs during puberty, pregnancy, or at menopause. Endemic goiter is caused by an inadequate intake of dietary

---

Box 4.1

Predisposing Factors for Hyperthyroidism

- Heredity
- Female gender
- Recent adverse life events causing psychological stress
- Smoking
- Pregnancy
- Parity
- Viral and bacterial infections that cause subacute thyroiditis
- Iodine supplementation or exposure to an iodine load
- Lithium, amiodarone, or antiretroviral therapy
- Type I diabetes

iodine. Other causes of goiter include foods containing goitrogens (e.g., turnips) and such medicines as sulfonylureas, lithium, iodine, and aminosalicylic acid.

Signs and Symptoms

In the early stages, the thyroid becomes symmetrically enlarged and smooth. Later, multiple nodules and cysts may develop.

Diagnostic Studies

An RAI uptake test may be normal or may show high uptake. The thyroid scan will show an enlarged, but smooth, symmetrical thyroid gland. The serum T_4 and thyroid hormone–binding ratio are usually normal.

THYROID CANCER

Patients are often asymptomatic with thyroid cancer, and it is commonly found, by the patient or practitioner, as a nontender nodule. Most thyroid nodules are benign adenomas, but evaluation is necessary. Predisposing factors include young age; female gender; family history; and a history of radiation exposure to the head, neck, or chest. There are four main types: papillary, follicular, medullary, and anaplastic; the papillary type accounts for 60% to 70% of all thyroid cancers.

Signs and Symptoms

Clinical signs are usually absent except for a painless enlargement of the thyroid gland. Anterior cervical lymph nodes may be enlarged. A history of rapid enlargement and a hard consistency should raise the index of suspicion for carcinoma. Radiographic evidence of a stippled calcification or a dense, homogeneous calcification warrants an FNA. Thyroid function tests are usually normal.

Diagnostic Studies

A thyroid scan is necessary to differentiate cold nodules from hot nodules. A solitary cold nodule on RAI uptake scanning is suspicious for carcinoma. Ultrasound of the neck is helpful to determine size, location, and metastases. FNA with histologic or cytologic tissue examination is necessary to confirm the diagnosis.

LYMPHADENOPATHY

Lymphadenopathy in the head and neck has numerous causes but is generally caused by either infection or malignancy. Figure 4.3 illustrates exact locations of the lymph nodes. Lymphadenopathy resulting from infection produces enlarged, tender, smooth, mobile lymph nodes, whereas lymphadenopathy resulting from malignancy produces enlarged, nontender, irregular, fixed nodes. Lymphadenopathy generally occurs in lymph nodes adjacent to or near the cause except in some malignancies where there is metastatic disease to distant

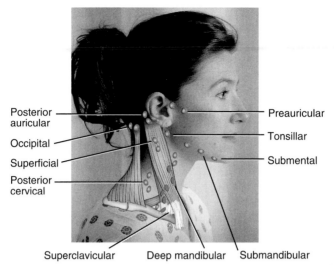

Posterior auricular

Occipital

Superficial

Posterior cervical

Preauricular

Tonsillar

Submental

Superclavicular   Deep mandibular   Submandibular

Figure 4.3 Cervical lymph nodes. (From Dillon, P.M. *Nursing Health Assessment: A Critical Thinking, Case Studies Approach.* Philadelphia: FA Davis, 2003, p. 199. Reprinted with permission.)

lymph nodes (see Fig. 4.3). The most common causes, signs and symptoms, and diagnostic studies are listed in Table 4.1.

■ Difficulty Swallowing

Dysphagia is an esophageal transport disorder and is caused by lesions of the pharynx and esophagus or by neuromuscular disorders that cause functional limitations. It is important to differentiate between pre-esophageal dysphagia, which occurs mostly in patients with neuromuscular disorders, and esophageal disorders, which can include obstructive or motor disorders. Neuromuscular disorders include myasthenia gravis, muscular dystrophy, dermatomyositis, and poliomyelitis. The obstructive disorders include cancer, peptic stricture secondary to gastroesophageal reflux disease (GERD), and esophageal rings. The obstructive esophageal disorders are often limited to solid food. Motor disorders can affect both solid and liquid intake and are caused by impaired esophageal peristalsis, which occurs with such conditions as achalasia and scleroderma.

History

The history is particularly important in these patients because physical examination is of little value in diagnosing dysphagia. Ask if the difficulty in swallowing occurs only with liquids or with both solids and liquids. Discern whether it is constant or intermittent. Ask about a history of cancer, neuromuscular or autoimmune diseases, or GERD. If the patient is elderly, inquire whether he or she has experienced frequent bouts of pneumonia, which might alert you to aspiration as a cause. Inquire about all medications. The bisphosphonates, a drug class used for treating osteoporosis, can cause esophagitis if not taken with a full glass of water. Ask about habits, such as smoking and alcohol intake, because cancers of the head and neck are more common in individuals with a history of tobacco or alcohol use/abuse.

Table 4.1

Lymphadenopathy: Causes, Signs and Symptoms, and Diagnostic Studies

Causes	Signs and Symptoms	Diagnostics
Pharyngitis/tonsilitis	Lymphadenopathy in the head and neck	Throat culture, specifically strep, viral if herpes simplex virus is suspected, and/or *Neisseria gonorrhoeae* or *Chlamydia trachomatis* if sexually transmitted disease is suspected.
Mononucleosis: Commonly caused by Epstein virus with cytomegalovirus being second	Lymphadenopathy is usually dramatic	Complete blood count and serologic testing for heterophil antibodies ("mono spot"). Treatment is supportive; steroids may improve symptoms; caution against contact sports because of splenomegaly.
Infections of the head, eyes, ears, nose, mouth, and throat: The head and cervical lymph nodes typically drain more than one area, and any infection in the area has the ability to cause lymphadenopathy	Fever may or may not be present	The health-care provider must determine the origin of the infection in order to treat it effectively.
Dental problems	Abscessed teeth are likely to cause lymphadenopathy of the tonsillar, maxillary, mandibular, or cervical nodes. Rarely do other diseases of the teeth and gums cause lymphadenopathy.	Prompt dental referral is necessary. Antibiotics and pain medicine may be necessary.

Table 4.1

Lymphadenopathy: Causes, Signs and Symptoms, and Diagnostic Studies—cont'd

Causes	Signs and Symptoms	Diagnostics
Neoplasms of the head and neck: The most common malignancies of the head and neck are squamous cell carcinomas of the larynx, palatine tonsil, and hypopharynx. Over 80% of patients with these cancers have a history of tobacco and/or alcohol abuse. Other causes include a history of radiation to the area, Epstein-Barr virus, poor dental hygiene or poorly fitting dental appliances, and dipping snuff.	Symptoms include a palpable mass, ulcerated lesion, edema, and pain at the primary site.	Biopsy is necessary for diagnosis, and referral to an ear, nose, and throat physician is warranted.
Leukemia: Malignant neoplasm of the blood-forming cells in the bone marrow. Besides being acute or chronic, leukemias are classified according to cell type: lymphoblastic or myeloid.	Lymphadenopathy may be present, although other symptoms are more common, including fatigue, weakness, anorexia, weight loss, fever, night sweats, bleeding, and easy bruisability.	Diagnosis is made through hematologic studies and bone marrow biopsy. Prompt referral to a hematologist and/or oncologist is warranted.
Lymphomas: This group of neoplasms arise from the lymphatic system and lymphoid tissues. The most common types are Hodgkin's lymphoma, which occurs more often in younger patients, and non-Hodgkin's lymphoma, which occurs more in the older population. Burkitt's lymphoma and mycosis fungoides are rare types.	Cervical and mediastinal lymphadenopathies are often the presenting complaints and generally precede systemic symptoms, which include fever, night sweats, weight loss, and fatigue.	Diagnosis is made through hematologic studies and bone marrow biopsy. If lymphoma is suspected, prompt referral to a hematologist and/or oncologist is warranted.

Physical Examination

Physical examination is not helpful other than as an observation of patient discomfort when swallowing or a regurgitation or cough following attempted swallowing. Definitive diagnosis requires swallow studies and/or endoscopy to determine the exact cause of the problem.

ACHALASIA

Achalasia is diffuse esophageal spasm involving the smooth muscle of the esophagus and is the most common cause of motor dysphagia. It occurs with both liquid and solid foods. It occurs more frequently in geriatric clients and is the most likely cause of aspiration pneumonia. GERD, strictures, and neoplasms are more common in the elderly, contributing to aspiration prevalence in this population.

Signs and Symptoms

With achalasia, the patient complains of discomfort or fullness in the throat and difficulty swallowing. In the elderly client who is nonverbal, aspiration may be the first sign.

Diagnostic Studies

The diagnosis of achalasia is made with endoscopy. Taking small amounts of food, eating a soft diet, and sitting while eating are helpful preventive measures.

ESOPHAGITIS

Esophagitis is an inflammation of the esophagus that can occur with GERD, certain medicines (especially when not taken with enough fluid), the ingestion of caustic substances, neoplasms, chemotherapy, or radiation.

Signs and Symptoms

The patient with esophagitis describes burning and pain in the esophagus with or without dysphagia. The symptoms may occur more with eating or drinking and at night when the patient is recumbent.

Diagnostic Studies

The diagnosis of esophagitis is made with endoscopy. Removal of the causative agent, if possible, helps toward healing. Medicines such as H_2 blockers and proton pump inhibitors may be necessary.

BARRETT'S ESOPHAGUS

This condition is typically associated with GERD or with mucosal damage secondary to chemotherapy or radiation; it is characterized by inflammation of the lower esophagus with possible ulceration.

Signs and Symptoms

As with esophagitis, patients may describe a burning sensation in the throat or difficulty swallowing.

Diagnostic Studies

The diagnosis is made via endoscopy with a biopsy of the mucosal tissue. Barrett's esophagus is associated with an increased frequency of squamous cell carcinoma, so regular follow-up is necessary.

SCHATZKI'S RING

Schatzki's ring is a mucosal narrowing of the distal esophagus at the squamo-columnar junction. It is thought to be congenital but may not manifest until later in life.

Signs and Symptoms

Dysphagia is the presenting symptom in patients with Schatzki's ring, especially with ingestion of solid foods.

Diagnostic Studies

The diagnosis is made via endoscopy, and the stretching of the stricture alleviates the symptoms. Recurrence is common, and repeat dilations or resection may be necessary.

SCLERODERMA

Scleroderma is a chronic disease of unknown etiology characterized by a progressive systemic fibrosis of the skin, joints, and internal organs, especially the esophagus, gastrointestinal (GI) tract, heart, lung, and kidney.

Signs and Symptoms

There is a wide range in the severity of the symptoms and the prognosis. It may affect only the skin and manifest as generalized thickening, or it may be systemic, involving the vital organs and resulting in death. The initial symptoms usually involve GI complaints, such as dysphagia or reflux; shortness of breath; polyarthralgia; or Raynaud's disease, causing a thickening and stiffening of the skin on the hands and feet. The symptoms may worsen with time and involve numerous systems: skin, musculoskeletal, GI, cardiorespiratory, and kidneys. It may take several years for these manifestations to occur, and the constellation of symptoms is often called CREST (Calcinosis, Raynaud's, Esophageal dysfunction, Sclerodactyly, and Telangiectasias) syndrome.

Diagnostic Studies

A positive antinuclear antibody (ANA) is present in over 90% of patients. An anticentromere antibody (ACA) is present in a high portion of patients who progress to CREST syndrome.

NEUROMUSCULAR DISEASES

Several neuromuscular disorders can cause pre-esophageal dysphagia, including myasthenia gravis, muscular dystrophy, dermatomyositis, and poliomyelitis.

Signs and Symptoms

Dysphagia is one of the common presenting symptoms in these neuromuscular diseases. Other symptoms vary according to the underlying disease but include proximal limb weakness, general muscle fatigability, ocular muscle weakness, quadriparesis, polyarthralgias, skin eruptions, muscle spasms, and loss of DTRs, to name only a few. Aspiration can be a risk in these patients.

Diagnostic Studies

Diagnosis depends on the underlying disease, which is beyond the scope of this text. These patients need to be immediately referred to a neurologist for diagnosis and follow-up.

SUGGESTED READINGS

Beers, M.H. (2006). *Merck Manual of Medical Therapeutics*, 18th ed. Rahway, NJ: Merck & Co.

Kasper, D.L., Braunwald, E., Fauci, A.S., Hauser, S.L., Longo, D.L., & Jameson, J.L. (Eds.). (2008). *Harrison's Manual of Medicine*, 17th ed. New York: McGraw-Hill.

Fitzgerald, P.A. (2009). Endocrinology. In McPhee, S.J., & Papadakis, M.A. (Eds.), *CURRENT: Medical Diagnosis & Treatment*. Stamford, CT: Appleton & Lange Medical Books.

Swartz, M.H. (2009). *Textbook of Physical Diagnosis: History and Examination*, 6th ed. Philadelphia: W.B. Saunders.

Venes, D. (Ed.). (2009). *Taber's Cyclopedic Medical Dictionary*, 21st ed. Philadelphia: F.A. Davis.

Chapter 5

THE EYE

Mary Jo Goolsby

Eye disorders are common in all age groups, although the nature of the problems varies across the life span. Of all eye disorders, those resulting in visual impairment are the source of greatest disability. The incidence of vision loss is rising, in spite of the fact that much blindness can be prevented. The most common forms of visual impairment are refractive errors. In fact, over 150 million Americans are reported to use corrective lenses for refractive errors.

Another extremely common cause of visual disturbance in adults is cataract. Over 20 million adults over 40 years of age have cataracts, and the majority of Americans over 80 years have cataracts. Other less prevalent but relatively common causes of visual impairment include advanced macular degeneration associated with age (1.7 million), diabetic retinopathy (about 5 million), and glaucoma (approximately 4 million, almost one-half of which are undiagnosed) (NEI, 2011). Figure 5.1 illustrates basic eye anatomy. Table 5.1 provides a summary of characteristics that help differentiate among the causes of visual change.

History

■ General Eye History

When a patient has concerns about the eyes and/or vision, it is necessary to obtain a thorough analysis of symptoms and a general history related to the eyes. Ask about symptoms such as scotoma; floaters; decreased, blurred, or double vision; eye pain, discharge, and redness; lid weakness; masses; or changes in vision. It is important to ask about previous eye disorders.

■ Past Medical History

Determine whether the patient uses corrective lenses and, if so, how they are worn and whether they successfully correct the vision. The history should include eye disorders such as glaucoma, strabismus, amblyopia, cataracts, retinopathy, and macular degeneration, as well as a history of eye surgery. Any current or previous diagnoses of systemic disorders that affect the eyes should be determined, including diabetes, hypertension, vascular disorders, infections,

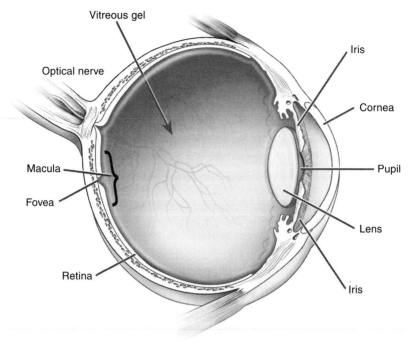

Figure 5.1 Basic eye anatomy. (From National Eye Institute, National Institutes of Health.)

and neuromuscular disorders. A history of all diagnostic procedures and results related to the eye and surrounding structures should be determined.

All medications should be identified. In addition to identifying drugs used to control diseases of the eyes or surrounding structures, the medication history also identifies agents that can alter vision. Box 5.1 includes a list of commonly prescribed drugs that affect the eyes or vision. Finally, knowing what medications the patient routinely takes may suggest the need for a more detailed medical history if it is found that the patient is taking drugs for disorders that were not disclosed earlier.

■ Family History

Identify the family history of eye disorders, including those conditions mentioned in the preceding paragraphs. Determine whether immediate relatives have refractive errors requiring correction.

■ Habits

Obtain a history of any recreational or occupational activities that expose the patient to trauma or to other contact that might place the eyes at risk, as well as the use of protective equipment. If the patient wears contact lenses, determine how long the lenses are worn, how often they are changed, and how they are cleansed and stored between wearings.

Table 5.1

Differentiating Among the Causes of Vision Changes

	Cataracts	Chronic Open-Angle Glaucoma	Acute Closed-Angle Glaucoma	Amaurosis Fugax	Retinal Detachment	Ischemic Ocular Neuropathy	Macular Degeneration
Onset	Gradual	Gradual	Sudden	Sudden	Sudden	Sudden	Gradual to sudden
Associated Symptoms			Head/eye pain, nausea, eye redness	Neurological deficits possible	Possible signs of trauma	Head, jaw, temple pain or soreness	
Severity of Vision Change	Ranges from cloudy, hazy to vision loss	Gradual darkening may range to complete vision loss	Blurring, halos; can range to total vision loss	Complete but transient loss initially; may lead to complete vision loss	Flash of light, darkened areas; may progress to complete loss	Affected portion lost	Blurring may progress to complete loss
Portion of Vision Affected	Unilateral or bilateral	Unilateral or bilateral; peripheral vision lost first	Unilateral	Unilateral	Unilateral, often specific fields affected; can be complete loss	Unilateral; may affect only portion but progress to complete loss	Unilateral or bilateral; starts centrally
Inspection	Clouding; loss of red reflex	Cup/disk ratio change; late afferent effect possible	Red eye, ciliary flush, fixed pupil, corneal edema	Pale retina with red fovea, embolus	Wrinkling and/or graying of retina, afferent pupil defect		Altered pigmentation; hemorrhage, exudates, microaneurysms, and/or neovascular

93

Box 5.1

Examples of Drugs With Oculotoxic Effects

- Amiodarone
- Gold salts
- Anticholinergic agents
- Hydroxychloroquine
- Antihistamines
- Isoniazid
- Chloramphenicol
- Phenothiazines
- Chloroquine

- Quinine
- Contraceptives (oral)
- Rifampin
- Corticosteroids
- Sympathomimetics
- Digitalis
- Tamoxifen
- Ethambutol

Physical Examination

■ Order of the Examination

The eye examination begins with determination of the patient's visual acuity. Next, the examiner typically inspects the external and accessory structures before concentrating inward to include the eye. Inspection is the primary technique used in the eye examination. However, when a mass or lesion is discovered, palpation of the area is indicated. If the patient has complained of discharge, palpation of the punctum, lids overlying meibomian glands, and in the region of the medial canthus may express the discharge. The globe also can be palpated gently to determine tone. If the patient has experienced sudden onset of eye pain, it is important not to dilate the eyes before determining whether acute angle glaucoma is present because dilating the eye may increase the intraocular pressure.

■ Visual Acuity

Visual acuity should be measured in a well-lighted area with and without corrective lenses, if lenses are worn. Testing the visual acuity assesses central vision and should be performed one eye at a time and then with both eyes simultaneously. Visual acuity is typically assessed with a Snellen chart, with the patient standing 20 feet from the chart. Some patients cannot read even the top line of the Snellen chart from 20 feet, so the examiner may have the patient move progressively closer to the chart and record the distance at which the top line can be read. If the patient cannot read the chart at a near distance, the examiner records whether the patient can count fingers, identify gross hand motion, or detect light. Near vision is tested using a handheld chart, such as a Rosenbaum chart, typically held 14 inches from the eyes. Color vision can be grossly tested using the color strips (green and red) on the Snellen chart or by asking the patient to identify the colors of other objects. Ishihara plates can be used for a more thorough assessment of color vision. Peripheral vision is tested separately.

■ Peripheral Vision

Peripheral vision is tested very grossly through confrontation with the examiner. Carefully identify the location of any visual defects. Alternatively, peripheral vision can be measured more objectively using equipment designed specifically for this purpose.

■ Alignment

Alignment is evaluated by observing eye motion, performing the cover/uncover test, and assessing the light reflex. Observe the position of the eyes as the patient follows an object as it is moved smoothly through the six cardinal positions, approximately 12 inches in front of the face. Perform the cover/uncover test, observing for movement as an eye is covered and uncovered. Ask the patient to focus on a distant object and observe one eye as the opposite eye is covered. If the visible eye, which is uncovered, moves as it fixates on the distant object as the opposite eye is covered, this is an abnormal finding indicating that the eye was not aligned prior to the opposite eye being covered. Next, uncover the opposite eye, as the patient continues to focus on the distant object. If this eye moves as it is uncovered, it indicates that the eye did not maintain alignment while it was covered and was unable to focus on an object. Repeat the same process, covering and uncovering the opposite eye. Later, as pupillary responses are assessed, alignment can be further evaluated by directing a penlight beam toward the bridge of the nose as the patient looks straight ahead and the examiner observes for symmetry of light reflex.

■ Accessory Structures

Inspect the eyebrows and lashes for symmetry and orientation. Inspect lids for symmetry and placement; palpate the lids for masses or tenderness. Observe for areas of discoloration, masses, and xanthomas.

■ External Eye Structures

Inspect the conjunctiva, cornea, and sclera, noting the condition of the surface, clarity, color, and vascularity. Examples of several abnormalities are identified in color plates. Box 5.2 reviews the procedure for performing a fluorescein stain to assess for potential corneal lesions.

■ Pupils

Observe the shape and symmetry of the pupils, including the response to light and accommodation. The pupils provide important indications of the cause for vision change. Examples of abnormal findings and causes are noted in Table 5.2. The cornea is also assessed during the pupil examination. Box 5.3 describes assessment of the pupils.

■ Anterior Chamber and Lens

Determine the approximate depth and clarity of the anterior chamber using oblique lighting. Also with the oblique lighting, assess the clarity of the lens.

Box 5.2

Special Procedure: Fluorescein Stain Technique to Assess Corneal Integrity

After determining that the patient has no relevant allergies, inspect the cornea and sclera without staining, if tolerated. A topical ocular anesthetic improves tolerance of further examination. Approximately 1 minute after installation of topical anesthetic, moisten the tip of a fluorescein stain strip with sterile saline. Holding the lids open with thumb and index finger, apply the stain by touching the moistened strip to the lower conjunctiva. Ask patient to blink to disperse the stain. If both eyes are being stained, use a separate strip for each eye to avoid cross-contamination.

Once the stain has been distributed by blinking, inspect the cornea and conjunctiva beneath the upper and lower lids using a cobalt blue light source, held obliquely to the structure being examined. Areas of stain uptake, indicating abrasion to the cornea, will fluoresce bright green. Any visible and superficial foreign body should be removed if possible.

Following inspection, flush the stain with sterile saline solution.

Table 5.2

Pupil Abnormalities

Horner's syndrome	Miosis is present unilaterally. Pupillary responses intact. Associated with ptosis and appearance that eye is "sunken" on affected side, with lack of sweating on opposite side. Cause by sympathetic lesion
Benign anisocoria	Some asymmetry of the pupil size is considered normal if the difference is less than 0.5 mm
Argyll-Robertson pupil	The pupil is small and may have an abnormal shape. Although the pupil does not respond to light, it exhibits a brisk response to accommodation (near vision). Usually bilateral involvement. Associated with neurosyphilis
Tonic pupil	No response to light (direct or consensual). Accommodation usually also affected. Most common in females. Unilateral. Caused by denervation of the ciliary muscle and sphincter

During the funduscopic examination, the clarity of the lens is also identified when the red reflex is noted.

■ Cranial Nerves

The eye examination includes an assessment of cranial nerves II, III, IV, and VI, which is accomplished during assessment of visual acuity, accessory structures, and pupils. The optic nerve is finally directly observed during the funduscopic examination.

Box 5.3

Special Procedure: Pupil Testing

The assessment of pupil shape, size, and reactivity provides much data. It is important to always assess direct and consensual pupillary response. If these are abnormal, you should then also assess for accommodation. By using the "swinging penlight" test in assessing the response to light, afferent defects—in which the consensual response is more pronounced than the direct response—are more easily detected. This method is performed by holding the light source in front of the patient so that it is directed toward one eye. At this point, observe both pupils, noting the direct response of the eye receiving the direct light and the consensual response in the opposite eye. Leave your attention on the opposite eye, continuing to note the consensual response as you briskly swing the light source in the direction of this eye. Note whether the pupil response is a slight constriction, slightly more pronounced with direct light, which is normal, or the pupil slightly relaxes so that the response is slightly less pronounced with direct light, which is an abnormal, Marcus-Gunn effect. Then observe the opposite eye, swinging the light back to that eye as you note any change between the indirect and direct responses. In some optic nerve disorders, such as ischemic optic neuropathy and optic neuritis, as well as other conditions that affect the pathway anterior to the optic chiasm, this afferent defect may be the only objective finding.

■ Funduscopic Examination

Funduscopic examination of each eye is performed in a darkened room. The sequence may vary by examiner preference, but this portion of the examination includes the identification of the red reflex and inspection of the lens, retinal background and vessels, optic disk, and anterior and posterior chambers (Box 5.4). The background and vessels should be assessed in four quadrants in each eye. It is important to recognize that there are limitations in the portion of the eye that is seen through an undilated pupil as performed in the typical primary care setting. Table 5.3 lists several abnormalities, with the related significance for each. Refer to Color Plates 42 through 47 illustrating the normal fundus and selected abnormal findings.

Differential Diagnosis of Chief Complaints

■ Visual Disturbances

Visual disturbances include a wide range of complaints, including blurred vision, loss of vision, blind spots, and altered color perception. When altered vision is the patient's chief complaint, it is crucial to be alert for indications of potential irreversible loss of vision. Sudden loss of vision is considered an

Box 5.4

Special Procedure: Funduscopic Examination

Successful use of the ophthalmoscope takes much practice and patience. The ophthalmoscope provides the ability to directly visualize both the external and internal structures of the eye. It is important that the examiner be familiar with adjusting the intensity of the light source, varying the apertures, and adjusting the diopters to best visualize the target structures. As the dial on the ophthalmoscope is moved counterclockwise, the diopters shift from positive to negative. Because the more negative diopters direct the focus posteriorly, by moving from the positive to negative diopters, your focus will shift from the anterior eye to the posterior eye, retina, and optic disk. Adjustment of the ophthalmoscope while inspecting the eye takes considerable practice and coordination. The newer panoptic ophthalmoscope provides a magnified view and is easier to manipulate than traditional equipment.

Table 5.3

Retinal and Background Abnormalities

Finding	Significance
Flame hemorrhages (superficial)	Linear hemorrhages, often associated with extreme elevation of blood pressure
Preretinal hemorrhages	Superficial hemorrhage, often characterized by a rounded inferior margin and a linear upper visible margin. Associated with both diabetic and hypertensive retinopathy and retinal tears
Microaneurysms	Tiny rounded dilations of retinal arteries, frequently associated with hypertension
Neovascularization	Proliferation of new, fragile vessels on the surface of retina, which have increased likelihood of bleeding. Associated with diabetes
Dot/blot hemorrhages (deep)	Deeper, rounded and/or irregularly shaped hemorrhages associated with diabetes
Cotton wool exudate	Yellow to white "fluffy" areas of ischemia. Associated with both diabetic and hypertensive retinopathy
Hard exudate	Very discrete yellow to white lesions, often distributed in a circular pattern. Associated with leakage of fluids into retinal tissue. Associated with both diabetic and hypertensive retinopathy

ocular emergency, regardless of whether the disturbance is partial or complete and whether or not it is accompanied by pain.

Altered vision can refer to decreased visual acuity with intact visual fields. This is a common complaint and, with age, is associated with the development of cataracts. It can also be associated with relatively benign refractive errors or with hyperglycemia and diabetes, macular degeneration, or glaucoma. In contrast, the loss of vision—whether limited to a specific visual field or area, one eye, or both eyes—typically indicates a very significant health problem that may result in permanent visual loss and disability.

History

When patients complain of altered vision, it is important to obtain a history of any other eye symptoms or disease, in addition to exploring the altered vision. Determine when the patient first noticed the altered vision and how, if at all, it has progressed since onset, as well as whether it has been transient or persistent. Ask whether the visual disturbance has affected the patient's ability to perform any normal activities and whether the patient has been exposed to chemicals or trauma. Always determine what the patient means if he or she complains of decreased or blurred vision; discriminate between decreased visual acuity and episodes of actual visual loss. Ask whether the alteration involves one or both eyes and is limited to central, peripheral, near, and/or distant vision. Figures 5.2 through 5.5 illustrate examples of normal and select types of altered vision. Establish the date and results of the patient's last visual examination and whether corrective lenses are prescribed and used. Find out whether there is history of systemic diseases, such as diabetes, and what medications the patient has recently taken. The family history of eye disease and other chronic diseases is important.

Physical Examination

The physical examination for altered vision starts with determination of visual acuity. Both far and near vision are tested in each eye alone and then in combination. Adaptations must be made for patients with very low vision. If applicable, vision should be tested with the patient wearing prescribed corrective lenses. Although it is tempting to go directly from testing visual acuity to the funduscopic examination, the assessment should next include inspection of the external structures, eye movement, peripheral vision/visual fields, and pupil reactions. Assess the appearance of the cornea and anterior chamber as well the quality of the red reflex. A funduscopic examination should be performed, with rare exceptions, such as when vision change is accompanied by severe eye pain and/or photophobia, as occurs with acute closed-angle glaucoma. Funduscopic examination also may be difficult with lens cloudiness, as occurs with advanced cataracts.

The decision to examine other systems should be determined in the context of the patient's history and general survey. For instance, if eye movement or

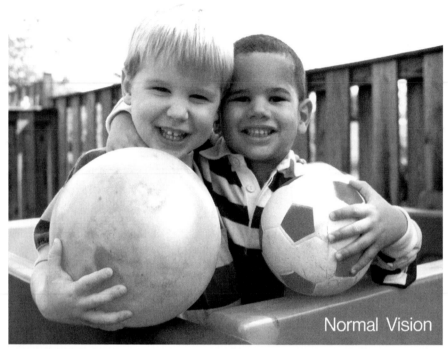

Figure 5.2 Normal vision. (From National Eye Institute, National Institutes of Health.)

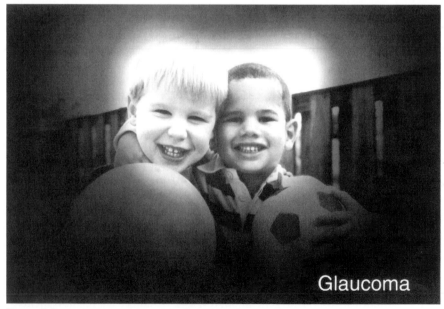

Figure 5.3 Glaucoma scene. (From National Eye Institute, National Institutes of Health.)

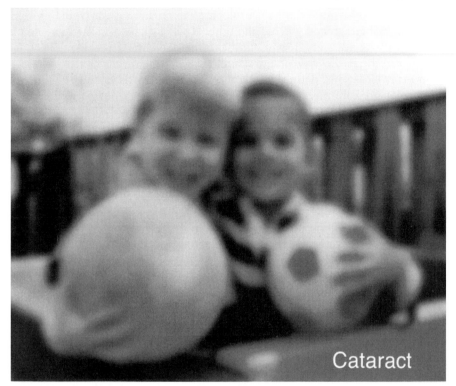

Figure 5.4 Cataract scene. (From National Eye Institute, National Institutes of Health.)

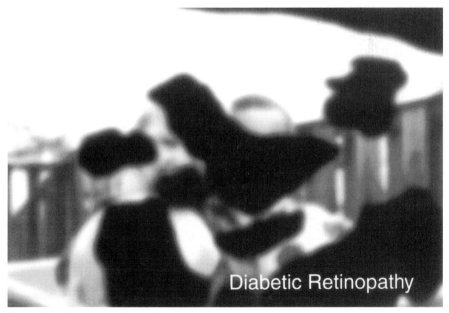

Figure 5.5 Diabetic retinopathy scene. (From National Eye Institute, National Institutes of Health.)

pupil reaction is asymmetrical, a neurological examination is warranted. With a history of diabetes, blood glucose and other signs of diabetes control should be determined. As necessary, the physical examination should include careful assessment of the cardiovascular and neurological systems.

In many situations, definitive diagnostic studies such as dilation of the eye, intraocular pressure measurement, and magnification are not performed at a general practice site but by a specialist to whom the patient is referred. The history taking and physical examination must be adequate to identify the need for prompt referral to another specialist, for instance, a neurologist. Although it is beyond the scope of this chapter to address the full range of disorders that could result in visual disturbance, many of the characteristic disorders are identified here.

CATARACTS

Cataracts are opacities of the optic lens and most typically occur as a disease of aging. However, cataracts can be caused or accelerated by conditions such as exposure to ultraviolet light and to certain drugs as well as systemic diseases such as diabetes.

Signs and Symptoms

Patients with cataracts generally describe a progressive and painless decreased visual acuity. The altered vision includes general blurring and haziness of vision as well as the development of halos and glares in response to bright lights as when driving in the dark. The opacities may be visible as gray or whitening areas over the pupil. The opacity makes ophthalmologic examination difficult, obscuring the visualization of the posterior chamber and retinal structures.

Diagnostic Studies

Early cataracts are best detected through ophthalmic examination of the dilated eye, using magnification.

CHRONIC OPEN-ANGLE GLAUCOMA

Glaucoma is characterized by increased intraocular pressure, which results in neuropathy of the optic nerve. This most common form of glaucoma results in a gradual and progressive altered vision. The incidence of chronic glaucoma is highest among African Americans, diabetics, and those over 35 years of age, particularly if they have a positive family history.

Signs and Symptoms

Patients with chronic open-angle glaucoma generally have no complaints until the disease progresses to the point that they perceive the decreased vision. The visual disturbance then progresses from blurring to complete vision loss if not recognized and treated. The patient may have required frequent corrective prescription changes up until definitive diagnosis. The vision loss begins peripherally; central vision is preserved until late in the disorder. The physical examination identifies an increased cup-to-disk ratio and elevated intraocular pressure.

Diagnostic Studies

A normal tonometric value is under 21, although the value can vary or fluctuate. Tonometry must be considered in combination with retinal signs of glaucoma and visual fields. Ophthalmologists perform additional tests, including gonioscopy, which assesses the drainage angle to determine whether it is open or closed.

ACUTE CLOSED-ANGLE GLAUCOMA

This less-common form of glaucoma results in acute visual disturbance. The increased intraocular pressure may be transient and triggered by conditions that cause pupillary dilatation, such as darkened rooms. As the intraocular pressure acutely increases, the patient typically experiences significant symptoms, which may resolve before the patient arrives for evaluation. It is very important that the examiner *not* dilate the eyes when a patient presents with a history of unilateral eye pain and visual disturbance because the dilation may further exacerbate the intraocular pressure increase.

Signs and Symptoms

During episodes of acute closed-angle glaucoma, patients usually experience severe, unilateral eye pain. Accompanying symptoms may include photophobia, headache, and nausea. The vision blurs, and patients may perceive halos around lights. Physical findings may include eye redness, ciliary flush, and a fixed and mid-dilated pupil. If the cornea becomes edematous, it may appear hazy and develop a "dewdrop" appearance.

Diagnostic Studies

Whenever acute closed-angle glaucoma is suspected, the patient must be immediately referred to an ophthalmologist, who can complete tonometry and further diagnosis, in order to provide prompt definitive treatment and to preserve vision.

AMAUROSIS FUGAX

Amaurosis fugax is a monocular, transient loss of vision. It stems from transient ischemia of the retina and presents an important warning sign for impending stroke. Depending on the circumstances reported, the patient should be immediately referred to either a cardiovascular or neurological specialist. Four broad causes of amaurosis fugax include emboli, retinal vascular insufficiency, arterial spasms, and idiopathy.

Signs and Symptoms

An episode of vision loss that accompanies amaurosis fugax may last from only seconds to minutes. The patient often describes the episode as if a shade had been pulled over one eye in a descending fashion and then, a short time later, the shade was raised and vision restored. Unlike acute glaucoma, there is no associated pain during the episode. Depending on the duration of the episode, the funduscopic examination may reveal the retina as whitened with a bright red fovea. If the occlusion is of the carotid, the patient may report or exhibit transient sensorimotor deficits consistent with a transient ischemic attack (TIA). The funduscopic examination may reveal emboli, altered vessels, microaneurysms, and blot hemorrhages. Carotid bruits may be present.

Diagnostic Studies

Depending on the setting, noninvasive carotid studies such as Doppler ultrasound or magnetic resonance angiography may be obtained before the patient is seen by the specialist. If valvular embolus has caused the disorder, the embolus may be visible.

RETINAL DETACHMENT

Retinal detachments are caused by trauma or by the traction caused by diabetic retinal disease. Regardless of the cause, patients suspected of having a retinal detachment should be immediately referred to an ophthalmologist.

Signs and Symptoms

The patient usually provides a history of trauma followed by a sudden visual disturbance, such as flashing light, floaters, or scotoma. The visual defect may advance or progress as the retinal detachment enlarges. Depending on the size of the defect, the patient may exhibit an afferent pupil defect, so that the pupil of the affected eye dilates rather than constricts when exposed to direct light. The affected retina appears wrinkled and gray.

ISCHEMIC OCULAR NEUROPATHY

The visual disturbances of ischemic ocular neuropathy stem from chronic ischemia, and resulting vision loss is irreversible. However, unilateral loss of vision in patients over 65 years may be caused by temporal arteritis; in this case, the patient is at risk for losing vision in the opposite eye.

Signs and Symptoms

The visual loss is unilateral and may be limited to either the upper or lower visual field. There is no associated pain of the eye. However, patients with temporal arteritis will have previously experienced pain of the head, temple, or face, as well as more generalized symptoms of polymyalgia rheumatica, including joint pain, malaise, weakness, fatigue, and even weight loss.

Diagnostic Studies

With temporal arteritis, the erythrocyte sedimentation rate (ESR) is often elevated. A temporal artery biopsy is diagnostic, although treatment must not be withheld pending the biopsy.

MACULAR DEGENERATION

Most commonly, macular degeneration is associated with aging and results either from atrophy of the macula or exudation and hemorrhage of the vessels in the macular region.

Signs and Symptoms

Visual alterations associated with macular degeneration are typically unilateral, vary from gradual to sudden in onset, and can range from blurring to complete blindness. The retina may show altered pigmentation, hemorrhage, or hard and soft exudates. In diabetics, neovascularization and microaneurysms may be visible.

Diagnostic Studies

An ophthalmologist will further evaluate the patient's central vision and perform fluorescein angiography. A commonly used test, the Amsler grid, assesses the patient's ability to accurately see a set of grids.

TRAUMA

Blunt trauma to the eye or orbit can be associated with altered vision. Depending on the type of trauma, the history should provide details of the event and the physical examination may allow detection of other signs of trauma.

■ Reddened Eye

Eye redness can be caused by a wide range of disorders, from conjunctivitis to acute closed-angle glaucoma. Eye redness may herald a disorder that has no associated visual impairment or others associated with complete loss of vision. Although most causes of eye redness are self-limiting, it is essential to perform a complete assessment when this is the presenting complaint.

History

When a patient complains of a reddened eye, first determine whether he or she has experienced eye trauma or any associated vision disturbance. Obtain a history of the redness and its progression, then ask about other symptoms such as eye itching, pain, swelling, discharge, or photophobia. Ask about exposures to chemical agents. If the patient wears contact lenses, determine the type and how the lenses are cared for. Ask about systemic symptoms such as general malaise, skin rashes, and cold or allergy symptoms. Ascertain whether the patient has had previous episodes of eye disorders or systemic problems, such as atopic or rheumatologic disorders. Identify any drugs or other products that have been used around or on the eyes. Old mascara has been shown to be full of bacteria. Determine whether there is a family history of eye conditions, such as glaucoma, iritis, or allergic conjunctivitis, as well as relevant systemic disorders. Autoimmune disorders and HIV are associated with certain eye diseases that may cause redness. If the patient has had eye trauma and/or corneal abrasion, determine his or her tetanus status.

Physical Examination

The physical examination must begin by determining the patient's corrected visual acuity, then observing the general characteristics of the redness, then finishing with a rapid assessment to rule out signs of trauma. Note whether there is any photophobia and adjust the light to the patient's comfort if possible. Assess the outer and appendage structures, looking for swelling, redness, discharge, or lesions. Next, focus on the eye itself, observing the cornea and conjunctiva for redness and noting the degree, pattern, and location of the redness. Identify any shadowing by passing oblique lighting over the anterior chamber. Assess the palpebral and tarsal conjunctiva beneath the lids; observe for foreign bodies or lesions. Assess the size, shape, and responsiveness of the pupils. If tolerated, perform a funduscopic examination. Depending on the history and examination of the eyes, it may be necessary to extend the assessment to the skin, ears, nose, throat, and joints to assess for infections, allergy, or rheumatic disorders.

Diagnostic studies are generally not warranted for eye redness. However, it may prove necessary to obtain a culture from the conjunctiva or to determine the intraocular pressure through tonometry. If foreign body or corneal abrasion is suspected, the examination should include fluorescein staining and examination of the eye with a Wood's lamp. If a foreign body is suspected, a slit lamp examination is necessary, and referral to an ophthalmologist is warranted.

CONJUNCTIVITIS

The most common cause of eye redness is conjunctivitis, which involves an inflammation of one or more areas of the conjunctiva. It is important to discriminate between allergic, viral, bacterial, and other causes of conjunctivitis in order to provide definitive treatment. Infectious conjunctivitis is usually caused by viral organisms, although bacterial infections are also common and can be secondary to viral infections. Allergies are the most frequent cause of noninfectious conjunctivitis. Other causes include chemical reactions.

Signs and Symptoms

The primary symptom of conjunctivitis, eye redness, is fairly consistent among the various causes. The degree of accompanying eye symptoms such as discomfort, itching, and discharge, as well as extraorbital symptoms, helps to define the problem. Examination of the eyes also provides important information to identify the cause. Table 5.4 differentiates among the signs and symptoms of viral, bacterial, and allergic conjunctivitis.

Diagnostic Studies

On occasion, diagnostic tests are helpful in assessing conjunctivitis. Studies can include viral and bacterial cultures of the conjunctiva or tests for atopy.

Table 5.4

Differentiating Conjunctivitis

Finding	Allergic Conjunctivitis	Bacterial Conjunctivitis	Viral Conjunctivitis
Pain/discomfort	Itchy sensation	Burning or gritty sensation	Foreign body or gritty sensation
Discharge	Watery, thin, clear	Mucopurulent, viscous	Mucoid
Preauricular nodes	Nonpalpable/ normal	Usually nonpalpable; palpable in hyperacute cases	Palpable
Accompanying symptoms	History of allergies, recurrent	May have URI symptoms	May have URI symptoms

URI: upper respiratory infection.

CORNEAL ABRASION

The cornea can become scratched or abraded by a variety of situations, including trauma and foreign bodies. A common foreign body involved in corneal abrasions is a contact lens. It is important to identify how the abrasion occurred in order to determine the risk of complications, including infection and ulceration. For instance, the abrasion is more likely to be contaminated and at risk for infection if caused by contact lenses or an animal scratch than if caused by a grain of sand.

Signs and Symptoms

The patient is likely to complain of "scratchiness," pain, or a foreign body sensation. The symptoms generally have a sudden onset after some exposure. Photophobia and significant tearing are common with abrasions. Decreased vision is likely to occur in the affected eye. The redness may be either diffuse or in a ciliary flush pattern. Fluorescein staining identifies an obvious break in the corneal surface with uptake of the stain. Examination of the fundus is normal. Unless the patient has delayed assessment, there should be no discharge or enlargement of the preauricular nodes, indicating infection.

Diagnostic Studies

Diagnostic study is not indicated unless signs of infection are evident. With appropriate treatment, abrasions generally resolve in 24 hours. Patients should be rechecked to ensure that the abrasion is resolving as anticipated. If not, the patient should be referred to an ophthalmologist because ulceration is common.

SUBCONJUNCTIVAL HEMORRHAGE

Subconjunctival hemorrhage, although an impressive sight, is usually a benign and self-limiting condition. Subconjunctival hemorrhage is caused by rupture of small capillaries and may follow trauma or an episode of coughing, sneezing, or rubbing of the eye. Scuba diving and childbirth are often associated with subconjunctival hemorrhage. Often, the cause is not determined. Always exclude other eye symptoms and signs to ensure that abrasion, perforation, or other conditions are not overlooked by the distraction associated with the very reddened eye.

Signs and Symptoms

Subconjunctival hemorrhage is not associated with vision loss, photophobia, or pain. The onset of the redness is sudden and typically limited to one eye; it may be localized to one region of the affected eye. With the exception of the deep redness, other findings are within normal limits.

UVEITIS

Uveitis involves inflammation of the uveal tract, including the iris, and thus includes iritis as well. The inflammation may be caused either by infection or as part of a reaction associated with a systemic disorder. For instance, an increased incidence of uveitis is associated with autoimmune disorders, such as Crohn's disease, ankylosing spondylitis, and HIV infection. It is important to identify any systemic source for the problem as well as to refer the patient for a thorough ophthalmic examination.

Signs and Symptoms

The vision changes associated with uveitis stem from altered responsiveness of the pupil and lens. Patients commonly experience both photophobia and eye pain. There is a ciliary flush and, usually, a constricted pupil. Precipitates may be visible on the posterior surface of the cornea. The patient may complain of other systemic symptoms, such as joint pain and altered bowel habits and abdominal pain, if an autoimmune disorder is involved.

Diagnostic Studies

The ophthalmologist will perform diagnostics related to the eye disorder, but if the uveitis is recurrent and/or has a suspected systemic cause, further diagnostic studies should be considered, including ESR, autoimmune panel, and HIV.

KERATITIS

Disorders in this category result in inflammation of the cornea and can lead to blindness in the affected eye. Keratitis can be caused by herpetic and other infections, ischemia, chemical exposures, foreign bodies, or corneal abrasions. It can be triggered by eye dryness or denervation; and it may also be secondary to conjunctivitis. Keratitis is noteworthy because it can lead to ulcerations, opacities, and blindness of the affected eye; thus, patients suspected of this disorder should be immediately referred to an ophthalmologist.

Signs and Symptoms

Patients with keratitis may complain only of a foreign body sensation or may complain of severe pain. Ask about trauma associated with contact lens wear.

Although vision may not be initially affected, it can be altered as the condition advances. Gray infiltrate may be visible on examination, and there may be a ciliary flush. If ulcerative keratitis is involved, perforations may be evident on staining. A hypopyon ulcer may develop, with pus collecting in the anterior chamber.

Diagnostic Studies

On referral, the ophthalmologist will perform a variety of studies to identify the causative agent of the situation, including bacterial, fungal, and viral cultures and slit lamp examination.

SCLERITIS AND EPISCLERITIS

Scleritis and episcleritis are inflammatory problems involving the sclera and episclera, respectively. Most cases of scleritis are associated with chronic autoimmune disorders, such as rheumatoid arthritis, systemic lupus erythematosus, and sarcoidosis. In contrast, episcleritis is self-limiting and not associated with chronic disorders. They are best differentiated by the degree of involvement. Although they do not typically affect the vision, both conditions are often chronic and warrant referral to an ophthalmologist. With time, scleritis can evolve to cause cataracts and/or glaucoma.

Signs and Symptoms

Visual acuity can be altered with advanced scleritis. While episcleritis is generally painless, scleritis may cause extreme pain. Although photophobia is not common with either disorder, it is more likely to occur with scleritis. Neither disorder is associated with altered pupils, and the redness may be localized or diffuse. However, the redness associated with scleritis may be intense—almost purple—and is darker than is typically seen with episcleritis. The discoloration lies immediately below the conjunctiva, and the sclera may develop inflammatory nodules and engorged vessels. Episcleritis, in contrast, is more localized but can also be associated with localized engorged vessels and nodular changes.

Diagnostic Studies

Episcleritis requires no specific diagnostic studies. However, if scleritis is suspected or the diagnosis is uncertain, the patient should be referred to an ophthalmologist for definitive diagnosis and treatment. Laboratory studies include complete blood count, ESR, and antinuclear antibody; in addition, rheumatoid factor should be considered.

■ Eye Pain

Eye pain can be caused by urgent problems that threaten vision, such as acute closed-angle glaucoma, various traumatic injuries, and infectious agents. There is a lot of overlap among the disorders that cause eye pain and those causing eye redness; thus, the history and physical examination are similar for both complaints.

History

When the chief complaint includes eye pain, first establish whether there is a history of chemical exposure or burn, trauma, or vision loss. In the case of chemical burn, further assessment must be delayed until the eye has been thoroughly irrigated. Once chemical exposure and/or trauma has been excluded, explore the onset and characteristics of the pain. For instance, determine whether the pain had sudden onset or developed gradually. Ask about the type of pain, for instance, whether it is sharp, dull, throbbing, or aching, as well as whether it is superficial, deep, or diffuse. Identify any associated symptoms, including malaise, vision change, discharge, photophobia, and redness.

Physical Examination

Test visual acuity, if tolerated, before proceeding with further examination. Carefully inspect the accessory and external eye structures. Note any lacerations, lesions, discolorations, swelling, redness, and discharge. Assess the size, shape, and responsiveness of the pupils. If there is a history of trauma to the eye, carefully assess the corneal surface. Grossly inspect for signs of perforation, such as bleeding or "leakage" from the globe, altered shape, and obvious entry points. If perforation can be excluded by history and examination, fluorescein stain should be applied so that the corneal surface can be inspected using Wood's lamplight. Assess the cornea for clarity, and note the anterior chamber depth. If tolerated, a funduscopic examination should be performed.

CHEMICAL BURNS

Chemical burns can occur from topical contact from many agents. Chemical burns make up the majority of ocular burns. Whereas acid burns do not penetrate the eye structures, alkali burns do cause penetrating injuries.

Signs and Symptoms

Inspect the face and periorbital region for blisters, redness, and other signs of a burn. The patient may not be able to hold the eye open. There may be significant redness, tearing, pain, and swelling of the eye and accessory structures. It is essential that the offending chemical be identified quickly, if possible, and that the appropriate decontamination measures be instituted immediately. It may be impossible to clearly assess visual acuity, owing to photophobia, pain, and tearing, which can blur vision.

Chemical ophthalmic burns represent an emergency situation. The patient should be referred immediately to an ophthalmologist to determine the severity of injury and to implement necessary treatment and follow-up.

HERPES ZOSTER

Herpes zoster is caused by the varicella-zoster virus and can affect the ophthalmic branch of the fifth cranial nerve. Ophthalmic involvement is often heralded by lesions on the tip of the nose.

Signs and Symptoms

The development of herpes zoster skin and mucous membrane lesions is usually preceded by a period of several days during which the patient experiences malaise and neuralgia along the affected nerve root. The pain is severe and often accompanied by systemic symptoms, including fever and fatigue. Photophobia may be present. Accessory structures may be inflamed and/or swollen. Vision may be altered in the affected eye. Inspection of the cornea following flourescein stain may reveal punctate or dentitic ulcerations.

Diagnostic Studies

Whenever eye involvement of herpes zoster is suspected, the patient should be referred to an ophthalmologist. Although the actual diagnosis may be evident, referral allows specialized examination—including slit lamp to assess the degree of involvement—and the timely initiation of appropriate and individualized treatment to minimize complications. Viral cultures may be obtained.

ACUTE CLOSED-ANGLE GLAUCOMA

Acute closed-angle glaucoma is described under Visual Disturbances, p. 103.

CORNEAL ABRASION AND EROSION

Corneal abrasions are discussed under Reddened Eye, p. 107.

CONJUNCTIVITIS

Conjunctivitis is discussed under Reddened Eye, pp. 106–107.

UVEITIS, IRITIS, AND SCLERITIS

Each of these inflammatory disorders affecting the eye is covered in the section on Reddened Eye, pp. 108–109.

TRAUMA

Trauma should always be considered with presentation of eye pain.

■ Eye Discharge

Eye discharge is most commonly associated with infectious disorders but can also be associated with other inflammatory conditions or systemic diseases affecting the eye. The most common causes of eye discharge are the various forms of conjunctivitis.

History

Ask about the onset of the discharge and whether the discharge is persistent or instead occurs in certain settings. Note associated eye symptoms, such as pain, altered vision, photophobia, or swelling. Ask about extraocular symptoms, such as sneezing, itching, fever, and malaise. Determine history of atopic disorders and exposure to infectious diseases.

Physical Examination

Test visual acuity, and then perform a general inspection, observing for the quantity and location of any discharge and noting the consistency and color.

Although not generally necessary, a culture of the discharge may be warranted. To obtain a culture, retract the lower lid and place a conjunctival swab in the palpebral space.

DACRYOCYSTITIS

Dacryocystitis is an infection of the lacrimal sac and is most common in infants, secondary to congenital stenosis of the lacrimal duct. In adults, it can be caused by hypertrophic rhinitis, polyps, or trauma. Older adults lose the elasticity of the drainage system, so that the duct is not flushed by tears, and dacryocystitis may result.

Signs and Symptoms

If the duct is occluded, constant tearing may occur. The lacrimal sac may be edematous, red, and tender. Pressure over the sac produces purulent discharge. The surrounding area can become inflamed, tender, and swollen. Associated conjunctivitis or blepharitis may be present.

Diagnostic Studies

Diagnostic studies are generally not warranted.

ERYTHEMA MULTIFORME—STEVENS-JOHNSON SYNDROME

Erythema multiforme involves inflammation of the mucous membranes and skin. It is often related to an infection or can be due to almost any medication. Often, no specific cause is identified. The most severe form is called Stevens-Johnson syndrome. Because the condition can be fatal, it is important to immediately recognize and treat.

Signs and Symptoms

In Stevens-Johnson syndrome, conjunctivitis with copious amounts of purulent discharge may occur. The eyes become painful. Conjunctival bullae and ulcerations may develop. Patients develop erythematous lesions and bullae over the skin and hemorrhagic lesions of the mucous membranes. The patient appears acutely ill and has systemic symptoms, including malaise, fever, and arthralgias.

Diagnostic Studies

The diagnosis is often made by identifying the classic skin lesions, which consist of red-centered bullae surrounded by white areas. In addition to the eye tissue, the palms, soles, anus, vagina, nose, and mouth are commonly affected.

CONJUNCTIVITIS

See the section on Reddened Eye, pp. 106–107, for differentiation of allergic, bacterial, and viral conjunctivitis.

■ Ptosis

Ptosis, or drooping of an eyelid, can be related to simple aging, with natural loss of elasticity and lid drooping, or it can result from a variety of other causes. The causes of ptosis are often categorized as congenital and acquired. Causes occuring after birth include trauma, conditions adding mass to the eyelid, and conditions that affect the nerves or muscles controlling the lid's position. In 75% of the cases, the first manifestation of myasthenia gravis is ptosis.

History

It is important to determine how and when the ptosis developed, including whether the onset was sudden or gradual. Identify any associated altered vision and whether the patient believes the vision has been obscured by the drooping eyelid. Ask about all other medical disorders and medications. Determine whether the patient has a history of hypertension, peripheral vascular disease or other risk factors for stroke, or a history of myasthenia gravis. Ask about any recent trauma to the head or eye region.

Physical Examination

Assess visual acuity. Closely inspect the lids, noting the degree of ptosis and location of the lid margin relative to other eye structures, such as the iris or pupil. Measure the palpebral fissure, comparing one eye with the other. While inspecting the lids and determining the degree of asymmetry, ensure that there is not merely an illusion of ptosis caused by a contralateral retraction of the opposite lid, as seen in conditions causing exophthalmos. Palpate the lids for masses or swelling; observe for redness and discoloration. Assess cranial nerve III and muscle function by testing extraocular movements. Perform a general assessment of the face and cranial nerves. Assess the pupils for symmetry, shape, and reaction to light.

HORNER'S SYNDROME

Horner's syndrome is caused by decreased sympathetic innervation to the structures of the eye. Horner's syndrome can be caused by a variety of lesions, including trauma, tumors, and ischemia.

Signs and Symptoms

The symptoms vary but usually include unilateral ptosis, reduced sweating of the face, and miosis. The ptosis is typically incomplete, and although there is no true enophthalmos, the eye appears to have receded. The pupil reaction to light and accommodation remain intact.

Diagnostic Studies

A complete history and physical examination should be performed to identify likely etiologies. Based on findings, referral and/or imaging studies should be ordered.

MECHANICAL PTOSIS

Lacrimal gland tumor is an example of a mechanical cause of ptosis, adding bulk to the upper lid. The degree of ptosis depends on the size of the tumor. Other causes of mechanical ptosis include chalazion and hordeolum.

Signs and Symptoms

Pain is often associated with a lacrimal gland tumor as well as with chalazion and hordeolum. When inflammation is involved, the abnormal lid may be reddened and tender. If lacrimal gland tumor is involved, there may be some degree of exophthalmos and deviation of the eye, depending on tumor size.

AGING

Senile involutional ptosis is a common cause of ptosis, particularly in patients with advanced age.

Signs and Symptoms

The lids and other accessory structures will have a thin, inelastic appearance. No masses, inflammation, or systemic signs will be evident.

MYASTHENIA GRAVIS

Myasthenia gravis causes skeletal muscle weakness owing to a dysfunction of the acetylcholine receptors; this dysfunction results in reduced muscle innervation. It is a common cause of ptosis. Ptosis is the most common initial sign of myasthenia gravis, which often occurs at an earlier age in women than in men.

Signs and Symptoms

In myasthenia gravis, patients often have intermittent diplopia in addition to the ptosis. The ptosis is often intermittent. The patient may attempt to compensate by raising the opposite lid. The ptosis of myasthenia gravis can be accentuated by having the patient maintain an upward gaze or forcibly blink for an extended time. Alternatively, the icepack test, where a bag of crushed ice is placed over the closed affected lid for 1 minute, may reveal a subsequent temporary decrease in the ptosis. The pupils are within normal limits and not affected by the disorder.

Diagnostic Studies

Myasthenia gravis is definitively diagnosed by the Tensilon test, which involves administration of edrophonium chloride, which counteracts acetylcholine. If myasthenia gravis is present, any mild weakness will rapidly become exaggerated for a brief period of time following the Tensilon test. Alternatively, serology studies, such as acetycholine receptor antibodies, may be ordered.

OCULOMOTOR NERVE DEFICIT

The third cranial nerve, the oculomotor nerve, stimulates most of the extraocular muscles, so this disorder was chosen as an exemplar of cranial nerve disorders. Deficits can be caused by a wide range of problems, including diabetes and tumors.

Signs and Symptoms

The affected eye may have a "down-and-out" deviation, and the pupil is dilated. The ptosis is significant: the lid occludes the pupil and the patient cannot see from the affected eye. Facial muscle movement and strength are affected, as is sensation. The exact findings depend on which cranial nerve(s) are affected; nerves III, V, and/or VII may be involved.

BOTULISM

Botulism is caused by toxins from the bacillus *Clostridium botulinum*, which can be either food borne or a wound contaminant. Following ingestion of the botulism toxin, the incubation period ranges from hours to several days. The incubation period following wound contamination may be as long as 2 weeks.

Signs and Symptoms

The earliest symptoms involve the cranial nerves, and neurologic involvement then follows a descending pattern. Symptoms are generally symmetrical. Ptosis is an early symptom and may be preceded by diplopia. When wound contamination is the source of the condition, symptoms are limited to the neurologic system. However, when ingested, systemic symptoms such as nausea, vomiting, and diarrhea occur. Immediate referral to a neurologist or emergency department should be made because botulism can be life threatening.

■ Double Vision

Double vision, or diplopia, usually occurs when the extraocular muscles do not work in a coordinated manner and the patient sees one object as two. There are a variety of causes for diplopia, including both neurological and muscular disorders. Only in rare circumstances is monocular diplopia a problem, as this typically stems from eye deformities or retinal abnormalities.

History

For the complaint of double vision, it is important to fully analyze the symptom, determining how severe the visual disturbance is, when it occurs, and so on. Ask about any associated symptoms, such as other weaknesses, headache, or pain. Explore whether the diplopia most commonly occurs in certain circumstances, including particular times of day. Ask about substance use and abuse, including alcohol intake. Identify any history of systemic disorders, including neuromuscular, endocrine, and neurological diseases.

Physical Examination

The physical examination should start with visual acuity testing. Determine whether the diplopia occurs only when the patient uses both eyes or is limited to only one eye. Carefully assess the placement and symmetry of the eyes, performing a cover/uncover test and observing for the corneal light reflex. Note any lack of conjugate movement as the patient follows an object through the six cardinal fields of gaze.

PROPTOSIS AND EXOPHTHALMOS

Proptosis is the general term for anterior displacement of the eye; *exophthalmos* specifically describes proptosis related to endocrinopathy, usually thyroid disease. In thyroid disorders, the eye muscles thicken and thereby move the eyes forward so that their ability to move conjugately is affected, and the lids may fail to close completely. Movement in all directions may be affected, although most commonly the patient finds it difficult to look upward. In addition to diplopia, patients may experience dry eyes, ulcerations, and diminished vision. Less common causes of proptosis include infections and tumors affecting the structures of or near the eye.

Signs and Symptoms

The patient may complain of signs of thyroid disease, primarily those of hyperthyroidism, such as nervousness, anxiety, weight loss, and so on. The thyroid may be nodular or enlarged, the heart rate elevated, and a fine tremor may be present. A fever may accompany the proptosis, regardless of whether the cause is from thyroid disease or infection. There may also be complaints of visual disturbances in addition to the diplopia, a dry or gritty sensation, and eye tenderness.

Diagnostic Studies

The initial tests are to assess thyroid function, with complete blood count and other studies obtained subsequently, as needed. A Hertel exophthalmometer can be used to measure the degree of anterior displacement.

OCULOMOTOR NERVE DISORDERS

Lesions of the third, fourth, or sixth cranial nerve may result in diplopia, either vertical or horizontal. The third, fourth, or sixth cranial nerve palsies are usually benign, self-limited, and resolve in weeks to months. They commonly occur in patients who have hypertension and/or diabetes. However, a mass-occupying lesion should be excluded.

Signs and Symptoms

If the third cranial nerve is affected, accompanying ptosis usually occurs, so that the lid obscures the vision in the affected eye and the patient's main complaint may not be double vision. If the fourth nerve is involved, the diplopia will be vertical, whereas sixth cranial nerve palsy results in horizontal diplopia. Depending on the cause, the patient may exhibit signs or complaints consistent with herpes zoster, other infections, or neurological involvement.

Diagnostic Studies

The patient who experiences new onset of diplopia related to nerve disorder should be promptly referred to an ophthalmologist for further evaluation and determination of subsequent assessment needs.

MYASTHENIA GRAVIS
See pp. 114–115.

BOTULISM
See p. 115.

REFERENCES

NEI (2011). Statistics and data: Prevalence of blindness data. www.nei.nih.gov/eyedata/pbd_tables.asp (accessed March 7, 2011).

SUGGESTED READINGS

Bickley, L.S., & Szilagyi, P.G. (2004). *Bates' Guide to Physical Examination and History Taking.* Philadelphia: Lippincott, Williams, & Wilkins.

Crouch, R., Crouch, E., & Gran, T. (2007). Ophthalmology. In Rakel, R.E. (Ed.), *Textbook of Family Practice.* Philadelphia: Saunders.

Dillon, P.M. (2003). *Nursing Health Assessment: A Critical Thinking, Case Studies Approach.* Philadelphia: F.A. Davis.

Horton, J.C. (2004). Disorders of the eyes. In Kasper, D.L., Baunwald, E., Fauci, A.S., Kasper, D.L., Longo, D.L., & Jameson, J.L. (Eds.), *Harrison's Principles of Internal Medicine.* New York: McGraw Hill.

Jacobs, D. (2008) Evaluation of the red eye. UpToDate. http://www.uptodate.com/index (accessed March 7, 2011).

Swartz, M.H. (2005). *Textbook of Physical Diagnosis: History and Examination.* Philadelphia: Saunders.

Yanoff, M., & Duker, J. (2004). *Ophthalmology.* Philadelphia: Mosby.

Chapter 6

EAR, NOSE, MOUTH, AND THROAT

Mary Jo Goolsby

Upper respiratory complaints make up a significant component of the primary care provider's daily patient encounters. Figures 6.1, 6.2, and 6.3 identify the major landmarks of the upper respiratory system. The most common complaints of childhood include earache, sore throat, and symptoms of allergy and common cold. Elderly clients frequently present with complaints of hardened cerumen and decreased hearing resulting from cerumen impaction aggravated by hearing aid wear. All ages have significant sensory compromise associated with complaints of the ear, nose, mouth, and throat. The ability to maintain homeostasis related to breathing and nourishment

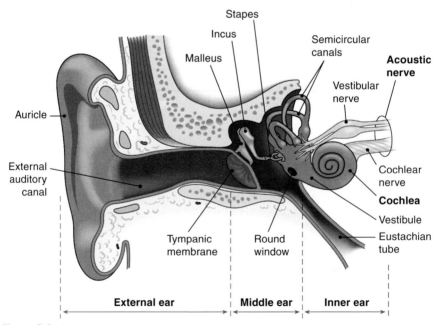

Figure 6.1 Anatomy of the ear. (From Dillon, P.M. *Nursing Health Assessment: A Critical Thinking, Case Studies Approach*. Philadelphia: F.A. Davis, 2003. Reprinted with permission.)

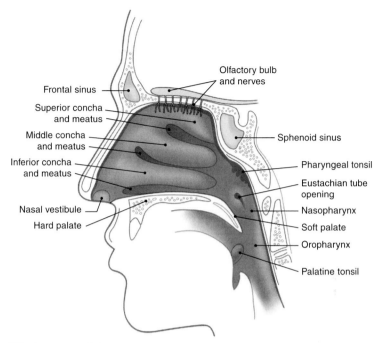

Figure 6.2 Anatomy of the nose. (From Dillon, P.M. *Nursing Health Assessment: A Critical Thinking, Case Studies Approach*. Philadelphia: F.A. Davis, 2003. Reprinted with permission.)

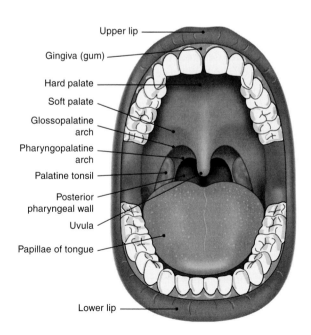

Figure 6.3 Anatomy of the mouth and oropharynx. (From Dillon, P.M. *Nursing Health Assessment: A Critical Thinking, Case Studies Approach*. Philadelphia: F.A. Davis, 2003. Reprinted with permission.)

may also be affected. Other issues are frequency of lost days of work or school related to allergies and upper respiratory infections.

History

■ General History

A general history of the ear, nose, mouth, and throat should include current or recent exposure to respiratory infections, such as flu or colds; complaints of ear, sinus, or throat pain; nasal or ear discharge, including color changes; changes in hearing, taste, or smell; and tinnitus. A history of nausea and vomiting, cough, or elevated temperature is relevant. A history of flu, upper respiratory infection, frequent sinus infections, allergies, and dental care is also important. A history of exposure to mononucleosis or strep and a history of smoking are also important.

■ History of the Present Illness

When a patient presents with a complaint related to the ears, nose, mouth, or throat, a symptom analysis is indicated. Ask what, if anything, has been noticed to make the symptoms worse or better. Ask about any self-treatment the patient may have attempted and the response. Determine whether exposure to potential allergy triggers, such as dust or pets, is related to symptoms. Have the patient quantify or rate the severity of the symptoms. When pain is present, determine its exact location as well as any areas of radiation. With ear, nose, and throat conditions, patients commonly experience multiple complaints. Ask about any associated symptoms. Ask about pain or discomfort (mouth, nose, sinus, ear, throat, etc.); nasal congestion or discharge; sinus pressure; postnasal drainage; ear fullness, drainage, or tinnitus; ulcerations of the lips, mouth, or throat; swollen or tender nodes; hoarseness; cough; and/or sneezing. In addition to symptoms of the ears, nose, mouth, and throat, ask about systemic symptoms such as fatigue, fever, myalgia, malaise, and headache. Finally, determine when the complaints were first noticed and how they have progressed.

■ Past Medical History

Ask about recent exposure to others with similar symptoms or potentially contagious conditions. Determine history and frequency of upper respiratory infections, such as strep throat, sinusitis, and otitis media. Establish whether the patient has ever had surgery or other procedures performed on the ears, nose, mouth, or throat; include cosmetic/aesthetic procedures as well as therapeutic ones. Identify any other major medical conditions. Ask about history of rhinitis or other atopic conditions, such as asthma, allergic conjunctivitis, and atopic dermatitis. Determine whether the patient has a prior history of skin or other malignancies. Ask about disorders that would affect the immune system, including HIV/AIDS. Obtain a history of all current and recent medications as well as immunizations/vaccinations. Prior diagnostic studies such as audiology and other hearing tests, along with the results, should be determined. The use of hearing aids should be noted.

■ Family History

Obtain a family history of hearing disorders and conditions, such as tinnitus, Ménière's disorder, allergies, malignancies, and asthma. Determine whether others in the family are ill with similar symptoms.

■ Habits

Exposure to recreational and occupational noise is important. Assess whether the patient works in an area that requires hearing protection and the type of protection used. Ask about activities that involve barometric pressure changes, such as scuba diving and flying, which may affect ear equilibrium. Determine whether the patient's activities involve exposure to toxins, trauma, or chemicals and any protection used. Ask about the use of smoked and smokeless tobacco, alcohol, and recreational drugs. Establish the patient's living conditions, including the method of cooling and heating the home and any exposure to pets or dust. Determine how often the patient sees a dentist, and identify any dental conditions.

■ Review of Systems

Based on the initial history, complete a review of other systems.

Physical Examination

■ Order of the Examination

Note the patient's vital signs, and complete a general survey. Develop a systematic approach to examining the ear, nose, mouth, and throat. These components are often incorporated into the examination of the head, face, and neck, described in Chapter 4.

Examination of the Ears

The ear examination begins with inspection of the external ear. Note the placement and symmetry of the ears. Inspect the external ears, noting the condition of the skin and the integrity of the structures. Assess any skin changes as described in Chapter 3. Identify any deformities, lesions, areas of enlargement, or other abnormalities. Observe for inflammation, signs of a foreign body, and drainage. Assess any piercings for healing and signs of tearing. Palpate the external ear, noting any areas of tenderness or deformities. Palpate the preauricular and postauricular lymph nodes for size, tenderness, consistency, and mobility.

The otoscope is then used to examine the canal and middle ear. If symptoms are unilateral, assess the asymptomatic ear before proceeding to the area of complaint. Use the largest ear speculum that is comfortable. Inspect the canal and associated structures for patency, erythema, tenderness, exudate, deformity, and drainage. Note the integrity of the tympanic membrane (TM) and the quality of the light reflex. Observe the visibility and placement of the bony landmarks posterior to the TM. Evaluate the TM for inflammation, retraction, or bulging. In children, observe for the presence of pressure-equalizing tubes. Look for any bubbles behind the eardrum, air-fluid level, and/or discoloration. A pneumonic otoscope may be used to evaluate TM motility. Color Plate 48 depicts a normal TM. Table 6.1 lists some abnormalities detected on the ear examination. Also see the Red Flags for presentations related to the ear.

Hearing can be grossly assessed using the whisper test, watch ticking, and tuning forks (see next subsection). If screening indicates a deficit or if the patient complains of hearing loss, an accurate assessment of hearing requires audiogram with proper equipment.

Special Maneuvers
Weber Test
The Weber test is performed with a tuning fork (500–1,000 Hz). The test measures the patient's ability to hear sound bilaterally. The tuning fork is tapped gently, and the base of the tuning fork is placed on the midline of the patient's head. The patient should hear the vibration equally in both ears.
Rinne's Test
This test uses the tuning fork to assess and compare the patient's ability to hear both through bone and air conduction. The vibrating tuning fork is placed on

Table 6.1	

Abnormalities of Inspection: Ear

Finding	Significance
External swelling and redness	Malignant otitis externa or mastoiditis
Light yellow to dark brown matter that occludes the eardrum	Cerumen impaction
Bloody discharge	External ear canal wound, skull fracture, traumatic perforation of the tympanic membrane
Purulent discharge	Infection or a foreign body
Whitish plaques on the eardrum	Scars from earlier infection
Dark area on the eardrum with drainage	Old or current perforation
Diffuse light reflex	Bulging eardrum
Bubbles on the eardrum	Serous fluid in the middle ear
Erythema of the tympanic membrane	Otitis, crying, or fever

> **RED Flag** ◀ Warnings for the Ear
>
> - *Red, warm, and very painful auricle.* Such a condition can be associated with malignant otitis externa and/or mastoiditis and warrants immediate referral.
> - *Auricular lesions.* Cancerous lesions are most often found in the helix of the auricle. They are associated with sun exposure and should be assessed using the ABCD cancer-screening criteria. Tophi are auricular lesions associated with gout.
> - *Clear fluid.* Clear fluid emitting from the ear may be associated with cerebral injury.

the patient's mastoid bone (bone conduction). When the patient indicates the tuning fork is no longer heard, the examiner positions the tines of the fork in front of the ear (air conduction) until the patient signals that the sound is no longer heard in that manner. The amount of time the patient hears the vibration in both positions is noted, and the maneuver is repeated on the opposite side. Air conduction should be twice as long as bone, and the results should be similar for both ears.

Hearing Tests

A skilled examiner using a soundproof booth should conduct audiometry. Before the audiogram is performed, ears should be examined for any cerumen buildup. Patients should be free from upper respiratory infection and the exacerbations of allergies. Patients should not have been exposed to loud noise activities for several days before the examination.

Tympanocentesis

Tympanocentesis, which involves aspiration of middle ear fluid by a specialist, should be considered in patients with recurrent otitis media to identify the causative organisms.

Pneumatic Otoscopy

Pneumatic otoscopy should be used to determine whether the TM is mobile.

Examination of the Nose and Sinuses

The examination of the sinuses begins with inspection of the face, noting any swelling or edema. Palpate over the frontal and maxillary sinuses, noting any tenderness. Unless tenderness is elicited by palpation over the sinuses, proceed with percussion of the sinuses. Ask the patient to notify you of tenderness and observe the facial expression for signs of discomfort. A sinus that is thickened or full may percuss dull, compared with the resonant tones usually associated with percussion of the sinuses. If sinus thickening or fullness is suspected, attempt transillumination using a penlight, otoscope, or transilluminator.

Observe the external nose for placement and any obvious deformity or discharge. Observe the patient's respiratory pattern, noting whether the patient is mouth breathing or is able to breath through the nose. Identify any flaring of the nostrils. Note the color, amount, and consistency of any drainage. Palpate the external nose, noting any deformities, masses, or tenderness. If the patient is experiencing significant nasal symptoms, the internal examination of the nose is best accomplished after asking the patient to blow his or her nose. Examine any discharge for color, consistency, and odor. To observe the internal structures, the patient's head should be tilted backward. The examiner's nondominant hand and thumb can be used to stabilize the nose and forehead with slight pressure of the thumb upward on the nose tip as a nasal speculum is gently inserted to observe the nasal mucosa and turbinates.

Assess the mucosa for integrity, color, moistness, and edema/lesions and the nasal septum for patency. The turbinates should be assessed for color and size. Pale, boggy turbinates suggest allergies; erythematous, swollen turbinates are often seen with infection. Any discharge should be noted. Clear, profuse discharge is often associated with allergies. Table 6.2 lists several abnormalities that can be identified during examination of the nose. See the Red Flag presentations for the nose.

Olfactory sensation is typically a component of the cranial nerve examination. However, depending on the patient's complaints, it may be part of the limited ear, nose, and throat (ENT) examination.

Special Maneuvers

Transillumination of the sinuses is accomplished in a slightly darkened room. A bright, focused light—an otoscope can be used—is placed directly on the cheek over the maxillary sinuses. The patient's mouth is opened, and the

Table 6.2	
Abnormalities of Inspection: Nose	
Finding	Significance
Transverse nasal crease	Allergic salute
Skin lesions	Skin cancer
Redness, papules, hyperplasia	Rosacea
Telangiectasia	Alcohol abuse, Rendu-Osler-Weber disease
Crooked or asymmetric nose	Past or recent trauma
Erythematous turbinates	Infection
Pale boggy turbinates	Allergies
Clear copious discharge	Allergies

> ### RED Flag Warnings for the Nose and Sinuses
>
> - *Epistaxis*—persistent, recurrent, or profuse.
> - *Severe maxillary pain.*
> - *Thin, honey-colored sinus drainage following head trauma* may indicate skull fracture.

examiner looks for a light glow on the roof of the mouth. Diminished light may indicate full sinus cavities. Unequal light may indicate unilateral sinus fullness.

Examination of the Mouth and Throat

The examination of the mouth and throat should begin with an inspection of all the structures that can be readily observed, followed by an examination that requires touching and moving the structures in order to facilitate the examination. The examination should end with palpation of the structures, paying particular attention to observed abnormalities. Gloves should always be worn during palpation. Ask the patient to remove any dental appliances; then systematically examine the mouth and the pharynx. The use of a tongue depressor facilitates examination of the inner cheeks/buccal mucosa, the floor and roof of the mouth, the gums, posterior mouth, and tongue.

Inspect the size, shape, and symmetry of the lips. Obvious lesions should be noted and their characteristics recorded. To inspect the oral cavity and the pharynx, use a good light source.

First, note the general condition of the internal structures of the mouth, including the tongue, buccal mucosa, hard and soft palates, gums, and teeth. Observe any abnormalities, such as lesions, ulcers, masses, exudate, inflammation, and missing or decayed teeth. Identify any tongue or lip piercings, which may cause microscopic enamel cracks to teeth as a result of constant abrasion. Using a tongue depressor to displace the lips and cheeks, inspect areas of the buccal mucosa that are not otherwise visible, including the sites of the Stensen's and Wharton's ducts. As the patient lifts the tongue to touch the palate, sticks it out, and moves it side to side, observe the lateral and ventral surfaces of the tongue as well as the sublingual mucosa and the frenulum. As the oral cavity is inspected, the general integrity of the mucosal coverings and structures should be continually noted.

Inspect the oropharynx, tonsils, and uvula, taking care not to trigger an unwanted gag reflex. Observe the mucosa to identify any inflammation, petechia, ulcerations, discolorations, edema, swelling, asymmetry, lesions, and exudate or postnasal drainage. Observe the movement of the uvula as the patient says "ah." Identify whether the tonsils are present and, if present, their size, symmetry, color, and presence of exudate. Smell the breath for acetone, ammonia, or foul breath (fetor oris).

RED Flag ◀ **Warnings for the Mouth and Throat**

- *Persistent, painless mouth lesions or lesions* consistent with malignancy require referral.
- *Sore throat associated with drooling or stridor* indicates potential epiglottitis or peritonsillar abscess.
- *Sore throat lasting more than 1 week* suggests untreated streptococcal pharyngitis and/or tonsillitis.

Finally, accessible structures should be palpated, including the tissue between the cheeks and buccal mucosa, the floor of the mouth, and the tongue. To palpate the floor of the mouth, use both hands, with one hand placed externally below the area being palpated and applying upward pressure so that any masses will be displaced upward and toward the palpating hand. Use a similar technique to apply external, lateral pressure when palpating the buccal mucosa so that masses are not pushed away by the examining hand. Note any areas of tenderness and masses. Masses should be assessed for consistency, dimensions, mobility, tenderness, and shape.

Differential Diagnosis of Chief Complaints: Ear

■ Ear Pain (Otalgia)

Ear pain is one of the most common complaints seen in primary care practice. It is most often seen in children and is usually associated with bacterial or viral upper respiratory infection. Complaints of ear pain in the summer are often associated with otitis externa owing to swimmer's ear. Complaints of primary ear pain decline with age and, in adults, are more likely associated with secondary conditions, such as sinus infection; dental disease; malignancy; other disorders of the head, face, and neck; and nervous and vascular symptoms.

History

The history should include information related to the pain's location, quality, quantity and/or severity, onset, timing, and duration. The presence of sinus and nasal congestion is relevant because otitis media is typically secondary to a cold or sinus infection. Other historical information includes air travel and deep-sea diving. In adults, possible underlying conditions, such as diabetes mellitus, and chronic inflammatory conditions, such as psoriasis, should be considered. A child's history should include exposure to secondhand smoke, day care, and swimming. A compromised immune status should be considered in those patients with atypical otitis media or who do not respond to therapy.

Physical Examination

The physical examination should include inspection of the external auditory structures, palpation and manipulation of the tragus and auricle, and otoscopic inspection of the canal and TM. Attention should be paid to detecting inflammation and/or exudate in the canal and the condition of the TM, noting color, light reflex, translucency, and perforation. The examination should also include screening for hearing acuity.

Diagnostic Studies

Diagnosis is based on findings from the physical examination. A culture and sensitivity test should be considered if there is a purulent discharge. If a complete blood count (CBC) is done, there may be an associated leukocytosis and elevated erythrocyte sedimentation rate.

ACUTE OTITIS MEDIA (PLATE 49)

Acute otitis media (AOM) involves infection of the fluid in the middle ear space. The three bacterial organisms most often associated with AOM include streptococcal pneumonia, *Haemophilus influenzae*, and *Moraxella catarrhalis*. Frequently, viral organisms coexist with one of the preceding bacterial causes.

Signs and Symptoms

The patient often complains of unilateral ear pain, which may radiate to the neck or jaw. There is commonly a current or recent history of symptoms consistent with an upper respiratory infection, including nasal congestion, sinus pressure/fullness, or sore throat. General hearing acuity may be diminished on the affected side, with bone conduction enhanced on that side. The external ear has a normal appearance unless there is drainage from perforated TM. The TM is typically dull, may be inflamed, and bulges so that the posterior landmarks are obscured. The light reflex is distorted or obscured. If myringitis (inflammation of the TM) is present, the TM is reddened. Purulent or yellow fluid may be evident posterior to the TM, with diminished TM mobility. The examination is associated with increased pain. There are often other findings of upper respiratory infection. With eustachian tube dysfunction, otitis media with effusion (OME) may result, and this condition is discussed under "Decreased Hearing or Hearing Loss."

Diagnostic Studies

Usually no diagnostic studies are indicated. However, tympanocentesis can be performed to alleviate discomfort and/or obtain culture in recurrent disease or when anticipated response to therapy is not achieved.

OTITIS EXTERNA (PLATE 50)

Otitis externa (OE) is inflammation of the canal. Frequent causes include pseudomonas and fungal organisms. It is frequently associated with swimming, as well as trauma, which may occur through attempts to clean the ear with cotton-tipped swabs or other objects. In immunocompromised patients, necrotizing otitis can occur and extend to the temporal bone, so it is important to monitor response to therapy.

Signs and Symptoms

There is often pain, which may be exacerbated when the auricle or tragus is touched or moved. In addition to the pain, which can be very severe, itching may occur. Depending on the amount of edema and exudate, there may be a significant sensation of stuffiness and/or decreased hearing. The examination may be quite uncomfortable, and the pain is often increased pain as the tragus is manipulated. The canal is inflamed and often edematous. Drainage or exudate may be present, ranging in consistency from cheesy to serous. Depending on the amount of swelling and exudate, the distal portion of the canal may not be visible. An odor may be present.

Diagnostic Studies

There is usually no indication for diagnostic studies, although exudate can be cultured, along with a sensitivity test. With failure to respond to treatment, referral to a specialist should be considered.

BAROTRAUMA

Barotrauma is injury to the structures of the ear resulting from extremes of atmospheric pressures, such as those associated with flying or deep-sea diving. Onset typically occurs within 24 hours of the exposure.

Signs and Symptoms

Complaints include ear pressure, pain, altered acuity of hearing, tinnitus, sinus pain/pressure, and headache. Vertigo may be present. The TM is often inflamed and may be perforated. A hemorrhagic collection may be present posterior to the TM. Benign positional vertigo and/or sinus tenderness may be evident.

Diagnostic Studies

No specific diagnostics are warranted unless the patient also has symptoms of decompression sickness.

TRAUMA

Direct trauma as a cause of ear pain is most commonly seen in children, who frequently insert foreign objects into their ears. However, it may occur in adults as the result of overzealous ear cleaning. Indirect trauma can be associated with blunt blows to the head, jaw, or ear.

Signs and Symptoms

The signs and symptoms depend on the type of trauma and structures injured. In direct trauma, the pain is consistent with OE or perforated TM. In blunt trauma, the signs and symptoms are consistent with the history of the injury. The actual findings may be from a source of referred pain (a fractured jaw, for instance) or from resultant perforation of the TM. The history of the traumatic event is important.

Diagnostic Studies

Often no diagnostic studies are warranted. However, in the case of trauma to the head, diagnostics should be accomplished as recommended in Chapter 4.

MASTOIDITIS

Mastoiditis refers to infection of the mastoid bone, which is almost always a complication of AOM.

Signs and Symptoms

The patient complains of radiating ear pain and fever. The pain is persistent (for days to weeks), severe, deep, and often worst at night. The hearing on the affected site is usually significantly diminished. As the condition progresses, there is swelling, erythema, and tenderness over the mastoid bone. The swelling can be so advanced as to displace the auricle; complications include paralysis resulting from facial nerve involvement and infection of the labyrinth or cerebrospinal fluid (CSF), causing meningitis or brain abscess.

Diagnostic Studies

The patient should be referred to a specialist for definitive diagnosis and treatment. On referral, diagnostics will likely include CBC, culture of fluid, and computed tomographic (CT) scan to determine the degree of involvement.

FOREIGN BODY

Any foreign body in the ear canal, such as beads, cotton, insects, or toys, can cause pain. The presence of a foreign body is most common in young children.

Signs and Symptoms

Pain is often the presenting complaint and may be associated with unilateral, purulent discharge from the canal. Other symptoms include altered hearing acuity. Physical findings often include tenderness on manipulation of the ear and with the examination, as well as the foreign body. Depending on the amount of trauma caused by the offending object, the canal may be inflamed, edematous, and have exudate consistent with a resultant OE.

Diagnostic Studies

Diagnostic studies are typically not warranted.

A variety of conditions can result in pain that is referred to the ear. These include temporomandibular joint pain, dental pain, neck mass/pain, carotodynia, tonsillitis, temporal arteritis, and trigeminal neuralgia. The variety of conditions are beyond the scope of the discussion for ear pain but can be found in other chapters, particularly Chapter 4.

■ Ear Discharge (Otorrhea)

Discharge emanating from the ear often indicates a condition warranting urgent diagnosis and treatment. In addition to stemming from conditions affecting the external and middle ear, otorrhea may indicate leakage of CSF. Purulent discharge is most often related to an infectious process or a foreign body. Bloody discharge associated with recent head trauma may indicate a skull fracture.

History

Immediate proximal causes for ear discharge, such as OM with perforation, OE, mastoiditis, and a foreign body, should be investigated. Consider more serious conditions such as head trauma if an immediate proximal cause is ruled out. Ask about how and when the discharge was first noticed as well as the patient's perceived health preceding that event. Explore the possibility of direct or indirect trauma as well as secondary or complicated infections. Obtain a history of previous episodes of ear discharge, ear infections, or other conditions. A thorough review of systems is warranted, particularly as related to other components of the upper respiratory and neurological systems.

Physical Examination

Examination usually includes the head, ears, nose, and throat. Begin by assessing the patient's general health and mental status. If there is no history of head trauma and the patient's general neurological status is intact, proceed to examination of the ears. Observe both external ears, comparing for symmetry of appearance. Identify areas of inflammation, swelling, deformity, or distortion of landmarks, signs of trauma. Note the color, odor, and consistency of any visible discharge. Palpate the structures of the external ear, noting any tenderness or palpable abnormalities. Observe the distal portion of the canal for swelling, erythema, discharge, or obvious foreign body. Complete the otoscopic examination, noticing the condition of the canal walls, TM, and visible portion of the middle ear structures.

Diagnostic Studies

Diagnosis is usually based on history and physical examination. Some specific diagnoses and other conditions that can be associated with discharge are discussed in preceding sections.

AOM WITH PERFORATION (PLATE 51)

Particularly in children, spontaneous rupture of the TM may occur owing to the pressure in the middle ear, resulting in a white or purulent discharge from the ear. In addition to the typical findings of AOM, there may be a visible perforation. See preceding section on AOM.

CEREBROSPINAL FLUID LEAKAGE

CSF leaks are associated with head trauma or surgery. If the history and/or physical examination suggest the potential for leakage of CSF, the drainage can be tested for glucose. Providing the patient is stable, a referral is warranted for definitive diagnosis, because CSF leakage indicates a heightened potential for the development of meningitis. Further diagnostic studies, including imaging, will be completed following referral.

CHOLESTEATOMA (PLATE 52)

A cholesteatoma is an abnormal growth of epithelial tissue in the middle ear. The tissue can grow to invade surrounding bone and/or extend into the inner ear. Surgical excision is usually indicated, so the patient should be referred when this is suspected.

Signs and Symptoms

The patient often complains of drainage from the ear. An associated sense of aural fullness and/or decreased hearing may be experienced in the affected ear. Over time, pain and dizziness can develop. The examination will reveal drainage and/or granular tissue in the canal. The drainage is often mucopurulent. If infection is present, inflammatory changes may be evident, as seen with AOM. The cholesteatoma may be visible behind the TM. Because of the risk of permanent hearing loss and invasiveness, the patient should be referred for definitive diagnosis and surgical intervention.

Diagnostic Studies

No studies are indicated in a primary care setting.

OTITIS EXTERNA

See pp. 127–128.

MASTOIDITIS

See p. 129.

FOREIGN BODY

See p. 129.

■ Decreased Hearing or Hearing Loss

A decreased ability to hear is most often associated with aging, with onset noticed in the sixth decade. In children, hearing deficits are often associated with middle ear effusions. Other reasons for decreased hearing include repetitive exposure to loud noise, which may occur with both occupational and recreational activities. Mechanical obstruction of the ear canal by cerumen or a foreign body may cause hearing impairment. The list of conditions and factors that can result in an altered sense of hearing is extensive. It includes a variety of infectious diseases, autoimmune disorders, chronic systemic diseases (diabetes, thyroid disease, and vascular and neurological conditions), and many more. Types of deafness can be categorized as conductive (e.g., perforated TM, serous otitis, and cerumen impaction), nerve (e.g., presbycusis, acoustic neuroma, and medication-related changes), and central (e.g., stemming from infections, such as meningitis, and stroke).

History

It is essential to explore the onset and progression of the hearing loss, determining whether the onset was progressive over a period of time or was acute and, regardless of the onset, how it has progressed since first noticed. Ask what the patient means by hearing decrease or loss and whether the symptom involves one ear or both. Investigate the severity with questions regarding the impact of the hearing loss on the patient's ability to communicate. Identify associated symptoms, including ringing in the ear(s), pain, fullness, or drainage. Have the patient identify all prescribed, over-the-counter (OTC), and recreational substances used before and since onset as possible causative agents. Medications with ototoxic effects include aminoglycoside antibiotics; platinum-based antineoplastics and methotrexate; loop diuretics; salicylates and anti-inflammatories; and quinine-based medications such as quinine, chloroquine, hydroxychloroquine, and mefloquine.

Explore the patient's general state of health from the period just before and since the altered sense of hearing was noticed, asking about other conditions and infections, including upper respiratory infections, Ménière's disease, OE, and OA. Identify the history of systemic disorders, such as diabetes, malignancies, hypertension, and vascular disorders. Ask about recent barotrauma as well as other trauma to the head or ear.

Physical Examination

An audiogram is required to quantitatively assess hearing acuity. However, it is reasonable to first grossly test hearing with the whisper test, ticking watch, or fingers being rubbed together. The type of loss (sensorineural or conductive) may be only grossly evaluated using tuning fork techniques. Evidence supports that these hearing tests have good specificity but poor sensitivity (see Box 6.1). Based on the results to these gross screenings, an audiogram can be obtained and/or the patient referred for more comprehensive hearing tests if a self-limited condition is not identified.

A complete examination of the ears should be performed, along with assessment of the other upper respiratory structures, particularly in younger patients.

Box 6.1
Accuracy of Gross Hearing Tests

In a study by Boatman, Miglioretti, Eberwein, Alidoost, and Reich (2007), each of the following tests was performed on 107 adults, 50 to 88 years of age, and compared to audiogram results. The sensitivity and specificity are based on patients with hearing loss >25 dB/>40 dB.

Test	Sensitivity	Specificity
	(Hearing Loss: >25 dB/>40 dB)	
Finger rub	0.27/0.35	0.98/0.97
Whispered speech	0.40/0.46	0.83/0.78
Watch tick	0.44/0.60	1.0/0.99
Rinne (256 Hz)	N/A	1.0/1.0
Weber (256 Hz)	0.30/0.26	0.74/0.74

As indicated by the patient's age and presenting history, general appearance, and ear findings, consider expanding the examination to include neurological, cardiovascular, and other systems.

Diagnostic Studies

As noted earlier, audiometric examination is essential to objectively measure hearing acuity and to determine affected frequencies. Other diagnostic procedures will depend on the suspected cause of hearing loss and can include vascular studies or neurological imaging as well as laboratory studies, including serum glucose, thyroid studies, tests for autoimmune diseases, CBC, and others.

CERUMEN IMPACTION

Cerumen impaction is a common cause of altered hearing, particularly in older patients.

Signs and Symptoms

The patient typically complains of progressive decreased hearing acuity, although onset may be sudden. The cerumen may cause discomfort and/or itching in the canal. In older patients, there is often a history of previous impactions. Hearing loss is conductive. The examination reveals the mass of cerumen within the canal. On occasion, the cerumen causes excoriation of the canal walls.

Diagnostic Studies

No studies are indicated.

PRESBYCUSIS

Presbycusis is an age-related cause of sensorineural hearing loss and involves diminished hairy cell function within the cochlea as well as decreased elasticity of the TM. Although the changes associated with presbycusis often start in early adulthood, the decreased hearing acuity is usually not noticed until the individual is older than 65. In addition to age-related changes, onset can be associated with exposure to environmental noise and influenced by genetic predisposition. When presbycusis is suspected, the patient should be referred to a specialist for definitive diagnosis and assessment for use of hearing aid(s).

Signs and Symptoms

Onset is usually gradual. There may be a family history of hearing loss and/or a personal history of atherosclerosis and/or diabetes. The physical examination is normal, with the exception of audiometric studies, which quantify the hearing loss and affected ranges. Presbycusis is a condition diagnosed by exclusion.

Diagnostic Studies

Audiometric studies identify the degree of hearing loss, usually affecting the higher frequencies.

OTOSCLEROSIS

Otosclerosis involves degenerative changes to the bony structures of the middle ear and results in gradual onset of hearing deficit as the bones lose their vibratory ability. It occurs most frequently in women and Caucasians. It seems to be related to estrogen and can be accelerated by pregnancy. Risk factors include family history. Onset is earlier than presbycusis, and lower frequencies are affected first.

Signs and Symptoms

The patient typically complains of painless, progressive changes in hearing. Symptoms are usually bilateral, and tinnitus may be present. The physical examination is usually normal, with the exception of the hearing acuity test. The ear has a normal appearance, and the TM mobility is normal.

Diagnostic Studies

Audiometry quantifies the deficit, which usually involves the lower frequencies. A referral to a specialist is warranted, as surgical intervention is often successful. The specialist may order images to determine the degree of change.

OTITIS MEDIA WITH EFFUSION (OME) (PLATE 53)

Otitis media with effusion, or serous otitis media, results from dysfunction of one or both eustachian tubes and may follow or contribute to the development of AOM. The presence of residual middle ear fluid can cause significant conductive hearing loss. This condition is most common in children.

Signs and Symptoms

Parents and/or teachers often relate that the patient does not listen well. There is a sense of ear fullness and a need to "pop" the ear(s). Hearing acuity is decreased on the affected side. The external ear and canal are normal in appearance. The TM may be bulging, with a yellowish hue from the fluid collected posteriorly in the middle ear chamber. The TM mobility is diminished or absent on pneumatic otoscopy.

Diagnostic Studies

A tympanogram reveals decreased compliance.

INFECTIOUS DISEASE

A variety of infectious conditions can affect hearing acuity. These include the conditions that are usually responsible for AOM and OE (described earlier in this chapter) as well as herpes simples, herpes zoster, syphilis, meningitis, mononucleosis, mumps, rubella, and rubeola. Infections are responsible for both conductive and sensorineural hearing loss.

Signs and Symptoms

Complaints and findings are consistent with the specific infection and may include malaise, fever, myalgia, headache, and pain. Physical examination should reveal findings consistent with AOM or OE if either is present. In addition to physical ear findings, there may be generalized signs of upper respiratory infection, skin rash or lesions, lymphadenopathy, and other changes. Tuning fork tests may reveal either conductive hearing loss (associated with bacterial or viral AOM) or sensorineural loss (syphilis, meningitis, herpes zoster). It is possible that the signs of a causative infection may have resolved by the time the patient presents with hearing loss; thus, the history will be important in identifying this as a possible etiology.

Diagnostic Studies

The selection of diagnostic studies will be guided by the history of exposure, symptomatology, and risk factors, as well as the physical findings.

ACOUSTIC NEUROMA

Acoustic neuromas are nonmalignant tumors affecting the acoustic nerve (cranial nerve [CN] VIII). The onset of symptoms usually occurs after age 30. Therapeutic interventions include surgery and radiation.

Signs and Symptoms

Symptoms depend on the size of the tumor. Early complaints include unilateral hearing loss, tinnitus, and vertigo. As the tumor advances, symptoms may include headache, facial pain, ataxia, nausea/vomiting, and lethargy. The ear structures appear normal. Audiogram will reveal diminished hearing acuity.

Diagnostic Studies

The patient should be referred for definitive diagnosis and treatment. Magnetic resonance imaging (MRI) is useful in identifying the tumor.

MÉNIÈRE'S DISEASE

Ménière's disease commonly involves a triad of symptoms: severe vertigo, tinnitus, and hearing loss, as described in Chapter 15, p. 475.

MEDICATIONS

A variety of medications can potentially affect hearing acuity. The most common are antibiotics (aminoglycosides); quinine derivatives; antineoplastics (platinum-based and methotrexate); loop diuretics; and nonsteroidal anti-inflammatories, both salicylate-based and others. When hearing loss is identified, a list of all agents taken by the patient may identify a potentially ototoxic drug. Medication-related ototoxicity can be permanent or reversible depending on the agent.

CHOLESTEATOMA

See p. 131.

■ Ringing (Tinnitus)

Ringing in the ears (tinnitus) is most often related to the use of ototoxic drugs. It is also associated with continued exposure to loud noise and environmental chemical exposure. Tinnitus refers to a wide range of sounds mimicking whistles, crickets, ringing, buzzing, and the like. It is typically persistent and bilateral. Tinnitus is associated with many of the causes of hearing loss.

History

Obtain a list of current medications and the amount and frequency of dosing. Ask about recent exposure to loud noise or chemical agents through activities, including work, hobbies, and recreation. A history of other ear disorders and symptoms, including labyrinthitis, Ménière's disease, or progressive hearing loss, should be obtained. Ask about ear pain, pressure, and drainage.

Physical Examination

A thorough ENT and neurological examination should be performed. In the absence of a structural abnormality of infection the physical examination should be normal. There may be a decrease in gross hearing acuity and in performance during a tuning fork examination because tinnitus is associated with the causes of hearing loss.

Diagnostic Studies

Diagnostic studies are related to the specific suspected etiology associated with the tinnitus but should include audiometry. The major causes of tinnitus are listed in Box 6.2.

■ Ear Fullness

The etiology of ear fullness is multidimensional. Fullness can be related to fluid in the middle ear as a result of otitis media or changes in barometric pressure. The most common causes vary by age; children are more likely to experience ear fullness associated with OME; older adults are more likely to have cerumen impaction.

History

Complete a symptom analysis, especially noting the timing of the symptom. Ask whether the onset was gradual or sudden. Determine whether the fullness is affected by the patient's position. Identify any concurrent or recent other ENT symptoms or respiratory conditions.

Physical Examination

Examine the external ear structures. Manipulate the external ear to identify any tenderness before inserting the otoscope speculum. Examine the canal for masses or swelling. Observe the TM to detect any dullness, decreased light reflex, bulging, retraction, or inflammation, which may indicate fluid or infection.

Diagnostic Studies

Pneumatic otoscopy will assist in determining the presence of fluid in the middle ear. The common causes of complaints of ear fullness are listed in Box 6.3.

Box 6.2	
Common Causes of Tinnitus	
Ménière's disease	Cerumen or foreign body
Acoustic trauma	Infections
Neoplasms	Ototoxic medications

Box 6.3

Common Causes of Ear Fullness

Ménière's disease
Infections (acute otitis media, otitis externa)
Otitis media with effusion
Allergies
Cerumen impaction or foreign body

Differential Diagnosis of Chief Complaints: Nose

■ Bleeding (Epistaxis)

Nosebleeds are a common complaint, with a variety of possible causes, and can occur at any age. Bleeding from the nose is bright red and often profuse but can usually be controlled within a few minutes after applying pressure and cold. Bleeding deep in the inferior meatus may be more difficult to manage. Nasal polyps rarely cause profuse bleeding, which is more likely to be vascular or tumor related. Nasal packing, and occasionally artery ligation, may be necessary to control the bleeding. Any unexplained, recurrent epistaxis warrants investigation and possible referral to an ENT specialist.

History

The history will often explain the bleeding. The past medical history should include medications the patient is taking that could be contributing, such as anticoagulants, aspirin, or NSAIDs, and the presence of other medical problems, such as hematologic, liver, or vascular disease. Cocaine abuse, which is more common than might be expected and frequently causes epistaxis, may need to be explored. A complaint of recent trauma is a straightforward cause of epistaxis. Ask about frequent sinus infections and the use of nasal sprays, obtained by prescription or OTC; steroid or antihistamine nasal sprays can cause dryness, irritation, and bleeding. Ask whether this is the first episode of bleeding, and, if not, ask about the frequency at which it has occurred. Chronic epistaxis warrants referral to an ENT specialist to determine a structural or vascular cause.

Physical Examination

The physical examination should start with an inspection of the external nose for alignment and the presence of any skin lesions. If possible, visualize the nasal mucosa for redness, purulent discharge, or lesions, although visualization is difficult to accomplish with active bleeding.

Diagnostic Studies

X-rays or CT scanning of the nose and/or sinuses assists in the diagnosis of fracture, infection, tumor, and polyps. Culture and sensitivity of nasal discharge can be taken for resistant infections. CBC with differential, platelet count, and coagulation studies might be needed to rule out hematologic or vascular causes. A liver profile might be needed to identify a hepatic cause of the epistaxis.

TRAUMA

Bleeding accompanied by edema and asymmetry of the nose indicates a possible fracture, and x-rays of the nose are warranted. Ice and pressure on the sides of the nose usually will control the bleeding, at least temporarily. If not, packing or cautery may be necessary.

Signs and Symptoms

There is a history of a blow to the nose. If the cause of apparent trauma is not reported by the patient, be alert for and inquire about any signs of abuse, particularly in women and children. Edema occurs rapidly after a blow to the nose and is obvious on visual inspection. There may be abrasions or lacerations present, and asymmetry is seen with fracture.

Diagnostic Studies

An x-ray should be done to look for fracture. If the x-ray is positive for a fracture, the patient should be referred to the ENT and/or plastic surgeon.

MEDICATION

Anticoagulant medications such as warfarin (Coumadin), heparin, or enoxaparin (Lovenox) are the most common medications to cause epistaxis. Other drugs that might cause bleeding include aspirin, NSAIDs, nasal sprays, and Ginkgo biloba.

Signs and Symptoms

A thorough medication history identifies prescription, OTC, or herbal preparations associated with epistaxis. In addition to the nasal bleeding, an over-anticoagulated patient may have bruising over the body from everyday minor contusions, particularly on the limbs. Bleeding from the gums also is commonly seen with over-anticoagulation.

Diagnostic Studies

If the patient is taking anticoagulants, a prothrombin time with international normalization ratio should be done.

HEMATOLOGIC DISORDERS

Hematologic disorders likely to cause increased bleeding include thrombocytopenia, leukemia, aplastic anemia, and hereditary coagulopathies. Multiple hematologic disorders can be seen with liver disease, including anemia, thrombocytopenia, leukopenia, leukocytosis, and impaired synthesis of clotting factors causing increased prothrombin time.

Signs and Symptoms

A history of hematologic disorders will quickly point toward the cause of the bleeding. There may be a history of easy bruisability, fatigue, shortness of breath, fever, or frequent infections. The patient may have a personal or family history of liver disease and/or alcohol use or abuse. Risk factors for hepatitis may be present. Except for the epistaxis, the physical examination may be unremarkable. Fever, bruising, or petechiae may indicate leukemia, thrombocytopenia, or coagulopathies. A rapid heart rate and/or heart murmur may be present with longstanding anemia, as may cyanosis around the lips or nails. Capillary refill may be altered. Hepatomegaly or ascites may be present in liver disease.

Diagnostic Studies

If hematologic disorders are suspected, a CBC, platelet count, liver profile, and coagulation studies should be done. A bone marrow aspiration may need to be performed by the hematologist or oncologist to confirm the diagnosis.

INTRANASAL DRUG USE

Cocaine abuse runs the gamut of socioeconomic class, age, and gender. It is important to not stereotype individuals who may or may not be at risk for cocaine abuse.

Signs and Symptoms

A history of any kind of illegal drug use or alcohol abuse should alert the practitioner to the possibility of cocaine use. Typical symptoms associated with cocaine use are tachycardia, tachypnea, elevated blood pressure, arrhythmias, dilated pupils, nervousness, euphoria, hallucinations, and friability of the nasal mucosa leading to epistaxis. An overdose may lead to tremors, seizures, delirium, respiratory failure, and cardiovascular collapse.

Diagnostic Studies

A drug screen should be performed for suspected cocaine abuse. Electrocardiogram, blood pressure monitoring, and pulse oximetry may be necessary until the heart and respiratory rates and blood pressure return to a normal range.

MUCOSAL DRYNESS, IRRITATION, AND INFECTION

Dry climates, especially during the winter months, may cause nasal mucosal irritation and bleeding, which is usually scanty. OTC nasal sprays and corticosteroid or antihistamine nasal sprays may dry the mucosal lining of the nose and cause bleeding. Infection, particularly recurrent or chronic infection, can lead to sinus and mucosal inflammation and irritation resulting in bleeding, which is usually scanty unless the infection is severe enough to erode the mucosal surface.

Signs and Symptoms

A history of a dry environment or recent sinus infections, fever, sinus pressure or pain, and purulent nasal discharge may be present. Bleeding may be aggravated by blowing the nose. Dry crusting found in the nares, along with areas of irritation, may indicate the etiology of the bleeding. Infections cause the nasal mucosa to look beefy red; some areas may be raw and bleeding. Infection is usually accompanied by fever, sinus tenderness on palpation and/or percussion, decreased or absence of light with transillumination, and purulent discharge.

Diagnostic Studies

Diagnostic studies are usually not warranted. Sinus x-rays or CT scanning may be necessary with treatment failure.

VASCULAR DISORDERS

The most serious vascular etiology of epistaxis is Rendu-Osler-Weber disease, also known as hereditary hemorrhagic telangiectasia, an autosomal dominant disease caused by vascular malformation. It affects both men and women. It can cause severe, recurrent epistaxis resulting from arteriovenous aneurysms in the mucous membranes. A less common vascular cause is hypertension, particularly uncontrolled or episodic hypertension.

Signs and Symptoms

A thorough family history is essential to uncover Rendu-Osler-Weber disease. The patient may give a history of recurrent, profuse nosebleeds. In hypertension, the patient may give a family or personal history of elevated blood pressure. The patient may either admit to nonadherence with the prescribed regimen or be unaware of the hypertension. Symptoms may include headache, lightheadedness, and pounding or swishing sounds in the ears. Hypertension is easily uncovered with blood pressure measurement. In Rendu-Osler-Weber disease, small telangiectatic lesions on the face, lips, oral mucosa, nasal mucosa, fingertips, and toes are characteristic, and the nosebleeds are profuse. Similar lesions occur internally in the mucosa of the gastrointestinal (GI) tract, which can cause major GI bleeding.

Diagnostic Studies

Diagnosis is usually made by history and physical examination. In Rendu-Osler-Weber disease, laboratory studies are normal except in iron-deficiency anemia, which may be severe. For hypertension, blood chemistries and renal studies, including 24-hour urine for catecholamines, should be done to rule out kidney or adrenal disease.

MALIGNANT NASAL AND SINUS TUMORS

The most common cancers seen in this area are squamous cell carcinomas. Less-common types in this area include adenocarcinoma, melanoma, sarcoma, and lymphoma. Neoplasias are most commonly seen in the nasopharynx, causing nasal obstruction and otitis media, but are also seen in the paranasal sinuses. Patients are often asymptomatic until late in the course.

Signs and Symptoms

Patients often complain of persistent unilateral nasal, sinus, or ear congestion and/or pain that have failed symptomatic and antibiotic treatment. This is a red flag and warrants further investigation. Nasal discharge is common and may be unilateral. Sinus pain with bleeding from the nose, particularly if it is unilateral, indicates the need for diagnostic studies. In advanced disease, there may be obvious swelling of the cheek or around the eye.

Diagnostic Studies

MRI or CT scanning is needed to define the extent of the tumor. Biopsy is necessary to confirm the diagnosis and the type of neoplasm.

■ Congestion and/or Drainage

Nasal congestion with associated drainage is one of the common complaints seen in the family practice setting. It is common in the winter months with the concomitant increase in upper respiratory infections. Complaints of congestion and drainage in the fall and spring may be due to allergies, and a thorough history and physical examination will assist in differentiating infection from allergy.

History

As with any history, start with the onset of the symptoms, their frequency, persistence, and progression. Ask about the presence of fever and about the color and consistency of the mucous drainage. Persistent fever and thick, yellow-green mucus indicate bacterial infection. Inquire about allergies to plants and animals and about environmental exposures to chemicals or noxious fumes. Explore related symptoms, such as sore throat, ear pain, headache, or cough. Ask about facial and/or sinus pain, which might indicate impacted sinuses. Some patients complain that their upper teeth hurt, which may indicate dental disease or sinus infection because the maxillary sinuses are located just above the upper teeth. Include questions regarding exposure to family members or coworkers with similar symptoms and whether they are being treated. A history of honey-colored sinus drainage following head trauma is a red flag warning because it may indicate a skull fracture.

Physical Examination

Vital signs are a good place to start, looking for fever, which would indicate infection. Inspect the nasal mucosa with the nasal speculum as you look for septal deviation or lesions, redness, irritation, friability, and discharge. Nasal discharge should be assessed for its amount and color and any associated symptoms. Clear, profuse discharge is allergic in nature; yellow-green purulent discharge indicates infection. Percuss the sinuses for tenderness. Impacted sinuses may require referral to the ENT. Examine the pharynx, ears, lungs, and lymph system in the head and neck.

COMMON COLD

Differentiating a viral cold from a bacterial infection of the sinuses is one of the more challenging diagnostic exercises for any practitioner. The similarity of symptoms between viral and bacterial illnesses, accompanied by the patient expectation that antibiotics will cure all things, can make management difficult.

Signs and Symptoms

If the patient experienced malaise and fever initially but feels well aside from the congestion, then the cause is likely viral in nature. The viral illness will usually run its course in 5 to 7 days. A physical examination that reveals no fever, TM dullness or redness, sinus pain, sinus tenderness, or chest congestion is likely viral.

Diagnostic Studies

Sinus x-rays may be helpful to rule out sinusitis, but otherwise the diagnosis can usually be made with history and physical.

SINUSITIS

Bacterial sinusitis is more common in persons with a long-term history of sinusitis, allergies, and asthma, with or without a history of smoking.

Signs and Symptoms

There is a history of fever, frontal headache, severe sinus congestion, sinus and ear pain and/or pressure, difficulty breathing, sore throat, purulent nasal discharge, and malaise. Unlike a virus, bacterial infection often worsens with time. The examination may reveal fever; inflamed nasal mucosa; thick, colored discharge; sinus tenderness; an accompanying dull or inflamed tympanic membrane; and perhaps cervical lymphadenopathy. A recent review of clinical decision rules regarding diagnosis of acute bacterial sinusitis and the supporting evidence determined that while no set of criteria were consistent, bacterial sinusitis was best predicted by unilateral nasal discharge paired with unilateral pain. When accompanied by purulent rhinorrhea and maxillary tooth pain, the likelihood of sinusitis increases (DeAlleaume & Parker, 2003).

Diagnostic Studies

Usually diagnostic studies are unnecessary. Recurrent sinusitis or persistent sinusitis after a course of antibiotics should be further investigated with sinus x-rays or CT scanning of the sinuses. CBC may confirm a bacterial cause, and a culture and sensitivity test of the nasal discharge may identify the organism responsible for chronic infections. Often, polyps are present, causing recurrent or prolonged symptoms. Tumor may be present, requiring prompt referral to the ENT specialist. In extreme cases, chronic sinus infection can cause bone erosion and sinus or brain abscess.

ALLERGIES

Allergies are more common in the fall and spring, especially in damp, warm climates where foliage is thick and present year around. In tropical climates, mold may be present in homes and buildings. Pets, especially cats, are commonly responsible for allergy symptoms, especially if they are new pets.

Signs and Symptoms

The history will identify seasonal symptoms or symptoms associated with exposure to allergens, including plants, foods, and animals. The patient may complain of fatigue but will not have fever. The nasal mucosa will be boggy and pale. The nasal discharge will be clear and watery. The patient may complain of sore throat resulting from postnasal drip, and there may be a cobblestone look to the posterior pharynx. Ear congestion may be present. Sinus tenderness should not be present.

Diagnostic Studies

RAST (radioallergosorbent test) studies performed on the blood will indicate the increased eosinophilia associated with allergies, and skin testing will identify specific allergens.

■ Loss of Smell

History

A change in olfaction can accompany any of the conditions related to nasal congestion, or it can be a more serious problem related to CN I injury from trauma or tumor. A closed head injury coupled with loss of smell may indicate an injury in the area of CN I. Other neurological complaints will likely be present: It is rare for a head injury to result in injury only to this small portion of the brain. In a patient without a history of trauma, an isolated complaint of olfactory changes without any accompanying symptoms of cold, allergies, or sinus congestion is a red flag suggesting a brain tumor. Brain tumors can cause either a decrease in olfaction or, in some cases, olfactory hallucinations. Headache along with olfactory changes increases the index of suspicion for a tumor etiology.

Diagnostic Studies

A CT or MRI of the head is necessary to determine the presence of a tumor. A thorough neurological examination should be performed to detect other neurological abnormalities. See Chapter 15 for a more in-depth discussion.

Differential Diagnosis of Chief Complaints: Mouth

■ Mouth Sores (Painful and Painless)

Many conditions manifest with lesions on the lips and/or oral mucosa. Most are self-limiting conditions, such as aphthous ulcers; others, such as Behçet's syndrome and oral cancers, can result in significant morbidity if not recognized and treated promptly. Oral lesions associated with pain can be very distressing to patients. Labial lesions (those on the lips) cause distress because they are obvious and difficult to conceal. Painful lesions, both on the lips and in the mouth, can significantly impair a patient's ability to take food and fluids by mouth. A diagnosis of herpes simplex can be very upsetting to a patient because of the association with herpes simplex and genital findings as well as the chronicity of the condition.

History

When a patient presents with a mouth sore (or sores), it is helpful to determine early in the history whether the lesion is painful: certain conditions are more likely than others to cause painful lesions. It is important to obtain a thorough analysis of the symptoms, including when the lesion was first noticed, whether the lesion was preceded by other symptoms, and whether there is a history of similar symptoms in the past. Identify any associated symptoms, including fever, malaise, joint pain, shortness of breath, nausea, vomiting, diarrhea, photosensitivity, and so on. Identify any chronic or coexisting conditions, as well as any prescribed or OTC medications taken.

Physical Examination

The physical examination should include measurement of vitals signs, particularly noting the presence of fever. A thorough assessment of the specific lesion should be performed, noting the type of lesion involved (ulcer, vesicle, papule, and so on) as well as the dimensions, coloring, shape, distribution, and other details. The surrounding tissue should be closely inspected, noting edema, erythema, or pallor. A thorough examination of the entire oral mucosa is necessary, with careful palpation of all accessible areas to note indurations, thickenings, nodules, or other palpable changes. Cervical lymph nodes should be palpated. Depending on the patient's presenting history and findings, examination may include other systems.

Diagnostic Studies

For most mouth sores, diagnostic studies are not indicated. However, lesions can be cultured to provide definitive diagnosis of candida, herpes simplex, or other infectious causes. Biopsies may be indicated to diagnose or rule out malignancy.

APHTHOUS ULCERS (PLATE 54)

The cause of aphthous ulcers is unclear. A number of theories exist, including infection, stress, and food sensitivities. They recur in some individuals. Episodes are self-limited. Onset is often in childhood.

Signs and Symptoms

The ulcers are painful and usually small (less than 1 cm). The patient often has had previous ulcers, which healed in approximately 1 week. The ulcer is shallow, surrounded by erythema and mild edema. The base of the ulcer is pale yellow or gray. Often only one ulcer is present, although patients may have multiple ulcers. On occasion, patients experience larger ulcers, which take longer to heal and are associated with increased pain.

Diagnostic Studies

None are warranted. Occasionally, the ulcers can be cultured to rule out herpes simplex.

HERPES SIMPLEX (PLATE 55)

Orolabial ulcers are often caused by herpes simplex type 1 virus.

Signs and Symptoms

The patient often complains of a history of intermittent mouth sores, with onset as a youth. The ulcers are typically preceded by a prodromal phase of tenderness, followed by edema at the site where an individual or cluster of vesicles forms and progresses to ulceration. The prodromal phase may also include malaise and fever. The vesicles have an erythematous base, and the ulcerated lesion often becomes crusted.

Diagnostic Studies

None are usually warranted. The vesicles can be cultured for definitive diagnosis; a Tzanck smear can be performed in the office for rapid diagnosis.

HERPES ZOSTER

Herpes zoster is described in Chapter 3, pp. 51–52. Compared with other painful mouth lesions, herpes zoster typically occurs in older individuals. Because the virus affects a dermatome, there are usually extraoral findings and complaints.

CHEMICAL AND THERMAL BURNS

As with any of the integument, the oral mucosa is at risk for chemical and thermal burns. The history is extremely important to identify whether the patient has been exposed to chemical agents or to a thermal source that resulted in the painful lesion. The distribution of the lesion(s) should be consistent with the history of exposure.

HAND-FOOT-AND-MOUTH DISEASE

Hand-foot-and-mouth disease is caused by a coxsackievirus. Outbreaks are most common in the summer and fall months. The condition is occasionally associated with meningitis.

Signs and Symptoms

Painful skin and oral lesions are often preceded by a period of malaise and fever. The patient often presents once the lesions appear on the lips and/or oral mucosa. The lesions erupt as vesicles, which later ulcerate. Multiple lesions are located on the lips and oral mucosa. As the condition's name implies, the lesions often appear on the hands and feet, as well as in the mouth. Lesions may also be evident on the genitalia and buttocks.

Diagnostic Studies

Diagnostic studies are not usually warranted. The patient's hydration status should be monitored if the lesions impair ability to take food and/or fluids by mouth.

CANDIDIASIS (PLATE 56)

Candidiasis is caused by a species of the fungal genus *Candida*. Risk factors for candidiasis include an impaired immune system, antibiotic therapy, malignancy, and recent surgery or trauma. Candidiasis affects a variety of systems and tissues, including the oral mucosa.

Signs and Symptoms

Candidal infections of the oral mucosa take several forms. Thrush, or pseudomembranous candida, results in white patches or plaques overlying a very red base. Erythematous candida results in erythematous lesions and, on occasion, ulcerative lesions. Angular stomatitis results in lesions at the corners or angles of the mouth. The amount of associated pain is variable.

Diagnostic Studies

Studies are not usually necessary because the diagnosis is based on the findings. Fungal cultures can be used to isolate specific organisms.

BEHÇET'S SYNDROME

Behçet's disease is considered a syndrome because it involves a variety of problems, including oral lesions. Other characteristic findings include uveitis, arthralgia, genital lesions, and nongenital skin lesions. The condition affects males more often than females and is more common in young adults. Although rare, Behçet's syndrome can lead to significant morbidity, and the patient should be referred to a specialist for definitive diagnosis and treatment if the condition is suspected.

Signs and Symptoms

The patient complains of recurrent episodes of oral lesions that are consistent with aphthous ulcers. The number of lesions ranges from one to several; the size of the ulcers varies from less than to greater than 1 cm. Like aphthous ulcers, the lesions are well defined, with a pale yellow or gray base surrounded by erythema. The majority of patients also develop lesions on the genitals or other skin. Eye findings are varied and include conjunctivitis, keratitis, uveitis, and others. The condition can, over time, lead to decreased visual acuity and blindness. A number of other miscellaneous findings and/or complaints may include the GI, musculoskeletal, neurological, and cardiovascular systems.

Diagnostic Studies

There is no definitive laboratory test specific to Behçet's syndrome. Patients may have anemia, leukocytosis, elevated sedimentation rate, or elevated C-reactive protein. Rheumatoid factor and/or antinuclear antibody tests are negative.

ORAL LICHEN PLANUS (PLATE 57)

The exact cause of lichen planus is not known. The condition causes inflammatory changes in the mouth, with the development of mucosal changes that are primarily white in color. The condition is most common in adults older than 40 years of age. Although the relationship between lichen planus and oral cancers is not clear, there is a slight increased risk of malignancy in patients with lichen planus.

Signs and Symptoms

The oral mucosa develops a variety of white lesions, ranging from papules, plaques, and patches. Erythemic and/or erosive lesions develop, often affecting the buccal mucosa. Although pain is not always an early symptom, many patients complain of discomfort at the affected sites when, for instance, spicy foods are eaten. The more inflammatory and erosive lesions are usually painful. Episodes of lichen planus are often recurrent. Some patients develop extraoral pruritic skin lesions of the extremities, genitalia, and/or scalp, as well as nail changes.

Diagnostic Studies

Diagnostic studies are often not required. However, biopsies can be performed to rule out malignancy and to provide definitive diagnosis.

ERYTHEMA MULTIFORME

Erythema multiforme is described in detail in Chapter 3, p. 54. Oral lesions are common manifestations of erythema multiforme, ranging from shallow, crusted lesions of the lips to deeper ulcerations of the lips and oral mucosa. Depending on the severity, lesions may have a necrotic appearance.

INFECTIOUS CAUSES OF ORAL LESIONS

In addition to the infections noted previously, many others have painful oral mucosal manifestations. These include gonorrhea and chickenpox.

NONINFECTIOUS SYSTEMIC CONDITIONS

A wide range of systemic conditions, including Crohn's disease, ulcerative colitis, anemia, and sarcoidosis, are associated with oral lesions. It is important to explore the potential other symptoms when the patient presents with unexplained oral lesions.

LEUKOPLAKIA

The cause of most episodes of leukoplakia is not determined. However, this condition, which results in the development of white patches on the oral mucosa, is associated with an increased risk of oral squamous cell cancer. Risk factors for the development of leukoplakia include chronic/recurrent trauma to the affected site and the use of smokeless and smoked tobacco and alcohol.

Signs and Symptoms

The lesions are painless, so the patient will usually have noticed the lesion after looking in the mouth. Some lesions become rather "warty" and raised, and thus a patient can feel the lesion's presence. However, most are flat and smooth. Unlike thrush, these lesions cannot be rubbed or scraped away.

Diagnostic Studies

The diagnosis is usually based on the history and physical examination. However, biopsy should be considered to rule out dysplasia.

ERYTHROPLAKIA

Because erythroplakia is so frequently associated with malignancy, its causes are believed to be the same as those of oral squamous cell cancer. These lesions often coexist with leukoplakia, either in the form of "speckled leukoplakia," where leukoplakia lesions are superimposed on larger erythemic lesions, or the two lesions coexist.

Signs and Symptoms

These lesions are painless, so the patient may not notice the lesion unless she or he has inspected the oral mucosa for some reason. The lesions are usually flat and often have a velvety texture. Some erythroplakia lesions are "pebbly," with raised areas. The red lesions vary in size and are often very well demarcated.

Diagnostic Studies

Biopsies are obtained on referral to a specialist for definitive diagnosis and removal or destruction of the lesion.

MALIGNANCY

The most common form of oral cancer is squamous cell cancer. Most lesions occur on the lips or along the lateral aspects of the tongue. However, other forms of malignancy, including malignant melanoma, do affect the oral mucosa, and any of the tissue in the oral cavity can be involved. Because many oral cancers are not diagnosed until they are quite advanced, the prognosis can be poor.

Signs and Symptoms

Most oral malignancies are painless until quite advanced, so patients are often unaware of the lesion unless the lip or anterior portion of the tongue is involved. The patient may become aware of the lesion if it bleeds. Squamous cell cancer lesions vary in appearance, from the reddened patches of erythroplakia to areas of induration/thickening, ulceration, or necrotic lesions. Lesions of malignant melanoma have varied pigmentation, including brown, blue, and black. Even lesions that appear flat and smooth may be nodular, indurated, or fixed to adjacent tissue on palpation. Even though patients with squamous cell malignancies often have a history of heavy alcohol use, tobacco use, or poor dentition, these are not risk factors for malignant melanoma. The regional lymph nodes may be enlarged and/or nodular.

Diagnostic Studies

Oral malignancy is diagnosed by biopsy.

KAPOSI'S SARCOMA

Kaposi's sarcoma is a vascular tumor often associated with HIV. It is believed that herpes virus is implicated in the development of this condition.

Signs and Symptoms

Like the other oral malignancies described in the preceding subsections, the lesions of Kaposi's sarcoma are usually painless. The lesions most commonly occur on the palate, which is not easily seen by the patient, although it can occur on any of the oral mucosa. Initially flat, the lesions often become nodular with time. The coloring of the lesions is consistent with a vascular tumor and range from deep reddish brown to purple. The patient may provide history of HIV.

Diagnostic Studies

Diagnosis is made by biopsy.

DENTURE OR ORTHODONTIC DERMATITIS

Individuals wearing dentures and orthodontic devices are at risk for developing oral lesions, which may be related to an allergic reaction to a component of the device or to chronic rubbing and irritation from the device.

Signs and Symptoms

These lesions may result in mild discomfort or be painless. The history and physical findings should be consistent with use of the appliance that has caused the irritation.

Diagnostic Studies

No diagnostic studies are indicated.

■ Mouth Pain Without Obvious Lesions

On occasion, patients present with mouth pain yet have no visible lesions. In this case, the history should be directed to a careful analysis of the pain from the time it was first noticed. A thorough review of systems and a history of present illness and medications taken are necessary. Ask the patient about recent trauma or previous episodes of similar pain.

A careful examination of the mouth should be conducted. Most patients experiencing mouth pain without the clinical signs to guide diagnosis should be referred to a dentist for dental imaging and assessment.

TOOTHACHE

Toothache can result from periodontal inflammation, lost filling, tooth decay, infection, fracture, and/or related abscess. The pain is related to nerve irritation, pressure, and inflammation or to periodontal injury.

Signs and Symptoms

The patient typically complains of unilateral mouth pain and/or toothache. The pain may be worsened by hot or cold food or by chewing. The source of the discomfort may be evident on examination. The affected tooth may be loose. If abscess is involved, marked edema and inflammation of the surrounding gum is usually evident. Cervical lymphadenopathy may be present.

Diagnostic Studies

No diagnostic studies are indicated. Dental images will usually be obtained by a dentist on referral.

HERPES

Both herpes simplex and herpes zoster affect the oral mucosa. The appearance of skin lesions is often preceded by a prodromal phase that may include significant pain.

Signs and Symptoms

The patient with herpes simplex may report a history of recurrent painful mouth sores, often preceded by discomfort, before an eruption of herpetic lesions. A patient who is developing herpes zoster may describe pain distributed along a specific dermatome. There may be some palpable induration and lymphadenopathy, particularly with herpes simplex infections. Mouth pain may be the presenting complaint in a patient who is experiencing postherpetic neuralgia after the visible signs of herpes zoster have resolved.

Diagnostic Studies

There are no diagnostic studies warranted if either early herpes simplex or early herpes zoster is suspected. Follow-up should be arranged to confirm diagnosis.

PAROTITIS

Parotitis involves inflammation of the parotid salivary glands. The condition most commonly affects children, who often have recurrent episodes. The etiology is often uncertain, although some cases, particularly in adults, are caused by salivary stones, which obstruct the outflow of saliva from the affected duct.

Signs and Symptoms

The patient complains of painful swelling that is worsened by chewing. Fever may be present. There is an area of fullness or edema and often obvious redness and/or warmth. The parotid gland is extremely sensitive, and any manipulation triggers pain. The patient's ability to fully open the mouth is often limited by swelling and pain. Pressure over the parotid gland may result in purulent matter expressed from duct.

Diagnostic Studies

Diagnostic studies are usually not necessary. If the condition fails to respond to initial treatment, imaging should be performed for definitive diagnosis.

BURNING MOUTH SYNDROME

Burning mouth syndrome is characterized by burning pain of the oral structures. The onset is typically sudden and is sometimes variable through the day. The cause is uncertain, although there are several theories under consideration, including nutritional deficit, dry mouth, and emotional disorders.

Signs and Symptoms

The patient complains of significant burning pain that may affect the ability to sleep or to focus on normal daily activities. Many patients also complain of altered taste. There are no visible clinical signs or abnormalities.

Diagnostic Studies

The condition is a diagnosis of exclusion. The patient should be referred for specialist assessment.

Differential Diagnosis of Chief Complaints: Throat

■ Sore Throat or Throat Pain

Sore throat is a very frequent complaint in primary care settings. Most episodes of sore throat are associated with self-limited viral upper respiratory infections, although there are a number of more serious causes.

History

The history should begin with a thorough analysis of the throat pain, including determining what is meant by "sore throat," which may be used to describe sensations ranging from a mild, scratchy sore throat to excruciating throat pain. In addition to determining the characteristics of the pain, identifying all associated symptoms is helpful in narrowing the differential diagnosis. It is important to identify any other recent illnesses as well as recent exposures to others who are ill. Determine whether the patient is experiencing any dysphagia or respiratory difficulty.

Physical Examination

The physical examination for sore throat should include comprehensive assessment of the upper and lower respiratory systems, including ears, nose, mouth, throat, and lungs. The neck assessment should include, at a minimum, assessment of the cervical lymph nodes. A more thorough neck assessment is indicated if carotidynia or thyroiditis is suspected.

Diagnostic Studies

Strep screens, throat cultures, and mononucleosis screens are common diagnostic studies used to narrow the differential diagnosis of sore throat. A CBC with differential count is helpful in determining the cause of sore throat.

INFECTIOUS PHARYNGITIS

Most cases of pharyngitis are viral in origin, and any number of the respiratory viruses can cause inflammation of the throat. The majority of viral pharyngitis cases are self-limited. Herpes infections can also affect the pharynx. Group A beta-hemolytic streptococcal (GABHS) pharyngitis is a bacterial infection of the pharynx, commonly called strep throat. Complications of GABHS pharyngitis, although rare, include rheumatic heart disease and glomerulonephritis, and the condition requires prompt diagnosis and definitive treatment. Most patients with GABHS pharyngitis are children and youths. Other bacterial causes of pharyngitis include mycoplasmal pneumonia, gonorrhea, and diphtheria.

Signs and Symptoms

Complaints typically include malaise, headache, rhinitis, and/or cough in addition to the throat pain, which can range from mild scratchy discomfort to severe pain. The onset can be sudden, as with influenza, or may develop over many hours. Fever and chills may be present. In all cases of pharyngitis, the pharynx is reddened, and tender lymphadenopathy is often present. The findings associated with varied causes of non-GABHS pharyngitis are summarized in Table 6.3.

The classic symptom of GABHS is a severe sore throat with sudden onset. The patient often also complains of nausea, vomiting, fever, headache, and malaise. Unlike other forms of pharyngitis, the patient does not usually experience rhinitis or cough. The patient often appears quite ill and lethargic. The findings of GABHS include very inflamed pharynx, uvula, and tonsils. The tonsils are enlarged, usually with a white or gray-white exudate. There is tender cervical lymphadenopathy. Although some patients with viral pharyngitis may have an exanthem, GABHS can present with a fine scarlatinal rash, often described as "sand paper" rash owing to the tiny, punctate pink-red lesions.

A clinical decision rule exists to guide diagnosis of GABHS (McGinn, Ahlawat, Mobo, & Wisnivesky, 2003). The formula assigns one point each for temperature above 100.9°F, recent exposure to person with GABHS, exudates on pharynx or tonsils, and enlarged or tender nodes. A point is deducted for cough. Patients with two or more points are presumed to have GABHS and should be treated without culture. Patients with one or zero points should have rapid strep test.

Diagnostic Studies

With GABHS pharyngitis, a throat culture and/or rapid strep assay is positive. If monospot is performed to rule out mononucleosis, it is negative.

MONONUCLEOSIS

Mononucleosis is usually caused by the Epstein-Barr virus (EBV), although it can result from other viruses. Even though complications are rare, they can lead to significant morbidity or death. The potential list of complications is broad and includes hepatitis, splenic rupture, myocarditis, meningitis/encephalitis, and hemolytic anemia.

Table 6.3

Differential Diagnosis of Infectious Pharyngitis

Cause	Onset	Associated Symptoms	Pharyngeal Signs	Anterior Lymphadenopathy
Respiratory viruses	Variable	Headache, fever, chills, malaise, rhinitis, conjunctivitis, cough, nausea, diarrhea	Inflamed pharynx	Present
Herpes pharyngitis	Evolves with prodromal phase	Malaise, fever	Inflamed with ulcerative lesions	Present
Herpangitis or hand-foot-and-mouth disease	Evolves over few days	Malaise, lesions in mouth, on hands, feet, buttocks, and/or genitalia	Inflamed with ulcerative lesions	Present
Diphtheria	Evolves over 1–2 days	Headache, rhinitis, fever/chills, dysphagia, difficulty breathing	Inflamed pharynx with thick, gray membrane	Present
Group A beta-hemolytic streptococcal (GABHS)	Sudden onset	Malaise, nausea/vomiting, headache, sand-paper rash; no rhinitis, cough, conjunctivitis, diarrhea	Inflamed uvula, pharynx, tonsils; white-gray tonsillar exudate	Present

Signs and Symptoms

The patient often complains of an onset over several days or more than a week. The sore throat may be preceded by prodromal symptoms that include malaise, generalized aches, and headache. Throat pain is usually severe and is associated with lymphadenopathy of the posterior cervical nodes in addition to generalized lymphadenopathy. The pharynx is inflamed, and the tonsils are usually involved, with inflammation and exudate that ranges from white to yellow or green. The pharynx is often similar in appearance to GABHS. Petechiae over the palate are often identified. A maculopapular generalized rash frequently occurs. Other skin changes may include jaundice. Splenomegaly is common, and hepatomegaly may also be present.

Diagnostic Studies

The white blood cell count is increased, with an increased ratio of lymphocytes. A rapid monospot is often positive in the clinical setting. Liver function tests are often elevated. Depending on the degree of findings suggesting one of the previously listed potential complications, consultation of or referral to the appropriate specialist should be completed.

TONSILLITIS (PLATES 58 AND 59)

Tonsillitis involves infection of the tonsils, usually by GABHS, although viral tonsillitis (often associated with EBV) is more common in very young children. Most cases of tonsillitis are diagnosed in school-aged children and adolescents. Patients can develop chronic tonsillitis and/or have frequent recurrences of the condition.

Signs and Symptoms

The patient complains of severe sore throat pain and difficulty swallowing. A fever is present, and the patient appears ill. The patient is usually mouth breathing, has a deepened voice, and may have difficulty articulating and moving the mouth because of the swelling and pain. The tonsils are edematous and have exudate that varies in color. If EBV is present, palatal petechiae may be visible. If herpes virus is present, tonsillar ulcerations are visible. Lymphadenopathy is present, and the patient limits neck motion owing to pain. The history may reveal previous episodes.

Diagnostic Studies

Definitive diagnosis is made by throat culture, rapid strep, and/or monospot test.

PERITONSILLAR ABSCESS

Peritonsillar abscesses may occur at any age, although most cases involve adults. Many cases evolve as a complication of tonsillitis, but others develop as peritonsillar abscess without a history of tonsillitis. The condition involves infection of the peritonsillar space. A number of pathogens cause peritonsillar abscesses, although the most common cause is GABHS.

Signs and Symptoms

The patient describes onset over several days of sore throat, fever, and malaise. Over time, the sore throat becomes severe and localized to one side. It becomes increasingly difficult to move the neck, speak, and swallow. The patient's breath is fetid, and the patient often drools, unable to swallow saliva. Fever is present, and respiratory distress is possible. Pharyngeal examination can be difficult, as the patient may have trismus, an inability to move the jaw because of the swelling. On examination of the pharynx, the area adjacent to the tonsil is swollen, the tonsil is often displaced, and the uvula is deviated away from the site. The patient's voice is muffled. The tonsil may be enlarged, with exudate. There may be signs consistent with dehydration, including dry skin and tachycardia.

Diagnostic Studies

The patient should be referred to a specialist, who may aspirate the abscess to obtain a culture or obtain a culture at the time of therapeutic incision and drainage. White blood count is elevated. An ultrasound or CT scan are used to confirm diagnosis.

EPIGLOTTITIS

Epiglottitis is rare, but it can cause significant respiratory obstruction and death. The condition can occur at any age.

Signs and Symptoms

The patient presents with rapidly developing sore throat, fever, cough, and difficulty swallowing. The patient's voice is muffled, and there is drooling. Stridor and/or varying signs of respiratory distress may be evident. The patient often leans forward while sitting to maximize airway opening. The patient has a very ill appearance, and gentle palpation over the larynx causes significant pain.

Diagnostic Studies

The patient should be closely monitored for complete airway obstruction, but urgent referral for emergency care via an ambulance is indicated prior to performing any diagnostic evaluation, because the potential exists for sudden loss of airway. An ENT specialist should be informed to meet the patient at the emergency department.

THYROIDITIS

Painful subacute thyroiditis involves inflammation of the thyroid gland. It is a self-limiting condition. The condition includes a hyperthyroid phase, followed by a period of hypothyroidism, before the patient regains a euthyroid state. More women than men are affected. A variant, postpartum thyroiditis, occurs within 6 months of giving birth and is generally painless. Although the etiology of painful subacute thyroiditis is not clear, it may have a viral trigger.

Signs and Symptoms

Patients commonly complain of pain in the throat and/or neck, with radiation to an ear. Onset is described as relatively sudden, and associated symptoms include fever, malaise, and achiness. The throat pain may be associated with dysphagia. The patient may not complain of symptoms of hyperthyroidism or hypothyroidism during those phases; however, the severity of metabolic symptoms is quite variable. On physical examination, the thyroid region is very tender and enlarged.

Diagnostic Studies

Depending on the phase during which diagnosis is made, thyroid studies may indicate an increase or decrease. Sedimentation rate is usually elevated. If radioactive iodine uptake is performed, uptake will be low. Thyroid antibodies may be elevated in painful thyroiditis.

CAROTIDYNIA

Carotidynia is a self-limiting condition with unknown origin.

Signs and Symptoms

The patient presents with sudden onset of sore throat and/or unilateral neck pain. The pain may radiate to the jaw or ear on the affected side. The pain may be worsened or triggered by exposure to cold temperature or by chewing or neck movement. The patient is afebrile, and physical findings include a normal oropharynx. The thyroid is nonpalpable, and there is no lymphadenopathy. However, palpation along the course of the carotid is quite painful.

Diagnostic Studies

No studies are indicated.

■ Hoarseness

While the causes of hoarseness are typically self-limiting, it is important to consider a range of potential causes: laryngeal growths; gastroesophageal reflux; vocal cord paralysis; and tumors of the larynx, lung, or mediastinum.

History

When a patient presents with hoarseness or voice alteration, it is important to obtain an explanation of how the voice has changed—in tone, volume, and so on. Determine whether the onset was sudden or gradual and whether the change has been constant or intermittent. Also determine the patient's typical pattern of voice use and whether any unusual use (e.g., singing, lecturing, shouting) occurred before the onset of hoarseness. The presence of associated symptoms, such as sore throat, neck pain, postnasal drainage, heartburn, and/or cough, is important. Identify use of alcohol and tobacco. Identify past medical history of such conditions as thyroid disorders, pulmonary disease, gastroesophageal reflux, and malignancy. Ask about previous surgical history as well as any trauma to the neck or chest.

Physical Examination

The physical examination specific to a complaint of hoarseness should include the ears, nose, throat, neck, lungs, and cranial nerves (particularly CN IX and CN X). When hoarseness is persistent or laryngeal structural disorders are considered, laryngoscopy should be performed to view any redness, edema, motion, and masses or polyps.

Diagnostic Studies

Diagnostic studies are not warranted for most cases of hoarseness, but chest radiographs are recommended to rule out pulmonary or mediastinal masses when the symptom persists or in individuals with history of smoking.

OVERUSE

Voice overuse/stress is a common cause of hoarseness. It can occur at any age and may be a recurrent problem for patients who use their voice extensively in lecturing, singing, or speaking in loud environments.

Signs and Symptoms

The patient provides history consistent with voice overuse or abuse. The hoarseness may tend to occur toward the end of the day and be better the next morning after some period of rest. The hoarseness may be associated with a sensation of muscle tension and/or discomfort in the neck. The physical findings are benign.

Diagnostic Studies

None are warranted.

POSTNASAL DISCHARGE

Postnasal discharge (PND) associated with allergies or upper respiratory infections can cause hoarseness. Hoarseness associated with PND is usually relieved by clearing the throat.

Signs and Symptoms

The patient complains of intermittent hoarseness with associated sensation of mucus or matter in the back of the throat. There may be mild to moderate throat discomfort associated with the drainage. The physical examination is usually benign, although there may be mild erythema and/or cobblestoning of the posterior pharynx, and the PND may be present.

Diagnostic Studies

None are warranted.

GERD

Gastroesophageal reflux can result in reflux laryngitis. GERD is described in Chapter 10, pp. 261–262.

INFECTIOUS LARYNGITIS

A number of pharyngeal and upper respiratory infections can also involve the larynx, resulting in hoarseness. Findings will be consistent with the descriptions in the previous sections.

VOCAL CORD PARALYSIS

Vocal cord paralysis can be caused by malignancies, trauma, surgery, infections, and neurological conditions.

Signs and Symptoms

The patient may complain of a change in the character of the voice or in the intensity or volume. In addition to hoarseness, the patient may experience associated painless difficulty swallowing and respiratory stridor or dyspnea. The pharynx will appear within normal limits.

Diagnostic Studies

The patient should be referred to a specialist for diagnostic studies and definitive diagnosis. In addition to laryngoscopy, other diagnostic studies may include imaging, bronchoscopy, and/or esophagoscopy.

TUMOR AND MALIGNANCY

Hoarseness may result from squamous cell cancer of the larynx as well as from malignancies within the pulmonary tree, neck, and throat. The risk of malignancy as a cause for hoarseness is greatest in patients with a history of cigarette smoking and/or alcohol abuse.

Signs and Symptoms

The history usually reveals a progressive onset of hoarseness that has persisted for weeks. There is usually no associated pain. Other associated symptoms and physical findings depend on the type of malignancy, although no abnormal findings may be evident on routine examination.

Diagnostic Studies

The patient with persistent hoarseness should be referred to a specialist for laryngoscopy, other diagnostic studies, and definitive diagnosis.

REFERENCES

Boatman, D., Miglioretti, D., Eberwein, C., Alidoost, M., & Reich, S. (2007). How accurate are bedside hearing tests? *Neurology, 68,* 1311–1314.

DeAlleaume, L., & Parker, S. (2003). What findings distinguish acute bacterial sinusitis? *Journal of Family Practice, 52*(6), 563–565.

McGinn, T., Deluca, J., Ahlawat, S., Mobo, B., & Wisnivesky, J. (2003). Validation and modification of streptococcal pharyngitis clinical prediction rules. *Mayo Clinic Proceedings, 78,* 289–293.

SUGGESTED READINGS

Bickley, L.S., & Szilagyi, P.G. (2003). *Bates' Guide to Physical Examination and History Taking.* Philadelphia: Lippincott, Williams, and Wilkins.

Dillon, P.M. (2003). *Nursing Health Assessment: A Critical Thinking, Case Studies Approach.* Philadelphia: F.A. Davis.

Rubin, M.A., Gonzales, R., & Sande, M.A. (2005). Infections of the upper respiratory tract. In Kasper, S.L., Braunwald, E., Fauci, A.S., Hauser, D.L., Longo, D.L., & Jameson, J.L. (Eds.), *Harrison's Principles of Internal Medicine.* New York: McGraw-Hill.

Isaacson, J.E., & Vora, N.M. (2003). Differential diagnosis and treatment of hearing loss. *American Family Physician, 68,* 1125–1132.

Lalwani, A.K., & Snow, J.B. (2005). Disorders of smell, taste, and hearing. In Kasper, S.L., Braunwald, E., Fauci, A.S., Hauser, D.L., Longo, D.L., & Jameson, J.L. (Eds.), *Harrison's Principles of Internal Medicine.* New York: McGraw-Hill.

Shohet, J.A., & Scherger, J.E. (1998). Which culprit is causing your patient's otorrhea? *Postgraduate Medicine, 104*(3), 50–55.

Steyer, T.E., & Hueston, W.J. (2003). Otitis media and otitis externa. In Hueston, W.J. (Ed.), *20 Common Problems: Respiratory Disorders.* New York: McGraw-Hill.

Swartz, M.H. (2005). *Textbook of Physical Diagnosis: History and Examination.* Philadelphia: Saunders.

Temte, J.L. (2003). Pharyngitis. In Hueston, W.J. (Ed.), *20 Common Problems: Respiratory Disorders.* New York: McGraw-Hill.

Vincent, M.T., Celestin, N., & Hussain, A.N. (2004). Pharyngitis: Problem oriented diagnosis. *American Family Physician, 69*(6), 1465–1470.

Chapter 7

CARDIAC AND PERIPHERAL VASCULAR SYSTEMS

Laurie Grubbs

Cardiac System

Cardiovascular disease (CVD) is the leader in all-cause morbidity and mortality across ages and genders. It accounts for approximately 5 million hospital admissions and over 800,000 deaths annually, not to mention lost work and reduced quality of life. Men are affected more than women, especially before age 50 years. CVD often goes undetected, especially among females. Early detection and intervention can save many lives and advanced practice nursing can have a significant impact in terms of prevention, early detection, and treatment.

The New York Heart Association classifies heart disease into four functional categories according to the limitation on activity (Hurst, Morris, & Alexander, 1999):

Functional Classification of Heart Disease

Class I	No limitation. Ordinary physical activity does not cause undue fatigue, dyspnea, palpitation, or anginal pain.
Class II	Slight limitation. Comfortable at rest, but ordinary physical activity results in symptoms of fatigue, dyspnea, palpitation, or anginal pain.
Class III	Marked limitation. Comfortable at rest, but less than ordinary activity causes symptoms of fatigue, dyspnea, palpitation, or anginal pain.
Class IV	Unable to engage in any physical activity without discomfort, and symptoms of cardiac insufficiency are present at rest.

Anatomy and Physiology

Figure 7.1 illustrates the anatomy of the heart.

■ Heart Sounds

S_1, the closing of the mitral valve (in the following diagram, M_1) and the tricuspid (T_1) valve, together are known as the atrioventricular valves.

S_2, the closing of the aortic (A_2) and pulmonic (P_2) valves, together are known as the semilunar valves.

S_1 represents the beginning of systole; S_2 represents the beginning of diastole.

S_1 systole	S_2 diastole	S_1 systole	S_2 diastole
M_1T_1	A_2P_2	M_1T_1	A_2P_2

Normally, the S_1 and S_2 occur as single sounds. In some conditions, these sounds may be split and occur as two sounds. In healthy young adults, a physiologic split of S_2 may be detected in the second and third left interspaces during inspiration as a result of changes in the amount of blood returned to the right and left sides of the heart. During inspiration, there is an increased filling

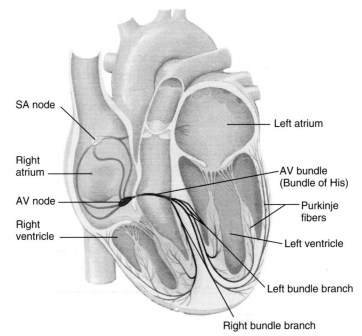

Figure 7.1 **Anatomy of the heart.** (From Scanlon, V.C., & Sanders, T. *Essentials of Anatomy and Physiology*, 4th ed. Philadelphia: F.A. Davis, 2003. Reprinted with permission.)

time and therefore increased stroke volume of the right ventricle, which can delay closure of the pulmonic valve, causing the second heart sound to be split. This physiologic split differs from other splits that are pathologic in origin in that it occurs with inspiration and disappears with expiration.

Pathologic split heart sounds include the following:

- **Split S₁** may occur in right bundle branch block (RBBB), and with premature ventricular contractions (PVCs).
- **Fixed splitting of S₂** occurs with ASD and right ventricular failure.
- **Wide splitting of S₂** is associated with delayed closure of the pulmonic valve and can be caused by pulmonic stenosis and right bundle branch block or by early closure of the aortic valve in mitral regurgitation.
- **Paradoxical splitting of S₂** occurs only on expiration and is associated with delayed closure of the aortic valve, usually as a result of left bundle branch block (LBBB).

In addition to the first and second heart sounds are S₃ and S₄, heard both in normal and pathologic conditions. Both S₃ and S₄ occur during diastole: An S₃ is heard in early diastole right after S₂, and an S₄ is heard in late diastole just before S₁. An S₃ can occur physiologically or pathologically depending on the age and disease status of the patient; an S₄ usually occurs under pathologic conditions.

- **Physiologic S₃** is generally confined to children, young adults, and pregnant women as a result of rapid early ventricular filling. It is low pitched and is heard best at the apex or left sternal border with the bell of the stethoscope.
- **Pathologic S₃**, also called a ventricular gallop, is heard in adults and is associated with decreased myocardial contractility, heart failure, and volume overload conditions, as can occur with mitral or tricuspid regurgitation. The sound is the same as a physiologic S₃ and is heard with the patient supine or in the left lateral recumbent position.
- **S₄**, also called an atrial gallop, occasionally occurs in a normal adult or well-trained athlete but is usually due to increased resistance to filling of the ventricle. Possible causes of a left-sided S₄ include hypertension, coronary artery disease (CAD), cardiomyopathy, and aortic stenosis. Possible causes of a right-sided S₄ include pulmonic stenosis and pulmonary hypertension. S₄ is heard with the patient supine or in the left lateral recumbent position.

Other heart sounds may occur in pathologic conditions and include opening snaps and pericardial friction rubs.

- **Opening snap** is caused by the opening of a stenotic mitral or tricuspid valve and is heard early in diastole along the lower left sternal border. It is high pitched and heard best with the diaphragm of the stethoscope.
- **Friction rubs** occur frequently after a myocardial infarction (MI) or with pericarditis. The sound is a high-pitched grating, scratching sound—resulting from inflammation of the pericardial sac—that issues from the parietal and visceral surfaces of the inflamed pericardium as they rub together.

■ The Cardiac Cycle

The cardiac cycle is diagrammed in Figure 7.2. Blood is returned to the right atrium via the superior and inferior vena cavae, and to the left atrium via the pulmonary veins. As the blood fills the atria during early diastole, the pressure rises until it exceeds the relaxed pressure in the ventricles, at which time the mitral and tricuspid valves open and blood flows from the atria to the ventricles. At the end of diastole, atrial contraction produces a slight rise in pressure termed the *atrial kick*. As ventricular contraction begins, the rise in pressure in the ventricles exceeds that of the atria, causing the mitral and tricuspid valves to close. This closure produces the first heart sound (S_1). As ventricular pressure rises, it exceeds the pressure in the aorta and pulmonary artery, forcing the aortic and pulmonic valves to open. As the blood is ejected from the ventricles, the pressure declines until it is below that of the aorta and pulmonary artery, causing the aortic and pulmonic valves to close and producing the second heart sound (S_2). As the ventricles relax, the pressure falls below the atrial pressure, the mitral and tricuspid valves open, and the cycle begins again.

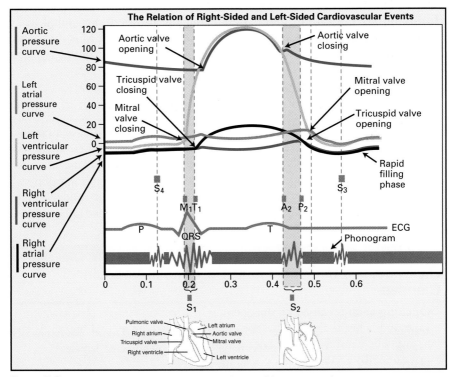

Figure 7.2 The cardiac cycle and mechanisms of heart sounds. (From Dillon, P.M. *Nursing Health Assessment: A Critical Thinking, Case Studies Approach.* Philadelphia: F.A. Davis, 2003. Reprinted with permission.)

History

■ General History for the Cardiac and Peripheral Vascular System

In many instances, the history may be more telling than the physical examination. It is important to take a thorough history for signs and symptoms of heart disease but also to alert the clinician to the need for lifestyle education or further evaluation regarding smoking, hypertension, exercise habits, diet, and professional and personal life behavior. Investigate complaints of chest pain, pressure, or heaviness; left arm or jaw pain or numbness; dyspnea on exertion; cough; paroxysmal dyspnea; hemoptysis; syncope; palpitations; fatigue; or edema. Complaints indicating peripheral vascular disease, such as claudication, skin changes especially in the lower extremities, dependent edema, or pain, also should be investigated. Determine the date of the last chest x-ray and electrocardiogram (EKG). Inquire about comorbid conditions or other factors that may increase the patient's risk for heart disease and peripheral vascular disease (see Box 7.1).

■ Past Medical History

History of heart disease includes any previous diagnoses of congenital heart disease, murmurs, palpitations, arrhythmias, abnormal EKGs, unstable angina, MI, angiography, angioplasty, stent placement, or coronary artery bypass graft.

■ Family History

Family history is particularly important for cardiac assessment because CVD, hypertension, hyperlipidemia, and other vascular diseases often have a familial association that is not easily ameliorated by lifestyle changes. If there are deaths in the family related to CVD, determine the age and exact cause of death because CVD at a young age in the immediate family carries an increased risk compared with CVD in an elderly family member. Ask about sudden death, which might indicate a congenital disease such as Marfan's syndrome. This is

---

Box 7.1

Risk Factors for Heart and Peripheral Vascular Disease

Hypertension	Hostility
Smoking	**Age:** >45 years for males and >55 years for females
Diabetes	**Gender:** males and postmenopausal females
Obesity	Positive family history
Dyslipidemia	Increased C-reactive protein
Sedentary lifestyle	

especially important to ask for pre-sports physicals because sudden death in athletes is often related to congenital or familial heart disease. Familial hyperlipidemia is autosomal dominant, and often leads to CAD and MI at a young age. Family history of obesity and type 2 diabetes are also secondary risk factors for heart disease because the familial tendency for these is strong. Ask about smoking in the house because secondhand smoke is a risk factor for respiratory and cardiac disease.

▪ Habits

The social history should include habits or behaviors that increase the risk for heart disease, include smoking, sedentary lifestyle, high-fat diet, drug or alcohol abuse, and stress.

Physical Examination

▪ General Assessment

General signs of heart or circulatory disease include pallor, cyanosis, diaphoresis, edema, restlessness, and confusion. Vital signs should be thoroughly assessed. Blood pressure readings in the prehypertensive stage of 120–139/80–89 mm Hg (Chobanian et al., 2003) should be further evaluated, and patients should be educated on lifestyle modifications. Heart rates above 90 bpm may be seen in noncardiac conditions, such as fever, anxiety, pain, medication, thyroid disease, dehydration, anemia, or pulmonary disease, but if other clinical signs or symptoms are present, an EKG is warranted. Heart rates below 50 bpm can be seen in young trained athletes, but otherwise, there should be a high index of suspicion for other causes, such as heart block, and an EKG is recommended. Diminished or accentuated peripheral pulses, pulsus paradoxus (decreased pulse amplitude at the end of inspiration, associated with pericarditis), pulsus alternans (alternating weak and strong pulsation, associated with left ventricular failure), and a bisferious pulse (having two systolic peaks, associated with aortic regurgitation or hypertrophic cardiomyopathy) are indicative of valvular heart disease or tamponade. Jugular venous distention and hepatojugular reflux suggest an increase in right ventricular pressure. Wheezes, rhonchi, crackles, or significant increase in respiratory rate should alert the examiner to the possibility of pulmonary disease or heart failure.

▪ Inspection

A general inspection of the patient is necessary, noting particularly short or tall stature, which may be associated with Turner's or Marfan's syndrome—both linked to congenital heart defects. Inspect the skin for changes in temperature, color, and ulcerations or sores that will not heal. Pallor, coolness, ulcerations, or hyperpigmentation of the extremities suggests arterial or venous insufficiency. Cyanosis of the nail beds or, in more severe cases, circumoral cyanosis suggests hypoxia. A red, ruddy complexion can be seen in hypertension and in alcohol abuse. Inspect the skin around the eyes for xanthelasma seen in hyperlipidemia.

Inspect the configuration of the chest, noting thoracic scoliosis or pectus excavatum that may be associated with restrictive lung or cardiac disease. Inspect the respiratory rate and effort, looking for dyspnea. Inspect the point of maximal impulse (PMI) and the precordium for visible heaves or lifts, seen in ventricular hypertrophy. The apical impulse is easily observed in the pediatric client but not always visible in the adult. An accentuated or displaced apical impulse may indicate ventricular hypertrophy. Inspect the neck for the jugular venous distention seen in right-sided heart failure.

■ Auscultation

Auscultation is generally the most useful part of the cardiac examination. First, identify the rate and rhythm of the heart. Identify S_1 (heard louder at the apex) and S_2 (heard louder at the base). Determine if these are heard as single sounds or if there are splits. A physiologic split of the second heart sound is common and varies with respiration in that S_2 splits on inspiration and is heard as a single sound on expiration. This is due to changes in intrathoracic pressure during inspiration that cause increased filling time of the right ventricle and therefore increased stroke volume and a slightly later closing of the pulmonary valve (P_2). Note any fixed splitting of the first and second heart sounds, which can occur in a variety of pathologic conditions, including RBBB, LBBB, premature ventricular contraction, right ventricular failure, atrial septal defect, pulmonic stenosis, and mitral regurgitation. Next, identify any extra sounds, such as an opening snap heard early in diastole in mitral or tricuspid stenosis, an early systolic ejection click heard in aortic or pulmonic stenosis, the midsystolic ejection click of mitral valve prolapse, a ventricular gallop (S_3), an atrial gallop (S_4), or a systolic or diastolic murmur. Auscultating the carotid arteries for bruits and amplitude is an important part of the cardiovascular examination. Audible bruits should be further evaluated with a carotid duplex scan to assess the amount, if any, of carotid artery stenosis or occlusion. Occlusion of the carotid artery should alert the examiner to the increased risk of stroke, and prompt referral should be made to the surgeon.

■ Palpation

It is important to palpate the precordium because palpation of a sustained apical or ventricular impulse can give information about heart size. A lift or heave caused by right ventricular hypertrophy can be palpated along the left sternal border, and a left ventricular lift or heave can be palpated at the apex. Thrills associated with grade IV, V, and VI murmurs are palpated over the precordium and are vibratory in nature. Palpate the carotid, femoral, and dorsalis pedis arterial pulses for amplitude and regularity.

■ Percussion

Percussion of the heart borders is not often performed owing to its low sensitivity, however, it may be useful in some conditions—such as in pericardial effusion with or without cardiac tamponade—and especially in emergency situations when x-ray is not readily available. In addition, when the heart is either located or displaced to the right of the sternum, as in dextrocardia or tension pneumothorax of the left chest, percussion can be helpful.

Cardiovascular Laboratory Tests

Table 7.1 presents normal values for common laboratory tests used in assessment of the cardiovascular system, along with the significance of each test.

Table 7.1		
Cardiovascular Laboratory Tests		
Lab Test	Normal Value	Significance
Lactate dehydrogenase (LDH)	45–90 U/L	An enzyme released when organ or tissue is destroyed, particularly myocardial tissue. Can also be elevated in hemolytic states, hyperthyroidism, renal disease, gastric malignancy, and megaloblastic anemia
Creatine phosphokinase (CPK)	5–75 mU/mL	CPK is elevated in MI but not specific to myocardial damage. Also seen with skeletal muscle damage owing to excessive exercise or rhabdomyolysis
Myocardial band creatine kinase (MB CK)	0–3 µg/mL	This cardiac isoenzyme is most sensitive in detecting myocardial injury within the first 4 hours after onset of chest pain
Troponin I (cTnI)	<0.35 ng/mL	This index is useful in the diagnosis of acute myocardial injury. After 4 hours, it is equally as sensitive as MB CK for up to 48 hours. Troponin I remains elevated longer than MB CK and is more cardiac specific
Troponin T (cTnT)	<0.2 µg/L	The sensitivity of cTnT for detecting acute MI is 100% from 10 hours to 7 days after onset. The sensitivity begins to decrease after 7 days
Potassium (K+)	3.5–5.0 mEq/L	Most importantly, elevated K+ levels can cause ventricular fibrillation. Other changes in the EKG include widened P waves, peaked T waves, widened QRS complex, depressed ST segment, and heart block. Decreased K+ can cause inverted T waves, U waves, and depressed ST segment

Continued

Table 7.1

Cardiovascular Laboratory Tests—cont'd

Lab Test	Normal Value	Significance
Sodium (Na+)	135–145 mEq/L	Na+ is important for fluid balance particularly, when dehydration may be an issue or in heart failure
Calcium (Ca+)	8.5–10.6 mg/dL	The hypercalcemic effects on the heart include shortening of the QT interval and atrioventricular block. The effect of hypocalcemia is prolongation of the ST segment
Glucose	70–100 mg/dL	Changes in blood glucose can have indirect effects on the heart. Diabetes significantly increases the risk for MI and hyperlipidemia
Creatinine	0.6–12 mg/dL	Renal disease may elevate blood pressure, which, over time, will increase the risk for CVD. Creatinine level is also important when prescribing certain medications for hypertension and CHF, particularly ACE inhibitors and diuretics.
Cholesterol	Total, <200 mg/dL LDL, <130 mg/dL HDL, >40 mg/dL	Increased total and LDL cholesterol and decreased HDL increase the risk for CAD. Cause may be inherited or acquired, secondary to obesity, thyroid disease, or high-fat diet
Triglycerides	<200 mg/dL	Elevated levels increase the risk for heart disease
Thyroid-stimulating hormone (TSH)	0.4–4.2 mIU/L	In the elderly, hypothyroidism may contribute to the development of CHF. Hyperthyroidism may present as atrial fibrillation or other arrhythmias in patients over 50 years
Hemoglobin (Hgb)	11.5–15.0 g/dL	Anemia may be a cause or a result of many forms of heart disease
Hematocrit (Hct)	34.0%–44.0%	Anemia may be a cause or a result of many forms of heart disease
Oxygen saturation	95%–97%	Pulse oximetry can be helpful in patients with severe myocardial damage and CHF to evaluate clinical status

CAD = coronary artery disease; CHF = congestive heart failure; CVD = cardiovascular disease; HDL = high-density lipoprotein; LDL = low-density lipoprotein; MI = myocardial infarction.

Differential Diagnosis of Chief Complaints

■ Palpitations or Arrhythmia

The Conduction System

The conduction pathway of the heart begins in the sinoatrial (SA) node, travels through the atria to the atrioventricular (AV) node, the bundle of His, the bundle branches, the Purkinje fibers, and finally to the ventricular muscle. When the electrical impulse travels normally through this pathway, it is considered a normal sinus rhythm (NSR), with a rate of 60 to 100 beats per minute, but perhaps lower in patients taking beta-blockers or in athletes.

The EKG

Following are the elements of the EKG (also see Figure 7.3).
* *P wave*—Represents depolarization of the atria. The absence of P waves may indicate atrial fibrillation or an idioventricular rhythm.
* *P-R interval*—0.12 to 0.20 second, measured from the beginning of the P wave to the beginning of the QRS. Prolongation of the P-R interval indicates a conduction delay producing first-, second-, or third-degree heart block. A shortened P-R interval is seen in Wolff-Parkinson-White and Lown-Ganong-Levine syndromes.

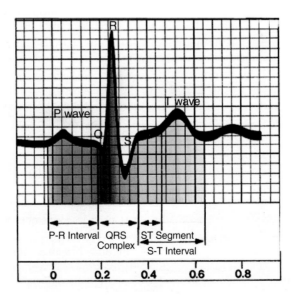

Figure 7.3 The electrocardiogram. (From Scanlon, V.C., & Sanders, T. *Essentials of Anatomy and Physiology*, 4th ed. Philadelphia: F.A. Davis, 2003. Reprinted with permission.)

- *QRS duration*—0.08 to 0.12 second. The QRS represents depolarization of the ventricles. A wide QRS is seen in conduction delays in the ventricles, such as with bundle branch blocks and complete heart block, and in ventricular ectopic beats, such as with PVCs.
- *T wave*—Represents repolarization of the ventricles. Repolarization of the atria is not represented on the EKG tracing because it takes place within the QRS complex. Configuration should be upright. Myocardial ischemia, injury, and necrosis cause inversion of the T wave as a result of altered repolarization. Hyperventilation may also cause flipped T waves.
- *QT interval*—Less than 0.05 seconds. Prolongation may result in syncope and sudden death.
- *QRS complex*—The amplitude of the R wave is decreased in MI owing to altered depolarization, decreased myocardial contractility, or in pericardial effusion.
- *S-T segment*—Should be isoelectric. Myocardial injury causes elevations in the S-T segment in the leads that reflect the area of injury and reciprocal S-T depression in the leads opposite the area of infarct.
- *Q wave*—Represents death (infarction) of the muscle and is due to the absence of depolarization in dead tissue. A pathologic Q wave measures greater than 0.04 second and is greater than one-third the height of the QRS.

Each small block on the EKG represents 0.04 second, and each large block represents 0.20 second.

History

Occasional palpitations occur physiologically in the majority of the population or as a result of other noncardiac conditions, such as anxiety, exercise, hyperthyroidism, and anemia. They can also occur with valvular heart disease, increased or decreased stroke volume, and arrhythmias. The patient may complain of palpitations or skipped beats, or an arrhythmia may be seen on EKG. Patients are often aware if their heart rate is slower or faster than normal or if it is irregular. With some arrhythmias, patients may complain only of fatigue, shortness of breath, weakness, or syncopal episodes. These are common symptoms in patients who have atrial fibrillation, and if the ventricular response is slow, the patient may be unaware of the arrhythmia. Ask the patient about the frequency and duration of the palpitations and the presence of associated symptoms, such as loss of consciousness, lightheadedness, chest pain, shortness of breath, nausea, or vomiting.

Ask about history of MI or valvular heart disease. In young women, mitral valve prolapse is a common cause of palpitations, which are benign in nature but unsettling to the patient. Ask patients how long they have had the symptoms and whether they are constant or intermittent. Paroxysmal supraventricular tachycardia (PSVT) occurs intermittently and lasts anywhere from several seconds to several hours. Determine whether there is chest pain because myocardial ischemia predisposes the patient to ventricular arrhythmias. Age and other risk factors are important to the history. Occasionally, young, healthy patients will have fairly frequent PVCs that are benign in nature but warrant investigation to rule out serious causes.

Physical Examination

Although the EKG remains the major diagnostic tool, a thorough cardiac examination, including vital signs and carotid and jugular venous pulsation, as well as an examination of the extremities and peripheral vascular system, are necessary.

BRADYARRHYTHMIAS

A pulse rate lower than 60 bpm is considered bradycardia, although many trained athletes normally have a sinus bradycardia. In an elderly or untrained individual, it is more concerning. The underlying cardiac history is of utmost importance. Sinus node pathology and heart blocks should be suspected in the elderly or in patients with underlying heart disease. A thorough medication history is also imperative because many medications, including many heart medications, can cause arrhythmias. Electrolyte imbalance, particularly potassium (K^+), should be excluded. See Table 7.2 for common causes of bradyarrhythmias.

Table 7.2

Common Causes of Bradyarrhythmias

Cause	Description
Sick sinus syndrome	This term describes sinus arrest, sinoatrial block, and persistent sinus bradycardia of unknown origin. Often caused or exacerbated by drugs, particularly digitalis, calcium-channel blockers, beta-blockers, and antiarrhythmics
First-degree heart block	This rhythm is characterized by a lengthening of the P-R interval greater than 0.20 second
Second-degree heart block: • Mobitz type I or Wenckebach • Mobitz type II	In Mobitz type I, the P-R interval progressively lengthens until a QRS complex is completely dropped, and the pattern is repeated. In Mobitz type II, there is a regular P-R interval, and a QRS is absent on a regular interval
Third-degree (complete) heart block	There is a complete dissociation between the atrial and ventricular rhythms. None of the electrical activity originating in the sinoatrial or atrioventricular node is being conducted through the ventricles. The atria continue beating at the normal rate, while the ventricles are beating at rate of 30–40 bpm
Interventricular conduction defect/bundle branch block	Electrical impulse is slowed or blocked in one of the branches of the bundle of His. The right and left ventricles will not beat in complete synchronization, causing a widened and slightly delayed QRS

Signs and Symptoms

Fatigue and shortness of breath are common symptoms of bradyarrhythmias. In the elderly, weakness, confusion, and syncope may occur as cerebral perfusion is decreased due to decreased cardiac output. Congestive heart failure may ensue in elderly patients or patients who already have some degree of cardiac compromise.

Diagnostic Studies

- *EKG*—An EKG is the first step in diagnosing arrhythmias. If the problem is intermittent, however, it may not show on a single EKG.
- *Holter monitor*—This device gives a continuous EKG reading for 24 hours or more and is useful in identifying paroxysmal arrhythmias.
- *Electrolytes*—An electrolyte panel, particularly to obtain the K^+ level, is necessary because problems with potassium balance can cause arrhythmias. Medications such as diuretics can lead to hypokalemia.
- *Thyroid functions*—A low level of thyroid-stimulating hormone (TSH), or an elevated level of triiodothyronine (T_3), and thyroxine (T_4) may indicate thyroid disease as a cause for the arrhythmia.
- *Cardiac enzyme studies*—Elevations in myocardial band creatine kinase (MB CK) and/or troponin levels suggest myocardial ischemia/injury as a cause of the arrhythmia.
- *Medication levels*—It may be necessary to measure blood levels of medications such as digoxin and theophylline that can cause arrhythmias. Many other medications may affect cardiac rhythms, and patients' medication lists should be carefully reviewed.

TACHYARRHYTHMIAS

A pulse rate over 100 bpm is considered tachycardia. Pulse rates increase with age, but a rate over 100 bpm should be investigated. Tachycardia can result from many noncardiac conditions, including hyperthyroidism, respiratory disease, anemia and blood loss, illegal drugs, prescription medications, heat exhaustion, emotions, and exercise. The underlying cardiac history is also important to rule out a cardiac origin. See Table 7.3 for common causes of tachyarrhythmias.

Signs and Symptoms

The symptoms vary greatly depending on the cause of the arrhythmia, the ventricular rate, and the cardiac output. Those with mild to moderate increases in ventricular rate may be asymptomatic. With higher rates, patients will complain of weakness, dizziness, syncope, and shortness of breath, and they may lose consciousness.

Diagnostic Studies

See Diagnostic Studies under Bradyarrhythmias.

Table 7.3

Common Causes of Tachyarrhythmias

Cause	Description
Sinus tachycardia	When the heart rate is greater than 100 bpm but the impulse is via the normal sinus pathway, it is a sinus tachycardia. This is due to outside influences, such as fever, pain, anemia, volume depletion as in shock, or volume overload as in congestive heart failure, thyrotoxicosis, drugs, fear or other emotions, and exercise
Supraventricular tachycardia (SVT)	The heart rate ranges from 140–240 bpm, and SVT may last a few seconds to several hours. The usual mechanism is reentry, which is initiated by a premature atrial or ventricular beat involving dual pathways within the atrioventricular node. Most do not involve structural heart disease. SVT may be a result of digitalis toxicity. Patients may complain of dizziness, shortness of breath, or mild chest pain, or they may be asymptomatic except for the sense of a racing heart rate
Ventricular tachycardia	The usual ventricular rate is 160–240 bpm and results in syncope owing to decreased stroke volume. The usual mechanism is reentry, which is initiated by a premature atrial or ventricular beat. Causes include myocardial infarction, cardiomyopathy, myocarditis, and, occasionally, mitral valve prolapse
Atrial fibrillation	Atrial fibrillation may or may not result in tachycardia. Although the atria are not beating regularly, there may be a controlled ventricular response. In some cases, there is a rapid ventricular response resulting in tachycardia
Atrial flutter	In atrial flutter, the atrial rate is often over 250 bpm, but there is a variable ventricular response. In 2:1 or 3:1 flutter, the ventricular response may be close to normal, and the patient may have few or no symptoms

■ Chest Pain

The coronary arteries supply blood to the heart muscle. A blockage in one of the coronary arteries results in decreased blood supply, and when the lesion becomes significant, myocardial ischemia and chest pain occur. Blockage in the right coronary artery (RCA) results in damage to the posterior/inferior area of the heart. Blockage in the left main coronary artery (LCA) results in damage to the atrial, apical, lateral, and septal areas and is usually fatal. Blockage in the left anterior descending artery (LAD) results in damage to the anterior portion of the heart. Blockage in the circumflex branch (CFX) results in damage to the posterior and lateral areas.

History

Any complaint of chest pain should be thoroughly investigated in all patients. Initially, determine whether the patient is having an acute episode of cardiac chest pain and the need for emergent referral. Although it may be a low likelihood in seemingly young, healthy patients, a cardiac origin for the chest pain should always be kept on the list of differential diagnoses. Start by asking the patient about current medicines and comorbidities. Ask whether this is the first episode of chest pain or a recurrent attack. Ask how long the pain has been going on, whether it is constant or intermittent, and whether it radiates to either arm, back, neck, or jaw. Ask how long the pain lasts, what the pain is like, and where the level of pain lies on a scale of 0 to 10. Inquire about associated symptoms, such as shortness of breath, sweating, dizziness, syncope, nausea, vomiting, palpitations, or cough. Determine if the pain has a trigger or is associated with certain activities, such as exercise, sexual intercourse, eating, sleeping, stress, or strong emotions. Be sure to inquire about sports or exercise activities that could have resulted in injury to the intercostal muscles, ribs, or chest wall. Ask about alleviating or aggravating factors and whether the patient is taking any kind of medicine for the pain, either prescription or over the counter, or other alternative treatment.

Strong suspicion of a cardiac origin of the pain warrants prompt evaluation by a cardiologist or a referral to the emergency department. Characteristics that indicate angina include crushing, substernal pain with radiation to the neck or left arm, a score of greater than 7 on the pain scale, an association with exertion or stress with relief on rest, a duration of minutes and associated symptoms of nausea, diaphoresis, weakness, or shortness of breath.

Physical Examination

The physical examination is not definitive for ruling out myocardial infarction as the cause of the chest pain. Assess the patient's pain level and associated signs, such as changes in color (paleness or cyanosis), and the presence of dyspnea, diaphoresis, nausea, or vomiting. Listen to the heart and note any murmurs, arrhythmias, bradycardia, or tachycardia. Auscultate the lungs for rales/crackles or decreased breath sounds that might signal a pulmonary origin for the chest pain. If a pulmonary origin is suspected, percuss the lungs for areas of dullness and assess for voice sounds. For patients with obvious dyspnea, a pulse oximetry reading provides useful information. Palpate the chest wall for tenderness. The EKG, chest x-ray, and cardiac enzymes are most helpful in determining a cardiac origin for the chest pain.

With angina and MI, changes can be seen on the EKG. Each lead reflects an area of the heart, and EKG can determine the location of the ischemia. The lateral wall of the heart is reflected in Leads I, aVL, V_5, and V_6. The inferior wall is reflected in Leads II, III, and aVF. The anterior wall is reflected in Leads V_1, V_2, V_3, and V_4. The posterior wall is reflected in Leads V_1, V_2, and V_3. Reciprocal EKG changes can be seen in the area of the heart opposite the injured area.

Diagnostic Studies

- *MB CK*—The serum level of myocardial band creatine kinase is elevated 10 to 25 times above normal in the first few hours after MI and returns to normal within 2 to 4 days. The levels can also be elevated following trauma or with progressive muscular dystrophy.
- *Troponin*—An inhibitory protein found in muscle fibers, troponin is elevated within 4 hours of an MI and stays elevated for several days. It is more specific than creatine kinase for cardiac muscle.
- *EKG*—The practitioner should look for signs of MI, such as ST-segment elevation or depression, arrhythmias, and conduction delays. EKG is minimally helpful in diagnosing pericarditis except in the case of tamponade or constrictive pericarditis where decreased amplitude may be seen.
- *Graded exercise test (GXT)*—The stress test can assist in diagnosing CAD and angina and establishing safe exercise levels. The addition of the radioactive substance thallium helps determine the extent of coronary artery blockage and blood flow both at rest and with exercise.
- *Imaging*—Studies such as computed tomography (CT) scan, electron beam computed tomography (EBCT), positron emission tomography (PET), magnetic resonance imaging (MRI), and single photon emission computed tomography (SPECT) can assist in diagnosing CAD, aortic aneurysms, cardiac masses, myocardial disease, and pericardial disease.
- *Arterial blood gases (ABGs)*—These measures evaluate oxygenation and acid–base balance and can assist in ruling out pulmonary disease.
- *Chest x-ray*—Pneumonia, pulmonary masses or other pulmonary disease, heart size, and aortic aneurysms can be identified on x-rays.
- *Echocardiography*—There are currently three types of echocardiography: transthoracic (TTE), transesophageal (TEE) and 3-dimensional. TTE is noninvasive and is used for simple assessments of overal cardiac health including aneurysms, pericardial effusion, and other structural abnormalities in the chest. TEE and 3-d echocardiography are more invasive, but give a more detailed analysis of anatomical cardiac pathology particularly type and severity of valvular disease, and cardiomyopathy.
- *Cardiac catheterization*—If the chest pain is due to MI, cardiac catheterization can assess the need for revascularization or coronary artery bypass graft. Revascularization must be performed promptly, within a few hours

of onset of the MI, in order to minimize the amount of cardiac muscle damage.

- *Endoscopy*—Once a cardiac origin is ruled out, endoscopy can rule out a gastric cause for the pain.
- *Amylase/lipase*—Once a cardiac origin is ruled out, blood laboratory tests for GI causes should be initiated. Amylase/lipase measures will assist in the diagnosis of pancreatitis and cholecystitis.
- *Complete blood count (CBC), erythrocyte sedimentation rate (ESR), and chemistry panel*—These tests should be done if pericarditis is suspected.

ANGINA AND MYOCARDIAL INFARCTION (MI)

With a complaint of chest pain, the most life-threatening diagnosis should be ruled out first. A thorough history identifying the quality and quantity of the pain, alleviating and aggravating factors, and associated symptoms assists in raising or lowering your index of suspicion for a myocardial origin of the pain. Age, gender, weight, vital signs, family history, and medical history also assist in diagnosis.

Signs and Symptoms

Signs and symptoms that are suspicious for myocardial ischemia include crushing substernal chest pain that may radiate into the neck or left arm, diaphoresis, nausea, shortness of breath, and perhaps weakness. Pain that increases with physical activity and disappears at rest can indicate myocardial ischemia. Pain that occurs in the early morning or wakes a patient at night can also be cardiac in origin. Pain at rest is worrisome because it may signify unstable angina.

PERICARDITIS

Pericarditis, inflammation of the pericardium, is usually not seen as a solo disease process but in conjunction with other diseases or conditions. Pericarditis may occur as a complication of MI (Dressler's syndrome) or coronary artery bypass surgery. It is also more commonly seen in patients with connective tissue disorders such as rheumatoid arthritis, systemic lupus erythematosus (SLE), scleroderma, and sarcoidosis. Bacterial, viral, or fungal infections, including HIV, are risk factors for pericarditis. Pericarditis can occur with kidney failure, metastatic neoplasias, or as a reaction to medication, particularly phenytoin, hydralazine, and procainamide. Rarely, it is idiopathic and the cause is unknown, although a common viral infection is suspected. Cardiac tamponade can occur as a serious complication, and it is an emergency requiring immediate pericardiocentesis. Constrictive pericarditis can occur over time due to scarring of the pericardial sac.

Signs and Symptoms

Unlike the crushing, steady pain of angina and MI, the pain associated with pericarditis is sharp and stabbing; it may worsen with inspiration or when lying flat or leaning forward. Associated symptoms may include shortness of breath, fever, chills, and malaise.

THORACIC/ABDOMINAL AORTIC ANEURYSM

Thoracic aneurysms account for less than 10% of aortic aneurysms, are rarely symptomatic, and are usually found in routine examinations for other reasons. The history should include any chest trauma; hereditary connective tissue disorder, especially Marfan's or Ehlers-Danlos syndrome; congenital cardiac anomalies, such as coarctation, patent ductus arteriosus, or bicuspid aortic valve; and severe, longstanding hypertension.

Signs and Symptoms

Symptoms may include substernal or back pain as well as symptoms related to pressure on the trachea or esophagus, such as dyspnea, cough, hoarseness, and dysphagia. Superior vena cava syndrome may accompany thoracic aneurysm. The systolic murmur of aortic regurgitation may be heard in aneurysms of the ascending aorta. The risk of rupture depends on the diameter of the aneurysm. The long-term prognosis is generally poor. Surgical intervention is also risky, with a high rate of morbidity and mortality. Control of hypertension is imperative to prevent progression of the aneurysm.

GASTROESOPHAGEAL REFLUX (GERD) AND PEPTIC ULCER DISEASE (PUD)

It is often difficult to differentiate the pain of GERD or PUD from cardiac pain. A good history and diagnostic tests are necessary. Patients with a history of GERD or PUD should still be worked up for a cardiac origin, particularly if the characteristics of the pain or the history have changed to raise the index of suspicion for cardiac disease.

Signs and Symptoms

The pain of GERD and PUD can be severe and anxiety provoking. It is substernal and may be accompanied by nausea and diaphoresis if severe enough. Unlike cardiac pain, GERD tends to be worse at night when the patient is lying down, which is helpful in differentiating it from cardiac pain. Pain relieved with nitroglycerin or a "GI cocktail" cannot rule in or rule out a cardiac origin because GERD, PUD, and angina often respond to either or both treatments.

CHOLECYSTITIS

The history and location of the pain are good indicators for differentiating cholecystitis from angina. Cholecystitis is more common in young to middle-aged women and is seen more in those with a positive family history.

Signs and Symptoms

The pain of cholecystitis is generally colicky in nature and localized to the right upper quadrant. It is often accompanied by nausea and vomiting, and Murphy's sign is positive. Often there is fever and an elevated white count. Attacks are intermittent and are usually related to large or fatty meals. See Chapter 10 for further detail.

PANCREATITIS

Alcohol abuse accounts for more than 80% of pancreatitis, making the history most helpful. Other causes include hyperlipidemia, drugs, toxins, infection, structural abnormalities, surgery, vascular disease, trauma, hyperparathyroidism and hypercalcemia, renal transplantation, and hereditary pancreatitis.

Signs and Symptoms

The pain of pancreatitis is severe, steady, and "boring"—radiating from the epigastric region through to the back. It is often accompanied by nausea and vomiting, tachycardia, hypotension, and diaphoresis. The above symptoms are also seen in MI, however, the exquisite abdominal tenderness present in pancreatitis assists in differentiating it from cardiac pain. See Chapter 10 for details.

CHEST WALL PAIN AND COSTOCHONDRITIS

Chest wall pain can often be differentiated from cardiac pain through history. A history of injury; heavy lifting; contact sports; excessive coughing; or even late-stage pregnancy, which stretches the intercostal muscles, leads the examiner to consider chest wall pain. This often occurs in a younger population with no cardiac risk factors.

Signs and Symptoms

One of the most helpful differentiating symptoms is that the pain is increased with movement, cough, or in some cases, respiration. The pain tends to be less severe than with other causes and, generally, no accompanying symptoms occur.

PULMONARY DISEASE

Several pulmonary conditions can cause chest pain, most commonly, pulmonary embolism, pneumonia, pleurisy, and tumor. The symptoms vary widely depending on the underlying disease. See Chapter 8 for details.

Signs and Symptoms

Except in the case of pulmonary embolism, in which the pain can be sudden and severe, the pain accompanying pulmonary disease is often more insidious in onset, localized to the area of disease, less acute in nature, and less severe than the pain of myocardial ischemia. Shortness of breath is almost always an accompanying symptom, and, in some cases, cough is present. For details, see Chapter 8.

■ Patient History of Heart Murmur

Heart murmurs fall into two general categories: systolic and diastolic. Systolic murmurs are further categorized into pathologic, functional, and innocent murmurs. Diastolic murmurs are generally not considered to be functional or innocent. The following are the broad categories of the causes of murmurs with parenthetical examples:

- Flow across a partial obstruction (valvular stenosis)
- Flow across a valvular irregularity (bicuspid aortic valve)
- Increased flow through normal structures (anemia, pregnancy)
- Flow into a dilated chamber (aneurysm)
- Backward or regurgitant flow across an incompetent valve (valvular incompetence)
- Shunting of blood out of a high-pressure chamber through an abnormal passage (atrial or ventricular septal defect)

Grading of murmurs is based on a scale of I through VI. Grading murmurs is an experiential process, but the following characteristics can be used as a guide:

- Grade I—very faint, not heard in all positions
- Grade II—soft, but easily heard
- Grade III—moderately loud
- Grade IV—loud and may be associated with a thrill
- Grade V—very loud, may be heard with the stethoscope barely on the chest, associated with a thrill
- Grade VI—may be heard with the stethoscope off the chest, associated with a thrill

Murmurs should be described according to grade (intensity), location, radiation, pitch (high, medium, low), quality (blowing, rumbling, harsh, musical), and where they occur in the cardiac cycle.

History

One of the first questions to ask when a murmur is heard on examination is whether the patient has ever been told that he or she has a murmur and if any diagnostic testing has been done, particularly an echocardiogram. Inquire about palpitations, weakness or syncope, cough, exercise intolerance, endocarditis, and respiratory problems. A medical history is important for congenital anomalies or rheumatic fever.

Physical Examination

A thorough cardiac examination is performed with the patient sitting, leaning forward, lying, and in the left lateral recumbent position. Some murmurs are heard better in different positions. Listen over the carotids for radiation of an aortic or pulmonic murmur, in the left midaxillary line for radiation of a mitral murmur, and in the epigastric area for a bruit indicating an aneurysm. Assess the peripheral vascular system for bruits, pulses, and edema. Auscultate the lungs for crackles, which might indicate respiratory involvement.

SYSTOLIC MURMURS

Systolic murmurs occur between S_1 and S_2 and are broken down into ejection murmurs and regurgitant murmurs. Ejection murmurs are the most common type of systolic murmurs and are associated with forward flow through the semilunar valves. They have a crescendo–decrescendo pattern. Because systolic ejection murmurs are often physiologic, especially in children and pregnant women, they are further classified as pathologic, functional, or physiologic/innocent. Pathologic murmurs result from obstruction to forward flow through the semilunar valves (aortic stenosis, pulmonic stenosis, and hypertrophic cardiomyopathy [HCM]) or backward flow through the atrioventricular valves (mitral regurgitation, tricuspid regurgitation).

AORTIC STENOSIS

Aortic stenosis is heard best in the second right intercostal space with the client leaning forward. The murmur is harsh, loud, and often associated with a thrill. It may radiate to the neck, left sternal border, and in some cases, to the apex.

Associated physical findings include the following: an early ejection click, a diminished S_2, a heave or sustained apical impulse with left ventricular hypertrophy (LVH), crackles at the lung bases with left ventricular failure, jugular venous distention, hepatomegaly, and peripheral edema with right ventricular failure.

Signs and Symptoms

Syncope, angina, and dyspnea on exertion are the classic symptoms of aortic stenosis. If syncope occurs with exertion, the aortic stenosis is severe. Angina may be present because of decreased perfusion of the left ventricle due to LVH rather than CAD, but both exist in many cases. Treatment includes medical and/or surgical intervention.

Diagnostic Studies

- *Chest x-ray*—X-ray is helpful for outlining the heart border in LVH. Calcification of the aortic valve may be visible on x-ray.
- *EKG*—EKG may show evidence of LVH. On examination, look for other signs of LVH, such as a left ventricular heave and an S_4.
- *Echocardiography*—This diagnostic can determine the presence or absence and the severity of aortic stenosis.
- *Graded exercise test*—GXT is helpful in determining the severity of aortic stenosis.
- *Cardiac catheterization*—The definitive study for the severity of aortic stenosis, cardiac catheterization measures systolic blood flow across the aortic valve along with pressure differences between the left ventricle and the aorta.

PULMONIC STENOSIS

Pulmonic stenosis, less common than aortic stenosis, is heard best at the third left intercostal space. The quality of the murmur is harsh, of medium pitch, and, if loud, may be associated with a thrill. It is the second most common form of congenital heart disease. It is more common in women, and about two-thirds of adults are hemodynamically insignificant.

Signs and Symptoms

In patients with severe pulmonic stenosis, dyspnea, cyanosis, syncope on exertion, palpitations, and right heart failure can occur.

Diagnostic Studies

- *Chest x-ray*—Unless right ventricular failure occurs, the heart may not appear enlarged on x-ray. Pulmonary artery dilatation is commonly seen but does not reflect the severity of the disease.
- *EKG*—EKG changes in mild pulmonic stenosis are minimal, but in severe obstruction to right ventricular flow, peaked P waves can be seen and sometimes right bundle branch block.
- *Echocardiography*—This study can be helpful in determining the degree of right ventricular hypertrophy and in distinguishing pulmonic stenosis from other lesions.
- *Cardiac catheterization*—As in aortic stenosis, cardiac catheterization is the definitive diagnostic test for the presence and severity of pulmonic stenosis.

HYPERTROPHIC CARDIOMYOPATHY (HCM)

Hypertrophic cardiomyopathy has also been termed idiopathic hypertrophic subaortic stenosis or asymmetrical septal hypertrophy. Clinical findings include a grade 4/6 systolic murmur heard at the left sternal border that increases when upright and decreases with squatting, and an S_4. The cause of HCM is unknown but is thought to be genetic. Manifestations may not be apparent until adulthood, and it is generally seen in conjunction with essential hypertension.

Signs and Symptoms

The most common presenting symptoms are dyspnea on exertion and chest pain. Although the chest pain mimics that of angina, it is not relieved by nitroglycerin. Syncope is also a common complaint and may be more severe after exertion. Both atrial and ventricular arrhythmias can occur and are problematic. Atrial fibrillation may occur as a result of a chronic elevation of left atrial pressure. Ventricular arrhythmias can cause sudden death especially after extreme exertion. This illuminates the importance of a good history and physical for athletic screening. Questions regarding a family history of sudden death, dyspnea on exertion, syncopal episodes during or after exercise, and chest pain warrant diagnostic testing.

Diagnostic Studies

- *Echocardiography*—In the case of HCM, electrocardiography is diagnostic, and more invasive studies generally are not necessary. Echocardiogram findings include asymmetric LVH, a hypercontractile left ventricle, and delayed diastolic filling of the left ventricle.
- *Cardiac catheterization*—This diagnostic procedure may be helpful but generally is not necessary for diagnosis.

MITRAL REGURGITATION

The murmur of mitral regurgitation is heard best in the apex, often with radiation to the left axilla. It is pansystolic, high pitched, and blowing and may be associated with a thrill. There may be a decreased S_1, an S_3, and a sustained apical impulse owing to LVH. Secondary left atrial enlargement results from systolic backflow into the left atrium.

Signs and Symptoms

Dyspnea is the most common presenting symptom. Palpitations are common, and atrial fibrillation may develop. Complications include embolism, usually secondary to the atrial fibrillation. Bacterial endocarditis occurs most frequently (20%) in patients with mitral incompetence.

Diagnostic Studies

- *Chest x-ray*—The left atrium and left ventricle are enlarged proportionate to the severity of the disease.
- *EKG*—Atrial arrhythmias are common, particularly atrial fibrillation. Right and left bundle branches are uncommon. The main change seen is higher voltage.
- *Echocardiography*—In addition to visualizing the diseased valve, echocardiography can assist in determining the size of the left atrium and left ventricle.
- *Cardiac catheterization*—In patients with hemodynamically significant mitral regurgitation, cardiac catheterization is the definitive choice for determining the need for surgical intervention.

MITRAL VALVE PROLAPSE (MVP)

MVP, also termed *click-murmur syndrome*, is a variant of mitral regurgitation and occurs in approximately 10% of young women. MVP generally is hemodynamically insignificant and characterized by normal heart size and dynamics, although the process can progress to hemodynamically significant mitral regurgitation. Characteristically, a portion of the mitral valve balloons into the left atrium, giving rise to a midsystolic click followed by a soft grade I murmur that crescendos up to S_2. It is high pitched and is heard best at the apex or left sternal border. Some patients with MVP have only a murmur and no click, and others have only a click and no murmur.

Signs and Symptoms

Patients are usually asymptomatic but may complain of palpitations. It is of concern only in that antibiotic prophylaxis is needed in some cases for surgical and dental procedures to avoid the rare chance of subacute bacterial endocarditis.

Diagnostic Studies

* *Echocardiography*—In addition to visualizing the diseased valve, echocardiography can assist in determining the size of the left atrium and left ventricle. No other diagnostics should be necessary for diagnosing MVP.
* *Holter monitor*—If the patient complains of frequent palpitations related to MVP, a Holter monitor might be indicated to determine if the palpitations are benign, and the patient can be reassured.

TRICUSPID REGURGITATION

The murmur of tricuspid regurgitation is heard best at the left sternal border and may radiate to the right of the sternum. It is pansystolic, high pitched, and blowing, and it increases with respiration. Tricuspid regurgitation may be associated with right ventricular hypertrophy resulting in a right parasternal lift. When right ventricular failure occurs, jugular venous distention occurs with a prominent *v* wave, and liver enlargement may be present. There may be secondary right atrial enlargement owing to backflow into the right atrium. The most common initiator is pulmonary hypertension; it may also be a secondary result of left ventricular failure.

Signs and Symptoms

Symptoms are consistent with the right ventricular low-output state (i.e., fatigue, fullness in the abdomen, ankle swelling, and in late stages, ascites). Right upper quadrant discomfort may be present due to liver congestion. Atrial fibrillation or flutter occurs as the right atrium enlarges, giving rise to right ventricular failure.

Diagnostic Studies

* *Chest x-ray*—The right atrium and right ventricle are enlarged proportionate to the severity of the disease.
* *EKG*—Atrial arrhythmias, particularly atrial fibrillation are common. Bundle branch blocks are uncommon. The main change seen is higher voltage.
* *Echocardiography*—In addition to visualizing the diseased valve, echocardiography can assist in determining the size of the right atrium and right ventricle.
* *Swan-Ganz pressure readings*—The *v* peak and the *y* trough are exaggerated during inspiration.

PHYSIOLOGIC OR FUNCTIONAL MURMURS

Physiologic or functional murmurs are systolic murmurs caused by a temporary increase in blood flow rather than by a structural abnormality and include such conditions as anemia, hyperthyroidism, pregnancy, and fever.

INNOCENT MURMURS

This type of systolic murmur results from turbulent blood flow and is not associated with heart disease. Innocent murmurs occur commonly in children and young adults and reflect the contractile force of the heart resulting in greater velocity of flow during early systole. They are heard best in the second and third left interspaces along the left sternal border or at the apex. They are short, heard in early systole, and are less than grade III. Innocent murmurs often disappear with the patient in a sitting position.

DIASTOLIC MURMURS

Unlike some physiologic causes of functional or innocent systolic murmurs, diastolic murmurs almost always indicate pathology.

MITRAL STENOSIS

Mitral stenosis results from thickening and stiffening of the mitral valve, usually secondary to rheumatic fever. The murmur is generally grade I to IV and low pitched; therefore, it is heard better with the bell at the apex in the left lateral recumbent position. The first heart sound (S_1) is loud, followed by S_2 and a loud opening snap that precedes the murmur.

Signs and Symptoms

The most common presenting symptoms are dyspnea on exertion and hemoptysis due to pulmonary congestion. The pulmonary congestion is caused by increased left atrial pressure related to the decrease in left atrial emptying. Crackles may be heard at the lung bases but are not present in all patients with pulmonary congestion. Orthopnea may be present because the lungs become more congested in the recumbent position. When the heart rate is increased as a result of fever, exertion, anxiety, or infection, congestion worsens and pulmonary edema may result. In addition, atrial fibrillation often develops in patients with mitral stenosis, which in turn worsens the pulmonary congestion. Over time, increased pulmonary vascular resistance may lead to right ventricular hypertrophy.

Diagnostic Studies

- *EKG*—Broad, notched P waves will provide evidence that mitral stenosis exists, but the EKG is not helpful in determining the severity. If right ventricular hypertrophy is present, it is manifested by right axis deviation.
- *Chest x-ray*—The heart size may be normal, or the left atrium may be enlarged, but enlargement of the pulmonary artery is usually not seen until the pressures in the pulmonary artery are high. Radiographic changes in the chest that signify chronic pulmonary congestion are Kerley B lines, which are seen as thickened, interlobular septa, particularly at the outer edges of the lungs.

- *Echocardiography*—In addition to visualizing the diseased valve, echocardiography can assist in determining the size of the left atrium and left ventricle.
- *Cardiac catheterization*—Heart catheterization is the definitive diagnostic study to determine the severity of the mitral stenosis.

TRICUSPID STENOSIS

Tricuspid stenosis is most often caused by rheumatic fever and almost always accompanies the dominant mitral stenosis. The right atrium becomes hypertrophied with a small right ventricle. Physical examination findings include a low-pitched, rumbling middiastolic murmur, heard at the left sternal border in the fourth interspace, that increases with inspiration. The duration of the murmur is related to the severity of the stenosis and the stroke volume.

Signs and Symptoms

Patients complain of fatigue and possibly right upper quadrant discomfort related to an enlarged liver. There is an accentuated *a* wave in the jugular venous pulse.

Diagnostic Studies

- *EKG*—The EKG will show peaked P waves in the inferior leads because of an overload of the right atrium.
- *Chest x-ray*—An enlarged superior vena cava and enlarged right atrium are revealed.
- *Echocardiography*—In addition to visualizing the diseased valve, echocardiography can assist in determining the size of the left atrium and left ventricle.
- *Cardiac catheterization*—Catheterization is helpful in determining the pressure gradients across the tricuspid valve and the severity of the valvular stenosis.

AORTIC INSUFFICIENCY/REGURGITATION

Aortic regurgitation results from failure of the leaflets of the aortic valve to close completely during diastole. This causes a backflow of blood from the aorta into the left ventricle. The murmur of aortic regurgitation is heard best in the second, third, and fourth interspaces, just to the left of the sternum. The quality is blowing, high pitched, and usually grade III or less. It may radiate to the apex, and having the patient sitting and leaning forward aids in hearing the murmur. Volume overload of the left ventricle occurs owing to the backflow of blood, which can lead to LVH. In this case, the apical impulse is accentuated, and a left ventricular heave is seen. An accompanying S_3 or S_4 indicates significant regurgitation. There may be an associated midsystolic murmur caused by the increased volume of blood flowing through the aortic valve. The most common cause of aortic insufficiency is infective endocarditis associated with rheumatic fever. In acute infectious destruction of the aortic valve, dyspnea, orthopnea, and cough are the most common presenting cardiac symptoms, resulting from pulmonary edema. This is often life threatening, and prompt treatment is necessary.

Signs and Symptoms

In chronic aortic regurgitation, patients often complain of palpitations. If these are caused by ventricular arrhythmias, a thorough investigation is necessary to avoid a lethal ventricular arrhythmia. If LVH and failure develop, the symptoms typically are dyspnea and chest pain. An unexplained symptom of patients with aortic incompetence is increased sweating, which is thought to involve the cholinergic sympathetic vasodilator fibers. The greater volume of blood being pumped out of the ventricle increases the systolic pressure, causing a widened pulse pressure.

Diagnostic Studies

- *EKG*—In patients with hemodynamically significant aortic regurgitation, LVH is reflected on the EKG by increased height of the R waves in the left-sided chest leads, increased depth of the S waves in the right-sided chest leads, and associated S-T changes.
- *Chest x-ray*—In chronic, severe aortic regurgitation, the chest x-ray shows an enlarged left ventricle and aortic dilatation. Confirmation with EKG is prudent.
- *Echocardiography*—In addition to visualizing the diseased valve, echocardiography can assist in determining the size of the left atrium and left ventricle.
- *Cardiac catheterization*—Catheterization is preferred over echocardiography for definitive diagnosis of aortic valve disease causing rapid aortic runoff. It is also useful in determining heart pressures and pulmonary vascular resistance.

PULMONIC INSUFFICIENCY/REGURGITATION

Pulmonary insufficiency rarely occurs in patients without pulmonary hypertension and is usually seen in conjunction with right ventricular hypertrophy. This diastolic murmur is high pitched, heard best at the base, and difficult to distinguish from aortic incompetence.

Signs and Symptoms

Pulmonary regurgitation rarely occurs except in conjunction with pulmonary hypertension, and the symptoms are consistent with cor pulmonale. Progressive exertional dyspnea is present in the majority of cases.

Diagnostic Studies

See Diagnostic Studies under Aortic Insufficiency/Regurgitation.

VENTRICULAR SEPTAL DEFECT (VSD)

VSD is a congenital heart defect in which oxygenated blood is shunted from a higher-pressured left ventricle to a lower-pressured right ventricle through an abnormal opening in the ventricular septum. This left-to-right shunt causes an increased blood flow across the pulmonic valve. The signs and symptoms depend on the size of the defect and the age of the patient. Characteristic of a VSD is a loud, harsh, pansystolic murmur at the lower left sternal border usually accompanied by a thrill. If the shunt is large, there is a middiastolic murmur of mitral flow heard at the apex, elevated pulmonary artery pressure, and possible heart failure.

Signs and Symptoms

Adult patients with large defects usually complain of dyspnea on exertion. In children, VSDs are often accompanied by other congenital anomalies and can be life threatening if not surgically repaired. Small defects can be clinically insignificant and may become smaller or even close as the child grows.

Diagnostic Studies

- *EKG*—The EKG initially shows signs of LVH (tall R waves and inverted T waves in leads II, III, aVF, and V_6), but as right ventricular and pulmonary artery pressures increase, changes consistent with right ventricular hypertrophy are seen (tall R wave in V_1, small R wave in V_6, prominent S wave in V_6, and right axis deviation).
- *Chest x-ray*—Left and right ventricular enlargement, cardiomegaly, and an enlarged pulmonary artery are seen on x-ray.
- *Echocardiography*—In addition to visualizing the diseased valve, echocardiography can assist in determining the size of the left atrium and left ventricle.
- *Cardiac catheterization*—A heart catheterization is necessary prior to corrective surgery to determine the size and location of the VSD, the severity of pulmonary vascular resistance, and the presence of other congenital anomalies, such as patent ductus arteriosus or coarctation of the aorta.

ATRIAL SEPTAL DEFECT (ASD)

Atrial septal defect (ASD) is a congenital abnormality in which oxygenated blood is shunted from a higher-pressured left atrium to a lower-pressured right atrium through an abnormal opening in the atrial septum. This causes an increased blood flow across the tricuspid valve and to the lungs. A visible pulsation over the second and third left intercostal space may be seen because of an increased right ventricular stroke volume. A pulmonic systolic ejection murmur is present owing to the increased blood flow through the pulmonary valve. Tricuspid stenosis likewise develops as a result of the increased diastolic flow across the tricuspid valve, producing a diastolic murmur. There is fixed splitting of the second heart sound. Atrial arrhythmias, especially atrial fibrillation, are common in the adult population with ASD.

Signs and Symptoms

ASDs are often accompanied by other congenital heart defects, but in an uncomplicated lesion, patients are often asymptomatic until early adulthood, when they present with dyspnea on exertion or palpitations resulting from atrial arrhythmia. Because patients may be asymptomatic for many years, right heart failure can be the first sign, and patients may present with edema and ascites.

Diagnostic Studies

- *EKG*—A majority of patients with ASD have a right ventricular conduction defect, and in older patients, a prolonged P-R interval is also common. Evidence of right ventricular hypertrophy may be present.
- *Chest x-ray*—The heart is usually enlarged, and the pulmonary artery and branches are dilated. The right atrium and ventricle are enlarged, although right atrial enlargement can be difficult to determine.
- *Echocardiography*—These studies are helpful to visualize right ventricular enlargement and movement of the mitral and tricuspid valves.
- *Cardiac catheterization*—Although the preceding studies are helpful in diagnosis, cardiac catheterization is essential for confirmation of ASD.

■ Elevated Blood Pressure

From The Seventh Report of the Joint National Committee on Detection, Education, and Treatment of High Blood Pressure (Chobanian et al., 2003), the classification and follow-up of blood pressure measurements are as follows.

Category	Systolic Blood Pressure, mm Hg*	Diastolic Blood Pressure, mm Hg*	Follow-Up
Normal	Less than 120	Less than 80	Recheck in 2 years
Prehypertension	120–139	80–90	Recheck within 2 months; lifestyle modifications
Hypertension Stage 1	140–159	90–99	Confirm within 2 weeks; single drug treatment necessary
Stage 2	≥160	≥100	Two-drug combination for most patients; recheck 1–2 weeks

*Classification is based on the average of two or more readings on two or more occasions after initial screening.

History

It is important to determine whether there is a medical history or family history of hypertension. Identify the medications the patient is taking. Ask about lifestyle behaviors including smoking, alcohol, drugs, and exercise. Inquire about the presence of chronic disease in the patient or family that may cause or contribute to hypertension. The subjective complaints depend on the type of hypertension.

Physical Examination

The blood pressure should be measured in both arms and lying, sitting, and standing. Measure temperature, pulse, and respirations, and note fever, tachycardia, or tachypnea. Upper and lower extremity pulses should be compared to look for coarctation. The abdomen should be auscultated for aortic and renal artery bruits. The heart should be examined for an S_3 or S_4 indicating decreased compliance of the left ventricle and ventricular hypertrophy, a systolic ejection murmur that might indicate aortic stenosis, or the diastolic murmur of aortic insufficiency. The eyes should be examined for exophthalmos and the retinas inspected for such hypertensive changes as hemorrhages, exudates, A-V nicking, copper or silver wire appearance, or papilledema, which might point to a more serious neurologic cause.

PRIMARY (ESSENTIAL) HYPERTENSION

Approximately 10% to 15% of Caucasians and 20% to 30% of African Americans in the United States have primary hypertension. The pathophysiology of primary hypertension is varied. Genetic factors are significant contributors, especially if both parents are hypertensive. Other factors include sympathetic nervous system hypersensitivity, decreased ability to balance sodium and calcium, and a renin-angiotensin-aldosterone imbalance. Factors that may exacerbate the predisposition to develop hypertension include a sedentary lifestyle, obesity, smoking, alcohol, sodium intake in some individuals, low potassium intake, polycythemia, and long-term use of NSAIDs.

Signs and Symptoms

In primary hypertension, symptoms may be absent. Some patients complain of a throbbing headache that is usually worse in the morning. Some patients state that they can hear their heart beating in their ears when it is quiet or when they go to bed at night.

Diagnostic Studies

- *TSH, T_3, and T_4*—These hormones are measured to identify thyroid disease.
- *Electrolytes*—K^+ is decreased and Na^+ increased in hyperaldosteronism.
- *Fasting blood glucose*—Hyperglycemia is seen in pheochromocytoma.
- *Renal chemistries*—These studies identify renal parenchymal disease.

- *Urinalysis*—This test is used to determine specific gravity, proteinuria, hematuria, or casts that might indicate renal parenchymal disease.
- *24-Hour urine for catecholamines*—The presence of urine catecholamines assists in the diagnosis of pheochromocytoma.
- *Echocardiography*—Heart defects are identified by echocardiography studies.
- *Renal Doppler ultrasound*—This procedure identifies renal vascular disease.
- *Renal arteriography*—Renal arteriography is used to identify renal vascular disease.
- *CT or MRI*—These procedures can identify renal vascular disease, adrenal adenoma, adrenal hyperplasia, or pheochromocytoma.
- *Chest x-ray*—Coarctation of the aorta is revealed on x-ray.
- *EKG or echocardiography*—These procedures can identify ventricular hypertrophy or valvular disease in patients with known cardiac disease.

SECONDARY HYPERTENSION

A small percentage of patients have specific, identifiable causes of hypertension, particularly those who develop hypertension at an early age with no family history, those whose previously controlled hypertension suddenly becomes uncontrolled, and those who first develop hypertension after age 50. There are several causes of secondary hypertension, including renal parenchymal disease, such as glomerulonephritis, pyelonephritis, tuberculosis of the kidney, or scarring from trauma; renal arterial disease, such as renal artery stenosis, aneurysm, embolism, or infarction; renal tumors; coarctation of the aorta; endocrine disorders, such as pheochromocytoma, primary aldosteronism, Cushing's syndrome, thyroid disease, or acromegaly; hypercalcemia; pregnancy; neurological disorders, such as tumor or trauma causing increased intracranial pressure; and medications, such as hormone replacement therapy, oral contraceptives, prolonged use of corticosteroids, NSAIDs, theophylline, or cold preparations containing ephedrine.

Signs and Symptoms

In secondary hypertension, the symptoms are consistent with the underlying etiology. Listen for complaints such as nervousness, diaphoresis, palpitations, dyspnea, tremor, muscle weakness, polyuria, nocturia, nausea, or vomiting.

Diagnostic Studies

See Diagnostic Studies under Primary Hypertension.

■ Elevated Lipids

Dyslipidemia is a disproportionate amount of deleterious lipids in the blood leading to an increase in atherosclerotic heart disease. The amount of high-density lipoprotein (HDL) and low-density protein (LDL) seem to be most important for both primary and secondary prevention of heart disease. The aim for primary prevention is to keep LDL levels below 130 mg/dL (less than 100 is optimal) and HDL levels above 40 mg/dL. Although primary prevention lowers a person's risk of heart disease and MI, it has shown only small, if any, effect on all-cause mortality. In patients with known coronary disease or diabetes, the target cholesterol levels are more stringent, aiming for an LDL level below 100 mg/dL and an HDL level above 60 mg/dL. Raising HDL may be more important than lowering LDL to protect against heart disease, and this may be particularly true for women. The complete guidelines for management of hyperlipidemia can be found in the National Heart, Lung, and Blood Institute ATP III Guidelines (2003).

Patients over the age of 40 years should be screened every 1 to 2 years and elevated lipids treated aggressively with diet and exercise, weight loss, and lipid-lowering drugs when necessary. The relationship of hyperlipidemia to heart disease lessens with age and, therefore, patients over 75 years of age without heart disease or other risk factors are treated less aggressively.

History

The history includes screening for the risk factors listed in Box 7.2 in addition to any history of elevated lipids.

Physical Examination

The physical examination includes measurement of height and weight to calculate body mass index (BMI). The formula for calculating BMI is $wt(kg)/ht(m^2)$. A waist/hip ratio is also an indicator for risk of heart disease. A ratio greater than 0.85 for women and greater than 0.95 for men is considered to place individuals at increased risk, especially if accompanied by hyperinsulinemia or diabetes. These are part of a constellation of symptoms, termed syndrome X or metabolic syndrome, that indicate the greatest risk for the development of heart disease.

SYNDROME X OR METABOLIC SYNDROME

A cluster of risk factors known as syndrome X, or metabolic syndrome, when occurring together, seem to dramatically increase the risk for CAD, diabetes, and stroke. Lack of physical activity and poor dietary habits lead to a

---

Box 7.2

Risk Factors for Dyslipidemia

Obesity	Hypothyroidism
Sedentary lifestyle	Chronic renal disease
Diabetes	Obstructive liver disease
Positive family history	Cushing's disease
High-fat diet	Medications, particularly progestins, androgenic
Alcohol use	steroids, β-blockers
Tobacco	

positive energy balance, increased body fat, and insulin resistance. Therefore, obesity may be the underlying factor causing the regulation defect in the insulin receptor, thus promoting insulin resistance. The more calories consumed, the more insulin is needed to store the glucose and break down protein and fat. As fat cells become full, they become less sensitive to insulin, increasing the amount of insulin needed to perform the same work. Eventually, the body loses its ability to increase insulin secretion. Decreased secretion and insulin resistance impair sugar storage, leading to increased circulating glucose and a tendency for the increased sugar to be converted to fat, thus increasing the risk for type 2 diabetes and dyslipidemia, which leads to atherosclerosis.

Characteristics of Metabolic Syndrome

Hypertension
Dyslipidemia
Central obesity
Glucose intolerance with hyperinsulinemia (insulin resistance)

Treating only one of these risk factors does not lower morbidity and, in some cases, makes other risk factors worse. Weight loss through diet and exercise has been found to be the most important factor in the prevention of the progression of this syndrome. Insulin sensitivity increases with weight loss and is thought to be due to the loss of visceral fat. The target BMI is less than 22 kg/m^2 for women and less than 27 kg/m^2 for men. Weight loss will also reduce hypertension and improve the lipid profile. Aerobic and resistance exercise assists in weight loss and improves carbohydrate and lipid metabolism. Medication for hypertension and dyslipidemia may be necessary in patients who do not make necessary lifestyle changes or who are slow to make significant improvement.

GENETIC HYPERLIPIDEMIA

Two genetic disorders that result in dyslipidemia are familial hypercholesterolemia and familial hyperchylomicronemia, which cause extremely high levels of LDL and triglycerides respectively. Persons with familial hypercholesterolemia may develop atherosclerotic disease in childhood and CAD by age 30 to 40 years. Persons with familial hyperchylomicronemia may develop recurrent pancreatitis and hepatosplenomegaly in childhood.

Signs and Symptoms

Generally, patients are made aware of their hyperlipidemia only from laboratory blood tests. Occasionally, lipid plaque, called xanthelasma, develops around the eyes, but it is not apparent until hyperlipidemia has been present for some time.

Diagnostic Studies

- *Lipid panel*—The lipid panel measures triglycerides, total cholesterol, HDL, LDL, and a total cholesterol/HDL ratio as a risk for heart disease. More sophisticated lipid profiles measure particle size, which gives a more accurate picture of cardiac risk.
- *Glucose*—Fasting glucose should be measured because type 2 diabetes is often responsible for hyperlipidemia.
- *Insulin*—Insulin levels are not part of a routine workup, although they are helpful in detecting hyperinsulinemia and early type 2 diabetes.
- *Thyroid panel*—Hypothyroidism affects lipid levels and should be ruled out before placing a patient on lipid-lowering drugs.
- *Genetic testing*—Children with significant hyperlipidemia may warrant genetic testing.

■ Difficulty Breathing and Shortness of Breath

Dyspnea, or shortness of breath, has many causes, including cardiac or pulmonary disease, anxiety, obesity, and anemia. Patients with a cardiac cause may also complain of increased symptoms with exertion and dyspnea that wake them up at night and are relieved by sitting up. This paroxysmal nocturnal dyspnea (PND) is one of the early signs of heart failure and therefore is more specific for cardiac disease. Dyspnea caused by cardiac disease results most commonly from left ventricular dysfunction and/or valvular disease.

History

The history should include history of respiratory disease, heart failure, MI, heart murmur, arrhythmias, rheumatic fever, angioplasty, or cardiac surgeries. Inquire about other serious illnesses or hospitalizations and about current medicines, both prescription and over the counter. The review of systems should include chest pain, hypertension, palpitations, dyspnea on exertion, PND, cough, fatigue, weight gain or loss, and last EKG. A thorough respiratory review of systems should also be done, which includes history of productive cough, asthma, wheezing, pleurisy, bronchitis, pneumonia, hemoptysis, tuberculosis, last chest x-ray, and purified protein derivative (PPD) tuberculin test. A smoking history is also essential.

Physical Examination

The general survey includes any acute respiratory distress at rest, cyanosis, anxiety, restlessness, or confusion. Monitor vital signs for tachycardia, tachypnea, hypotension, or narrow pulse pressure, which could indicate ventricular dysfunction. A thorough examination of the lungs, heart, neck, abdomen, and extremities should be done. Auscultate the lungs for adventitious sounds, particularly crackles at the bases, which might indicate heart failure. Other adventitious sounds could indicate a respiratory rather than cardiac cause. Keep in mind that obstructive lung disease is often complicated by cardiac disease, so there may be more than one disease process occurring. Percuss the lungs for areas of dullness, indicating fluid or solid mass, such as pneumonia, pleural effusion, cancer, or pulmonary fibrosis. If possible, pulse oximetry provides valuable information about oxygenation. Inspect the precordium for a parasternal lift or accentuated apical impulse indicating ventricular hypertrophy. Palpate the precordium for a thrill indicating at least a grade IV murmur. Auscultate all cardiac areas for murmurs indicating valvular heart disease, an S_3 related to volume overload and heart failure, an S_4 usually heard in diastolic failure, and any arrhythmias that could be either a cause or a result of heart failure. The neck should be examined for jugular venous distention with the patient's head elevated to 30 degrees. This is a sign of right-sided heart failure. Auscultate the carotids for bruits or murmurs that may radiate into the neck, usually aortic in origin. Palpate the thyroid for enlargement or nodules because hyper- and hypothyroidism can both cause heart failure. The abdomen should be examined particularly for right upper quadrant discomfort related to hepatic congestion and enlargement, secondary to right heart failure. Check for hepatic jugular reflux by placing sustained pressure on the liver while observing for jugular venous distention. In right heart failure, ascites may also be present. Examine the extremities for pitting edema seen in heart failure.

Diagnostic Studies

- *CBC*—A CBC should be done to check for anemia, which could cause or worsen dyspnea and heart failure.
- *Chemistry panel*—A chemistry panel should be ordered to check renal function, liver function, and electrolyte balance—particularly hypokalemia, which can cause arrhythmias.
- *Thyroid profile*—It is wise to rule out hyper- or hypothyroidism.
- *Pro-brain natriuretic peptide (pro-BNP)*—For patients with comorbid respiratory disease, this blood test can help differentiate a cardiac from a respiratory etiology of dyspnea.
- *Chest x-ray*—Most importantly, the x-ray reveals the presence of cardiomegaly, which can assist in the diagnosis of heart failure as a cause of the dyspnea. Look for fluid at the bases, flattening of diaphragms in chronic obstructive pulmonary disease (COPD), tumors in cancer, increased markings, interstitial edema, atelectasis, or pneumonia. Pulmonary vasculature may be normal, especially in chronic heart failure. Pleural effusions indicate heart failure or metastatic cancer, and thoracentesis is indicated to examine the fluid for malignant cells.
- *Echocardiography*—These diagnostics show the size and function of the ventricles if heart failure is thought to be the cause of the dyspnea. They can also be helpful in detecting shunts and pericardial effusion and for visualizing the heart valves for abnormalities.
- *Cardiac catheterization*—This procedure may be necessary only when valvular disease is thought to be the cause of the dyspnea or if left

ventricular dysfunction is caused by myocardial ischemia and revascularization is a treatment consideration.

CONGESTIVE HEART FAILURE

Congestive heart failure (CHF) can occur at any age depending on underlying diseases, but as a primary diagnosis, it is more common in the elderly. There are four main determinants of systolic function:

1. *Myocardial contractility*—A decrease in contractility can result from a loss of functional muscle caused by MI or other diseases affecting the myocardium. A decrease in contractility results in decreased stroke volume.

2. *Heart rate*—When the stroke volume decreases, the heart attempts to compensate by increasing heart rate. When increased heart rate cannot compensate, cardiac output decreases, leading to heart failure. Bradycardia can occur in a number of cardiac conditions, which are outlined in this chapter under Bradyarrhythmias. Also, bradycardia in a nonathlete can lead to decreased cardiac output and ensuing heart failure.

3. *Preload*—Preload is determined by the end-diastolic stretch of the ventricular muscle fibers. This is equal to the end-diastolic volume or pressure. If preload is excessively elevated, pump failure can result. This occurs with valvular regurgitation. Starling's law states that the force of the heartbeat is determined by the length of the fibers constituting the muscular wall; that is, an increase in diastolic filling increases the force of the heartbeat.

4. *Afterload*—Afterload is the ventricular wall tension during systole, which determines the impedance to ejection of blood from the left ventricle. If afterload is excessive, the heart cannot pump adequately against increased resistance. This can be seen in severe hypertension or aortic stenosis.

Heart failure also can occur when supply cannot meet demand as a result of high output states, such as severe anemia and thyrotoxicosis. Other, less common causes of high output states are arteriovenous shunting and Paget's disease of the bone.

Signs and Symptoms

One of the early signs of CHF is paroxysmal nocturnal dyspnea. Patients also may complain of dyspnea on exertion, nonproductive cough, and fatigue. Signs include ankle or pretibial edema, rapid weight gain caused by fluid retention, bibasilar crackles, tachycardia with a gallop rhythm, and hypoxia. By symptom, left ventricular failure is most commonly characterized by dyspnea on exertion, cough, fatigue, orthopnea, paroxysmal nocturnal dyspnea, cardiac enlargement, crackles, gallop rhythm, and pulmonary congestion. Right ventricular failure is more commonly characterized by dependent edema, elevated venous pressure, hepatomegaly, and possibly ascites. Although left and right failure can occur independently, they often occur together, and left ventricular failure is the most common cause of right ventricular failure.

RESPIRATORY DISEASE

Dyspnea is a symptom in many respiratory diseases, which are covered in Chapter 8. A holistic look at the patient—including age, history, such habits as smoking and alcohol use, and comorbid conditions—can assist the practitioner in differentiating a cardiac from a respiratory origin for dyspnea.

LIVER DISEASE

Severe liver diseases, resulting in ascites, can cause venous congestion and dyspnea. These symptoms generally occur in end-stage liver disease and are secondary to the more serious symptoms of liver disease, such as jaundice, bleeding, right upper quadrant pain, and encephalopathy. Liver disease is easily diagnosed by laboratory tests, ultrasound, and biopsy. See Chapter 10.

RENAL DISEASE

As in liver disease, dyspnea is a secondary symptom in renal failure as a result of fluid retention. Renal failure can be a cause of heart failure, and dyspnea is one of the early symptoms. Laboratory testing for renal function, as well as urinalysis, will assist in diagnosis. See Chapter 11.

■ Acute and Subacute Bacterial Endocarditis

Bacterial endocarditis is a microbial infection of the endocardium. The most common causative organisms are *Staphylococcus aureus*, group A streptococcus, pneumococcus, and gonococcus. Although the incidence of subacute bacterial endocarditis has been fairly stable over the last few decades, it has increased in the elderly owing to stiff, sclerotic valves. Other risk factors include intravenous drug use, dental disease, and invasive diagnostic procedures. Nosocomial infections have increased in open-heart surgery patients. The disease may be acute or subacute, and recurrences are not uncommon. If untreated, bacterial endocarditis is fatal because of a variety of complications. Prompt referral and hospitalization are necessary for antibiotic therapy and other supportive measures. As prevention against bacterial endocarditis, patients with valvular disorders or septal defects should have antibiotic prophylaxis prior to dental or surgical procedures.

Signs and Symptoms

Initially, the signs and symptoms are similar to those of other systemic illnesses, including fever, chills, arthralgias, malaise, and fatigue. Petechiae, anemia, weight loss, new or worsening heart murmur, and emboli alert the examiner to a more serious disease process. Emboli may cause life-threatening events such as stroke or myocardial infarction. Hematuria or proteinuria may result from a renal embolism or acute glomerulonephritis. Endocardial vegetation may occur, causing valvular incompetence or obstruction.

Diagnostic Studies

- *Blood cultures*—Cultures will confirm the diagnosis. Three blood cultures should be taken, 1 hour apart, before starting antibiotics.
- *Chest x-ray*—Underlying cardiac disease and/or pulmonary infiltrates are revealed on x-ray.
- *Echocardiography*—Echocardiography is helpful to identify which valves are affected and the presence of valve vegetations and valve ring abscesses.

Peripheral Vascular System

The assessment of the peripheral vascular system includes the following.

- Inspection and palpation of the peripheral pulses for strength and quality.
- Inspection and palpation of the skin for color, texture, and temperature changes.
- Inspection of the extremities for edema, open sores, ulcers, and pressure areas.
- Auscultation of the arteries for bruits.
- Questioning the patient for subjective complaints of discomfort or pain at rest and with exercise.

Note that arterial and venous insufficiency present with different signs and symptoms. See Table 7.4.

Differential Diagnosis of Chief Complaints

■ Peripheral Edema

In ambulatory patients, fluid collects dependently in the lower extremities; in nonambulatory patients, it collects in the sacral area. Nonpathologic causes of edema include poor venous return in prolonged standing or sitting.

Table 7.4

Differentiation of Arterial and Venous Insufficiency

Sign	Arterial Insufficiency	Venous Insufficiency
Pulse	Decreased/absent	Normal
Edema	Absent or mild	Significant
Pain	Severe	Absent/mild
Temperature	Cool	Normal
Color	Pallor with elevation; dusky red on dependency	Hyperpigmented; cyanotic on dependency
Skin	Thin, atrophic; risk of gangrene	Thick; risk of stasis ulcers

Pathologic causes of edema result from right and left heart failure, kidney disease, liver disease, or tumors that obstruct venous return. One of the early signs of congestive heart failure is pretibial and ankle edema. Renal failure causes fluid retention, and hepatic disease may cause ascites, which contribute to peripheral edema.

History

The age and general health of the patient can lead to either a high or low index of suspicion for cardiac causes of edema. Older patients and those with comorbid conditions have a greater risk of a cardiac cause for the edema. Ask the patient about history of respiratory, cardiac, renal, liver, or vascular disease. A history of heart failure makes a recurrence likely. Ask about any history of cancer, particularly abdominal or genitourinary. Ascites can occur with these cancers, causing lower extremity edema. Determine how many pillows the patient sleeps on at night, and ask about the presence of paroxysmal nocturnal dyspnea, another early sign of CHF. Inquire about daily activities, exercise, and occupation to determine a simple, mechanical cause of the edema. Psychosocial data is important, such as alcohol intake and sexual practices, which might lead to suspicion of a possible hepatic cause. A positive smoking history is a significant contributing factor in peripheral vascular disease. Note any symptoms of intermittent claudication, such as complaints of cramping, aching, or pain in the ankle, calf, or thigh that occur with exercise and are promptly relieved with rest.

Physical Examination

Assess the extent and magnitude of the edema. Is it confined to the ankles, or does it extend up the leg to include pretibial edema or higher? Grade the edema on a scale of 1+ to 4+, or mild to pitting. Assess the peripheral pulses and major arteries—the abdominal aortic, renal, iliac, and femoral arteries—for bruits. Stenosis or occlusion of any of these arteries can affect distal pulses. Assess capillary refill time and pallor or rubor of the skin on elevation and dependence.

Assess the skin integrity as you look for thinning, ulcers, or necrosis, which often occur in peripheral vascular disease. Hyperpigmentation and atrophic skin changes are common in venous insufficiency. Note any change in temperature of the skin. Cellulitis can sometimes mimic peripheral vascular disease and causes increased temperature. Coolness of the skin suggests circulatory impairment. Ulceration or necrosis are serious signs of circulatory impairment and must be promptly treated to avoid amputation.

Many people have dependent edema in the absence of heart disease that is due to prolonged sitting and standing or poor venous return, but a thorough examination of the heart, lungs, and abdomen is warranted. If the edema is accompanied by congestive heart failure, crackles may be heard at the lung bases. Listen for other adventitious sounds, such as wheezes or decreased breath sounds that might indicate obstructive lung disease, often complicated by right heart failure. Auscultate all cardiac areas for murmurs that would indicate valvular heart disease, an S_3 related to volume overload and heart failure, an S_4 usually heard in diastolic failure, and any arrhythmias that could be either a cause or a result of heart failure. Palpate the precordium for a thrill that would indicate at least a grade IV murmur. Inspect the precordium for a parasternal lift or accentuated apical impulse indicating ventricular hypertrophy. The neck should be examined for jugular venous distention with the patient's head elevated to 30 degrees. This is a sign of right-sided heart failure. Auscultate the carotids for bruits or murmurs that may radiate into the neck, usually aortic in origin. Palpate the thyroid for enlargement or nodules because hyper- and hypothyroidism can both cause heart failure. The abdomen should be examined particularly for right upper quadrant discomfort related to hepatic congestion and enlargement secondary to right heart failure. Check for hepatic jugular reflux by placing sustained pressure on the liver while observing for jugular venous distention. In right heart failure, ascites may also be present.

Diagnostic Studies

- *CBC*—A CBC should be done to check for anemia, which could cause or worsen heart failure, of which edema is a symptom.
- *Chemistry panel*—This study should be ordered to check renal function, liver function, and electrolyte balance.
- *Thyroid profile*—It is wise to rule out hyper- or hypothyroidism.
- *Chest x-ray*—Most importantly, the x-ray reveals the presence of cardiomegaly, which can assist in the diagnosis of heart failure as a cause of the edema. Look for fluid at the bases, flattening of diaphragms in COPD, pleural effusion, tumors in cancer, increased vascular markings, interstitial edema, atelectasis, or pneumonia. Pulmonary vasculature may be normal, especially in chronic heart failure. Pleural effusions indicate heart failure or metastatic cancer, and thoracentesis is indicated to examine the fluid for cancer cells.
- *Echocardiography*—These studies show the size and function of the ventricles if heart failure is thought to be the cause of the edema. Echocardiography can also be helpful in detecting shunts and pericardial effusion and for visualizing the heart valves for abnormalities.

CONGESTIVE HEART FAILURE
See the section on Dyspnea/Shortness of Breath, p. 197.

RENAL DISEASE
See the section on Dyspnea/Shortness of Breath, p. 198.

LIVER DISEASE
See the section on Dyspnea/Shortness of Breath, p. 198.

PERIPHERAL VASCULAR DISEASE

See further discussion under Leg Pain (next) and later in this section.

■ Leg Pain

Consider a vascular origin for leg pain that is not musculoskeletal in nature. Pain or weakness that occurs in the calves, and sometimes thighs or buttocks, with exercise and dissipates at rest is most likely related to peripheral vascular disease. If it is related to arterial insufficiency, the pain comes on rapidly during exercise, is quickly relieved by rest, and usually increases as the intensity and duration of the exercise increases. This is termed *intermittent claudication*. If the leg pain is due to venous insufficiency, the picture is quite different. The onset of the pain is gradual and may not even occur until some time after exercise. There is greater variability of the pain in response to duration and intensity of exercise. The pain tends to be a constant ache that may last hours to days. A potentially life-threatening complication of venous insufficiency is thrombophlebitis.

History

The most important question to ask is if there is a history of previous blood clots in the lower extremities. Also inquire about other blood clotting disorders. Ask about recent trauma to the lower extremities, history of abdominal cancers, prolonged immobility or travel, CVD, chronic spinal conditions, paresthesias, weakness in the lower extremities, or calf pain during walking or exercise.

Physical Examination

The physical examination should include temperature, color, condition of the skin, and presence of arterial pulses in the lower extremities. Note any calf redness or edema. Evaluate sensory response to sharp and dull in the lower extremities, as well as deep tendon reflexes. Note any weakness or evidence of discomfort with ambulation.

THROMBOPHLEBITIS

In addition to arteriovenous insufficiency, other risk factors for thrombophlebitis include immobility, orthopedic surgery, malignancy, CHF, smoking, pregnancy, oral contraceptive use, advanced age, and clotting disorders. The majority of cases occur in the deep veins of the calf, and the remainder occur in the iliac or femoral veins. The prognosis of thrombophlebitis is good unless the patient develops pulmonary embolism. Recurrent pulmonary embolism may occur. Deep vein thrombosis (DVT) can be a result or a cause of chronic venous insufficiency. Anticoagulant therapy should be instituted to avoid the complication of chronic venous insufficiency.

Signs and Symptoms

The signs and symptoms of DVT include swelling, tenderness, and inflammation of the calf and often pain with ambulation. In about 50% of the cases, symptoms are absent and pulmonary embolism may be the first sign.

Pulmonary embolism should be suspected with a complaint of acute onset of shortness of breath, chest pain, or hemoptysis in a person with any of the above risk factors. Preventive measures include early mobilization of postsurgical patients, raising the foot of the bed, and antiembolism hosiery, especially for patients who have a history of venous insufficiency and for people traveling long distances by plane.

Diagnostic Studies

- *Calf measurement*—A simple measurement with a measuring tape of both calves for comparison should always be performed in the clinical setting. DVT causes swelling and redness of the affected leg.
- *Duplex Doppler ultrasound*—Because of its sensitivity, specificity, and noninvasive method, duplex ultrasound is the recommended diagnostic test for venous thrombosis. It gives segmental readings on blood flow both distal and proximal to the thrombus. It is most accurate for clots in the veins proximal to the popliteal; however, it is not a reliable indicator of small thrombi in the calf veins.
- *Venography*—Contrast venography remains the most accurate diagnostic procedure for DVT. It gives information regarding location, extent, and degree of attachment of the thrombus. Venography is particularly useful when there is a strong clinical suspicion of a calf thrombosis and when Doppler ultrasound has not given adequate information.

ARTERIAL INSUFFICIENCY

Patients with peripheral arterial disease often have underlying atherosclerosis. Other diseases, such as diabetes, hypertension, and obesity, should also raise the index of suspicion for arterial insufficiency. Smoking is a risk factor for all vascular disease. A history of significant trauma or surgeries may be a risk factor.

Signs and Symptoms

See Table 7.4 for the signs and symptoms of arterial insufficiency.

Diagnostic Studies

The ankle-brachial index (ABI) is currently the easiest, least expensive noninvasive method for diagnosing peripheral vascular disease and is particularly helpful in the office and home settings. The ABI is obtained by the following steps:

1. Obtain brachial systolic pressure in both arms. Select the higher of these two values.
2. Use Doppler stethoscope to obtain systolic pressure in the dorsalis pedis or posterior tibialis vessel.
3. Divide ankle pressure by the higher brachial pressure.
4. The index should be 1.00 or higher. If it is less than 0.5, impairment to blood flow is significant. An abnormal ABI indicates the need for a vascular consult.

5. The ABI may be falsely elevated in diabetic patients because calcification of the vessels raises the pressure, especially in the ankle. Doppler ultrasound is also helpful but requires specialized equipment.

Duplex Doppler ultrasound is a relatively inexpensive, accurate method for the diagnosis of arterial insufficiency, often making arteriography unnecessary. Flow velocity can be measured, and arterial stenosis and occlusion can be detected.

CHRONIC VENOUS INSUFFICIENCY

Chronic venous insufficiency can be a long-term complication of venous thrombosis owing to the destruction of valves in the deep veins. The calf muscle pump that returns blood from the lower legs is damaged, increasing ambulatory pressure in the calf veins. A constellation of symptoms is set up: aching or pain in the lower legs, edema, thinning and hyperpigmentation of the skin, superficial varicosities, venous stasis, and ulceration. Ankle edema is often the earliest sign. Other causes of chronic venous insufficiency include trauma, pelvic neoplasm, and occasionally secondary to superficial venous disease. Prompt treatment of DVT with anticogulants decreases the risk for chronic venous insufficiency. General measures for symptom management include the following: elevation of the legs intermittently during the day and at night, avoidance of prolonged sitting or standing, and support or compression stockings. Wearing an Unna boot is valuable and successful in the treatment of stasis ulcers.

Signs and Symptoms

Stasis dermatitis and stasis ulcers are common in chronic venous insufficiency. See Table 7.4 for signs and symptoms of venous insufficiency.

Diagnostic Studies

* *Duplex Doppler ultrasound*—Owing to its sensitivity, specificity, and noninvasive method, duplex ultrasound is recommended for the diagnosis of venous disease. It gives segmental readings on blood flow and is accurate for the diagnosis of occlusion. It is most accurate for clots in the veins proximal to the popliteal; however, it is not a reliable indicator of small thrombi in the calf veins.
* *Venography*—Contrast venography remains the most accurate diagnostic procedure for venous disease. Venography is particularly useful when there is a strong clinical suspicion of a calf thrombosis and when Doppler ultrasound has not given adequate information. It gives information regarding location, extent, and degree of attachment of the thrombus.

VARICOSE VEINS

Often a precursor to chronic venous insufficiency, varicose veins are usually caused by occupations that involve prolonged standing or sitting in one place, overweight, pregnancy, or a familial tendency. They may increase the patient's risk for DVT, or they may occur secondary to a DVT. Blockage to lymphatic flow can cause varicosities as seen with pelvic neoplasm. They appear as long, dilated, tortuous veins in the lower extremities.

Signs and Symptoms

Although cosmetically unsightly, varicose veins may be completely asymptomatic, or the patient may complain of aching or fatigue in the legs, particularly with standing. The same general measures should be applied that are used with chronic venous insufficiency.

Diagnostic Studies

Usually the physical examination is enough for the diagnosis, but ultrasound or venography may be warranted if thrombosis is suspected. Excision of the varicosity and ligation of the vein are possible for symptom relief or for cosmetic reasons and rarely to prevent complications. For small varicosities, compression sclerotherapy is helpful.

REFERENCES

Chobanian, A.V., et al. (2003). The seventh report of the Joint National Committee on prevention, detection, evaluation, and treatment of high blood pressure (JNC 7). *JAMA, 289,* 2560–2572.

Hurst, J.W., Morris, D.C., & Alexander, R.W. (1999). The use of the New York Heart Association's classification of cardiovascular disease as part of the patient's complete problem list. *Clinical Cardiology, 22,* 385–390. http://www.medicalcriteria.com/criteria/nyha.htm (accessed March 9, 2011).

National Heart, Lung and Blood Institute Third Report of the Expert Panel on Detection, Evaluation, and Treatment of High Blood Cholesterol in Adults (ATP III). http://www.nhlbi.nih.gov/guidelines/cholesterol/atglance.pdf (accessed March 8, 2011).

SUGGESTED READINGS

Bickley L.S., & Szilagyl, P.G. (2007). *Bates' Guide to Physical Examination and History Taking,* 9th ed. Philadelphia: J.B. Lippincott.

Beers, M.H. (2006). *Merck Manual of Medical Therapeutics,* 18th ed. Rahway, NJ: Merck & Co.

Sokolow, M., & McIlroy, M.B. (1986). *Clinical Cardiology,* 4th ed. Los Altos, CA: Lange Medical Publications.

Tierney, L.M., McPhee, S.J., & Papadakis, M.A. (Eds.). (2008). *CURRENT Medical Diagnosis & Treatment.* New York: Lange Medical Books/McGraw Hill.

Chapter 8

RESPIRATORY SYSTEM

Mary Jo Goolsby

Respiratory complaints are commonly encountered in most health-care settings. Chronic obstructive pulmonary disease (COPD) affects over 12 million adults in the United States and is now the fourth leading cause of death (National Heart, Lung and Blood Institute [NHLBI], 2006). Pneumonia, with influenza, is currently the eighth leading cause of death in the United States and the greatest cause of infection-related deaths (Centers for Disease Control and Prevention [CDC], 2010). The prevalence of asthma is also increasing. The number of individuals diagnosed with asthma doubled from 7 million in 1980 to over 14 million in 1996 (NHLBI, 2002). There are now over 22 million people affected by asthma in the United States (NHLBI, 2006).

Respiratory complaints, such as dyspnea and cough, can be vague and quite nonspecific. In addition to potentially stemming from many extrapulmonary systems, including cardiac, neurological, and upper respiratory, they may be psychogenic in origin. A careful and detailed history and physical examination, with attention first to the respiratory system, enable accurate diagnosis. For instance, the history of uncontrolled hypertension and previous myocardial infarction (MI) in a nonsmoker, paired with the complaint of cough or sudden onset of dyspnea, direct the examiner to consider the potential for congestive heart failure (CHF), whereas a similar complaint in an otherwise healthy-appearing teen is more likely to suggest asthma or bronchitis.

History

■ Symptom Analysis

Regardless of the chief complaint, a thorough symptom analysis is warranted. It is important to get an understanding of when the complaint started and how the onset occurred. Determine how it has evolved, starting with the initial episode or awareness of the problem. Ask whether the problem is constant or intermittent. Determine whether a similar problem has been experienced in the past. It is important to learn whether anything in particular, such as emotions, exposure to outdoor allergens, or fatigue, tends to precipitate or accelerate the complaint. Also determine whether the symptoms tend to be tied to any particular time of day, such as the night, early morning, or immediately following a meal. Another timing-related issue involves whether the complaint has continued essentially unchanged, worsened, or improved since first noticed.

The quality of the symptom is important. For chest discomfort, it is important to determine whether the pain or discomfort is sharp, dull, or aching. If the complaint is a cough, the potential qualities include whether the cough is mild and tickling or sharp and paroxysmal. For some complaints, such as wheezing and tightness or pain, it is also necessary to determine the exact location of the symptom as well as whether the patient has noticed any radiation to other sites and how it relates to respirations. The severity is always important to establish.

As with other symptoms, it is always important to ask about self-treatment the patient may have tried and the response. For instance, determine what the patient has done to minimize the symptoms, including whether he or she has altered normal activity or taken any medications (prescribed or over the counter). Include questions to identify herbal agents, illicit drugs, and/or complementary therapies tried.

When asking about the existence of associated symptoms, the pulmonary review of symptoms should be performed. There is a long list of symptoms that should be explored during this part of the history. Determine whether the patient has experienced any shortness of breath and, if so, record the amount of work or effort that causes this symptom. Ask about nocturnal orthopnea or related difficulty sleeping. Specifically, ask about the number of pillows the patient uses to sleep and about the sleeping position. A patient may use no pillows but rest comfortably only in a recliner. Determine whether the patient has had a cough and whether any cough has been associated with the production of sputum or with hemoptysis. Also ask about wheezing, chest tightness, and sense of congestion. Ask whether the patient has had a fever, chills, or night sweats. In addition to asking about symptoms related to the lower respiratory tract, other systems should be explored on the basis of the presenting symptom and symptom analysis.

■ Past Medical and Family History

The past medical history should identify history of allergies, emphysema, bronchitis, asthma, pneumonia, recent or recurrent upper respiratory infections, and tuberculosis. Ask about the history of malignancy. Conditions stemming from other systems are often important to specifically address, including heart failure, gastroesophageal reflux disease (GERD), and allergies. During this part of the history, determine the approximate date of the patient's last chest x-ray and skin test for tuberculosis and the results of the tests. The family history should be explored. Ask whether there is a family history of the conditions just mentioned.

■ Habits

The patient's habits are important in the assessment of respiratory complaints. Always establish the patient's smoking history, calculating pack years. Also determine any occupational or recreational exposures to toxins. Travel history is often significant, particularly for exposure to various infectious disorders affecting the lungs. Knowledge of the patient's exposure to pets is important because it can suggest exposure to infectious diseases or allergens. Identify all medications/drugs taken, including prescribed, over the counter, and recreational drugs, as well as any herbal or alternative therapies.

Physical Examination

The history should guide attention within the physical examination. However, regardless of the complaint, a thorough and orderly approach is recommended. In addition to the respiratory examination, a more comprehensive approach is usually necessary, regardless of whether the symptoms are mild or severe, acute or chronic. Other systems that should often be included are cardiac, musculoskeletal, neurological, and upper respiratory (ear, nose, throat).

The examination actually starts during the history, as the examiner observes the patient's general condition. For instance, note whether the patient is able to provide a history without shortness of breath. Notice the patient's demeanor and apparent energy level. Assess the patient's breathing pattern and general coloring as he or she talks.

In assessing the lungs and chest, it is important that the patient be disrobed from the waist up and examined in an area with good lighting. The assessment of the chest involves all four components of physical assessment: inspection, palpation, percussion, and auscultation.

■ Inspection

Start by observing the patient's quiet respirations. Notice the rate, rhythm, depth, and amount of effort required. Check for obvious use of accessory muscles, as might be seen in a number of pulmonary conditions, including asthma, COPD, and pneumonia. Notice the movement of the chest and whether it is symmetrical. Identify any intercostal inspiratory retractions or expiratory bulges, which may indicate asthma, a tumor, tracheal/bronchial occlusion, or COPD. The chest configuration should be determined, including whether the chest is symmetrical and noting the ratio of the anterior-to-posterior (AP) diameter compared with the transverse chest diameter. An asymmetric configuration is often seen in scoliosis or kyphosis, both of which may restrict respiratory effort. Increased AP diameter is indicative of COPD as well as pectus carinatum.

■ Palpation

Following inspection, gently palpate any area of discomfort or pain. Examples include intercostal tenderness, which could indicate inflamed pleurae, and costal-sternal border pain, which could indicate costochondritis. Next palpate any area of visible deformity. The respiratory excursion, or expansion, is determined by placing hands around the patient's posterior rib cage with the thumbs at the level of the 10th rib and sliding them together so that a "pinch" or "pucker" of skin is raised between the thumbs, and then asking the patient to take a deep breath and observing the movement of the hands. The motion should be symmetrical. Less than anticipated movement occurs with COPD and pleural effusions. Asymmetry of movement occurs with atelectasis, pneumothorax, and fibrosis.

The quality of tactile fremitus is determined by palpating symmetrical areas with the palmar surface of the hands and fingers, as the patient is directed to speak, usually repeatedly saying "99" or "one, two, three" in a loud and a low-pitched voice. This maneuver provides only a rough estimate of lung condition but is useful in guiding further assessment. Areas of increased fremitus should raise the suspicion of conditions resulting in increased solidity or consolidation in the underlying lung tissue, such as in pneumonia, tumor, or pulmonary fibrosis. Conversely, areas of decreased fremitus raise the suspicion of abnormal fluid- or air-filled spaces, such as occurs with pleural effusion, pneumothorax, or emphysema. In the instance of an extensive bronchial obstruction, no palpable vibration is felt in the related field.

■ Percussion

Percussion provides an estimate of the relative amounts of air, fluid, and solid matter in a space and is helpful in identifying the margins of organs, including the lungs. The lung fields should be percussed starting from the superiormost areas at Kronig's isthmus, the area superior to the clavicles that connects the anterior and posterior aspects of the chest. Percussion proceeds downward to the level of the diaphragm. Areas of hyperresonance suggest air trapping, which occurs with COPD and may occur superior to an area of atelectasis or pleural effusion. Dullness is detected over the actual site of atelectasis and pleural effusion and over tumors or the consolidation/pneumonia.

■ Auscultation

The most helpful assessment maneuver involves auscultation of the lung fields. The general lung fields should be auscultated, with special attention paid to any areas where previous abnormalities were detected. With the patient breathing fully through an open mouth, a full inspiratory and expiratory cycle should be assessed at each site. During auscultation, the examiner should first notice the qualities associated with the breath sound, then assess for the presence of any adventitious lung sounds.

Breath sounds vary in intensity, volume, and duration depending on the site along the tracheobronchoalveolar system. In the upper part of the respiratory tree, over the trachea, breath sounds should be "bronchial," meaning they are loud and the inspiratory component is shorter than the expiratory component. Over the bronchi, the bronchovesicular sounds are of a medium intensity, and the inspiratory and expiratory components are of equal duration. Finally, the vesicular sounds over the peripheral lung tissue are, by comparison, softer in volume and have a shorter expiratory phase. Increased breath sounds over peripheral lung regions indicate consolidation, which may occur with tumor, pneumonia, or atelectasis. Decreased, or softer, peripheral breath sounds indicate bronchial obstruction or shallow breathing.

Adventitious breath sounds are extra and abnormal sounds detected in addition to the expected breath sounds. Terms such as rales, rhonchi, wheezes, and crackles are used to describe these adventitious sounds. The terms *rales* and *rhonchi* are confused by some people and are more or less synonymous with crackles and wheezes respectively. Regardless of the terminology used, it is important to provide as many descriptors as possible relative to the adventitious sound. Descriptors can include details of the detected pitch, amplitude, and quality of the sound. For instance, crackles can be described as loud or soft, coarse or fine. Wheezes, or rhonchi, can be described as loud or soft, high- or low-pitched, coarse/sonorous, squeaking, or hissing/sibilant. Another important characteristic to note is whether adventitious lung sounds occur early or late in the respiratory cycle. All of these characteristics are helpful in determining the cause. Table 8.1 describes potential adventitious sounds tied with some respiratory disorders.

Because mobile bronchial secretions can cause both crackles and wheezes, ask the patient to take a deep breath and cough if these sounds are detected. This often clears the airway and eliminates or changes the adventitious sounds. The effect of cough (or lack of cough) on the adventitious sounds is important to record. Failure to have the patient clear the airway of mobile secretions could result in a misdiagnosis.

A final adventitious sound is the pleural friction rub, typically a loud, grating sound produced when the two inflamed and roughened surfaces of the

Table 8.1

Adventitious Sounds

Description	Significance
Crackles (Rales)	
Low-pitched, coarse, early inspiratory	Bronchial; bronchitis
Medium-pitched, mid-inspiration	Smaller bronchial branches; bronchiectasis
High-pitched, fine, late inspiration	Bronchioles/alveoli; emphysema, atelectasis, pneumonia, congestive heart failure, pulmonary fibrosis
Wheezes (Rhonchi)	
Low-pitched, early, deep	Bronchi; bronchitis
High-pitched, hissing	Smaller airways; asthma
Friction Rub	
Loud, grating; late inspiratory–early expiratory	Inflamed pleura; pneumonia, pleuritis, malignancy

visceral and parietal pleurae rub together. A friction rub is usually noted in the late inspiratory and early expiratory phases and in the lower anterolateral lung fields. Examples of conditions that result in a pleural rub include pneumonia and malignancy.

Depending on the findings associated with the examination up to this point, the examiner can decide whether to proceed with auscultated spoken sounds: bronchophony, egophony, and/or whispered pectoriloquy. If the examination is normal up to this point, there is no need to proceed with spoken sounds. However, if an abnormality is detected, this maneuver may provide valuable data that will help to narrow the assessment. As with tactile fremitus, the patient is again directed to repeatedly say "99" or "1-2-3" as the examiner auscultates the lung fields. The expected norm is that the volume and clarity of the transmitted speech sounds are uniform throughout the lung fields. An increased volume in one area is called bronchophony, suggesting an area of consolidation or effusion. Whispered sounds are also auscultated as the patient whispers "99" or "1-2-3." Any area of increased clarity is positive for whispered pectoriloquy, another indication of consolidation. Finally, the lung fields can be auscultated as the patient repeats "E-E-E." If the detected sound is heard as "A-A-A" with a nasal quality over a particular area, indicating egophony, this is a final indication of consolidation.

■ Diagnostic Studies

Diagnostic studies are often helpful in making definitive diagnosis for pulmonary conditions. Spirometry provides a range of information about the lung function and is important in differentiating among causes of respiratory complaints. A number of portable and accurate devices are available. Arterial blood gases provide data on a patient's acid–base balance and whether or not disturbances stem from respiratory or metabolic derangements. Pulse oximetry provides a portable, simple method to determine the percentage of hemoglobin saturated with oxygen.

■ Imaging Studies

A wide range of imaging studies are useful in assessing respiratory complaints. In addition to plain films, computed tomography (CT), magnetic resonance imaging (MRI), and positron emissions tomography (PET) scans provide noninvasive ways to assess pulmonary tissue and space.

Differential Diagnosis of Chief Complaints

■ Cough

Cough is an extremely common and potentially nonspecific complaint. Whereas the cough serves as an important defense mechanism, it is often the major reason a patient seeks diagnosis and treatment of many self-limiting and minor complaints as well as many life-threatening ones. Cough is classified as acute (less than 3 weeks in duration) and chronic (3 or more weeks in duration), and this distinction helps to narrow the potential differential diagnoses. However, patients with chronic cough may present acutely, as some component of their problem is exacerbated.

The history and physical are essential in eliminating potential causes and identifying the most likely causes of cough. For instance, when a person presents with a cough after being prescribed an angiotensin-converting enzyme (ACE) inhibitor, a thorough history and physical help the provider ensure that there is no other likely coexisting problem triggering and/or causing the cough.

History

The history should include a thorough analysis of the cough, including a determination of how long it has persisted. It is essential to determine any associated symptoms, including shortness of breath, wheezing, orthopnea, fever, chills, chest pain or discomfort, sputum production, postnasal drainage, and hemoptysis. The past medical history should be comprehensive, with a particular focus on the potential for asthma, emphysema, chronic or acute bronchitis, heart failure, GERD, recent upper respiratory infections, or atopy. The medication history will not only exclude the potential for ACE inhibitor–induced cough but also identify other problems for which medications are taken. The patient's prior self-treatment or prescribed treatment of cough should be explored, including the response and tolerance of the treatment. Family history should be established.

Physical Examination

A thorough examination of the lungs should be performed as described earlier in this chapter. Note the patient's general appearance and any distress as the history is provided. Vital signs should be evaluated for respiratory rate, pulse, and temperature. Note the respiratory excursion as deep breaths are taken and whether or not cough is triggered. If tactile fremitus is conducted, be attentive to areas of increased or decreased vibration. Carefully assess breath sounds and note the characteristics of any adventitious sounds. Observe any sputum that can be produced for color and consistency. Depending on the history and physical findings to this point, additional assessment may be warranted and may include the upper respiratory, cardiac system, or gastrointestinal systems, for instance.

Diagnostic Studies

Diagnostic studies are often not indicated. Depending on the presentation, chest or spirometry are the studies most likely to be indicated.

POSTNASAL DISCHARGE SYNDROME

Postnasal discharge is the most common cause of chronic cough.

Signs and Symptoms

The patient complains of a chronic cough often associated with a sensation of drainage in the back of the throat and/or the need to clear the throat frequently.

There may be accompanying hoarseness. Depending on the cause of the post-nasal discharge syndrome (PNDS), the patient will have symptoms consistent with allergic rhinitis, chronic sinusitis, or other condition, such as cold or viral upper respiratory infection (URI). Although no sputum is produced, there is a potential that secretions will be cleared from the posterior pharynx by the coughing effort. Common signs include throat clearing, drainage on the posterior pharynx, and hyperemia and/or cobblestoning of the posterior pharynx, with a negative chest examination.

Diagnostic Studies

No studies are usually warranted initially. Response to treatment for PNDS provides presumptive diagnosis. Depending on the patient's risk factors, specific diagnostic studies can be considered to rule out other causes, which could coexist with PNDS, and/or contributing factors. These include allergy testing and radiographs of the sinuses or chest.

ASTHMA

Asthma is a chronic condition that involves inflammation of the airways, with varying degrees of airway obstruction and hyperresponsiveness. The incidence of asthma is increasing in the United States, and it affects people of all ages. Although typically associated with wheezing, a cough may be the primary complaint associated with asthma.

Signs and Symptoms

The patient complains of intermittent sensation of chest tightness, cough, shortness of breath, and/or wheezing. The cough is nonproductive. The symptoms may become relatively persistent and affect quality of life. Symptoms often worsen with activity, viral infections, exposure to allergens, or other triggers. The Expert Panel Report 3 (NHLBI, 2007) provides a number of tables defining the characteristics to stage asthma according to levels of severity. The history is an important aspect because the frequency of various symptoms, night-time awakenings, use of short-acting beta agonist, and interference with activities are used, along with spirometry, in staging asthma. Examination may reveal wheezes. Deep respiratory effort may trigger paroxysmal coughing. Respiratory effort may require use of accessory respiratory muscles. However, absence of physical findings does not rule out the presence of asthma. In addition to respiratory findings, patients with asthma often have other signs of atopy, including allergic rhinitis or atopic dermatitis.

Diagnostic Studies

Pulmonary functions provide diagnosis, with the forced expiratory volume in 1 second (FEV_1) diminished, indicating restricted outflow. Some degree of reversibility occurs with administration of bronchodilators. Chest films are generally within normal limits unless there is significant air trapping. Peak flow meters should not be used as diagnostic tools. They are appropriate for monitoring ongoing symptoms and determining the response to therapy, particularly once a patient's "personal best" is determined.

CHRONIC OBSTRUCTIVE PULMONARY DISEASE

COPD is most commonly caused by smoking, with the onset of symptoms typically beginning in middle age. When younger patients or nonsmokers develop findings consistent with COPD, alpha-1-antitrypsin deficiency should be suspected. COPD is actually made up of two related and often coexisting problems: chronic bronchitis and emphysema. The condition is progressive and, overall, irreversible.

Signs and Symptoms

The symptoms of COPD include chronic cough usually following years of smoking and with sputum production. The symptoms are worse on exertion and are usually progressive over time. There is often a history of exacerbations, during episodes of acute bronchitis. On physical examination, lung sounds are diminished. Crackles are more common than wheezes. The patient develops a "barrel chest" in which the AP chest diameter is greater than the lateral diameter. Progressive disease results in right heart failure with abdominal distention, liver tenderness, and edema.

Diagnostic Studies

Spirometry should be performed to confirm diagnosis. The GOLD staging system (2007) categorizes COPD into four stages ranging from mild to very severe. Each stage is characterized by a decreased ratio of FEV_1 to forced vital capacity to less than 70%. The percentage of predicted FEV provides further differentiation; this value varies from greater than 80% for stage I to less than 80%, less than 50%, and less than 30% for stages II, III, and IV, respectively. Alternatively, stage IV or very severe COPD can be diagnosed with a percentage predicted FEV less than 50% if there is also chronic respiratory failure. Unless there is some degree of asthma, postbronchodilator spirometry does not improve more than 12%. Chest radiographs reveal hyperinflation of lungs with flattened diaphragm. If alpha-1-antitrypsin deficit is suspected, a qualitative serum should be performed as a screen, followed by quantitative study, as indicated.

PNEUMONIA

Pneumonia involves inflammation and consolidation of lung tissue. Pneumonia is broadly categorized by whether it occurs outside of the hospital (community-acquired pneumonia) or within the hospital (nosocomial, or hospital-acquired, pneumonia). The cause is most often *Streptococcus pneumoniae, Haemophilus influenzae,* or *Staphylococcus aureus.* Atypical pneumonia involves infection of mycoplasma, legionella, or chlamydia. However, pneumonia can be caused by a wide range of microorganisms, including other bacteria, viruses, and fungi.

Signs and Symptoms

The symptoms of pneumonia are quite varied. Commonly, the patient complains of cough associated with fever, malaise, shaking chills, rigors, and/or chest discomfort. The patient often appears ill. Abnormal vital signs include tachycardia and tachypnea and fever. There is uneven fremitus, and the area over the consolidation percusses dull. On auscultation, there are bronchial breath sounds, often with crackles. Bronchophony, egophony, and whispered pectoriloquy are often present.

Diagnostic Studies

Chest film typically reveals an area of infiltrate. Cultures and Gram stains of sputum are usually not ordered for outpatients. The white blood cell count is often elevated.

ACUTE BRONCHITIS

Acute bronchitis is commonly encountered in ambulatory care and affects persons of all ages. It involves inflammatory processes of the bronchial smooth muscles and is associated with a wide range of microorganisms.

Signs and Symptoms

Cough is the most common symptom of bronchitis and may persist for several weeks after the initial infection is resolved. During the acute phase, the cough may be productive. There may be associated symptoms including fever, malaise, chest discomfort, chills, and headache. The chills and chest discomfort are mild in comparison to the symptoms of pneumonia. There may be wheezes and/or crackles on auscultation, which disappear or alter with cough effort. Fremitus is equal, and there is no egophony.

Diagnostic Studies

No studies are necessary unless chest radiology is needed to rule out pneumonia. Spirometry can be performed to rule out asthma and/or monitor response to therapy.

CONGESTIVE HEART FAILURE

CHF often results in cough associated with the other symptoms and findings common to CHF. See Chapter 7, p. 197.

GASTROESOPHAGEAL REFLUX DISEASE

GERD is a common cause of chronic cough. The mechanism by which GERD causes cough usually involves vagal stimulation rather than aspiration. Although cough may be the only symptom of GERD, patients usually also complain of heartburn or other GI symptoms. See Chapter 10, p. 261.

BRONCHIECTASIS

Bronchiectasis involves dilation of one or more bronchi. Congenital bronchiectasis affects infants and children. Acquired bronchiectasis involves older children and adults and stems from infections, bronchial obstruction, and cystic fibrosis.

Signs and Symptoms

There is usually a history of chronic, productive cough. Sputum is typically mucopurulent. Other common findings include hemoptysis, shortness of breath, wheezing, fatigue, pleuritic pain, and weight loss. Physical examination reveals crackles and/or wheezing. In advanced disease, clubbing and cyanosis may be present.

Diagnostic Studies

Chest films reveal linear markings, atelectasis, and/or pulmonary cysts. To confirm diagnosis, CT scan is used. Sputum studies may include positive cultures. Complete blood count may identify either anemia or polycythemia and increased white blood cell count. Pulmonary functions vary. Diagnostic studies are further needed to identify the cause of the condition.

TUBERCULOSIS

Tuberculosis is caused by a mycobacterium and frequently affects the lungs, although other organs may be involved. Risk factors include low socioeconomic status, impaired immune system, and crowded conditions. Tuberculosis presents a significant public health threat, and early diagnosis and treatment are important.

Signs and Symptoms

Many times, patients with active tuberculosis are essentially symptom free. Some complain of malaise and/or fevers but have no significantly disruptive complaints. When respiratory symptoms occur with tuberculosis, cough is common; the cough is nonproductive at first and is later associated with sputum production. Additionally, patients with tuberculosis may experience progressive dyspnea, night sweats, weight loss, and hemoptysis.

Diagnostic Studies

Plain chest films reveal hilar adenopathy and/or multilobular granulomas, particularly of the upper lungs. For this reason, it is important to include a lordotic view with the usual AP and lateral views. Tuberculin skin testing is positive. Sputum reveals acid-fast bacilli. Sputum culture requires up to 3 weeks for definitive diagnosis but should identify *Mycobacterium tuberculosis*.

MALIGNANCY

Pulmonary malignancies may arise anywhere from the tracheobronchial tree to peripheral lung tissue.

Signs and Symptoms

There may be few symptoms until the condition is advanced. Common complaints include dyspnea, cough, hemoptysis, fatigue, wheezing, and chest discomfort. Suspicion of potential malignancy should be heightened in patients who present with cough and hemoptysis paired with history of recurrent respiratory infections. Physical signs depend on the area of involvement, and the examination may be entirely normal. However, patients with pulmonary malignancy may appear ill, have unexplained weight loss, and have a variety of abnormal pulmonary findings, including asymmetrical breath sounds, adventitious sounds, and/or stridor.

Diagnostic Studies

Pulmonary functions vary depending on the location and size of mass. Chest films are often nondiagnostic, although they may reveal a nodule, mass, or other abnormality. A CT scan of the chest is typically used diagnostically and can be followed by MRI if the CT does not identify a mass. Diagnosis is made on biopsy and histopathology, with samples obtained by fine needle aspiration, bronchoscopy, mediastinoscopy, or thoracentesis.

PHARMACOLOGIC AND ACE INHIBITOR–INDUCED COUGH

Although cough can be associated with a variety of other medications, including aspirin, ACE inhibitors are a common cause of chronic cough. ACE inhibitors allow kinins to accumulate in the respiratory tract, causing a cough in 10% to 20% of patients who are prescribed these agents.

Signs and Symptoms

The cough associated with ACE inhibitors is dry and intractable and often worst at night. Aspirin is a common trigger of asthma, and a cough due to aspirin or NSAIDs is often tight and dry, accompanied by wheezing. The history is of cough onset soon after a newly prescribed agent.

Diagnostic Studies

No studies are warranted except to rule out other causes. Diagnosis is typically made by discontinuing the offending agent. Aspirin-associated cough may persist for a considerable time following elimination of the agent.

PSYCHOGENIC COUGH

The term psychogenic cough is used to describe the situation in which no organic cause for a cough is apparent. This may be associated with psychological disorders. Sometimes, patients develop a nervous habit cough. These causes must be considered after other organic causes have been ruled out.

Signs and Symptoms

Patients may complain of chronic cough, or family members may complain that the patient has persistent cough. There are usually no other related symptoms, and the physical examination is negative.

Diagnostic Studies

Based on the patient's risk factors and exposures, diagnostic studies may be necessary to exclude other causes. The results of diagnostic studies should be within normal limits.

■ Shortness of Breath and Dyspnea

Dyspnea is the subjective sense of discomfort or difficulty breathing. Commonly, patients with dyspnea may present with complaint of shortness of breath, chest tightness, or simply difficulty breathing or catching the breath. In addition to the history and physical specific to the respiratory system, a comprehensive assessment must be included, because the causes of dyspnea may stem from many extrapulmonary conditions.

History

It is essential that the symptom be thoroughly explored in order to help the patient definitively define the complaint. The setting in which the dyspnea occurs is important, including whether it occurs in specific situations or activities, is persistent or intermittent, and has any associated symptoms. The duration and progression are important to identify. Ask about how, if at all, the patient's routines have been affected by the dyspnea.

A variety of measures can be used to assess dyspnea. For instance, the patient can be asked to identify the point along a 10-cm visual analog scale that best depicts the dyspnea experienced, with one pole representing absence of shortness of breath or dyspnea and the other pole representing the worst dyspnea imaginable. Other scales depend on numerical rating and/or are specific to dyspnea related to a particular condition, such as asthma or cancer. A thorough medication history must be obtained along with a medical and family history. Habits such as tobacco use are important.

Physical Examination

A thorough respiratory and cardiac examination should be performed. Be attentive to signs of shortness of breath during the history or in response to the various maneuvers associated with the examination. Note any signs of anemia or edema.

Diagnostic Studies

The need for diagnostic studies is indicated by the patient's presentation. Examples of studies that might be warranted include chest films, complete blood count, and spirometry.

PNEUMONIA

Pneumonia often causes acute dyspnea. See previous discussion on pneumonia, pp. 214–215.

CONGESTIVE HEART FAILURE

Dyspnea is associated with CHF. See Chapter 7, p. 197.

PLEURAL EFFUSION

Pleural effusions involve an abnormal collection of fluid in the pleural space. Effusions are usually secondary to another condition, such as malignancy, heart failure, cirrhosis, trauma, and infections.

Signs and Symptoms

Dyspnea is the most common symptom associated with pleural effusion, but effusion may be accompanied by cough, pain, and systemic symptoms, such as malaise and fever. Abnormal physical findings become evident as the effusion increases in volume. These include decreased lung sounds, dullness over the effusion, decreased fremitus, egophony, and whispered pectoriloquy. With extremely large effusions, the mediastinum and trachea may shift to the opposite side. The exception involves effusion related to malignancy, in which case the mediastinum and trachea may be pulled toward the malignancy.

Diagnostic Studies

Chest films reveal the fluid collection as an increased area of density, blunting of costophrenic angle, and/or elevation of the hemidiaphragm. Plain films may also reveal a potential cause, including a mass or malignancy, infiltrates of pneumonia, or cardiomegaly of heart failure. A consultant may perform a thoracentesis to remove the effusion for observation and therapy. Observations include determining whether the fluid is purulent, bloody, milky, and/or malodorous. Testing could involve Gram stain, cultures, pH, cytology, and chemical studies.

PULMONARY EMBOLISM

Pulmonary emboli (PE) are life-threatening events stemming from venous thrombi. The symptoms associated with pulmonary emboli range from very dramatic to nonspecific, making them sometimes difficult to diagnose.

Signs and Symptoms

A history of immobility, surgery, pregnancy, hypercoagulability, deep venous thrombosis, or other conditions may be associated with the development of emboli. Dyspnea is common to PE, as is pain. Patients may have no symptoms at all or only nonspecific dyspnea. However, in severe cases, the patient presents with a sudden onset of severe dyspnea, associated with cough, chest pain, and, potentially, hemoptysis. Physical findings also vary. The patient is often tachycardic and tachypneic. Crackles and chest tenderness are common. There may be findings consistent with pleural effusion on the affected side (see preceding subsection).

Diagnostic Studies

Plain chest films are usually normal but may reveal atelectasis, pleural effusion, or infiltrates. Ventilation/perfusion (V/Q) scanning reveals a perfusion defect. Arterial blood gases are nonspecific but reveal respiratory alkalosis with hypoxemia and hypocapnia. Spiral CT with contrast has high sensitivity and specificity for PE.

RESTRICTIVE LUNG DISEASE

Both pulmonary and extrapulmonary disorders can result in diminished lung capacity and restrictive lung disease. Pulmonary disorders that affect the compliance of the lung tissue result in decreased ventilation, as do extrinsic conditions, such as kyphosis. Onset may be gradual for lung problems such as pneumonitis, pulmonary fibrosis, and sarcoidosis, as well as extrinsic causes, such as kyphosis or obesity.

Signs and Symptoms

There may be a family history of intrinsic restrictive lung disease or personal history of occupational exposure to toxins. Patients with neuromuscular disorders often have symptoms of generalized fatigue and weakness. With extrinsic conditions, such as kyphosis or obesity, physical findings are usually evident. Examination reveals restricted respiratory excursion and, often, crackles.

Diagnostic Studies

Appropriate studies vary depending on the suspected cause of restricted airway disease. Spirometry reveals decreased FEV_1, total lung capacity, and/or forced vital capacity.

PNEUMOTHORAX

Pneumothorax involves air in the pleural cavity. A pneumothorax can occur spontaneously in otherwise healthy individuals or be secondary to trauma or intrinsic lung disease.

Signs and Symptoms

There is history of sudden onset of shortness of breath associated with chest pain. The patient usually presents in great distress, with tachycardia and tachypnea, and is often splinting the chest. There is decreased fremitus and increased hyperresonance on the affected side. Lung sounds are diminished or absent. The trachea may shift away from the affected side if a large pneumothorax is present.

Diagnostic Studies

Plain chest films usually reveal the pneumothorax with an absence of lung markings in the affected area and shift of the mediastinum.

FOREIGN BODY ASPIRATION

Aspiration of a solid or semisolid object can be life threatening. Foreign body aspiration can occur at any age. However, young children, who have a tendency to put objects in their mouths, have the highest incidence of foreign body aspiration and associated mortality. Onset of symptoms may be sudden if the object obstructs airway. However, if the airway is not significantly obstructed, symptoms may develop more slowly, as the aspiration results in pneumonia.

Signs and Symptoms

There may be a witnessed episode of sudden difficulty breathing and/or choking accompanied by inability to speak, cyanosis, coughing, and/or loss of consciousness. If the airway obstruction is complete, respiratory arrest occurs. If obstruction is partial, there will be varying degrees of coughing, wheezing, and stridor. If the obstruction is not significant, the patient may present with complaints of cough, increasing dyspnea, fever, and symptoms consistent with pneumonia. Physical findings depend on the degree of obstruction and can include stridor, wheezing, diminished lung sounds, cyanosis, and/or findings consistent with pneumonia.

Diagnostic Studies

Plain chest films may reveal air trapping or atelectasis as well as the radiolucent object. A CT scan may be necessary to identify radiopaque objects. A bronchoscopy may be necessary to identify and/or remove a foreign object.

MALIGNANCY

Pulmonary and nonpulmonary malignancies may result in difficulty breathing. See previous discussion, pp. 216–217.

ASTHMA

Shortness of breath or dyspnea is extremely common in asthma. See previous discussion, pp. 213–214.

COPD

Progressive dyspnea is a common finding of COPD. See previous discussion, p. 214.

ANEMIA

Anemia can result in dyspnea or a sense of "air hunger." See the discussion of anemia in Chapter 16, pp. 481–482.

■ Wheezing and Chest Tightness

Wheezing is an audible respiratory sound often associated with a sense of chest tightness and/or dyspnea. Many of the conditions included in the preceding discussions of cough and dyspnea also cause wheezing and chest tightness. For this reason, the history and physical assessment for this complaint are the same as for the other respiratory complaints and should be thorough.

LARYNGEAL OR TRACHEAL OBSTRUCTION

Obstruction of the large airways can occur with many conditions, including inflammation, malignancy, laryngospasm, and foreign body aspiration.

Signs and Symptoms

The symptoms and signs vary depending on the condition responsible for the obstruction. The wheezing is evident over the major airways, and the sound is often more harsh and stridorous than typical wheezing.

Diagnostic Studies

Appropriate diagnostic studies depend on the suspected cause.

ASTHMA

Wheezing is commonly associated with asthma. See previous discussion, pp. 213–214.

ACUTE BRONCHITIS

See previous discussion, p. 215.

COPD

Wheezing often occurs with COPD, particularly chronic bronchitis. See p. 214.

MALIGNANCY

Bronchial and pulmonary tumors can present with wheezing. See pp. 216–217.

■ Hemoptysis

Hemoptysis can be associated with a wide range of pulmonary disorders, which have been described in this chapter. With presentation of a hemoptysis complaint, it is essential that the history identify associated symptoms in addition to the analysis of hemoptysis. Investigate recent exposures to other persons with infectious diseases. Patients living in close proximity to others are at increased risk for contracting infectious respiratory disorders. A history of smoking is important; history of tuberculosis or positive skin tests must be identified. A thorough examination of the respiratory system provides data important to narrowing the differential diagnosis. Diagnostic studies often include plain radiographs of the chest.

TUBERCULOSIS

Hemoptysis is a late symptom of tuberculosis, which is described on p. 216.

PNEUMONIA

Pneumonia may result in hemoptysis and is described on pp. 214–215.

MALIGNANCY

Malignancy should be considered for patients with hemoptysis. See pp. 216–217.

BRONCHITIS

Bronchitis can result in hemoptysis. See p. 215.

PULMONARY EMBOLISM

See p. 219.

■ Pleuritic Pain

Pleuritic pain is associated with respiratory movements and breathing. Although the cause is often respiratory in nature, pleuritic pain is also associated with chest trauma and inflammation as well as with gastrointestinal and cardiac disorders. Pleuritic pain can be very distressful and can also cause great anxiety. A thorough symptom analysis is necessary. Through the history, determine whether there have been recent symptoms of respiratory infection, trauma to the chest, or extrapulmonary symptoms consistent with musculoskeletal, gastrointestinal, or cardiac problems. A comprehensive physical assessment is necessary.

COSTOCHONDRITIS

Costochondritis is pain at a costosternal cartilage site. It can follow trauma to the chest wall, but the cause is often not identifiable. The symptoms may follow a period of strenuous exercise or coughing.

Signs and Symptoms

The patient reports pleuritic pain that is affected by breathing or chest motion. The site of tenderness is limited, and the pain is reproducible with firm pressure to the site. On occasion, there are signs of inflammation at the tender area, but generally the physical examination is otherwise negative.

Diagnostic Studies

Generally no diagnostic studies are warranted.

PLEURISY

Pleurisy involves inflammation of the pleura and is often related to underlying infectious process.

Signs and Symptoms

The patient complains of severe and sharp pleuritic pain with acute onset. The pain may be noted only with cough, respiration, or maneuvers causing chest motion. However, there may be a sense of vague consistent pain that becomes pronounced with respiratory motions. The patient often splints the chest and attempts shallow respirations to limit the discomfort. A pleural friction rub can be auscultated. Pleural effusion may develop, with physical findings of percussive dullness, decreased fremitus, egophony, and decreased breath sounds at the site.

Diagnostic Studies

The diagnosis is usually based on the history of definitive pleuritic pain and physical findings. However, chest films can be obtained and will vary from being within normal limits to revealing pleural effusion.

CHEST TRAUMA

Direct trauma to the chest can result in pain that is worsened with respirations owing either to rib fracture or injury to the intercostal muscles

Signs and Symptoms

The history should reveal the offending trauma, with physical findings consistent with the injury.

Diagnostic Studies

Diagnostic studies should be determined by the history of trauma.

PERICARDITIS

Pericarditis involves inflammation of the pericardium. Pericarditis can be associated with an infectious disorder and a variety of other conditions. See the discussion in Chapter 7.

PULMONARY EMBOLISM

See previous discussion, p. 219.

MALIGNANCY

See previous discussion, pp. 216–217.

REFERENCES

Centers for Disease Control and Prevention (CDC). (2010). Centers for Disease Control and Prevention. *National Vital Statistics Report, 58*(14), 17.

GOLD. (2007). "Global Strategy for Diagnosis, Management, and Prevention of COPD: Updated 2010." www.goldcopd.com (accessed March 10, 2011).

National Heart, Lung and Blood Institute (NHLBI). (2006). "COPD Essential Facts for Health Professionals." http://www.nhlbi.nih.gov/health/public/lung/copd/campaign-materials/html/providercard.htm (accessed March 9, 2011).

NHLBI. (2007). "Expert Panel Report 3 (EPR3): Guidelines for the Diagnosis and Management of Asthma." http://www.nhlbi.nih.gov/guidelines/asthma/ (accessed March 9, 2011).

SUGGESTED READINGS

Bickley, L.S. (2008). *Bates' Guide to Physical Examination and History Taking*. Philadelphia: Lippincott, Williams, and Wilkins.

Dillon, P.M. (2007). *Nursing Health Assessment: A Critical Thinking, Case Studies Approach*. Philadelphia: F.A. Davis.

Hah, D.L. (2003). Evaluation and management of acute bronchitis. In Hueston, W.J. (Ed.), *20 Common Problems: Respiratory Disorders*. New York: McGraw-Hill.

Hebbar, K. (2003). Pulmonary embolism. In Hueston, W.J. (Ed.), *20 Common Problems: Respiratory Disorders*. New York: McGraw-Hill.

Holmes, R.L., & Fadden, C.T. (2004) Evaluation of the patient with chronic cough. *American Family Physician, 69*(9), 2159–2166.

Hueston, W.J. (2003). Dyspnea and shortness of breath. In Hueston, W.J. (Ed.), *20 Common Problems: Respiratory Disorders*. New York: McGraw-Hill.

Kraft, M. (2007). Approach to the patient with respiratory disease. In Goldman, L., & Ausiello, D. (Eds.), *Cecil Textbook of Medicine*. Philadelphia: Saunders.

Swartz, M.H. (2004). *Textbook of Physical Diagnosis: History and Examination*. Philadelphia: Saunders.

Chapter 9

BREASTS

Mary Jo Goolsby

Women in the United States have a one-in-eight chance of being diagnosed with breast cancer during their lifetime. In 2007, the American Cancer Society (ACS, 2008) estimated the diagnosis of over 178,000 cases of invasive breast cancer in addition to over 62,000 cases of in situ cancer. Breast cancer is responsible for over 40,000 deaths each year. Whereas most breast cancer occurs in women, 1% of all breast cancer is diagnosed in men.

The role of mutations in the breast cancer susceptibility genes (including *BRCA1* and *BRCA2*) is being explored. Although fewer than 1% of women have mutations in these genes, between 5% and 10% of the women diagnosed with breast cancer are found to have a mutation (Burke et al., 1997). Genetic mutations must be considered with family and personal history in establishing risk for future development of breast cancer (Begg, 2002). Further discussion regarding the genetics of breast cancer is provided in Chapter 2.

It is important to remember that the majority of breast complaints and findings are related to benign conditions. It is crucial to recognize and respond appropriately to potential signs of malignancy and to recognize the range of other common breast conditions and their indications.

History

In addition to intrinsic breast disease, the function and structure of the breasts are influenced by changes in many other body systems. For example, disorders of the musculoskeletal, respiratory, cardiovascular, or neurological systems can result in chest discomfort that is perceived as mastalgia, having breast origin. Endocrine problems, both reproductive and nonreproductive, may result in changes to breast tissue, comfort, and/or secretions. When assessing problems related to the breasts, it is important to consider the range of disorders that may influence breast health. A number of risk prediction rules are available to estimate, based on her history, a woman's risk of developing breast cancer at some point in time. One such tool is available through the National Cancer Institute at www.cancer.gov/bcrisktool.

■ General History: Symptoms Analysis and Review of Systems

When obtaining a history related to a breast complaint, always complete a symptom analysis, using the PQRST (palliative/provoking, quality, radiation, severity, timing) sequence. The analysis of individual symptoms is addressed in detail later in this chapter. When a patient complains of one breast symptom, it is important to obtain a complete review of other possible symptoms, including pain, mass, nipple discharge, skin changes, and recent nipple inversion. It is also important to ask about the presence of general and nonspecific symptoms, such as fatigue, fever, appetite change, and weight loss. These will often be helpful in identifying potential endocrine problems or malignancy, which may present with nonspecific complaints.

■ Past Medical History

Ask about reproductive and menstrual history, including, as appropriate, age at menarche and at menopause. Ask about pregnancies, including the age at each pregnancy and whether the pregnancy resulted in a live birth. Assess the history of breastfeeding. Identify all previous breast surgeries or procedures, including breast augmentation or reduction, biopsies, and diagnostic studies. Determine the history of trauma to the chest/breasts. Obtain a history of chronic or current acute illnesses, particularly those of the reproductive or endocrine system. If the patient complains of breast pain, ask about musculoskeletal, cardiac, and neurological disorders. Obtain a history of all medications prescribed for and/or taken by the patient. Many pharmacological agents have the potential to affect breast function, including hormone replacements, contraceptives, antidepressants and psychoactives, and antihypertensives. The medication history may also help to identify a previously undisclosed health problem.

Box 9.1

Gail Model for Breast Cancer Risk Assessment

The Gail model is a clinical prediction rule used to estimate a patient's risk for breast cancer. The model identifies the relative risk associated with three factors obtained through history: age at menarche, number of previous breast biopsies, and the age at first live birth. The model combines the three risks to determine the woman's overall relative risk for her current age. Although applying the model is somewhat cumbersome, electronic calculators based on the model, some with slight adaptations, are readily available. One source is the calculator available at the National Cancer Institute's Web site, where individuals and providers can enter the information pertaining to each identified risk factor and receive the patient's risk for developing breast cancer within the next 5 years and by age 90.

■ Family History

The family history should identify any breast problems as well as disorders that might influence the breasts. Ask about the history of breast cancer, fibrocystic breasts, and any reproductive and endocrine disorders. Chapter 2 describes how to obtain a three-generation genetic history relevant to breast cancer.

■ Habits

Obtain a history of caffeine and alcohol intake as well as all over-the-counter and recreational drug use. Identify the level of physical activity and any occupational or recreational activities that might cause trauma to the chest area.

Physical Examination

Although the examination of the female breasts is described, the same assessment should be performed for both men and women, particularly when the male patient presents with any of the symptoms described under Differential Diagnosis of Chief Complaints.

■ Order of the Examination

Examination of the breasts typically includes only inspection and palpation. Inspect the breasts with the patient in both sitting and supine positions, and palpate once the supine position is assumed.

Inspection

Observe the breasts as the patient is at rest, comparing for symmetry of size and contour. While the breasts often differ in size, the difference is typically not excessive and is longstanding as opposed to a recent development. Continue to inspect the breasts as the patient moves her arms through various motions: raising the arms over head, lowering the arms so that she presses palms together in front of her, and then pressing the hands downward against the hips. Finally, observe as the patient leans forward at the waist. Through each motion, inspect the breast contours individually, observing for retractions, dimples, and irregularities of contour while also comparing the breasts with each other for symmetry. If normal, the breasts should move freely and the contours should remain smooth throughout the movement. The motions cause contraction of the breasts' underlying musculature, which may result in a "pulling" from any abnormal mass so that a retraction or dimple becomes evident.

Following this surface inspection, assist the patient in assuming a supine position. Inspect the breasts again for general symmetry, comparing one with the other. Then inspect each breast individually, noting the skin's color and apparent texture, the general contour and smoothness, vascular pattern, areola, and nipple. Carefully note any irregularities or suspicious areas for detailed palpation. Identify any areas of retraction, dimpling, swelling, skin lesions, or discharge. Recent nipple inversion, retraction, or excoriation should be identified.

Observe for other skin changes, including the peau d'orange condition in which the skin of the breast is swollen so that the hair follicles look like "dimples" and the skin develops the texture of an orange peel.

Palpation

Before palpating either breast, ask the patient to raise her arm on the side to be examined, placing her hand behind her head so that her shoulder is extended to approximately 90 degrees. This position provides better access to the breast region because it flattens the breast tissue across the chest wall. Examination of the breast should include the region from the midsternal line to the midaxillary line, from the subclavicular to approximately the 6th to 7th rib, or the "bra line." Palpation of the breast should also include attention to the axillary and subclavicular lymph nodes. Several systems provide good coverage of the breast region. The specific sequence of palpation is unimportant, although each practitioner should become comfortable and consistent with one sequence that seems logical for him or her and that ensures palpation of the full breast region.

Regardless of the approach used, light, medium, and deep pressure should be applied at each palpation point. Varying the palpation pressure is more likely to allow detection of masses—whether they are superficial or deep. Compress the area immediately beneath each areola, and gently squeeze each nipple. Ask the patient to inform you of any areas of tenderness or pain elicited with the examination.

Breast tissue may be normally somewhat nodular or irregular, but the texture should be generally consistent between the breasts. Note any masses, nodules, or areas of firmness. Any mass should be assessed for size, consistency, mobility, margins/borders, shape, and delineation. It is sometimes helpful to palpate symmetrical areas of breast tissue simultaneously to assess areas of thickening or fullness.

As you palpate each breast, identify any discharge, which is most likely to be produced with pressure over the areola and/or when the nipple is gently squeezed. If discharge is produced, notice whether it comes from one or multiple ducts. When there is discharge from multiple ducts, there is a higher likelihood of a cause such as fibrocystic change or galactorrhea. While malignancy should always be considered in the differential diagnosis for nipple discharge, the likelihood of malignancy increases when the discharge is from only one duct. Any discharge should be assessed for color, consistency, and odor. Collect the discharge by pressing a clean glass slide lightly against the nipple. In addition to facilitating the ability to judge the color and consistency of the discharge, the slide can also be used for cytology testing if warranted. The discharge should also be tested for blood, using a guaiac card.

■ Special Considerations

Women for whom special consideration is warranted include those who have had a mastectomy or breast-sparing surgery, cosmetic or postmastectomy augmentation, or breast reduction surgery. In these cases, careful history and examination relevant to the breasts are indicated. When mammograms or other imaging studies are ordered on a woman who has undergone any of these procedures, these details of the history should be clearly noted.

Women who have previously been diagnosed and treated for breast cancer may require more frequent clinical breast examinations than is usually recommended. The unaffected breast should be examined using standard technique. Any remaining tissue on the affected side, including the axilla, should also be carefully examined.

Following breast augmentation, the ability to examine the breast tissue is somewhat dependent on the type and placement of the implant or augmentation. Ask about any difficulty the woman may have experienced at the time of the procedure or implant as well as current symptoms. Access to certain tissues may be occluded by the implant.

Following breast reduction, deep scarring and adhesions may form, confounding the ability to palpate a mass. There may also be voids in the breast tissue, particularly in the tissue underlying the area of scarring, such that the normal and regular distribution of tissue is altered.

Differential Diagnosis of Chief Complaints

■ Breast Mass

Breast tissue is normally glandular and may have a rather nodular consistency. The degree of nodularity tends to fluctuate through the menstrual cycle in premenopausal women. A *dominant breast mass* is a mass that persists throughout a woman's hormonal cycles, is larger and firmer than any other irregularities, and differs from rest of the breast tissue. Dominant masses typically fall into the following categories: fibroadenomas, cysts, fibrocystic changes, fat necrosis, and malignancy. Whenever a breast mass is identified, it should be followed to diagnostic resolution. Breast cancer is always included in the differential diagnosis, and diagnostic efforts should definitely include either ruling out the existence of a malignancy or identifying it in a timely manner. Missed or delayed diagnoses can have catastrophic results and are, in fact, consistently among the most frequent causes of malpractice suits.

History

It is essential to obtain a complete reproductive and menstrual history and to ascertain the symptoms associated with the discovery of the mass. Determine how long the mass has been present and whether it has changed since first noticed. If present for a while, ask whether any of its characteristics fluctuate in relation to the menstrual cycle. Identify any accompanying symptoms, such as pain, nipple discharge, or skin changes. Ask about recent trauma to the breast. The presence of systemic symptoms, including loss of energy, altered appetite, weight loss, and fever, is important because they may be signs of advanced breast cancer. Determine family history of breast disease, malignancies, and related conditions.

Physical Examination

It is important to perform a complete breast examination for any complaint of breast mass. Throughout the examination, be attentive for changes in the skin; the contours of the breasts, including dimpling or retractions; nipple discharge; eczematous or similar rash or erosions around the nipple; and palpable axillary or subclavicular lymph nodes. It is crucial to confirm the presence of a palpable mass, carefully noting its location and other characteristics.

The dimensions, mobility, consistency, and texture of each palpable breast mass are important in determining further diagnostic work-up. For any mass, determine whether the consistency is soft, rubbery, firm, or hard; whether it is fixed and immobile or moves freely; whether it has smooth or irregular margins; and whether it is tender, painful, or painless. Determine whether the skin over-lying an identified mass moves independently of the mass or, instead, is con-nected to the mass so that they move together. As the mass is palpated, try to determine whether it is cystic or solid. Any patient with a dominant breast mass should be referred for definitive diagnosis.

Diagnostic Studies

All patients with a palpable dominant breast mass should be referred. Imaging and other studies, such as biopsies, are necessary to discriminate among poten-tial causes when a breast mass is detected either by the patient or the provider. Unfortunately, palpation and mammography, alone or together, are inadequate to definitively identify the cause of a breast mass and to rule out malignancy. The "triple test" recommended for evaluation of a breast mass involves clinical exam-ination, either ultrasound or mammogram, and aspiration and/or biopsy. The determination of whether an ultrasound or mammography is recommended is based on age and other situations. The American College of Radiology (2006) recommends that women under 30 years of age should be assessed through ultrasound, and women who are older than 30 years should be assessed with mammogram. Younger women have denser breasts, and ultrasound is therefore often more useful than a mammogram. Ultrasounds are helpful in determining whether or not a mass that feels potentially "cystic" is fluid filled or solid. It is crucial that the woman understand that the imaging procedure is a screening tool and is never diagnostic regarding the existence or absence of a malignancy.

The patient should be referred to a surgeon for definitive diagnosis through fine needle aspiration (FNA) or core biopsy. If an FNA reveals only nonbloody aspirate and the mass appears to be resolved following aspiration, the surgeon may decide to recheck the patient in approximately 1 month. If the mass is still resolved at the follow-up visit, a decision may be made to do no further follow-up at that time but instead to perform serial examinations over time. If an FNA reveals bloody aspirate or reveals a solid mass (suggested by inability to aspirate the mass), or if the cyst returns following aspiration, a biopsy is indicated.

MALIGNANCY

In the United States, breast cancer is responsible for over 40,000 deaths annually. It is the most common form of cancer among women and the second leading cause of cancer deaths. The differential diagnosis should include malignancy when a woman complains of or the practitioner identifies a breast mass. A thorough history and careful physical examination are essential if breast cancer is suspected.

Signs and Symptoms

A breast lump is the most common presenting complaint in breast cancer and is usually the only presenting complaint. More rarely, the presentation may include complaint of discomfort, skin change, or discharge. If the cancer is advanced, the patient may have extra-breast symptoms, such as fatigue, weight loss, and bone pain. The typical malignant mass is solitary, nontender, hard, immobile or fixed, and poorly defined. It may be accompanied by nipple erosion or other inflammatory skin changes, as seen in Paget's disease; nipple discharge; skin thickening or dimpling; retraction; and palpable axillary nodes. Although most malignant masses are painless, associated discomfort does not exclude the potential for breast cancer.

Diagnostic Studies

Any breast mass, particularly those that are solitary, noncyclic, and nontender, should trigger a mammogram or ultrasound as well as a consultation with a surgeon who will determine the need for FNA, biopsy, or other diagnostic studies.

FIBROADENOMA

Fibroadenomas are common, benign neoplasms that usually occur in premenopausal women, appearing in the second or third decade. Women with fibroadenomas have a slightly higher than average lifetime risk of developing breast cancer.

Signs and Symptoms

There are usually no complaints other than the mass. Although fibroadenomas are usually solitary, they can be multiple. The lump is generally mobile, rubbery, and nontender; has discrete and smooth borders; and is less than 5 cm in diameter. However, fibroadenomas may also have irregular borders.

Diagnostic Studies

A mammogram or ultrasound is usually ordered to confirm the diagnosis and rule out malignancy. Even when a newly identified mass is consistent with a fibroadenoma and imaging supports the diagnosis, a surgical consult should be considered for definitive diagnosis.

FIBROCYSTIC CHANGE

Fibrocystic breast changes include a variety of histopathological variations, with fibrotic thickening often paired with the development of cysts. This condition, however, is considered benign and/or physiologic rather than pathologic.

Signs and Symptoms

The nodularity is usually associated with tenderness. The nodularity and tenderness are both cyclic in nature, fluctuating with the menstrual cycle. The symptoms are usually most severe just before menses. The size and/or number of lumps or nodules may fluctuate during the cycle. The changes are usually bilateral. Breast discharge may also occur cyclically before menses and is usually serous.

Diagnostic Studies

Diagnostic studies are usually not warranted in young women who have lumpy breasts with multiple areas of thickening and a cyclic component, with or without tenderness. The patient should be instructed to complete a breast symptom calendar for at least 2 months, at which time the calendar can be studied to assess the cyclic nature of the symptoms. If there is a dominant mass identified or some other diagnostic uncertainty exists, a surgical consult should be obtained.

TRAUMA

Trauma to the anterior chest area may result in a palpable breast mass. An automobile accident with injury from contact with the seat belt, air bag, steering wheel, or dashboard is a common source of breast trauma. The trauma may result in a variety of injuries, and deeper damage should be considered, with assessment for musculoskeletal and lung injury. When a palpable mass results from chest trauma, it typically represents either a hematoma or area of secondary fat necrosis. Even when a mass is identified subsequent to direct trauma, the provider must remain suspicious for the possibility of malignancy that preexisted but was undetected before the accident.

Signs and Symptoms

A palpable mass due to trauma typically is associated with chest wall and breast discomfort. There may be an area of ecchymosis or discoloration in the distribution of trauma. Patients with large breasts are more likely to develop fat necrosis than are those with small breasts. A palpable mass associated with trauma is often poorly defined and immobile. An area of fat necrosis is typically superficial and may develop calcified margins. It can be difficult to differentiate between isolated trauma and a potential for malignancy. Serial examinations should demonstrate resolution of any hematoma and/or no increase in mass size.

Diagnostic Studies

Because the potential for malignancy is not easily excluded, an ultrasound or mammogram should be considered. Additional imaging may include plain films to assess the condition of ribs and other bones and to exclude pneumothorax or hemothorax resulting from trauma.

■ Breast Pain

Breast pain—mastalgia or mastodynia—is the most common breast complaint. The most common type of breast pain is cyclic mastalgia, which occurs in premenopausal women and is associated with hormonal fluctuations. In contrast, noncyclic breast pain is often unilateral and may be described in many ways, including sharp, burning, and aching. Many benign breast changes, including cysts, mastitis, trauma, abscess, duct ectasia, and fibroadenoma, are associated with noncyclic mastalgia. While breast pain tends most often to be mild, it can be quite severe. Both noncyclic and cyclic breast pain may be associated with certain variables, such as the intake of methylxanthine/caffeine-containing products. Although pain is not commonly associated with the diagnosis of breast cancer, it may accompany malignancy and is sometimes the presenting complaint. A complaint of breast pain may also represent pain referred from another origin, usually related to some musculoskeletal or neuropathic disorder.

History

It is important to have the patient describe the pain in detail, through a symptom analysis to identify palliative/provocative factors, the actual quality and type of pain, the primary region of pain and any radiation, the severity of the pain, any associated breast or systemic symptoms, and the timing. Any prior breast complaints, disorders, surgeries, and procedures should be determined. Ask whether the pain is associated with any particular physical activities. Determine whether there have been any other symptoms, such as fever or general malaise. The menstrual history is important. If the patient has an infant, determine the history of lactation. It may be appropriate to explore symptoms associated with other systems, including cardiac, neurological, and musculoskeletal. Identify any current medications, particularly hormonal contraceptives. The family history should include questions about breast cancer and fibrocystic breasts.

Physical Examination

A general survey should be completed to determine the patient's overall appearance. The examination should focus on the breasts and should be expanded as indicated. Observe for masses, skin texture changes, redness/inflammation, and discharge. Notice whether any of the motions involved in the inspection phase of the examination seem to elicit discomfort. Ask the patient to point to the area of discomfort. If the patient has complained of discomfort limited to a specific region, palpate the opposite breast first before proceeding to the nontender portion of the affected breast. Gently palpate the area of tenderness or pain, noting the boundaries of the discomfort, and assess the underlying tissue for any change in texture, or for masses.

Diagnostic Studies

A variety of diagnostic studies may be appropriate for the assessment of breast pain. If the pain is cyclic in nature and related to menses, there is generally no indication to order diagnostic studies. A diary of the breast discomfort may prove helpful, however. If the patient is over 30 and has not had a recent mammogram, it is appropriate to order a routine mammogram as a part of normal care. If a solid mass or cyst is suspected, the pain is noncyclic, or the patient is postmenopausal, a surgical consult should be obtained. If the patient is under 30, an ultrasound is appropriate in lieu of the mammogram. If mastitis is suspected, a white blood count is indicated.

HORMONAL, CYCLIC MASTALGIA

Although it is broadly assumed that cyclic mastalgia is related to fluctuating hormones, the mechanisms resulting in the discomfort are unknown. There does not seem to be a direct correlation between fluid retention, for instance, and breast tenderness or pain. Women who experience cyclic mastalgia usually have onset as a teen or young adult. It is important to determine menstrual and reproductive history and to identify all pharmacologic agents taken. A complete breast examination should be performed.

Signs and Symptoms

The pain associated with hormonal fluctuation most commonly occurs during the second half of the woman's cycle. The variability of the signs and symptoms is identified with a symptom calendar. The pain is typically poorly localized, bilateral, and nonspecific. It may be accompanied by a sense of breast fullness. The examination may identify the multiple, bilateral nodularities associated with fibroadenomas or fibrocystic changes.

Diagnostic Studies

The breast pain diary identifies the cyclic nature of the pain and its association with the menstrual cycle. A mammogram or ultrasound reveals no indication of malignancy or mass other than fibroadenomas or cysts.

FIBROADENOMAS AND FIBROCYSTS

Two benign causes of breast pain include fibroadenomas and fibrocystic breasts. Although fibroadenomas are not typically painful, they can be accompanied by discomfort. Both conditions are described in the previous section on breast masses.

MASTITIS

Mastitis is an inflammatory breast disorder, typically occurring in lactating women (puerperal mastitis) and caused by either a streptococcal or staphylococcal infection. The cause likely stems from altered nipple/areola skin integrity with retrograde infection. Mastitis occurs rarely in nonlactating females, and in this situation, it often stems from duct ectasia (see later discussion on breast discharge) with an anaerobic microbe. It is important to recognize mastitis so that it can be promptly treated. Because mastitis is rare among nonlactating women, providers should remain suspicious of the potential for inflammatory breast cancer in women who are not nursing, particularly if there are no systemic symptoms of infection.

Signs and Symptoms

The patient typically complains of unilateral pain, redness, and swelling of one breast. Systemic symptoms include fever, chills, and myalgia. The examination reveals a wedge-shaped area of redness that is swollen and very tender. The patient is typically nursing, and there is often visible discharge of milk, which may be spontaneous as the breast becomes engorged once the breast becomes too painful to nurse.

Diagnostic Studies

A white blood count should be obtained and is usually elevated. Even though the breast milk can be cultured, this is not generally recommended. If the presentation is atypical—that is, the patient is not lactating—and there are no associated systemic signs or symptoms, a consultation should be obtained and mammography ordered to determine the definitive diagnosis and rule out malignancy.

MALIGNANCY

Although pain is not a common complaint with breast cancer, the potential for a malignancy must always be considered in the differential diagnosis.

CHEST WALL PAIN AND COSTOCHONDRITIS

Costochondritis involves localized discomfort, often quite sharp in nature, along the costochondral and/or costosternal cartilages. Costochondritis is described in Chapter 8.

PENDULOUS BREASTS

Pain can be associated with pendulous breast, which cause strain on the underlying muscles and fibers.

RADICULAR NERVE PAIN

Nerve root inflammation or impingement can result in pain that radiates or is experienced in the region of breasts. Thoracic lesions may radiate to the chest. Nerve pain typically is sharp or burning in nature. Nerve pain is described in Chapter 15, and herpes zoster pain is described in Chapter 3.

CARDIAC PAIN

Ischemic heart pain can be misinterpreted as breast pain. When the presentation involves atypical breast pain and/or occurs in a patient at high risk for cardiac disease, cardiac pain should be strongly considered in the differential diagnosis. Cardiac pain is described in Chapter 7.

■ Breast Discharge

Although breast discharge may occur without pathology, it may be indicative of serious disorders. Categories of breast or nipple discharge include galactorrhea, physiologic discharge, and pathologic discharge. Galactorrhea can be caused by a variety of endocrine disorders. Causes of pathologic discharge include ductal papilloma, duct ectasia, and fibrocystic changes. Discharge may be present at the diagnosis of breast cancer. However, the vast majority (95%) of breast discharge cases are from benign causes. In over 50% of females, a very small amount of discharge (one or a very few drops) can be produced by manipulating the breast and nipple, but this is not considered spontaneous.

History

Determine whether the discharge is bilateral or unilateral and whether it comes from single or multiple ducts. Ask whether or not it comes from the same site on the nipple each time. Determine whether the discharge is spontaneous or comes after breast manipulation. The color and consistency of the discharge should be determined, as should the presence of any other breast symptoms, including pain, retraction, skin changes, or mass. The menstrual, reproductive, and lactation histories are important. A thorough medication and substance history is crucial, as breast discharge can be caused by several agents. Because discharge can be a sign of other conditions, including renal, endocrine, and idiopathic disorders, ask about a history of headaches, visual changes, recent trauma, and thyroid symptoms or disorders. Determine whether the patient participates in high-intensity exercise and, if so, what type of bra is worn.

Physical Examination

The breast examination should be thorough and include manipulation intended to produce discharge. If no discharge is produced by the general breast examination, depress the areolar region and note any discharge. The characteristics of the discharge should be noted, including color, consistency, and odor. If milky discharge is produced, milk production can be confirmed by microscopic identification of fat globules. Bloody discharge is often associated with malignancy but can stem from other conditions. If blood is not evident, the discharge should be tested for blood, using guaiac process. The assessment should also include a general physical assessment, noting facial features, skin, and visual fields because acromegaly, hypothyroidism, and pituitary tumors are commonly associated with galactorrhea. The examiner should also check for signs of other endocrine disorders, including Cushing's syndrome, and signs of renal failure, liver failure, and sarcoidosis.

Diagnostic Studies

Pregnancy should be excluded. Prepare a slide of the discharge for cytology if blood is detected. If pregnancy is excluded, additional studies should include a prolactin level and thyroid studies. Pituitary imaging should be considered if the prolactin level is elevated. If thyroid and pituitary studies are negative, renal and liver function tests should be ordered. A mammogram should be obtained to exclude malignancy even if a palpable mass is not identified.

GALACTORRHEA

Galactorrhea is characterized by bilateral and milky discharge from multiple ducts in a woman who is neither pregnant nor lactating. Causes of galactorrhea include a variety of drugs as well as an elevated prolactin level associated with pituitary tumor or hyperthyroidism. The drugs associated with galactorrhea include antidepressants (amitriptyline, imipramine), psychoactives (haloperidol, thioridazine), hormones (estrogens, progestogens), antiepileptics (valproic acid), and antihypertensives (verapamil). This list is not exhaustive.

Signs and Symptoms

If associated with prolactin elevation, there may be symptoms of a pituitary tumor, including headaches, vision change, relative infertility, and amenorrhea. The signs of thyroid disease or acromegaly may be present. If acromegaly is involved, the woman may admit to recent changes in shoe or ring size as well as other structural changes. The history may identify one or more of the medications commonly associated with galactorrhea. The breast examination is negative with the exception of possibly stimulating the production of milky, nonbloody discharge from multiple ducts.

Diagnostic Studies

Laboratory studies should include a pregnancy test, prolactin level, and thyroid functions.

PHYSIOLOGIC DISCHARGE

As noted earlier, physiologic discharge is not rare. Physiologic discharge may be associated with fibrocystic breasts or gynecomastia, or it may exist with no other breast complaints. In addition to squeezing of the breast, physiologic discharge may be caused by trauma or exercise. It may occur in response to hormonal changes at puberty or menopause.

Signs and Symptoms

Physiologic discharge is not spontaneous but is triggered by manipulation and/or excessive movement. It is bilateral, comes from multiple ducts, and is serous in appearance. The patient may complain of cyclic symptoms of mastalgia or lumpy breasts.

PATHOLOGIC DISCHARGE

Pathologic discharge is most often unilateral, spontaneous, and limited to one duct, although multiple ducts in a limited area may be involved. It can be intermittent and persistent. The color of pathologic discharge ranges widely and can be watery, cloudy, bloody, serosanguineous, green-gray, and multicolored. In spite of the term *pathologic,* the cause is usually benign and frequently includes duct ectasia or an intraductal papilloma. Duct ectasia results in dilation of one major breast duct and causes approximately one-third of the cases of pathological discharge. Papillomas are responsible for 44% of pathologic discharge. Papillomas can occur singly or in multiples; the intraductal papilloma is generally located proximal to the nipple.

Signs and Symptoms

Because the discharge associated with ductal ectasia is often stagnant, the discharge is cheesy in appearance. It is often associated with noncyclic breast discomfort and a subareolar lump at the site of the dilated duct. Because one major duct is involved, the discharge comes also from one duct or nipple area. However, in contrast to the discharge associated with duct ectasia, papillomas cause discharge that ranges from serous to serosanguineous to bloody. A clean glass slide is used to collect discharge for inspection and any subsequent analysis.

Diagnostic Studies

A mammogram should be ordered, and it will reveal the dilated duct or the papilloma. Surgical consultation is indicated to determine the need for excision.

MALIGNANCY

Breast discharge is also a potential sign of malignancy (11%). Up to 5% of women diagnosed with breast cancer have nipple discharge as part of their presentation, although it is rarely a solitary symptom or sign. Cytology of the discharge is diagnostic in only approximately 50% of cases in which cancer is present and is therefore not reliable in diagnosis. Mammography should be performed to begin discrimination among benign causes, such as mammary duct ectasia, cancer, and other possibilities. However, a negative mammogram does not exclude malignancy. In fact, of those women who presented with nipple discharge and were diagnosed with cancer, only approximately 50% had an abnormal mammogram. Thus, if a benign explanation is not identified for the discharge, the woman should be referred to a surgeon for further evaluation.

PAGET'S DISEASE

It is possible that spotting from nipple erosion of Paget's disease may be construed by a patient as discharge, which is described in the following section.

■ Skin Lesions of the Nipple and Areola

It is not common for skin conditions to involve the breast area, although it is possible for the skin overlying the breast to be involved with atopic rashes, herpes zoster, or other conditions. Paget's disease is a malignancy that involves skin changes of the nipple and, later, the areola and which should be considered when patients complain of a rash or other skin lesion on the breast.

History

The history for breast-related skin changes should include the analysis of the skin lesion. Ask when the patient first noticed the lesion and how, if at all, it has progressed since that time. Ask about associated symptoms such as pain, discharge, bleeding, or itching. Ask whether the patient has noticed any masses or other breast changes. Determine whether skin changes have been noticed elsewhere. Ask about any activities that might have caused the lesion. Explore whether the patient has experienced any general symptoms such as fatigue or fever. Ask about prior history of atopic diseases and malignancies. Similarly review the family history for atopic diseases and malignancies.

Physical Examination

A thorough breast examination should be performed with assessment of any masses, nodules, or discharge, as described earlier in this chapter. Any skin lesions should be evaluated as described in Chapter 3, noting particularly the location and whether or not the nipple and/or areola are involved.

Diagnostic Studies

If the lesion involves the nipple and/or areola, a surgical consult and mammogram should be arranged. Otherwise, if the physical examination does not cause suspicion for malignancy, the diagnostic studies are likely not warranted but would be consistent with the differential diagnosis.

PAGET'S DISEASE

Paget's disease is responsible for a small percentage of breast cancers. The typical presentation involves skin changes of the nipple and/or areola, with the nipple being involved first. The condition does not always involve a palpable mass or nodule. Any patient with unexplained skin changes to the nipple and areola area should be evaluated by a surgeon. Even with another potential explanation for the condition, a surgical consult should be considered, or the patient should be scheduled for a timely reevaluation.

Signs and Symptoms

The patient may describe the persistence of skin changes for several months. The skin changes involving the nipple and, potentially, the areola range from scaling redness to various degrees of ulceration. On occasion, the patient may provide a history of intermittent clearing with or without some prior self-treatment. There is often no palpable mass and there may be no mammographic abnormality.

Diagnostic Studies

A mammogram should be ordered and a surgeon consulted for definitive diagnosis.

SKIN MALIGNANCY

It is possible that a skin malignancy, such as malignant melanoma or Bowen's disease, could involve the skin overlying the breast. Skin malignancies are described in Chapter 3.

HERPES ZOSTER

Herpes zoster can affect the skin overlying the breast, depending on the nerve root involved. Herpes zoster is described in Chapter 3.

OTHER SKIN CONDITIONS

Atopic diseases such as eczema, contact dermatitis, and infectious skin conditions could involve the breast area. See Chapter 3.

▪ Male Breast Enlargement or Mass

As noted previously, although the risk for developing breast cancer is much lower in men than in women, 1% of all breast cancer is diagnosed in men. In addition to the potential for a malignancy, complaints of breast changes in men may indicate hormonal disturbances, adverse effects of medications, and systemic symptoms of liver or renal disease. Complaints of breast enlargement or mass should trigger careful investigation.

The general term for male breast enlargement is gynecomastia, which can be present in one or both breasts. Even though hormone-related gynecomastia is relatively common, particularly in pubertal and older adult males, it must be differentiated from adipose tissue, lipoma, hematoma, malignancy, and systemic conditions.

History

Obtain a full history of the breast enlargement, including when it was first noted, any subsequent changes in the area, and any associated symptoms. When asking about associated symptoms, include skin changes, discharge and pain or tenderness, and systemic symptoms that would indicate extramammary conditions. Identify any history of previous breast changes or procedures and the family history of breast disease. The medical history should be directed toward identifying all current and previous medical problems and a list of all medications/drugs currently taken.

Physical Examination

A complete examination of the breasts should be performed. The male breasts are best examined with the patient resting supine with his arm raised over his head. The same examination techniques used for women should be incorporated, including careful inspection for any skin changes, retractions, areas of thickening, bulges, or visible masses. The palpation should include comparison of breast tissue consistency between the breasts and identification of any palpable masses and their characteristics. The axillary nodes should be assessed. Obese men are more likely to have "fatty breasts" than true gynecomastia. It is often helpful to compare the consistency of the affected breast(s) with the consistency of the tissue in the anterior axillary fold region to determine whether adipose tissue is involved.

Diagnostic Studies

If a palpable mass is discovered that is not consistent with gynecomastia (see the following section), imaging studies (an ultrasound or mammogram) should be obtained to determine the cause. A surgical consult should be obtained if a benign diagnosis is not certain.

GYNECOMASTIA

Gynecomastia most often occurs during infancy, puberty, and senescence. It is caused by an altered balance between estradiol and testosterone levels. Although it can be an indication of primary hypogonadism (see Chapter 12), hyperthyroidism, cirrhosis, or renal disease, the majority of the cases are specific to hormonal changes of puberty, are drug induced, or are idiopathic. With the presentation of breast enlargement in a male, malignancy must always be considered.

Signs and Symptoms

The enlargement associated with gynecomastia presents as a disk-shaped rubbery area of tissue that is centered beneath the areola, extending out centrifugally. The thickened area of tissue may be tender, and there may be associated nipple discharge. Other times, there are no other findings or symptoms except for the area of enlargement. If drug induced, the patient may identify one of the many drugs known to cause gynecomastia, such as phenytoin, cimetidine, estrogens, calcium-channel blockers, ACE inhibitors, spironolactone, finasteride, methyldopa, or marijuana. If the drug is eliminated, the enlargement may resolve. If related to cirrhosis or renal failure, other physical signs of the etiologic condition should be evident. A mass that is located remote to the areola and/or is hard, irregularly shaped, or immobile is not consistent with gynecomastia.

Diagnostic Studies

If the mass or enlargement is consistent with gynecomastia, there is no need to perform diagnostic studies. However, ultrasound or mammography should be considered, if necessary, for either definitive diagnosis or reassurance of the patient. The provider should be alert to the remote potential that the gynecomastia stems from cirrhosis or renal disease and determine whether renal or liver function studies should be ordered.

PSEUDOGYNECOMASTIA

Pseudogynecomastia refers to fatty deposits and enlargements of the breast related to obesity.

Signs and Symptoms

The patient will have no tenderness, discharge, discrete palpable masses, or other symptoms related to the breast enlargement. The area of enlargement will have a consistency similar to the patient's other fatty areas, such as the tissue in the immediate region of the anterior axillary fold.

Diagnostic Studies

There are no diagnostic studies indicated for pseudogynecomastia.

MALIGNANCY

On average, 1,500 new cases of male breast cancer are diagnosed each year in the United States, and there are over 400 related deaths (ACS, 2008). Men develop the same types of breast cancer as women. Therefore, it is important to include malignancy in the differential diagnosis when a man complains of breast enlargement. Factors that increase the risk of breast cancer in men include a previous history of breast or testicular disease and Klinefelter's syndrome. A history of gynecomastia is not associated with an increased risk for breast cancer.

Signs and Symptoms

The man may complain of breast tenderness, skin changes, and/or nipple discharge. There may be associated systemic symptoms of fatigue, weight loss, and so on. The mass may be more evident in a male patient who has less breast tissue than a woman. The mass will usually lie in a location inconsistent with gynecomastia. However, regardless of the site, any firm or hard mass should trigger investigation for malignancy. Nipple discharge associated with malignancy is often bloody.

REFERENCES

American Cancer Society. (2008). *Breast Cancer Facts and Figures 2007–2008*. Atlanta, GA: America Cancer Society.

American College of Radiology. (2006). "ACR Appropriateness Criteria: Palpable Breast Masses." http://www.acr.org/SecondaryMainMenuCategories/quality_safety/app_criteria/pdf/ExpertPanelonWomensImagingBreastWorkGroup/PalpableBreastMassesDoc3.aspx (accessed March 14, 2011).

Begg, C. (2002). On the use of familial aggregation in population-based case probands for calculating prevalence. *Journal of the National Cancer Institute, 94*(16), 1221–1226.

Burke, W., et al. (1997). Recommendations for individuals with an inherited predisposition to cancer. *JAMA, 277*(12), 997–1003.

SUGGESTED READINGS

Bickley, L.S. (2008). *Bates' Guide to Physical Examination and History Taking*. Philadelphia: Lippincott, Williams, and Wilkins.

Bland, K.L., & Copeland, E.M. (2004). *The Breast: Comprehensive Management of Benign and Malignant Disorders*. Philadelphia: Saunders.

Dillon, P.M. (2007). *Nursing Health Assessment: A Critical Thinking, Case Studies Approach*. Philadelphia: F.A. Davis.

Grube, B., & Guiliana, N. (2007). Benign breast disease. In Berek, J. (Ed.), *Berek & Novak's Gynecology*, 14th ed. Philadelphia: Lippincott, Williams, & Wilkins.

Hall, J., & Kraus, J. (2003). *An Atlas of Breast Disease*. New York: Parthenon.

Klein, S. (2005). Evaluation of palpable breast masses. *American Family Physician, 71*, 1731–1738.

Swartz, M.H. (2005). *Textbook of Physical Diagnosis: History and Examination*. Philadelphia: Saunders.

Chapter 10

ABDOMEN

Mary Jo Goolsby • Laurie Grubbs

Digestive diseases encompass more than 40 acute and chronic conditions of the gastrointestinal tract. The average number of visits to physician offices, hospital outpatient and emergency departments for gastrointestinal diseases is 42.2 million annually (Centers for Disease Control and Prevention [CDC], 2006). Over 110,000 cases of digestive tract cancer are diagnosed each year. Colorectal cancer is the fourth most common cancer and the third most common cause of cancer deaths (2006), and chronic liver disease and cirrhosis together was ranked twelfth in leading causes of death (CDC, 2007). Digestive disease is the second leading cause of disability due to illness in the United States and the leading cause of lost work for male employees (Parker, 2008).

The causes of abdominal complaints can range from very mild, self-limited problems to those that can be disabling or result in mortality. In addition to digestive diseases, abdominal complaints may be indicative of musculoskeletal, neurological, genitourinary, reproductive, cardiovascular, or respiratory disorders.

History

■ General History

A general history for the abdominal examination should include any reports of nausea and/or vomiting; current bowel habits, including diarrhea, changes in bowel or bladder habits, or constipation; and pain, weight loss or gain, change in appetite, bloating, excessive gas or belching, dysphagia, heartburn or indigestion, rectal bleeding, or black stools. Ask about history of jaundice, liver disease, hepatitis, gallbladder disease, fever, or malaise. As specific complaints are discussed subsequently in the chapter, further symptom analysis is described.

■ Past Medical History

A general past medical history should include any history of jaundice, liver disease, hepatitis, gallbladder disease, infectious diseases, PUD, GERD, bleeding or platelet disorders, trauma, or previous surgeries with the emphasis on abdominal surgeries.

■ Family History

Identify any family history of liver or gallbladder disease, hepatitis, or cancer. There is a familial predisposition to certain diseases of the digestive tract, such as inflammatory bowel disease, polyposis, and cancer of the colon. The risk of hepatitis is increased among family members in the same household, especially hepatitis C.

■ Habits

Habits may be particularly important for certain abdominal complaints, especially the use of tobacco, caffeine, and alcohol. Also important are a list of all medications/drugs, activity, exercise, and sleep patterns. Identify usual dietary intake. Explore sexual habits. Ask about travel patterns and recent exposures.

Physical Examination

The abdominal examination begins with inspection, followed by auscultation, percussion, and palpation. Auscultating before percussion or palpation allows the examiner to listen to the abdominal sounds undisturbed. Moreover, if pain is present, it is best to leave palpation until last and to gather other data before possibly causing the patient discomfort. When examining the abdomen, it often helps to break the abdomen down into quadrants, or regions, in order to consider which organs are involved (see Fig. 10.1).

Abdominal Regions

RUQ	Epigastric	LUQ
Liver	Stomach	Spleen
Gallbladder	Pancreas	Pancreas
Tip of right kidney		Tip of left kidney
Diaphragm		
Right Lumbar	**Umbilical**	**Left Lumbar**
	Uterus	
	Bowel	
	Aorta	
RLQ	Suprapubic	LLQ
Appendix	Bladder	Left ovary
Right ovary	Uterus	Bowel
Bowel		

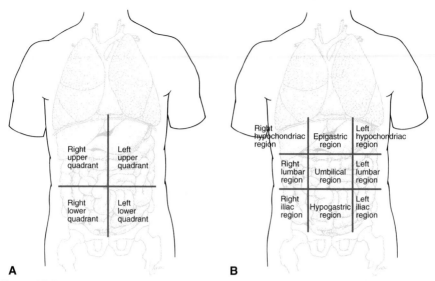

Figure 10.1 Areas of the abdomen: (A) four quadrants, (B) nine regions. (From Scanlon, V.C., & Sanders, T. *Essentials of Anatomy and Physiology*, 4th ed. Philadelphia: F.A. Davis, 2003. Reprinted with permission.)

■ Order of the Examination

Inspection

Inspect for scars, striae, venous pattern, rashes, contour, symmetry, masses, peristalsis, pulsations, or discolorations. Tangential lighting is helpful when observing for peristalsis and pulsations. See Table 10.1 for abnormalities found on inspection.

Auscultation

Perform auscultation before palpation so as to hear unaltered bowel sounds. Listen for bruits over the aorta and the iliac, renal, and femoral arteries. See Table 10.2 for abnormalities found on auscultation.

Percussion

Percuss for areas of dullness, indicating fluid or solid rather than air. See Table 10.3 for normal percussion tones.

Palpation

Both light and deep palpation are necessary to detect tenderness, tumors, or changes in underlying structures. Note areas of tenderness, changes in contour, and the presence of masses—and if masses are present, their consistency, size, shape, location, and delineation. See Table 10.4 for abnormalities found on palpation.

- Light palpation is helpful in detecting tenderness and guarding.
- Deep palpation is usually required in order to delineate masses.

Table 10.1

Abnormalities on Inspection

Physical Finding	Cause
Scars	Indicating past surgery or trauma
Striae	Includes obesity, ascites, pregnancy, tumor, Cushing's disease, and steroid use
Venous pattern	May be prominent in fair-skinned people or due to congested portal circulation
Discoloration	Consider jaundice, Addison's disease, von Recklinghausen's disease, trauma, or other rashes or lesions
Visible peristalsis	In an older adult, consider bowel obstruction. In newborns, upper abdominal peristalsis is diagnostic for pyloric stenosis
Pulsations	Visible aortic pulsations may be normal in thin individuals but in others may indicate aortic aneurysm
Distention	For changes in contour or symmetry, consider the Fs of abdominal distention: fat, fluid, feces, fetus, flatus, fibroid, full bladder, fatal tumor, false pregnancy

Table 10.2

Abnormalities on Auscultation

Physical Finding	Cause
Bruits	A swishing sound heard over the aortic, renal, iliac, and femoral arteries, indicating narrowing or aneurysm
Pops/tinkles	High-pitched sounds suggesting intestinal fluid and air under pressure, as in early obstruction
Rushes	Rushes of high-pitched sounds that coincide with cramping suggest intestinal obstruction
Borborygmi	Increased, prolonged gurgles occur with gastroenteritis, early intestinal obstruction, and hunger
Rubs	Grating sounds that vary with respiration. Indicate inflammation of the peritoneal surface of an organ from tumor, infection, or splenic infarct
Venous hum	A soft humming noise often heard in hepatic cirrhosis that is caused by increased collateral circulation between portal and systemic venous systems
Succussion splash	A splashing noise produced by shaking the body when there is both gas and fluid in a cavity or free air in the peritoneum or thorax
Decreased/absent sounds	Occurs with peritonitis or paralytic ileus

Table 10.3

Normal Tones Produced by Percussion

	Most Dense			Least Dense	
Tone	Flat	Dull	Resonant	Hyperresonant	Tympanic
Intensity	Soft	Medium	Loud	Very loud	Loud
Pitch	High	Medium	Low	Very low	High
Duration	Short	Medium	Long	Very long	Medium
Area	Muscle, bone	Liver, spleen	Lung	Emphysematous lung	Gastric air bubble

Table 10.4

Abnormalities on Palpation

Condition	Description	Characteristics
Hepatomegaly	Liver enlargement can be detected by percussion and/or palpation and can be caused by cirrhosis, hepatitis, right heart failure, cysts, and malignancy	Cirrhosis produces an enlarged, firm, nontender liver. Hepatitis and right heart failure are characterized by a smooth, tender liver. Cysts may not be palpable but will produce right upper quadrant pain and tenderness. A malignancy typically produces a firm, irregular liver surface
Splenomegaly	The causes of an enlarged spleen include infectious or inflammatory diseases, such as mononucleosis, infectious hepatitis, subacute bacterial endocarditis, psittacosis, tuberculosis, malaria, sarcoidosis, amyloidosis, systemic lupus erythematosus; lymphoproliferative and myeloproliferative diseases, such as lymphoma, leukemia, polycythemia, and myelofibrosis; hemolytic anemias and hemoglobinopathies; splenic cysts; and storage diseases, such as Gaucher's, Niemann-Pick, and Hand-Schuller-Christian diseases	In addition to an enlarged and usually tender spleen, other symptoms are early feeding satiety, splenic friction rub, epigastric and splenic bruits, and cytopenias

Continued

Table 10.4

Abnormalities on Palpation—cont'd

Condition	Description	Characteristics
Aortic aneurysm	Arteriosclerosis is the most common cause of aortic aneurysm. Aging, cigarette smoking, and hypertension are contributing factors. Trauma; syphilis; congenital connective tissue disorders, such as Marfan's disease; and positive history of aneurysm also increase the incidence	A prominent lateral pulsation suggests an aneurysm
Tumor	Caused by any benign or malignant growth in any of the abdominal organs	Variable according to the affected organ but include pain, bloating, obstruction, anorexia, and changes in bowel or genitourinary functioning

Rectal Examination

A digital rectal examination is included in the abdominal examination. Note skin changes or lesions in the perianal region or the presence of external hemorrhoids. Insert the gloved index finger into the anus with the patient either leaning over or side-lying on the examination table, and note any internal hemorrhoids or fissures. Check the stool for occult blood. For males, the rectal examination is necessary for direct examination of the prostate.

■ Special Maneuvers

Rebound Tenderness

Rebound tenderness is tested by slowly pressing over the abdomen with your fingertips, holding the position until pain subsides or the patient adjusts to the discomfort, and then quickly removing the pressure. Rebound pain, a sign of peritoneal inflammation, is present if the patient experiences a sharp discomfort over the inflamed site when pressure is released.

Rovsing's Sign

Appendicitis is suggested when there is referred rebound pain in the *right* lower quadrant when the examiner presses deeply in the *left* lower quadrant and then quickly releases the pressure.

Heel Strike

Ask the patient to stand with straight legs and to raise up on toes. Then ask the patient to relax, allowing the heel to strike the floor, thus jarring the body. A positive heel strike is indicative of appendicitis and peritoneal irritation. Alternatively, strike the plantar surface of the heel with your fist while the patient rests supine on the examination table.

Obturator Sign

Pain is elicited in appendicitis by inward rotation of the hip with the knee bent so that the obturator internus muscle is stretched.

Psoas Sign

Place your hand on the patient's thigh just above the knee and ask the patient to raise the thigh against your hand. This contracts the psoas muscle and produces pain in patients with an inflamed appendix.

Murphy's Sign

Pain is present on deep inspiration when an inflamed gallbladder is palpated by pressing the fingers under the rib cage. Murphy's sign is positive in cholecystitis.

Hepatojugular Reflux

The hepatojugular reflux is elicited by applying firm, sustained hand pressure to the abdomen in the midepigastric region while the patient breathes regularly. Observe the neck for elevation of the jugular venous pressure (JVP) with pressure of the hand and a sudden drop of the JVP when the hand pressure is released. The hepatojugular reflux is exaggerated in right heart failure.

Scratch Test

An alternative to palpation/percussion to determine hepatic size is the "scratch" test. It is performed by placing the stethoscope over the liver and then lightly scratching up the abdomen on the right side, using a fingertip or tongue depressor. The sound you hear through the stethoscope will be intensified over the liver.

Shifting Dullness

To differentiate ascites, test for shifting of the peritoneal fluid to the dependent side by rolling the patient side to side and percussing for dullness on the dependent side of the abdomen. Note: This maneuver is nonspecific and has, for the most part, been replaced by ultrasonography of the abdomen.

Differential Diagnosis of Chief Complaints

■ Abdominal Pain

Abdominal pain is one of the most common complaints in primary care and can be functional or organic in cause and acute or chronic in nature. Even though the causes of abdominal pain are often self-limiting, the pain can also indicate a life-threatening situation and must be carefully assessed.

RED Flag **Red Flags for Abdominal Pain**

- Pain that awakens patient
- Pain that persists more than 6 hours and progresses in intensity
- Pain that changes location
- Associated syncope
- Pain followed by vomiting or intractable vomiting
- Hematemesis
- Black, tarry stools
- Progressive abdominal distention
- Pain worsened by movement, respirations
- Radiation of the pain to shoulder (cholecystitis) or back (pancreatitis/aneurysm)
- Decreased urine output
- Fever, leukocytosis, granulocytosis
- Pain associated with signs of hypovolemic shock

When a patient complains of abdominal pain, it is essential to rule out indications for an emergency referral by carefully reviewing the history of the complaint, including the general description, quantity, quality, location, timing, and onset of the pain and associated symptoms. Although the physical examination may suggest the cause, the examination may be normal even with underlying pathology. Laboratory studies and diagnostic testing may be necessary to pinpoint the actual cause and rule out the more serious causes. Table 10.5 presents normal values for some of the laboratory tests commonly used in differential diagnosis of the abdomen.

There are three major categories used to classify abdominal pain: visceral, somatoparietal, and referred. Referred pain is simply pain radiating or referring from a site external to the abdomen. See Table 10.6 for differentiating common characteristics of visceral and somatoparietal pain.

■ Right Upper Quadrant (RUQ) Pain

A complaint of RUQ pain encompasses a variety of possible causes, most commonly diseases of the liver, gallbladder, pancreas, or lung. In the abdomen, it is important also to consider referred pain from a different area in the abdomen or from a different body system. Also consider diseases of the colon or kidney, or gynecological system for women, which are covered in this chapter under lower quadrant pain. Because the abdomen contains many structures and organs, a thorough history and physical examination is necessary with special maneuvers if warranted.

Table 10.5

Normal Laboratory Values for Differential Diagnosis of the Abdomen

Test	Normal Value
Aspartate aminotransferase (AST) (serum glutamic-oxaloacetic transaminase [SGOT])	42 units/L or less
Alanine aminotransferase (ALT) (serum glutamate pyruvate transaminase [SGPT])	Less than 48 units/L
Alkaline phosphatase	25–150 units/L
Albumin	3.5–5.0 g/dL
Globulin	1.5–4.5 g/dL
Albumin to globulin (A/G) ratio	1.1–2.5
Total serum protein	6.0–8.5 g/dL
Total bilirubin	Less than 1.3 mg/dL
Amylase	30–170 units/L
Lipase	7–60 units/L
Blood urea nitrogen (BUN)	7–30 mg/dL
Serum creatinine	1.2 mg/dL or less
Uric acid	Female: 2.5–7.5 mg/dL Male: 4.0–8.5 mg/dL
White blood count (WBC)	3.8–10.8 × 10^3/μL
Hemoglobin (Hgb)	Female: 12.0–15.6 g/dL Male: 13.8–17.2 g/dL
Hematocrit (Hct)	Female: 35%–46% Male: 41%–50%
Cancer antigen 125 (CA-125)	Less than 35 units/mL
Carcinoembryonic antigen (CEA)	Non-smoker: less than 2.5 ng/L Smoker: less than 5.0 ng/L

History

Begin with the exact location of the pain, onset, timing, quality and quantity, and alleviating or aggravating factors—particularly if the pain is related to meals or movement. Ask if there has been any fever, nausea, vomiting, diarrhea, constipation, anorexia, or change in urine or stool color/consistency, which may indicate liver or gallbladder disease. A pleuritic cause for the pain should be considered; inquire about cough, shortness of breath, or fever. Include a smoking history. Ask about diet history, particularly in regard to a high-fat diet or fad diets that might exclude food groups or be very low in calories. This may increase the likelihood of gallbladder disease. Inquire about

Table 10.6

Differentiating Types of Abdominal Pain

Visceral	Somatoparietal
Poorly localized	Localized
Vague	Intense
Often midline	Guarding
Crampy	Patient often still
Burning	
Patient often restless	
Associated with:	**Worsened by:**
Diaphoresis	Movement
Pallor	Respirations
Nausea	Cough
Caused by:	**Caused by:**
Inflammation or injury to solid or hollow organs	Inflammation of the parietal peritoneum

sexual practices, alcohol, and drugs (prescription and illicit) that might alert you to an increased risk for liver disease, particularly hepatitis. Ask about foreign travel because hepatitis is endemic in some areas, and often the standards for food preparation are not the same as in North America. Ask about patient and family history of breast or colon cancer, gallbladder or liver disease, and general disorders of the digestive tract.

Physical Examination

A thorough abdominal examination should be performed with particular attention to the RUQ, assessing for tenderness, rebound, masses, and organ enlargement or nodularity. A respiratory examination should include auscultation for adventitious breath sounds and the presence of friction rubs or voice sounds. Table 10.7 summarizes differential diagnosis for RUQ (and left upper quadrant) pain.

The conditions of the underlying organs are key to identifying the etiology of RUQ pain. Consider diseases of the gallbladder, liver, pancreas, or lung as the most likely cause of pain. In the case of the RUQ, laboratory testing can be most helpful and often diagnostic (see Table 10.8).

GALLBLADDER DISEASE

A mnemonic used to describe a common presentation for cholecystitis is "female, fat, and forty," although it can occur in much younger and older individuals after surgery, trauma, burns, sepsis, or critical illness. Young people have shown an increased incidence of cholecystitis if they are adhering to drastic weight-loss diets that are extremely low in fat and calories.

Table 10.7

Differential Diagnosis for Right and Left Upper Quadrant Pain

Disease	History	Diagnostic Studies	Physical Findings
Cholecystitis	RUQ pain, anorexia, nausea, vomiting, fever	CBC, LFTs, amylase, GB US, HIDA scan	↑ Neutrophilic leukocytes, ↑ AST/ALT, ↑ amylase with common duct obstruction; US will show nonvi-sualization of the galbladder and wall thickening
Liver disease	RUQ pain, sexual practices, travel, alcohol use, history of malignancy, nausea, vomit-ing, anorexia, drugs, raw shellfish inges-tion, change in color of urine or stools, weight loss, abdominal distention	LFTs, hepatitis profile, abdomi-nal US or CT	↑ LFTs, ↑ IgM, and specific antigens will be present for Hep-atitis A, B, and C; US or CT may show cysts or tumors, obstruction
Pancreatitis	Epigastric pain, alcohol abuse, liver or gallblad-der disease, jaundice, hyperlipidemia	Amylase, lipase, LFTs, plain abdominal films, abdomi-nal US or CT, chest x-ray	↑ Amylase and lipase, ↑ LFTs, ↑ WBC, epigas-tric tenderness, pancreatic or biliary obstruc-tion on US or CT
Pleurisy	Respiratory disease, such as upper respiratory infection or pneumonia, shortness of breath, chest trauma, other systemic disease	Chest x-ray	If there is air or fluid in the pleu-ral space, inves-tigate other more serious diagnoses

Continued

Table 10.7

Differential Diagnosis for Right and Left Upper Quadrant Pain—cont'd

Disease	History	Diagnostic Studies	Physical Findings
Hypersplenism	LUQ pain, anorexia, fever, fatigue, weight loss, recent infection, bruising or bleeding, lymphadenopathy, jaundice	CBC, platelet, SPE, amylase, B_{12}, uric acid, bone marrow aspiration, abdominal CT	Vary depending on underlying cause: cytopenias or myeloproliferation or lymphoproliferation, $\uparrow B_{12}$ in leukemias and polycythemia, $\uparrow$ uric acid in proliferative disorders, monoclonal gammopathy or $\downarrow$ immunoglobulins on SPE, abnormalities on CT and bone marrow aspirate

ALT = alanine aminotransferase; AST = aspartate aminotransferase; CT = computed tomography; HIDA = hepatobiliary iminodiacetic acid; IgM = Immunoglobulin M; LFT = liver function tests; LUQ = left upper quadrant; RUQ = right upper quadrant; SPE = serum protein electrophoresis; US = ultrasound.

Table 10.8

Laboratory Studies for Upper Abdominal Pain

Study	Description
Complete blood count (CBC)	CBC determines elevated white blood cells in infection; decreased hematocrit and hemoglobin, indicating the possibility of a gastrointestinal bleed; and cytopenic or myeloproliferative disorders, indicating hepatic or splenic involvement
Platelet count	Thrombocytopenia or thrombocytosis may indicate diseases involving the liver or spleen
Alanine aminotransferase (ALT)	ALT primarily helps diagnose liver disease, but also detects biliary obstruction
Aspartate aminotransferase (AST)	AST primarily helps diagnose liver disease; however, elevations are also associated with acute common bile duct obstruction. AST levels may be affected by statin drugs, acetaminophen, and alcohol

Table 10.8

Laboratory Studies for Upper Abdominal Pain—cont'd

Study	Description
Alkaline phosphatase	Alkaline phosphatase is used as a tumor marker and an index of liver and bone disease or metastasis in correlation with other findings
Gamma glutamic transpeptidase (GGT)	GGT determines liver cell dysfunction and detects alcohol-induced liver disease. The GGT can be helpful as a confirmatory test
Lactate dehydrogenase (LDH)	LDH is a widely distributed enzyme that is elevated with cellular damage of the liver, kidney, skeletal muscle, and heart
Bilirubin	Bilirubin evaluates liver function, biliary obstruction, and hemolytic anemia
Albumin	Albumin is influenced by nutritional state and hepatic and renal function
Amylase	Amylase helps distinguish pancreatitis from other causes of abdominal pain
Lipase	Lipase helps diagnose pancreatitis and stays elevated longer than amylase. However, lipase is not specific and may also be elevated in biliary and hepatic disease, diabetes mellitus, and gastric malignancy
Hepatitis profile	A hepatitis profile detects acute or chronic, active and previous disease, carrier state, and immunity to hepatitis A, B, C
Prothrombin time (PT)	An increased PT indicates clotting dysfunction, which may be attributed to liver disease.
Serum protein electrophoresis (SPE)	An SPE is an evaluation of proteins (e.g., albumin, alpha globulins, beta globulins, and gammaglobulins) present in the serum. SPE may help diagnose autoimmune liver disease, cirrhosis, and α_1-antitrypsin deficiency
Helicobacter pylori	*H. pylori* is a serum blood test that detects common bacteria causing peptic ulcer disease.

Signs and Symptoms

Initially, acute colicky pain is localized in the RUQ and is often accompanied by nausea and vomiting. Murphy's sign is frequently present. Fever is low grade, and the increase in neutrophilic leukocytes in the blood is slight. Acute cholecystitis improves in 2 to 3 days and resolves within a week; however, recurrences are common. If acute cholecystitis is accompanied by jaundice and cholestasis (arrest of bile excretion), suspect common duct obstruction.

Diagnostic Studies

Suggested laboratory tests include alanine aminotransferase (ALT), aspartate aminotransferase (AST), amylase and lipase. A diagnosis can usually be made with ultrasound or hepatobiliary iminodiacetic acid (HIDA) scanning.

Decision Rule for Gallbladder Disease

Ebell (2001) reports a decision rule for common bile duct lithiasis developed by Houdart, Perniceni, Dame, and colleagues. The prediction rule was developed on a sample of 503 patients and validated on a group of 279 patients. They found that patients were at low risk (0.6%) for common bile duct lithiasis if they presented with no jaundice and normal transaminases, had a common bile duct diameter of less than 8 mm, and had no ultrasound-demonstrated intrahepatic duct enlargement. In contrast, patients who had jaundice, abnormal transaminases, a common bile duct diameter of greater than 8 mm, and intrahepatic duct enlargement were categorized as "at risk" (39%).

If the signs and symptoms do not typically point to cholecystitis, an abdominal ultrasound or computed tomographic (CT) scan will allow visualization of the entire abdomen. A chest x-ray is recommended if respiratory involvement is suspected.

LIVER DISEASE

Liver diseases include viral hepatitis (hepatitis A, B, C, D, E), alcohol-related hepatitis, cirrhosis, hepatic cysts, and malignancy (primary or metastatic).

Signs and Symptoms

The major clinical manifestations of liver disease include jaundice, hepatomegaly, cholestasis, portal hypertension, ascites, and encephalopathy. Symptoms vary with the cause, but many are insidious, especially with hepatitis. Liver disease is often discovered on routine examination or laboratory testing.

Diagnostic Studies

If liver disease is suspected, begin with liver function tests (ALT, AST, alkaline phosphatase, albumin, bilirubin, and total protein) and a hepatitis profile.

These tests provide valuable information on most liver diseases, except hepatic cysts, which generally do not alter liver functions. If cirrhosis, malignancy, or a hepatic cyst is suspected or should be eliminated, include an abdominal ultrasound or CT scan.

Those found to have hepatitis B or C should be referred to a gastroenterologist or infectious disease specialist. Hepatitis A is usually self-limiting and can be managed by the nurse practitioner or family physician.

PANCREATITIS

Biliary tract disease and alcoholism account for 80% or more of the pancreatitis admissions. Other causes include hyperlipidemia, drugs, toxins, infection, structural abnormalities, surgery, vascular disease, trauma, hyperparathyroidism and hypercalcemia, renal transplantation, and hereditary pancreatitis. The most common cause of pancreatitis is alcohol abuse.

Signs and Symptoms

Pancreatitis is characterized by severe abdominal pain, often with radiation to the back and usually accompanied by nausea and vomiting. The pain is steady and boring (piercing, penetrating), often refractory to narcotic pain medicines, and persistent for many days. Fever is present within a few hours, and other signs include tachycardia, rapid and shallow respirations, postural hypotension, diaphoresis, blunted sensorium, abdominal distention, tenderness, hypoactive bowel sounds, and possibly ascites.

Diagnostic Studies

There is no single test to diagnose pancreatitis, but several tests support the clinical impression, including serum amylase and lipase, white blood count (WBC), supine and upright plain films of the abdomen, chest x-ray, and ultrasound. Lipase and amylase are usually quite elevated, as is the WBC. Ultrasound imaging will detect an enlarged pancreas as well as gallstones and biliary obstruction. A CT scan can be used in lieu of ultrasound to image the pancreas, but it is less helpful in identifying gallstones as the potential cause.

PLEURISY

Pleurisy may result from (1) an underlying lung process, (2) an infection or irritation in the pleural space, (3) the transport of an infectious or other disease agent or neoplastic metastases to the pleura, and (4) trauma, especially rib trauma. Basilar pleurisy may produce referred pain to the abdomen.

Signs and Symptoms

Pleurisy is differentiated from abdominal disease by chest x-ray or evidence of a respiratory origin, such as increased pain with deep breathing and coughing, shallow or rapid breathing, the absence of nausea or vomiting, or a tendency toward relief of pain with pressure on the chest wall or abdomen. A pleural friction rub is pathognomonic.

Diagnostic Studies

Pleurisy may not be evident on any thoracic imaging and may be a diagnosis made by history and physical examination. A chest x-ray or CT of the chest showing inflammation or pleural thickening is helpful in some cases.

■ Left Upper Quadrant (LUQ) Pain

Diseases and disorders of the spleen, stomach, and pancreas are the most likely causes of LUQ pain (see Table 10.7). Also consider colon and kidney disease, which are covered in this chapter under lower quadrant pain. For disorders of the spleen and pancreas, laboratory evaluation is helpful along with the history and physical. For the stomach, more definitive diagnostic tests may be needed.

History

LUQ pain is often associated with causes that are outside the abdomen. Hematopoietic malignancies, such as lymphomas and leukemias, and other hematologic disorders, such as thrombocytopenia, polycythemia, myelofibrosis, and hemolytic anemia, often cause enlargement of the spleen leading to LUQ pain. In addition to questions about the specific characteristics of the pain, it is important to ask the patient about fever, unusual bleeding or bruising, recent diagnosis of mononucleosis, fatigue, malaise, lymphadenopathy, cough, arthralgias, anorexia, weight loss, jaundice, high blood pressure, and headache.

Decision Rule for Pancreatitis

Ebell (2001) reports a prediction rule developed by Balthazar, Robinson, Megibow, and Ranson (1990) to determine the severity of acute pancreatitis. The rule is based on 88 patients and was not validated on a second group. The rule uses a score determined by CT scan results, with an index possible range of 0 to 10. A categorization of patients indicates the risk of both mortality and complication from the disease. Patients at the low end of the index (1–3) are predicted to have a low risk of mortality (3%) and complications (8%), whereas patients scoring at the high end (7–10) of the index are predicted to have a higher incidence of mortality (17%) and/or complications (92%).

Physical Examination

A thorough abdominal examination is necessary with special attention to the LUQ. A respiratory examination should be included to rule out referred pain. A hematopoietic cause can be explored only through laboratory tests (see Table 10.8).

HYPERSPLENISM

Abnormalities are almost always secondary to other primary disorders, most commonly cytopenic hematologic disorders, such as lymphoma, leukemia, thrombocytopenia, polycythemia, myelofibrosis, and hemolytic anemias. Other causes include portal or splenic vein thrombosis; infection, such as mononucleosis, infectious hepatitis, subacute bacterial endocarditis (SBE), psittacosis, miliary tuberculosis, malaria, brucellosis, and syphilis; sarcoidosis; amyloidosis; connective tissue diseases, such as systemic lupus erythematosus (SLE) and rheumatoid arthritis; lipoid and nonlipoid storage diseases; and splenic cysts. Splenomegaly results from an increase in splenic workload by the trapping and destroying of abnormal blood cells or diverse abnormal circulating organisms.

Signs and Symptoms

The signs and symptoms are highly variable and relate to the underlying cause. The patient may complain of early satiety or abdominal fullness and LUQ pain. If the cause is infectious, fatigue and/or fever are common. On physical examination, splenomegaly is present. An epigastric or splenic bruit may be present. The complete blood count (CBC) may identify anemia, leukopenia, thrombocytopenia, or any combination of the three.

Diagnostic Studies

Several laboratory studies may be needed to diagnose the numerous underlying causes of hypersplenism. Begin with a CBC and platelet count, which will likely provide the most information on how to proceed. If abnormal, a bone marrow biopsy is indicated. Other tests to consider are serum protein electrophoresis, liver function tests, B_{12}, amylase, and CT or magnetic resonance imaging (MRI) of the abdomen.

PLEURISY
See Right Upper Quadrant (RUQ) Pain, p. 250.

PANCREATITIS
See p. 257.

GASTRIC CONDITIONS
See Epigastric Pain in the following subsection.

■ Epigastric Pain

Epigastric pain can represent the heartburn or dyspepsia often associated with GERD, as well as several other diseases, including malignancies. The epigastric region is a very common site of discomfort stemming from many digestive structures. Heartburn, often from GERD, is a very common complaint; patients may use alternative terms to describe this sensation, including "indigestion" or "sour stomach." *Dyspepsia* covers a variety of complaints that include heartburn, fullness, bloating, and upper abdominal pain. Because pain in this region provides little specificity on its own, the history is crucial in narrowing the differential diagnosis.

The physical examination is most helpful in eliminating some of the rarer causes of epigastric pain; the common causes are typically associated with benign physical findings. A change in vital signs can point to cardiac or respiratory disturbances as well as to potential fevers and infections. A positive hemoccult on rectal examination may indicate an upper gastrointestinal (GI) bleed or malignancy. Malignancy should also be suspected if there is weight loss and/or a palpable abdominal mass. Listen for adventitious abdominal sounds, such as succussion splash, indicating air or fluid in the thorax or peritoneum, or aortic bruit heard with abdominal aneurysm. Be alert for a positive Murphy's sign, which is seen in cholecystitis. Note any abnormalities in skin tone and/or color that could indicate liver disease, cholecystitis, or hypoxia owing to respiratory or cardiac disease.

Common Causes of Epigastric Pain

- Gastroesophageal reflux disease (GERD)
- Gastric or duodenal ulcer
- Gastric or duodenal malignancy
- Esophageal spasm
- Cholecystitis
- Pancreatitis
- Hepatitis/liver disease
- Medication intolerance
- Ischemic heart disease
- Pregnancy

History

To differentiate among the causes of epigastric pain, have the patient clearly describe his or her complaint, particularly the characteristics (sharp, dull, nagging, burning, steady, cramping, boring, etc.), and point to the exact location of the pain. Discomfort stemming from a serious disorder is often constant and intense and may radiate to the back. Determine what factors worsen and/or improve the discomfort, particularly any relationship to meals or activity. When rating the severity of the pain, determine what, if any, behaviors the pain has limited, including intake or physical activities. Establish the type of onset and progression, including whether the discomfort is intermittent, gradually increasing in severity, and so on. Finally, determine what, if any, associated symptoms the patient has noticed. Important considerations include vomiting, regurgitation, diaphoresis, dysphagia, blood in the stool or emesis, shortness of breath, fatigue, weight loss, and radiation to other sites (intra- and extra-abdominal). Ask about any new or current medications.

Physical Examination

A thorough examination of the entire abdomen is necessary, with special attention to the epigastric area. Tenderness can be present with PUD and pancreatitis. Auscultating for bruits in this area is vital; abdominal aortic aneurysm may present with epigastric pain. It is a life-threatening and possibly emergent problem. Vital signs and weight need to be recorded looking for any signs of infection, blood loss, or weight loss in the case of malignancy. A rectal examination for occult blood can add important information. In addition, a thorough respiratory and cardiac history and examination should be performed because the pain may be referred. Depending on history and cardiovascular risks, consider an electrocardiogram (EKG) to rule out a cardiac source for the pain (see Table 10.8).

GASTROESOPHAGEAL REFLUX DISEASE

GERD is the most common organic cause of heartburn. Lower esophageal sphincter (LES) control can be decreased by several medications (e.g., theophylline, dopamine, diazepam, calcium-channel blockers), foods and/or beverages (caffeine, alcohol, chocolate, fatty foods), and tobacco use. When LES tone is lower than normal, secretions are allowed to reflux into the esophagus, causing discomfort. Reflux is also promoted by weight gain and other variables causing greater pressure against the LES.

Signs and Symptoms

The most common symptom of GERD is heartburn, which typically occurs after meals and is often relieved by antacids. Other symptoms include belching, regurgitation, and/or water brash. Respiratory and ear, nose, and throat symptoms may develop, including cough, wheeze, aspiration, hoarseness, and globus sensation (fullness in the throat). Symptoms may occur primarily at night, when patients recline following a meal. See Box 10.1 for common triggers of GERD.

Diagnostic Studies

Diagnosis can often be made by the history, although the degree of symptoms may not be consistent with the degree of esophageal injury. When gastroesophageal reflux is the most likely cause of acute epigastric discomfort, empiric treatment may include avoiding any triggers as well as prescribing antacids and/or antisecretory agents, particularly for a young, otherwise healthy patient without known risk factors for more serious disorders.

Box 10.1

Common Triggers for GERD

Tomato products
Citrus
Spicy foods
Coffee
Fatty foods
Peppermint
Chocolate
Alcohol
Smoking

However, the risk of delaying the definitive diagnosis and treatment must be weighed when considering this route. Endoscopy provides direct visualization of the esophagus and evidence to rule out other disorders. Ambulatory esophageal pH monitoring may help to identify association between symptoms and reflux. Barium swallows and upper GI x-ray have a high potential of missing esophageal damage.

PEPTIC ULCER DISEASE

PUD includes both gastric and duodenal ulcers. *Helicobacter pylori* and NSAIDs are common causes of both disorders, along with some probable genetic predisposition. Zollinger-Ellison syndrome commonly results in gastric ulcer development. The incidence of gastric ulcer is higher in persons who smoke and those with certain chronic disease, including cirrhosis, hyperparathyroidism, chronic renal failure, and lung disease.

Signs and Symptoms

Epigastric pain is common with both gastric and duodenal ulcers and is described as a gnawing or burning sensation. Whereas the pain of gastric ulcer is usually worsened by intake, a duodenal ulcer usually causes pain on an empty stomach. It is not uncommon for the pain of duodenal ulcer to awaken the patient from sleep at 1 to 2 a.m. Antacids typically offer relief for both types of ulcer. Pain may be episodic with symptom-free intervals. Pain may radiate to the back. Associated symptoms include bloating, belching, nausea, and loss of appetite. The physical examination is not usually positive other than potentially identifying some degree of abdominal tenderness. As the mucosa erodes, bleeding may occur. If rupture occurs, pain acutely changes character and is intractable.

Diagnostic Studies

Stool guaiac should be performed on any patient with epigastric pain. PUD should be suspected in any patient with dyspepsia/epigastric pain who does not fit the profile associated with GERD, is older than 50 years, and has associated weight loss or loss of appetite; direct endoscopy should be ordered. Biopsies will be taken of any erosive site to rule out gastric malignancy. If PUD is diagnosed, testing for *H. pylori* should be performed. When patients with gastric ulcers have neither *H. pylori* nor a history of NSAID use, serum gastrin level should be determined, assessing for Zollinger-Ellison syndrome.

GASTRIC MALIGNANCY

Although the incidence of gastric cancer is lower than in the past, it has remained relatively steady for several years. It is estimated that 21,000 adults would be diagnosed in the United States in 2010, with 10,570 deaths (American Cancer Society, 2010). Suspected contributing factors, including excess salt intake and chronic gastritis, as is seen with *H. pylori*, can lead to gastric cancer. The early stage of the disease is asymptomatic, and diagnosis is made usually only after significant advancement; the 5-year survival rate is 20.6%.

Signs and Symptoms

Cancers of the stomach are rarely symptomatic until the disease has progressed. Symptoms may be mild and consistent with heartburn or include more definite abdominal pain. Other symptoms include nausea and vomiting, diarrhea, constipation, fullness, anorexia, fatigue, and weight loss. Although the abdominal examination may be negative, tenderness and/or a palpable mass may be present.

Diagnostic Studies

The patient should be referred for endoscopy. A CBC should be ordered, anemia assessed, and stool guaiac performed.

PANCREATITIS
See p. 257.

CHOLECYSTITIS
See p. 252.

HEPATITIS
See p. 256.

■ Right and Left Lower Quadrant Abdominal Pain

Lower abdominal pain can have a multitude of causes, including diseases or disorders of the appendix, colon, kidney, bladder, ureter, ovary, uterus, and prostate. Pinpointing the specific location of the pain is crucial to beginning the differential diagnosis; however, caution is recommended because abdominal pain can be referred from areas of the abdomen other than the point of origin. Because of the complexity of the differential diagnosis for lower abdominal pain, diagnostic tests are often necessary to confirm the findings of the history and physical.

History

There are a multitude of etiologies for lower abdominal complaints. It is important to begin with a thorough history. Although abdominal pain can often radiate to other areas or can present a vague and confusing picture, pinpointing the location of the pain is a prudent place to start. Question the patient about the onset of the pain and whether it is accompanied by fever, anorexia, nausea, or vomiting, which might suggest appendicitis, gastroenteritis, or obstruction. It is imperative to ask about the last menstrual period (LMP) and about birth control methods in order to rule out ectopic pregnancy. A history of miscarriages and/or sexually transmitted diseases (STDs) can give more clues for the risk of ectopic pregnancy. Safe sex practices and the number of sexual partners can alert the practitioner to the risk for pelvic inflammatory disease (PID). Ovarian tumors can go undetected for months, and the examiner must be alert to vague symptoms that might indicate a need for further investigation, such as bloating, gas, dyspepsia, and pressure type pain. These complaints in a postmenopausal woman should not be trivialized. A positive family history of ovarian cancer in a patient presenting with these complaints is a red flag. Urinary symptoms such as dysuria, hematuria, and a history of kidney stones indicate a risk for kidney stones. If the patient complains of pain with movement or exercise and gives a history of heavy lifting, then hernia may be suspected. Sudden onset of severe lower abdominal pain, nausea, and vomiting in a young male should alert the examiner to the possibility of testicular torsion. A complaint of fatigue, weakness, weight loss, or change in bowel or bladder habits is worrisome, and a malignancy should be on the top of the list of differential diagnoses. Occasionally, hip disorders can present as lower abdominal pain.

Physical Examination

An entire abdominal examination is necessary with the addition of the genitourinary system. It is warranted in both males and females but is of particular importance in females. *No complaint of lower abdominal pain in a female should be evaluated without performing a pelvic examination.* A rectal examination should be performed for occult blood, for palpation of the uterus or prostate, and for the presence of masses or tenderness. Although an unusual cause of lower abdominal pain, a musculoskeletal history and examination should be included, particularly when the pain is in the groin or hip area.

For clarity, the lower abdominal complaints are broken down into the following regions: right lower quadrant (RLQ), left lower quadrant (LLQ), periumbilical, and suprapubic. For an overview and summary of the differential diagnosis of lower abdominal pain as well as laboratory studies, see Tables 10.9 and 10.10.

Table 10.9

Differential Diagnosis of Lower Abdominal Pain

Disease	History	Diagnosis	Findings
Appendicitis	Anorexia, nausea, vomiting, fever, midline or RLQ pain worsening with cough or walking	CBC, abdominal CT or US	+ Rebound tenderness, fever, leukocytosis of 10,000–20,000/µL, US or CT may be positive for perforation/abscess
Ectopic pregnancy	Amenorrhea, severe RLQ or LLQ pain	Pelvic US, urine and serum hCG	A pregnancy outside the uterus, usually the tube, + hCG, + US, + rebound tenderness
Colorectal cancer	Weight loss, fatigue, change in bowel habits, anemia, + hemoccult	Hemoccult, CBC, CEA, flexible sigmoidoscopy, colonoscopy	+ Hemoccult, ↑ CEA ↓ hematocrit and hemoglobin, + flexible sigmoidoscopy or colonoscopy

Table 10.9

Differential Diagnosis of Lower Abdominal Pain—cont'd

Disease	History	Diagnosis	Findings
Urinary calculi	+ History of stones, severe colicky flank pain	U/A, plain abdominal x-ray, renal US, IVP	Hematuria, + stone visualization with x-ray or US
Ovarian tumor	+ Family history, abdominal bloating, pain, or heaviness	Pelvic examination, pelvic US, CT, CA-125	↑ CA-125, mass on examination, CT, or US
Hernia	History of straining or heavy lifting, previous abdominal surgery, lower abdominal or groin pain	Physical examination or US	Palpable mass in the inguinal ring or femoral area
Intestinal obstruction	History of abdominal surgery or inflammatory bowel disease, radiation, or impaction; abdominal pain or distention, vomiting; obstipation	Flat and upright abdominal x-ray, BE, CBC, electrolytes, BUN, creatinine, U/A	+ Mass on examination, BE, or x-ray; tinkles, rushes, borborygmi, or absent bowel sounds, ↑ SG, ↑ BUN and creatinine; electrolyte imbalance; leukocytosis
Diverticulitis	+ History of diverticulosis	CBC, flexible sigmoidoscopy, BE, abdominal CT	Leukocytosis, abdominal mass, stricture, hypertrophy of colonic musculature, possible free air in the abdomen
Gastroenteritis	Sudden onset diarrhea, abdominal cramping, nausea, vomiting, fever	CBC, stool for ova and parasites, culture and sensitivity	Abdominal tenderness, borborygmi, possibly positive stool culture

BE = barium enema; BUN = blood urea nitrogen; ALT = alanine aminotransferase; AST = aspartate aminotransferase; CA125 = cancer antigen 125: CEA = carcinoembryonic antigen; CT = computed tomography; hCG = human chorionic gonadotropin; HIDA = hepatobiliary iminodiacetic acid; IgM = Immunoglobulin M; LFT = liver function tests; LUQ = left upper quadrant; RUQ = right upper quadrant; SG = specific gravity; SPE = serum protein electrophoresis; U/A = urinalysis; US = ultrasound.

Table 10.10

Laboratory Studies for Lower Abdominal and Suprapubic Pain

Study	Description
Complete blood count	White blood cells (WBCs) are elevated in appendicitis and diverticulitis, and the hematocrit and hemoglobin may be decreased in colon cancer
Serum/urine pregnancy	In ectopic pregnancy, human chorionic gonadotropin may not be at the levels appropriate for the number of weeks as estimated by last menstrual period
Urinalysis (U/A)	A dipstick or complete U/A identifies WBCs and blood indicating infection, renal calculi, or malignancy; increased specific gravity with dehydration
Prostate-specific antigen (PSA)	A PSA is a useful screening and diagnostic tool for prostate disease; if elevated, a prostate ultrasound and biopsy is recommended
Wet prep, gonococcal/ chlamydia culture	A wet prep can identify WBCs, but a culture is necessary to identify the offending organism. A gonococcal/chlamydial culture may be positive in salpingitis/pelvic inflammatory disease (PID). If positive for STD, other test considerations include RPR, HIV, and hepatitis profile
Carcinoembryonic antigen (CEA)	The CEA will be elevated in colon cancer
Cancer antigen 125 (CA-125)	A CA-125 is a tumor marker for progression or regression of ovarian tumors but can be helpful for initial diagnosis. False negatives occur in approximately 20% of patients with ovarian cancer. False positives can occur in patients with endometriosis, benign ovarian cysts, first trimester pregnancy, PID, cirrhosis, and pancreatic cancer. It is more specific in postmenopausal than premenopausal women

APPENDICITIS

Other than hernia, appendicitis is the most common cause of acute abdominal pain. It occurs most commonly between the ages of 10 and 30 years. Because gangrene, perforation, and peritonitis can develop within 36 hours if untreated, approximately 15% of patients sent to surgery with a diagnosis of appendicitis are falsely positive. Ultrasound and CT have decreased the incidence of overdiagnosis, but in some cases, laparotomy or laparoscopy are still required for a definitive diagnosis. Gynecologic disorders and gastroenteritis are the most common causes of misdiagnosis.

Signs and Symptoms

The pain of appendicitis usually evolves over a few hours and initially is poorly localized, midline, and vague; associated with some degree of nausea and/or loss of appetite. In a matter of hours, the pain migrates to the RLQ, becoming more intense and localized, and may increase with coughing or walking. Low-grade fever typically develops. The various tests for peritoneal irritation (rebound tenderness, Rovsing's, heel strike, psoas, and obturator) are positive.

Diagnostic Studies

An elevated WBC and the physical examination are the two most important diagnostic tools. If the diagnosis is still uncertain, an abdominal CT with contrast is helpful.

ECTOPIC PREGNANCY

A pregnancy is considered ectopic if implantation takes place outside the cavity of the uterus, with 98% of those being tubal. Conditions that predispose a woman to an ectopic pregnancy are those that prevent the migration of the fertilized ovum to the uterus, and approximately 50% are due to a previous tubal infection. Other risk factors include a history of infertility, PID, previous abdominal or tubal surgery, previous tubal pregnancy, and the use of an intrauterine device.

Signs and Symptoms

The most obvious sign of ectopic pregnancy is amenorrhea followed by spotting and sudden onset of severe lower quadrant pain. A stat pregnancy test should be performed. Backache may be present. There is tenderness on pelvic examination, and a pelvic mass may be palpated. Blood is present in the cul-de-sac. Shock and hemorrhage occur if the pregnancy ruptures. Abdominal distention with peritoneal signs will ensue. Immediate laparoscopy or laparotomy is indicated because this condition is life threatening.

Diagnostic Studies

The diagnosis of ectopic pregnancy can be made with urine human chorionic gonadotropin (hCG) or stat serum hCG, pelvic ultrasound, and, if necessary, culdocentesis to detect blood in the cul-de-sac.

COLORECTAL CANCER

Colorectal cancer is the second leading cause of death from malignancies in the United States. Over half are located in the rectosigmoid region and are typically adenocarcinomas. Risk factors include a history of polyps, positive family history of colon cancer or familial polyposis, ulcerative colitis, granulomatous colitis, and a diet low in fiber and high in animal protein, fat, and refined carbohydrates.

Signs and Symptoms

The cancer may be present for several years before symptoms appear. Complaints include fatigue, weakness, weight loss, alternating constipation and diarrhea, a change in the caliber of stool, tenesmus, urgency, and hematochezia. Physical examination is usually normal except in advanced disease, when the tumor can be palpated or if hepatomegaly is present owing to metastatic disease.

Diagnostic Studies

Stool for occult blood is recommended, and a colonoscopy is diagnostic. A barium enema may be helpful initially, but if positive, colonoscopy will be necessary for biopsies. Recommended laboratory studies include a CBC and carcinoembryonic antigen (CEA) test. A positron emission tomography (PET) scan may be valuable for tumor origin and metastasis.

URINARY CALCULI

Men are more frequently affected by urinary calculi, with a ratio of 4:1, until the sixth or seventh decade, when the risk equalizes. Many factors contribute to the formation of stones, including geographic, diet, genetic, and occupational factors. Stones occur more frequently in people living in hot, humid climates. Diets high in salt and protein and, in some cases, oxalate and purines can increase the risk of calculi. Despite previous beliefs, a diet high in calcium is a contributing factor only in some individuals. Some stones, particularly cystine stones, may be genetically linked, and persons in sedentary occupations are more likely to develop stones than are manual laborers. The most common types of stones are made of calcium (calcium oxalate and calcium phosphate); the other three types are struvite, uric acid, and cystine.

Signs and Symptoms

Urinary calculi can occur anywhere in the urinary tract and therefore pain can originate in the flank or kidney area and radiate into the RLQ or LLQ and then to the suprapubic area as the stone attempts to move down the tract. The pain is severe, acute, and colicky and may be accompanied by nausea and vomiting. If the stone becomes lodged at the ureterovesical junction, the patient will complain of urgency and frequency. Blood will be present in the urine.

Diagnostic Studies

The urinalysis typically shows hematuria. Infection must be ruled out because a combination of infection and obstruction requires prompt intervention to prevent pyelonephritis and kidney damage. A plain, flat plate of the abdomen or a renal ultrasound is the most helpful in diagnosing stones. If diagnosis remains uncertain, a noncontrast CT is indicated. Alternatively, an intravenous pyelogram (IVP) should be ordered if a CT is not available. Pain medicine is imperative if patients are to undergo lengthy diagnostic testing.

OVARIAN CYST AND TUMOR

Although there are no hard-and-fast rules, ovarian cysts are more likely to occur in the younger female, whereas ovarian cancer has a greater incidence in the postmenopausal female. Women with a positive family history of ovarian cancer have a 5% lifetime risk versus a 1.6% risk in those with no family history. The long-term use of oral contraceptives may decrease the risk of ovarian cancer.

Signs and Symptoms

Ovarian masses are often asymptomatic, but symptoms may include pressure type pain, heaviness, aching, and bloating. Cysts tend to be more painful than malignant tumors and often spontaneously resolve with the onset of the menstrual cycle. Masses are typically detected on pelvic examination. In advanced malignancies, ascites is often present.

Diagnostic Studies

An elevated cancer antigen 125 (CA-125) result indicates the likelihood that the mass is malignant. A transvaginal pelvic ultrasound has a higher diagnostic sensitivity than transabdominal ultrasound. If diagnosis is unclear, CT, MRI, or PET scan can be performed. A laparoscopy or exploratory laparotomy is necessary for staging, tumor debulking, and resection.

INGUINAL AND FEMORAL HERNIA

In the majority of hernia cases, a history of heavy physical labor or heavy lifting can be elicited. Young children and individuals with a history of abdominal surgery are also at increased risk.

Signs and Symptoms

Right or left lower quadrant pain that may radiate into the groin or testicle is typical. The pain is usually dull or aching unless strangulated, in which case the pain is more severe. The pain increases with straining, lifting, or movement of the lower extremities. Physical examination includes palpating the femoral area and inguinal ring for bulging or tenderness. Ask the patient to bear down against your hand.

Diagnostic Studies

The physical examination is often all that is necessary for diagnosis, but ultrasound may be helpful.

INTESTINAL OBSTRUCTION

The most common causes of mechanical obstruction are adhesions, almost exclusively in patients with previous abdominal surgery, hernias, tumors, volvulus, inflammatory bowel disease (Crohn's disease, colitis), Hirschsprung's disease, fecal impaction, and radiation enteritis. Additional information can be found under the sections on nausea and vomiting and diarrhea.

Signs and Symptoms

Initially, the patient complains of a cramping periumbilical pain that eventually becomes constant. Abdominal distention, vomiting that may lead to dehydration, diarrhea in partial obstruction, and obstipation occur when obstruction is complete. Physical examination reveals mild, diffuse tenderness without peritoneal signs and possibly visible peristaltic waves. In early obstruction, tinkles, rushes, and borborygmi can be heard. In late obstruction, bowel sounds may be absent. There is minimal or no fever. Carefully inspect and palpate for hernias and masses.

Diagnostic Studies

The diagnosis can be made with flat and upright abdominal films and with barium enema if the diagnosis is unclear. CT or MRI may also be necessary. CBC and electrolytes are recommended to look for leukocytosis and electrolyte imbalance; blood urea nitrogen (BUN), creatinine, and urinalysis are performed to detect extracellular volume loss.

DIVERTICULITIS

Diverticular disease is prevalent in patients over 60 years of age. It is seen more commonly in Western countries and is thought to be due to a diet deficient in fiber. It most often affects the sigmoid colon. Patients with connective tissue disease, such as scleroderma, Marfan's syndrome, and Ehlers-Danlos syndrome, are at increased risk.

Signs and Symptoms

Although the pain can be generalized, it is typically localized to the left lower abdomen and is accompanied by tenderness, fever, and leukocytosis. These symptoms in a person with a known history of diverticulosis make the diagnosis almost certain for diverticulitis. Other symptoms can include constipation or loose stools, nausea, vomiting, and positive stool occult blood. With diverticulitis, there is an increased risk of perforation which presents with a more dramatic clinical picture as a result of peritonitis. Look for signs of peritonitis, such as a positive heel strike test and/or rebound tenderness.

Diagnostic Studies

A CBC will show mildly elevated white blood cells. Plain abdominal films should be obtained to look for an ileus, a small or large bowel obstruction, and free air in the abdomen, indicating perforation. Acute medical management is indicated, and after 7 to 10 days, a flexible sigmoidoscopy and/or barium enema is recommended. These should not be done in the acute stage because the risk of perforation increases during the procedure. A CT without contrast may also be helpful.

GASTROENTERITIS

See sections on nausea and vomiting and diarrhea pp. 271, 278.

■ Pelvic or Suprapubic Pain

The following are covered in detail in Chapter 11:

1. Inguinal and femoral hernia
2. Testicular torsion

3. Prostatitis
4. Prostate cancer
5. Epididymitis
6. Urinary tract infection
7. PID/salpingitis
8. Renal calculi
9. Pyelonephritis

History

Ask about urinary symptoms, such as dysuria and frequency; heavy lifting; contact sports; sexual practices; the presence of vaginal or penile discharge; and a history of STDs, kidney stones, or prostate disease.

Physical Examination

The physical examination should include a thorough abdominal examination, a pelvic and genital examination, and a rectal examination including prostate for males.

■ Nausea and Vomiting

Nausea and vomiting usually stem from GI infections but may reflect many categories of problems, including other infections, actual or functional GI obstruction, metabolic disorders, central nervous system disorders, drugs, pain, pregnancy, and psychiatric disorders. A detailed list of potential causes is provided in Table 10.11. This section describes the basic approach to nausea and vomiting to differentiate among major potential causes. Table 10.11 summarizes common findings for each condition listed and will help narrow your diagnosis and limit your work-up appropriately. The approach to nausea and vomiting should be determined by the patient's age, overall health, and medical history.

History

A thorough symptom analysis should identify any triggering events, such as meals, offensive odors, motion, position changes, and pain. Determine what, if anything, relieves the symptoms, including any attempted self-treatments. Determine what is meant by a complaint of "nausea": loss of appetite, queasiness, sense of imminent vomiting, or retching. When vomiting has occurred, determine the color, amount, presence of bile or undigested food, and frequency/number of episodes. The severity of the nausea can be rated; the presence of associated symptoms is an important consideration: fever, diarrhea, diaphoresis, syncope, or pain. When determining the temporal sequence, establish the relationship to meals, activity, or travel; the time of day when symptoms are the worst; when the symptoms were first noticed; sudden or gradual onset; and whether the patient has been exposed to others who are ill. Whereas nausea is commonly intermittent in nature, medications can cause unrelenting symptoms. Because many substances can cause nausea, the complete drug history is essential and should include prescribed, over-the-counter, and recreational drugs and alcohol. Table 10.11 lists specific causes of nausea and vomiting and the common descriptions. The current and past health history may identify comorbid disorders that might cause nausea (renal failure with metabolic disturbances, diabetes with gastroparesis) as well as treatment modalities that might contribute to the nausea and/or vomiting.

Table 10.11

Causes of Nausea and Vomiting

Cause	Examples	Typical Signs and Symptoms
Infection	Gastroenteritis (viral or bacterial), hepatitis, pelvic inflammatory disease, viral syndrome, upper respiratory infection	Abrupt onset, spontaneous vomiting, often accompanied by fever, malaise, and diarrhea
Food poisoning	Bacterial sources: *Clostridium botulinum*, staphylococcus Nonbacterial sources: mushrooms, poisonous plants, fish, chemicals	Symptoms occur hours to days after exposure, severe nausea and vomiting often with diarrhea, neurological symptoms, liver involvement
Gastrointestinal obstruction	Gastric outlet obstruction related to peptic ulcer disease, gastroesophageal reflux disease, malignancy, esophageal stricture, pyloric stenosis, or intestinal obstruction related to malignancy, intussusception, adhesions, and motility disorders	Emesis containing undigested food, upper or lower abdominal pain and tenderness, absent bowel sounds, x-ray or computed tomography showing bowel loops, ileus, mass, or stricture
Metabolic disorders	Renal disease with uremia, hyperglycemia, ketoacidosis, Addison's disease, hyperthyroidism	Mild nausea rarely accompanied by vomiting; fatigue, weakness, muscle cramping, skin changes, hypotension or hypertension, neuropathic changes, abnormal renal or endocrine laboratory studies
Medication	Cardiac medicines, especially digitalis and quinidine; antihypertensives; antibiotics; bronchodilators, especially aminophylline; antineoplastic drugs; NSAIDs; monoamine oxidase (MAO) inhibitors; antidepressants; antiretrovirals; oral hyperglycemics	Symptoms may be from central trigger zone stimulation or irritation to the gastric mucosa. Reactions to medicine generally cause a persistent nausea. If from gastric irritation, the nausea will worsen soon after medication administration. With trigger zone stimulation, nausea is often delayed. If related to cardiac medicines or bronchodilators, there may be changes in heart rate and EKG readings

Table 10.11

Causes of Nausea and Vomiting—cont'd

Cause	Examples	Typical Signs and Symptoms
Central nervous system disorders	Meningitis, increased intracranial pressure, migraines, space-occupying lesion or fluid, Ménière's disorder, cerebellar disorders	Central nervous system–related vomiting is often projectile and not preceded by nausea. Vomiting caused by a space-occupying lesion is often worse upon arising due to a recumbent increase in intracranial pressure. Depending on the cause, accompanying symptoms include headache, visual disturbances, nystagmus, ataxia and, in meningitis, nuchal rigidity
Cardiac disease	Myocardial infarction, congestive heart failure	Often nausea only, but vomiting may occur in myocardial infarction with severe pain. In congestive heart failure, the nausea is vague and persistent, accompanied by pain, diaphoresis, shortness of breath, edema
Pregnancy	Due to either hormonal or emotional changes	Typically nausea without emesis often in the morning but may present with persistent or intermittent vomiting, missed or irregular menses, positive human chorionic gonadotropin
Psychogenic	Anorexia, bulimia, anxiety	Usually promptly follows eating, may remit on hospitalization, more common in young women
Cholecystitis/ pancreatitis	Due to infection, inflammation, or obstruction of the pancreas or gallbladder	Nausea and vomiting is intermittent and usually accompanied by right upper quadrant or epigastric pain

Physical Examination

The physical examination should start with a general survey and vital signs. Pulse and blood pressure provide important information about hydration status, and a fever may suggest infection; weight helps to determine any changes associated with decreased intake and/or significant vomiting. Even though the physical is guided by the history and initial observations, signs of obstruction should be determined, including altered bowel sounds or succussion splash; scars should be noted as signs of surgery; percussion and palpation should be adequate to identify any tenderness, masses, or organomegaly.

INFECTION (VIRAL)

Viral gastroenteritis is the most common cause of nausea, vomiting, and diarrhea. At least 50% of cases of gastroenteritis as foodborne illness are due to norovirus. Another 20% of cases, and the majority of severe cases in children, are due to rotavirus. Other significant viral agents include adenovirus and astrovirus.

Signs and Symptoms

Nausea and vomiting associated with acute infections (viral and bacterial) may be accompanied by fever and diarrhea as well as by other commonly associated symptoms, including malaise and fatigue. Nausea and vomiting from infections generally have a very abrupt onset; spontaneous vomiting may occur when the patient is unable to reach the toilet. The patient may be able to identify exposure to other persons with similar symptoms or other persons who ate the same meal and then developed nausea and vomiting. If hepatitis is involved, the predominant symptoms are usually nausea and/or anorexia, although vomiting may occur. Fever might be present. With dehydration, the patient may complain of lightheadedness or dizziness; the pulse may be elevated and the blood pressure positive for postural changes. Mucous membranes may be dry, and skin turgor is diminished. Bowel sounds are often exaggerated even without diarrhea; borborygmi may be present. The abdomen may be tender and/or distended.

Diagnostic Studies

Typically, common viral causes of nausea and vomiting require no diagnostic studies because they resolve within 72 hours. If the vomiting is severe, baseline laboratory tests such as CBC, urinalysis, and electrolytes are indicated to assess for infection, electrolyte balance, and hydration status. If the nausea is accompanied by severe or prolonged diarrhea, suspect a bacterial cause and obtain a CBC, stool cultures for ova and parasites (O&P), culture and sensitivity (C&S), and *Clostridium difficile*.

INFECTION (BACTERIAL)

Food poisoning can have either an infectious or a noninfectious cause. Noninfectious causes occur when one eats food contaminated with chemicals or food that contains naturally occurring toxins, such as mushrooms or fish. The range of infectious causes is broad and includes *Staphylococcus, Clostridium botulinum, Clostridium perfringens, Escherichia coli, Salmonella*, and *Yersinia enterocolitica. Shigella* can be contracted through food but generally is due to poor handwashing, since it is a fecal-oral transmission. Some sources of the infection are improperly prepared food, reheated meat dishes, seafood, dairy, and bakery products. Other risk factors include travel or residence in areas of poor sanitation. Onset of symptoms is hours to days, depending on the organism, and also include fever, headache, malaise, and diarrhea.

Signs and Symptoms

The presentation of food poisoning varies depending on the offending agent. Symptoms include headache and fever, abdominal pain, and diarrhea. Although the disturbance is usually self-limited, severe fluid and electrolyte disturbances may occur. In contrast, a botulism-related attack usually begins with severe nausea, vomiting, and/or diarrhea, but these symptoms are often followed by neurologic symptoms. Staphylococcal food poisoning may result in fever, whereas vital signs usually remain normal with botulism. When noninfectious poisons are involved, the symptoms may progress to profound neurological findings, liver damage, and even death, depending on the offensive toxin.

Diagnostic Studies

When food poisoning is suspected, serum or stool culture for the offending organism should be performed. The food may be tested, as might the vomitus.

GASTROINTESTINAL OBSTRUCTION (REAL AND FUNCTIONAL)

Gastrointestinal (GI) obstructions cause vomiting when contents cannot pass distally. Gastric outlet obstructions may be related to PUD. Intestinal obstructions often occur from adhesions from old surgical procedures; other causes include malignancy and intussusception. Functional obstruction can develop from motility disorders, such as gastroparesis, when smooth muscle contraction is diminished.

Signs and Symptoms

The contents of the vomitus commonly vary according to the level of obstruction. Gastric outlet obstruction is associated with emesis containing undigested food. Proximal small intestinal blockage is likely to be bile-stained. Distal intestinal blockage is more likely to contain fecal matter. Proximal blockage may result in a large volume of emesis, as the stomach produces up to 1.5 L of secretions/24 hours. When real obstruction is involved, pain often builds in a crescendo fashion and is then intermittently relieved or lessened following emesis. The degree of cramping and pain is often related to the proximity of the obstruction, so that obstructions of the lower intestines may have less-severe cramping, vomiting, and/or pain. Bowel sounds often are high pitched and metallic sounding but may later become absent. Tenderness may be localized or diffuse. Distention as well as a succussion splash may be present.

Diagnostic Studies

Flat and upright plain films of the abdomen typically depict dilated loops of bowels, free air, gas, or ileus. A CT scan or MRI would determine the presence of an ileus or mass. Endoscopy can identify strictures associated with PUD and esophageal disorders. A barium swallow can monitor motility.

PREGNANCY

Hormonal changes associated with pregnancy are believed to contribute to nausea and vomiting, although other theories suggest some degree of emotional etiology.

Signs and Symptoms

Although pregnant women may well present with persistent or intermittent vomiting episodes, pregnancy more commonly causes nausea without emesis. The nausea can occur at any time of the day but occurs most often in the morning and without regard to meals. Although this may be the presenting symptom of pregnancy, the patient will have recently missed or had an irregular period.

Diagnostic Studies

Perform urine or serum hCG.

METABOLIC DISORDERS

A variety of metabolic disorders can present with nausea and/or vomiting. Common examples include renal disease associated with uremia and many endocrine problems, such as hyperglycemia, ketoacidosis, Addison's disease, and hyperthyroidism.

Signs and Symptoms

Nausea is more common than vomiting with metabolic disorders. With uremia of renal failure, other common symptoms are muscle cramping, neuropathic changes, hypertension, and skin changes. With diabetes, the patient may present with the classic symptoms of hyperglycemia. With adrenal insufficiency, or Addison's disease, common early symptoms include fatigue, weakness, hypotension, and skin changes.

Diagnostic Studies

The diagnosis depends on the suspected metabolic disorder. Consider BUN/creatinine, which will be elevated in renal disease. Order blood glucose, serum bicarbonate, and urine ketones if diabetes is suspected with or without ketoacidosis.

CENTRAL NERVOUS SYSTEM DISORDERS

The range of neurologic disorders that result in nausea and/or vomiting is broad. Included are meningitis, increased intracranial pressure (ICP), migraines, a space-occupying lesion, and Ménière's disorder.

Signs and Symptoms

Central nervous system–related vomiting is often projectile and may not be preceded by nausea. Associated complaints/findings depend on the causative lesion. Papilledema may accompany increased ICP. Neurological deficits may be evident with increased ICP, space-occupying lesions, and meningitis.

Nuchal rigidity is a classic finding for meningitis. With Ménière's or other forms of labyrinthitis, nystagmus and/or ataxia may be present. Migraines may be preceded with the classic visual disturbance or other auras and are typically unilateral. See Chapter 16.

Diagnostic Studies

A CT scan of the head is warranted in most cases, and if meningitis is suspected, a lumbar puncture may be necessary.

MEDICATIONS

Drugs are very common causes of nausea and vomiting. The nausea associated with medications may stem from either central trigger zone stimulation or irritation to the gastric mucosa. Drugs commonly associated with nausea and vomiting are listed in Table 10.11.

Signs and Symptoms

Drugs, like other toxins, generally cause a persistent nausea. There may be associated findings related to the toxic level. For instance, with excessive levels of digitalis, vision may be altered and bradycardia evident. With excessive aminophylline, tachycardia and tremors may be manifested.

Diagnostic Studies

The primary diagnostic study would be a level of the suspected agent.

PSYCHOGENIC CAUSES

Emotional disturbances may result in either chronic or recurrent episodes of vomiting. Examples include bulimia and extreme anxiety responses.

Signs and Symptoms

Usually, psychogenic vomiting promptly follows eating and may occur during the meal; it is more common in young women. This vomiting is not urgent and can usually be suppressed; it may remit on hospitalization. The patient may show little concern regarding the vomiting. The patient may be very thin, but often in the case of bulimia, the patient is of normal weight. In other patients, vomiting occurs when there is acute anxiety associated with stressful situations or events, such as public speaking, interviews, and tests.

Diagnostic Studies

When no organic cause is found to explain recurrent or chronic vomiting, a psychiatric history should be performed.

CARDIAC CAUSES

Depending on the patient's health history and/or risk factors, you may include cardiac-related disorders in your differential diagnosis for nausea and/or vomiting. These can be associated with both myocardial infarction and congestive heart failure (see Chapter 7). Another potential cardiac-related source, mentioned previously, includes cardiac medications.

GERD

See pp. 261–262.

PEPTIC ULCER DISEASE, GASTRITIS

See pp. 259, 262.

CHOLECYSTITIS

See p. 252.

■ Diarrhea

The causes of diarrhea are numerous and include bacterial, viral, organic, and functional. The mechanisms are due to (1) abnormal transport mechanisms; (2) a change in the osmotic mechanism, resulting in variations in absorption; (3) increased motility; and (4) exudative blood or pus, which decreases absorption.

Most cases are self-limiting and resolve within days without medical intervention. When high fever, intractable vomiting, or severe dehydration is present, prompt attention is necessary, and hospitalization frequently is required—especially in children or geriatric patients.

History

Symptoms vary according to the cause of the diarrhea. A thorough symptom analysis should identify the time of onset, whether onset was sudden or gradual, and the duration of the symptoms. Determine severity according to whether the diarrhea is intermittent or persistent and according to the number of stools per day. Inquire as to associated symptoms, such as abdominal pain, fever, nausea, or vomiting, as well as whether there is any relation to meals. Ask the patient to describe the color of the stool, looking for reports of dark or bloody stools; consistency (formed, watery, fatty, or greasy); and the presence of mucus or odor. It is important to ask about recent meals or travel and if accompanying others may have similar symptoms; recent antibiotics or other new medications, either prescription or over the counter; and history of alcohol abuse or PUD that could indicate a GI bleed. Dehydration and electrolyte depletion are concerns, and the volume of fluid intake should be determined. If diarrhea has been chronic, changes in weight or appetite should be recorded. Stress or anxiety may be a causative factor; therefore, psychosocial issues should be investigated.

Physical Examination

The physical examination should begin with vital signs, particularly determining the presence of fever, which might indicate infection, and tachycardia or orthostatic hypotension, which might indicate dehydration. Other signs of dehydration include dry mucous membranes, lightheadedness, syncope, lethargy, and oliguria. If there is accompanying electrolyte imbalance, cardiac arrhythmias, muscle weakness, tetany, or vascular collapse may occur, particularly in young children, the elderly, or patients who are already debilitated. Listen for hypoactive or hyperactive bowel sounds, which could indicate early obstruction; palpate for abdominal tenderness, indicating infection or inflammation; perform a digital rectal examination, checking for heme-positive stool. A CBC showing anemia might indicate malignancy; leukocytosis might indicate inflammatory bowel disease. Significant unexplained weight loss should be investigated. Sigmoidoscopy or colonoscopy is warranted if symptoms persist.

INFECTIONS (VIRAL AND BACTERIAL)

For a general discussion on causes and risk factors, see earlier section on nausea and vomiting, pp. 271–274.

Signs and Symptoms

Diarrhea associated with acute infections (viral and bacterial) may be accompanied by fever, nausea, and vomiting; other commonly associated symptoms include malaise, fatigue, weakness, and lightheadedness. Diarrhea from infections generally has a very abrupt onset; spontaneous diarrhea may occur, and the patient is unable to reach the toilet. The patient may be able to identify exposure to other persons with similar symptoms or who ate the same meal or traveled to the same area and then developed the diarrhea. If the diarrhea is severe, dehydration may ensue, causing tachycardia and postural hypotension. Mucous membranes may be dry and skin turgor diminished. Bowel sounds are often exaggerated even without diarrhea; borborygmi may be present. The abdomen may be tender and/or distended. Several viruses have been identified as causing diarrhea: Norovirus, rotavirus, adenovirus, and enterovirus, with the latter two sometimes associated with respiratory symptoms. Common bacterial causes of diarrhea either from toxins or from mucosal invasion and ulceration include *Vibrio cholerae, Salmonella, Shigella, E. coli, Clostridium, Yersinia,* and *Campylobacter.* A botulism-related attack usually begins with severe nausea, vomiting, and/or diarrhea, but these symptoms are often followed by neurological symptoms, such as diplopia, loss of accommodation, diminished pupillary reflex, and dysphagia. *E. coli* infection is characterized by acute-onset, severe abdominal cramps and watery/bloody diarrhea. Fever may be present. *E. coli* infection can be complicated by hemolytic-uremic syndrome, which is characterized by hemolytic anemia, thrombocytopenia, and acute renal failure. The prognosis in these cases is grave. *E. coli* infection can result in death with or without these complications, especially in children and the elderly. When noninfectious poisons are involved, the symptoms may progress to profound neurological findings, liver damage, and even death, depending on the toxin.

Diagnostic Studies

Typically, common viral causes of nausea, vomiting, and diarrhea require no diagnostic studies and will resolve within 72 hours. If the diarrhea is severe or prolonged, baseline laboratory tests such as CBC, urinalysis, and electrolytes are indicated to assess for infection, electrolyte balance, and hydration status. If a bacterial cause is suspected, obtain stool cultures for O&P, C&S, and, specifically, the offending organisms.

PARASITIC INFECTION

Parasitic infections are common in rural or developing areas of Africa, Asia, and Latin America and less common in industrialized areas. In industrialized areas, parasitic infections also may affect immigrants and people who are immuno-compromised. The infections may occur in institutions with poor sanitation and unhygienic practices (day-care centers, nursing homes). Parasites causing diarrhea usually enter the body through the mouth. They are swallowed and can remain in the intestine or burrow through the intestinal wall and invade other organs.

Signs and Symptoms

Certain parasites, most commonly *Giardia lamblia*, transmitted by fecally contaminated water or food, can cause diarrhea, bloating, flatulence, cramps, nausea, anorexia, weight loss, greasy stools because of its interference with fat absorption, and occasionally fever. Symptoms usually occur about 2 weeks after exposure and can last 2 to 3 months. Often the symptoms are vague and intermittent, which makes diagnosis more difficult. There is no chemopro-phylaxis, but boiling water deactivates the *Giardia* cysts. Anti-infectives are available for treatment. Other parasites that cause diarrhea include tapeworm and roundworm, but they are uncommon in humans.

Diagnostic Studies

Serial stool samples for O&P should be ordered because a single sample may not re-veal the offending parasite. Duodenal contents can be sampled by the Entero-Test, which collects the sample by having the patient swallow a nylon string with a weight on the end and then removing the string after a certain amount of time. This is more reliable than stool cultures, but the procedure is not desirable to the patient.

AMEBIC DYSENTERY

This particular type of dysentery is common in tropical climates but rare in temperate climates.

Signs and Symptoms

It is characterized by semifluid stools containing mucus, blood, and active trophozoites. This form of dysentery may become chronic, and the symptoms are recurrent abdominal cramping and soft stools. In the chronic state, weight loss is significant and anemia is present.

Diagnostic Studies

The diagnosis is made by stool cultures, and three to six specimens may be needed before an accurate diagnosis can be made.

MEDICATION REACTION/SENSITIVITY

Drugs are a very common cause of diarrhea. The diarrhea associated with medica-tions may stem from either a generalized allergic reaction or irritation of the intes-tinal mucosa. Many drugs can cause diarrhea, but among the drugs commonly associated are quinidine, digitalis, antibiotics, metformin, and many selective serotonin reuptake inhibitors. A late sequela of antibiotic treatment—particularly with clindamycin, ampicillin, cephalosporins, erythromycin, tetracycline, and sulfamethoxazole/trimethoprim—is pseudomembranous colitis resulting from *C. difficile*. An antibiotic-induced change in the intestinal flora is the predisposing factor. *C. difficile* has been implicated in much of the nosocomial cases of diarrhea in hospitals and nursing homes. In some instances, necrotizing colitis may ensue.

Signs and Symptoms

Drugs, like other toxins, generally cause persistent diarrhea. Drugs that affect the lower GI tract often affect the upper GI tract as well, and it is common to find associated nausea or vomiting.

Diagnostic Studies

A history of a new medication gives a high likelihood of that being the causative agent. A stool culture specifically for *C. difficile* is necessary. Stopping the drug or replacing it with another category of drug should result in resolution of the diarrhea.

MUCOSAL DISEASES

Several diseases can cause mucosal inflammation and ulceration, resulting in intermittent and often severe diarrhea. These diseases include ulcerative colitis, Crohn's disease, regional enteritis, GI tuberculosis, and carcinomas.

Signs and Symptoms

The symptoms and severity of the diarrhea vary according to the underlying cause. The symptoms of carcinomas are generally insidious. The diarrhea is mild and intermittent. Often malignancies are found on routine hemoccults, sigmoidoscopy, or colonoscopy. There should be a high index of suspicion with unexplained weight loss or new-onset iron-deficiency anemia in a patient over 40 years old. With colitis, enteritis, Crohn's disease, and tuberculosis, the onset of the diarrhea may be sudden and severe with fever and significant abdominal tenderness, or it may be slow in onset with mild cramps and the urge to defecate. The stool is frequently bloody with pus and/or mucus. Malaise, fever, and weight loss are common. Initially, a history and stool examination are helpful in making a diagnosis. The stool is heavy with red and white blood cells, and usually overt blood and pus are present. Because bouts are recurrent, a positive history of these diseases supports an exacerbation. There is a risk of bowel perforation and resultant peritonitis, and in these cases, mortality may be as high as 40%.

Diagnostic Studies

A CBC and erythrocyte sedimentation rate (ESR) should be performed. Colitis is often accompanied by leukocytosis, anemia, and an elevated sedimentation rate. In malignancies, anemia is often the first sign found on routine laboratory studies. A variety of diagnostic tests may be helpful in making a definitive diagnosis, including abdominal CT, barium enema, sigmoidoscopy, or colonoscopy.

IRRITABLE BOWEL SYNDROME

IBS is a functional bowel disorder characterized by mild to severe abdominal pain, discomfort, bloating, and alteration of bowel habits. The exact cause is unknown. In some cases, the symptoms are relieved by bowel movements. Diarrhea or constipation may predominate, or they may be mixed (classified as IBS-D, IBS-C, or IBS-M respectively). IBS may begin after an infection (postinfectious, IBS-PI) or a stressful life event. There is no cure for IBS, and treatments focus on symptom management through dietary adjustments, medication, and psychological interventions. Other GI disorders may present with symptoms similar to IBS, including celiac disease, parasitic infections, several inflammatory bowel diseases, functional chronic constipation, and chronic functional abdominal pain. The exact cause of IBS is unknown, but it is hypothesized that it is a disorder of the interaction between the brain and the gut.

Signs and Symptoms

Irritable bowel syndrome is a motility disorder involving the upper and lower GI tracts that causes intermittent nausea, abdominal pain and distention, flatulence, pain relieved by defecation, diarrhea, and/or constipation. Symptoms usually occur in the waking hours and may be worsened or triggered by meals. It is three times more prevalent in women, accounts for more than half of all GI referrals, and is highly correlated with emotional factors, particularly anxiety and stress. These patients have a heightened sensitivity to food and parasympathomimetic drugs, which causes abnormalities in transit—increased in the diarrhea-predominant group and decreased in the constipation-predominant group.

Diagnostic Studies

Diagnostic studies include digital rectal examination and 3-day hemoccults for occult blood; stool for O&P and C&S; CBC to check for anemia, which might indicate a malignant cause of the symptoms; and ESR, chemistry panel, amylase, and urinalysis to rule out inflammatory, hepatic, pancreatic, or renal causes. More recently, blood tests have been developed for both celiac disease and IBS. Sigmoidoscopy or colonoscopy is recommended.

CARBOHYDRATE INTOLERANCE

More commonly known as lactose intolerance, this condition actually represents a symptom complex resulting from a lack of intestinal enzymes (usually lactase) necessary to break down disaccharides. Unsplit disaccharides in the intestine retain water and result in diarrhea.

Signs and Symptoms

Symptoms include nausea, diarrhea, abdominal cramps, borborygmi, bloating, and flatulence, which generally occur within 1 to 2 hours after eating the offending food, usually dairy products. Diarrhea may be severe, but the duration is relatively short.

Diagnostic Studies

Acid stools with a pH less than 6 are suspicious. The hydrogen breath test, if available, is easy and reliable. A lactose or glucose challenge is diagnostic when diarrhea occurs in about 30 minutes. Jejunal biopsies are generally not performed because they are invasive and expensive.

LAXATIVE USE AND ABUSE

Laxative abuse is often seen in the elderly, as caused by chronic or overtreatment of constipation. It is also seen in eating disorders, particularly bulimia, as a water and weight loss aid.

Signs and Symptoms

Misuse of laxatives may cause muscle weakness, lethargy, weight loss, electrolyte depletion, cardiac arrhythmias, changes in the intestinal mucosa, and bleeding.

Diagnostic Studies

The diagnosis of laxative abuse is made by history. Those treating constipation should be educated regarding dietary changes, adequate fluid intake, and the proper use of bulking agents so as to avoid the need for laxative use. Overdependence on laxatives for regular bowel movements only compounds the constipation problem. Rarely does this type of laxative use cause serious electrolyte imbalance. In clients with an eating disorder, however, the abuse is significant and can lead to serious complications. CBC and electrolytes will identify anemia or electrolyte depletion. Psychological counseling is necessary for patients with an eating disorder.

GASTROINTESTINAL SURGERY

Any surgery that affects intestinal transit, such as large bowel resection, gastric resection, gastric or intestinal bypass, pyloroplasty, or vagotomy, may cause diarrhea. A history of any of these procedures suggests the surgery as the causative factor. Because malabsorption, malnutrition, vitamin deficiency, and anemia may result, patients need education on vitamin and mineral supplementation.

■ Constipation

Constipation is a common complaint generally used to describe excessively dry, small, or infrequent stools. According to a more specific definition, constipation is the presence of more than one of the following conditions for at least 3 months:

- Straining with bowel movements more than 25% of the time.
- Hard stools more than 25% of the time.
- Incomplete evacuations more than 25% of the time.
- Fewer than three bowel movements per week.

The term constipation covers more than infrequent stools and must be addressed from the patient's viewpoint. Constipation is often a chronic condition. Patients often self-treat both real and perceived constipation; its presence may be identified when the history identifies frequent or chronic use of laxatives or cathartics. Lifestyle factors (nutritional and fluid intake, activity) often contribute to chronic constipation. The altered colonic transit time may also be associated with medications, endocrine disorders, neurological deficits, and various GI disorders; constipation may be one sign of an eating or psychiatric disorder. Acute-onset constipation may stem from bowel obstruction or ileus.

History

Establish what the term constipation means to the patient. Ask how long it has existed and whether it is constant or intermittent. Determine how, if at all, the patient's previous bowel patterns differed. Explore the current bowel history: frequency of bowel movements; changes in caliber, color, quantity, or consistency (are the movements hard?); the need to strain; and whether there is complete evacuation. Ask about associated symptoms: abdominal bloating/fullness, rectal pain or bleeding, blood or mucus in the stool, altered appetite, and abdominal pain. Establish whether the constipation alternates with normal bowel pattern or diarrhea or is progressive. Find out whether the patient has experienced a weight loss because the potential for a malignancy must be considered. Establish the presence of any associated complications: hemorrhoids, fissures, or fecal incontinence. Obtain a history of endocrine, neurological, or GI problems; abdominal surgeries; and currently prescribed or over-the-counter medications. Obtain a history of dietary and fluid intake, activity, and recreational drug use.

Physical Examination

The physical examination should start with a general survey—note the patient's overall appearance and whether she or he appears healthy or ill, has any obvious deficits, or exhibits physical signs of systemic disorders. Obtain a weight. Observe the skin and mucous membranes for signs of dehydration. Depending on the history and your general survey, you should examine other systems. Otherwise, the examination can focus on the abdomen and rectum.

Inspect and auscultate the abdomen first, noting any scars, distention, visible masses, and discoloration. If bowel sounds are not immediately evident, continue listening for at least 15 seconds in each quadrant before you conclude that they are absent; if sounds are present, determine the pitch and frequency. Identify areas of dullness over organs, and estimate organ size. Note any areas of dullness over the bowel. Palpate superficially at first, noting any guarding, rigidity, or tenderness. Palpate more deeply to assess organs and any other areas of firmness or mass. For any palpable mass, determine the consistency, size, shape, mobility, and margins. Perform an anorectal examination, inspecting the anus for tone, fissures, external hemorrhoids, or other defects. Palpate the rectum for masses and stool, noting the consistency of anything palpated; perform guaiac on any palpated stool.

COLONIC MOTILITY DISORDERS

Disorders of the smooth muscle of the colon can cause hypotonia and decreased motility; examples include congenital and acquired myopathies and enteric nerve disorders, such as Hirschsprung's disease. The result can be slowed transit time with greater intervals between evacuations, the development of bowel dilation, or pseudoobstruction.

Signs and Symptoms

The history may identify a familial tendency to constipation. The patient may have previously attempted increasing dietary fiber and fluids, as well as maintaining a reasonable activity level, without improvement.

Diagnostic Studies

A barium enema can identify areas of colon dilation. Measurements of whole-gut transit time are available; serial radiographs identify the position of ingested radiopaque marker(s) over time. A variety of specialized tests, performed by a gastroenterologist, provide information regarding bowel motility and tone.

INTESTINAL OBSTRUCTION

Obstructions of the colon cause a progressive constipation, which may be associated with pain, nausea, or other symptoms. In older patients, constipation may be the presenting symptom of obstruction. Malignancy must be considered.

Signs and Symptoms

There may be a history of the stool having become smaller in diameter, the term "pencil" stool, as well as a history of decreasing frequency of bowel movements and/or blood in the stool. Obstipation—extreme obstruction—leads to the failure to pass even gas. If a volvulus is the cause, the symptoms may or may not include pain and discomfort. Abdominal distention is marked in colonic obstruction. As the problem progresses, the patient may develop signs of shock. A palpable mass may be evident in volvulus or malignancy. The degree of tenderness is variable. There may be high-pitched bowel sounds or borborygmi until a late stage, at which time bowel sounds are absent.

Diagnostic Studies

Plain films of the abdomen should be ordered, looking for dilated loops of bowel, air-fluid levels, and the absence of colonic gas. The nature of an obstruction can be identified with a barium enema, CT scan, or colonoscopy/flexible sigmoidoscopy. If the obstruction is due to strangulation, the CBC may show a leukocyte shift to the left. Never order a barium upper GI series until colonic obstruction has been ruled out.

RECTOCELE AND PROLAPSE

Structural disorders of the anorectum and/or pelvic floor can cause constipation. A rectocele occurs when the rectovaginal septum bulges anteriorly. Weakness of the pelvic floor results in a widened anorectal angle and thereby a weakened perineal body. The pelvic floor may be weakened during childbirth, trauma, or repeated straining during bowel movements (thus, the cause and effect are blurred). Once weakened, the pelvic floor resistance is lessened and the stool is not directed/extruded through the anal canal. Both problems are more common among females.

Signs and Symptoms

Patients may complain of general constipation but may also note that the problem is more related to the act of defecation, which is difficult. Women who have developed a rectocele may perceive that there is weakness in the perineal area and that a mass is evident at the introitus when they strain; some learn to support the introitus to facilitate defecation. The physical signs of rectocele are determined during the vaginal examination; refer to Chapter 13, p. 384.

Diagnostic Studies

A barium enema provides evidence of rectocele with lateral view but is usually not warranted, as the physical examination identifies the change. When bleeding from a fistula or hemorrhoid occurs, a proctoscopic examination should be performed to ensure there is not also a malignancy or other mass.

MEDICATIONS

Many medications can cause or contribute to constipation. The medications most commonly associated with constipation are listed in the Medication Causing Constipation box.

MEDICATIONS CAUSING CONSTIPATION

Analgesics/narcotics
Antacids containing aluminum
Anticonvulsants
Antidepressants
Antihypertensives (calcium-channel blockers, beta-blockers)
Antiparkinsonism agents
Antispasmodics
Calcium supplements
Diuretics
Iron supplements
Sedatives/tranquilizers

Signs and Symptoms

Constipation related to medications can be acute or chronic, either following the initial introduction of a new drug or after some time period has elapsed. The appearance of the abdomen and presence of bowel sounds are usually not altered. Depending on the severity of the constipation, the abdominal examination may be within normal limits; however, feces may be palpable, and there may be some tenderness with deep palpation. The anorectal examination will typically be normal, although you may palpate hard, dry feces.

Diagnostic Studies

There are usually no studies necessary. A common diagnostic effort is to discontinue the suspected offending drug; however, it is not always possible to discontinue a medication in order to confirm the relationship (thus, other treatments/recommendations must be made to minimize the constipating effects of necessary drugs). If obstruction is suspected, refer to earlier section.

PSYCHIATRIC DISORDERS AND EATING DISORDERS

Constipation has been associated with depression. Patients with eating disorders commonly develop constipation unless they are also using laxatives. Patients with various psychiatric disorders may deny having bowel movements and fictitiously report constipation.

Signs and Symptoms

The history is very important in order to determine the actual pattern of bowel movements. Patients may give a history of frequency and characteristics of bowel habits that are well within normal range, but they may indicate dissatisfaction or concern over some specific characteristic, such as the color or caliber, in spite of no report of a recent change. When a psychogenic cause is suspected, a psychiatric history is warranted. Look for indications of depression or obsessive-compulsive disorder. Be sure to perform a thorough overall history and physical, however, to ensure that an organic cause is not missed. Recognize, also, that patients who initially develop real or perceived constipation associated with psychogenic causes often begin to use laxatives and cathartics progressively and develop a dependence on these agents.

Diagnostic Studies

A patient might underestimate the frequency of bowel movements. Consider having the patient monitor his or her bowel movements over several days, using a diary card. The patient should document each bowel movement and the volume and form of the stool. Although no specific diagnostic studies are necessary, you should, on the basis of presentation and history, order those necessary to exclude major organic causes. Possible studies include thyroid studies, electrolytes, CBC, abdominal imaging, sigmoidoscopy, and colonoscopy.

ENDOCRINE DISORDERS

Both hypothyroidism and diabetes can contribute to or cause constipation by decreasing motility. In hypothyroidism, myxedematous tissue may infiltrate the gut, resulting in megacolon. Diabetes should be considered as contributory to constipation when patients have other signs of autonomic neuropathy. The hypercalcemia associated with hyperparathyroidism may cause constipation. A thyroid profile and/or Hgb A1C are diagnostic for thyroid disease and diabetes mellitus respectively.

NEUROLOGICAL DISORDERS

Many neurological disorders, including Parkinson's disease, multiple sclerosis, and spinal cord injuries, can alter bowel patterns. It is unknown whether the neurological changes caused in the brain of a patient with Parkinson's disease also affect the enteric nerves or constipation is the result of increased pelvic floor muscle tone. Multiple sclerosis is believed to contribute to slow transit time as well as altered pelvic floor muscle tone. The degree to which a spinal cord lesion affects bowel function depends on the level of injury; injuries may alter distal transit time as well as sphincter responsiveness. See Chapter 14 for further discussion.

IRRITABLE BOWEL SYNDROME

See previous discussion, p. 282.

■ Jaundice

Jaundice, a yellow discoloration of skin and mucous membranes, stems from an elevation of either the unconjugated or conjugated bilirubin. Causes of unconjugated hyperbilirubinemia include both bilirubin overproduction, as occurs in several hemolytic disorders, and impaired bilirubin uptake, associated with inherited disorders. Conjugated hyperbilirubinemia is more common and stems from either impaired hepatic excretion or extrahepatic obstruction. Hepatitis is the most common cause of jaundice (75%) among persons younger than 30. Obstruction is the most common etiology of jaundice (60%) after age 60, and the causes include gallstones, tumors, or strictures from past surgeries. Other relatively common causes in older adults include congestive heart failure (10%) and metastatic malignancy (13%). Jaundice may be the presenting sign of serious disease in all age groups. With appropriate history, physical, and early diagnostic studies, the cause of jaundice usually can be correctly identified as either obstructive or nonobstructive.

History

The patient's age is an important consideration in differentiating among potential causes of jaundice. Find out when the discoloration was first noticed and whether other symptoms have developed or been associated with this finding. Important associated symptoms include pruritus, malaise, fever/chills, nausea, anorexia, change in the color of urine or feces, and abdominal pain. The medical history must address previous hepatic or biliary diseases, malignancy, hemolytic disorders, and surgeries, as well as other potential contributing disorders, including congestive heart failure. Obtain a family history of hemolytic, biliary, and hepatic disorders. Obtain a thorough medication history, including over-the-counter and herbal agents; determine the use of alcohol and recreational drugs, particularly IV drug use, and social risk factors for hepatitis, including sexual practices.

Physical Examination

The physical examination should include a general survey of the skin and mucous membranes, observing for discoloration, dryness, spider angiomas, petechiae, and xanthomas as well as excoriations indicative of pruritus (see also Chapter 3). The general survey should also consider the patient's mental status as an indicator of liver disease. The lungs and heart should be assessed briefly to identify overall health and indications of heart failure (see also Chapter 7). Unless otherwise indicated by the history, the remainder of the physical should focus on the abdomen. Carefully observe for scars from previous surgical procedures. Percuss to determine organ size and any unexpected areas of dullness indicative of a possible mass. As you percuss, note any areas of tenderness, particularly over the liver. Palpate to further assess abdominal organs. As you palpate for the liver, be attentive for a positive Murphy's sign. If the liver is palpable, note the consistency and margins in addition to the size.

HEPATITIS

Jaundice causing injury to the liver can have many potential sources; viruses and hepatotoxins are the most common causes. Viral diseases that can cause hepatitis include the identified hepatitis viruses (A, B, C, D, and E), Epstein-Barr, and cytomegalovirus. Hepatotoxins include numerous prescribed and over-the-counter medications, such as acetaminophen, methyldopa, isoniazid, and phenytoin; herbal remedies; alcohol; and, more rarely, chemical exposures.

Signs and Symptoms

Explore potential sources of viral illness, including exposures to blood and body secretions and toxins through occupational, sexual, and/or recreational activities. Obtain a complete list of all drugs and herbal agents ingested as well as the use of alcohol. Viral causes of hepatitis with jaundice often have accompanying symptoms of the virus, including malaise and myalgia, as well as RUQ discomfort and anorexia. Medical history should include any episodes of viral hepatitis or other hepatic injury. Assess for nonhepatic signs of viral illness, including fever, splenomegaly, and lymphadenopathy. Identify the size and condition of the liver and the presence of discomfort.

Diagnostic Studies

Obtain a CBC, liver functions including ALT and AST, a hepatitis screen, total and direct bilirubin levels, and prothrombin times. Consider abdominal/liver ultrasound or CT to evaluate organomegaly or mass. Referral for liver biopsy may be warranted.

HEPATIC AND PANCREATIC CANCERS

Primary or metastatic cancers of the liver and/or pancreas can cause obstructive hyperbilirubinemia and jaundice. Jaundice may be the initial sign of a malignancy or may follow the development of other symptoms.

Signs and Symptoms

Ask about associated symptoms such as RUQ discomfort, nausea, fever, back pain, weight loss, fatigue/weakness, and pruritus. None of these symptoms are specific to malignancy; however, other causes of jaundice are less likely to be associated with weight loss. Review medical history of malignancies and family history of cancer. A previous malignancy should raise suspicion for a recurrent malignancy in the differential diagnosis for unexplained jaundice. If hepatic or pancreatic cancer is suspected, a prompt, thorough physical examination is warranted owing to the potential for metastatic disease and the need to identify the primary site. During the abdominal examination, carefully palpate the area of the liver and the remainder of the abdomen, checking for masses or unexpected findings.

Diagnostic Studies

In addition to a CBC, liver functions, amylase, and bilirubin levels, abdominal CT and/or ultrasound should be ordered promptly.

CIRRHOSIS

Cirrhosis develops with the replacement of normal liver tissue by regenerative, fibrotic nodules and may occur in the late phase of a variety of disorders that damage the liver, such as chronic viral hepatitis, Wilson's disease, and drug and alcohol toxicity.

Signs and Symptoms

Symptoms may be subtle at first or dramatic. A patient may present with jaundice and describe an associated, progressive pattern of pruritus, weakness, anorexia, nausea, and weight loss. Alternatively, a patient with undiagnosed cirrhosis may present with jaundice and also with acute onset of ascites, bleeding varices, and/or severe RUQ discomfort. Include a mental status examination as well as an examination of the lung and heart. Assess for ascites. Determine the size and consistency of the liver as well as any tenderness.

Diagnostic Studies

In addition to AST and ALT, diagnostic studies should include a CBC, alkaline phosphatase, bilirubin, albumin, and prothrombin time. An ultrasound or CT of the abdomen should be done to further evaluate the liver size and structure.

CHOLECYSTITIS, CHOLELITHIASIS, AND CHOLANGITIS

Occlusion of the common bile duct may occur with disorders of the gallbladder and/or bile duct.

Signs and Symptoms

All three conditions are generally accompanied by RUQ discomfort, anorexia, and nausea. Charcot's triad, which includes jaundice, RUQ pain, and fever/chills is common to problems resulting in obstructions of the bile duct. Identify any history of biliary surgery. Assess the abdomen, noting the condition of the liver, and test for Murphy's sign. Observe the skin for xanthomas.

Diagnostic Studies

Obtain an ultrasound of the gallbladder and biliary structures. When there is a high index of suspicion for obstructive causes of jaundice, either endoscopic retrograde cholangiopancreatography (ERCP) or percutaneous transhepatic cholangiography (PTC) are appropriate initial imaging studies.

HEMOLYTIC DISORDERS

A variety of conditions causing hemolysis of the red blood cells can result in jaundice: acquired hemolytic anemia, sickle cell anemia, hemolytic drug reactions, and others.

Signs and Symptoms

If hemolytic anemia is involved, the history may also include weakness, fatigue, dyspnea, palpitations, or other symptoms common to anemia. Other symptoms may include abdominal pain, fever, and chills if hemolysis has been rapid. Patients with sickle cell disorder usually can provide a history of recurrent episodes of symptoms, including severe pain, weakness, dyspnea, swollen joints, and/or skin lesions—often requiring serial hospitalizations. The medication survey may identify medications with hemolysis as a potential adverse effect, such as sulfonamides and methyldopa. Assess for splenomegaly and hepatomegaly. Observe skin and mucous membranes for lesions, purpura, and/or pallor. Assess joints for swelling, inflammation, or tenderness. Assess heart and lungs; determine the presence of any associated cardiomegaly.

Diagnostic Studies

Order a CBC, noting the hematocrit, red blood count and indices, hemoglobin, and reticulocyte count. Tests for hemoglobinopathies may be indicated, as might an indirect Coomb's test for levels of antibodies to the red blood cells.

Serum studies that are less common but are appropriate for certain causes of jaundice, including iron, transferrin, ferritin, antimitochondrial antibodies, antinuclear antibodies, and ceruloplasmin.

PANCREATITIS

See earlier discussion, p. 257.

■ Gastrointestinal Bleeding

Patients with gastrointestinal (GI) bleeding may complain of hematemesis, melena, or hematochezia. Alternatively, they may have occult bleeding and be unaware of the problem. When a patient presents with GI bleeding, the first step must be to determine his or her hemodynamic stability. Stability is assessed, to a large extent, by consideration of the patient's vital signs and general appearance. This discussion does not apply to patients who present with significant, acute blood loss or who otherwise require urgent stabilization and treatment. Rather, this section describes the approach for patients who appear stable and who present with a history of blood in emesis or stool as well as those in whom occult bleeding is suspected or confirmed. It is important to narrow the differential diagnosis to allow for a focused approach.

History

It is important to obtain a thorough symptom analysis of any complaint of GI bleeding, including the timing, progression, and description of the blood. Whether the blood is noticed in emesis and/or in stool, determine the amount, color, odor, and any other characteristics of the emesis and/or stool. The ability to differentiate between melena and hematochezia is helpful. When melena is present, the blood is likely to have been present for over 14 hours; therefore, the site of bleeding is most likely distant from the rectum (upper GI). When hematochezia is present, the blood is less likely to have remained in the bowel long enough for the hemoglobin to have degraded it, and thus the source is more likely to be nearer the rectum, usually in the colon. However, rapid upper GI bleeding can result in hematochezia. Establish the history of bowel movements and previous episodes of emesis and/or retching. Identify other indications of bleeding, including bleeding gums, bruising, or epistaxis. Associated symptoms such as pain, weakness, constipation, or diarrhea must be identified. Prior GI conditions, malignancies, bleeding disorders, comorbidities, and current medications must be determined. A review of habits should include diet, alcohol intake, and tobacco use. A history of any prior GI diagnostic studies and their results should be determined.

Physical Examination

The physical examination must start with a general survey and accurate vital signs. Observe the patient's general overall appearance and any signs of pallor, weakness, or dyspnea. Obtain pulse and blood pressure lying, sitting, and standing, and note any postural changes. The heart and lungs, as well as any compensatory changes related to bleeding, should be assessed to determine general well-being. Finally, unless otherwise indicated, the examination should focus on the abdomen. Note any areas of discomfort, organomegaly, palpable masses, and unexpected dullness to percussion. A rectal examination must be performed, noting the presence of hemorrhoids or masses and testing for occult blood.

MALLORY-WEISS TEAR

Upper GI hemorrhage may result from a tear at the gastroesophageal junction, a Mallory-Weiss tear. A patient may develop more than one tear.

Signs and Symptoms

These tears are most common in alcoholic patients following an episode of vomiting or retching. If a laceration/tear of the mucosa causes GI bleeding, the patient may demonstrate alterations in hemodynamic status.

Diagnostic Studies

A stat CBC is necessary as a baseline. Consider ordering an ethanol level if alcohol is suspected as a contributing factor. The bleeding associated with a laceration is considerable, and the patient must be referred immediately for evaluation and endoscopic visualization of the lesion.

GASTRITIS

Although gastritis is not commonly associated with major GI bleeding, it may lead to chronic blood loss and anemia. More often, bleeding occurs after an area of gastric mucosal injury has ulcerated.

Signs and Symptoms

Explore symptoms of epigastric and/or periumbilical discomfort. Identify potential causes of gastric mucosal injury—the most common being NSAID use and stress. Stress-related mucosal damage may follow a major surgery, burn, or severe medical illness, that is, a disorder that has caused the patient to become extremely ill rather than a mild, transient condition. Recently, stress-related gastritis is less common because at-risk patients are often prophylactically treated with agents to alter the gastric pH.

Diagnostic Studies

A CBC is warranted to identify the amount of blood loss, if any. Upper endoscopy will illuminate the cause of the gastric symptoms and/or bleeding.

MALIGNANCY

Even though cancer can cause a major bleeding episode, it more commonly causes chronic, slower bleeding. When occult blood or other signs of GI bleeding are present, a malignancy must be considered in the differential diagnosis, with a likely site dependent on the presentation.

Signs and Symptoms

Determine the history of malignancies and risk factors for malignancy. Bleeding caused by cancer is usually painless but may have associated symptoms, such as altered bowel patterns, fatigue, and so on. A palpable mass may be present. There is usually no tenderness on examination. Rectal examination may detect a palpable mass. Consider the patient's overall appearance, and determine whether there has been significant weight loss.

Diagnostic Studies

A CBC should be drawn to check for anemia that may be the first sign of a malignancy, and a chemistry profile should be done for distant metastases. A CEA is an important marker for the diagnosis and treatment of colon cancer. Colonoscopy is necessary for diagnosis and biopsy. Upper endoscopy is necessary for diagnosis and biopsy of gastric malignancies. An ultrasound or abdominal CT with contrast will identify organ tumors. PET scan may assist in pinpointing the site of malignancy and presence of metastasis.

HEMORRHOIDS

The most common cause of lower GI bleeding is hemorrhoids. The bleeding associated with hemorrhoids is usually evident as red blood on the formed stool, in the toilet bowl, or on the toilet tissue following a bowel movement.

Signs and Symptoms

Patients with hemorrhoids often complain of rectal discomfort as well as the contributing factors for hemorrhoid development, including constipation. Inspect the perianal rectal tissue. Anoscopy may be indicated. Perform a digital rectal examination to assess internal hemorrhoids.

Diagnostic Studies

No diagnostic studies are generally indicated. Hemorrhoids can usually be visualized with anoscopy. Consider flexible sigmoidoscopy for internal hemorrhoids. The patient should be reassessed following treatment of the hemorrhoids to ensure there is no continued bleeding to investigate.

DIVERTICULA

Most diverticula do not commonly cause GI bleeding; however, diverticula are quite common. Because the incidence of diverticula is so high and they have the potential to bleed, diverticula actually account for a great percentage of lower GI bleeding that is not related to hemorrhoids.

Signs and Symptoms

Diverticular bleeding is usually painless. Diverticula should be considered if the patient gives the history of sudden onset of bright red blood in a large amount. Chronic, small bleeding is not associated with diverticula. The physical examination is usually unremarkable.

Diagnostic Studies

Because the amount of bleeding is significant, the patient should be referred, and a colonoscopy will likely be performed to identify the site of bleeding.

PORTAL HYPERTENSION

Patients with portal hypertension may develop GI bleeding from varices of the esophagus, stomach, intestines, or other sites. Portal hypertension is most commonly associated with cirrhosis, usually caused by alcohol abuse or hepatitis.

Signs and Symptoms

Because the incidence of esophageal and gastric variceal bleeding is greater than that associated with the intestines, it is important to assess the history of liver disease in any patient presenting with upper GI bleeding. Determine whether there have been previous episodes of variceal bleeding. Rule out risk factors for the development of liver disease and portal hypertension. Check for signs of liver disease, including jaundice, cirrhosis, telangiectasia, hepatomegaly, and RUQ tenderness.

Diagnostic Studies

Laboratory studies should include a CBC to assess for anemia and a pro-thrombin time and partial thromboplastin time to determine coagulation status. An CT or MRI and upper endoscopy will assist in the varices diagnosis.

OSLER-WEBER-RENDU DISEASE

Osler-Weber-Rendu disease, also known as hereditary hemorrhagic telangiecta-sia (HHT), is an autosomal dominant, hereditary disease caused by vascular malformation. It affects men and women equally. A thorough family history will aid in the diagnosis.

Signs and Symptoms

Arteriovenous malformations can occur at any age and affect the brain, liver, lungs, and bowel. Epistaxis usually begins in childhood, and telangiectases of the lips, tongue, and skin appear in late childhood and adolescence. Patients may have a family or personal history of hypertension. GI bleeding, caused by mucosal vascular malformations, generally does not occur until the middle-adult years.

Diagnostic Studies

Diagnosis is usually made by history and physical examination. MRI and CT arteriography will detect arteriovenous malformations. Molecular analysis to identify the gene mutations responsible for HHT is currently available.

PEPTIC ULCER DISEASE

PUD causes over 50% of GI bleeding, with the most common site being the duodenum. The use of NSAIDs is the most important risk factor for the development of bleeding from PUD, although the risk can be increased further by the use of anticoagulants, by *H. pylori*, and by increased acid in such conditions as Zollinger-Ellison syndrome. See p. 262 for more information.

ESOPHAGITIS AND HIATAL HERNIA

It is rare for patients to develop a significant bleeding episode related to esophagitis or a hiatal hernia. Either may cause a chronic blood loss with occult blood in the stool and anemia. For further information, see p. 261.

COLITIS

See p. 281.

REFERENCES

American Cancer Society (2010). *Cancer Facts and Figures 2010.* Atlanta, GA: American Cancer Society.

Balthazar, E., Robinson, D., Megibow, A., & Ranson, J. (1990). Acute pancreatitis: value of CT in establishing prognosis. *Radiology, 174,* 331–336.

Centers for Disease Control and Prevention (CDC). (2006). *National Ambulatory Medical Care Survey: 2001 Summary.* Hyattsville, MD: CDC/National Center for Health Statistics.

———. (2007). "United States Cancer Statistics." http://www.cdc.gov/Features/CancerStatistics/ (accessed March 16, 2011).

Centers for Disease Control and Prevention (CDC). (2007). National Vital Statistics Report, Deaths: Final data for 2007, Vol 58, No 19. http://www.cdc.gov/nchs/fastats/liverdis.htm (accessed March 16, 2011).

Ebell, M.H. (2001). *Evidence-Based Medicine.* New York: Springer.

Feldman, M., Friedman, L.S., & Sleisenger, M.H. (2002). *Gastrointestinal and Liver Disease.* Philadelphia: Saunders.

Parker, S. (2008). Digestive disease: The facts. *HealthGuidance.* http://www.healthguidance.org/entry/6328/1/Digestive-Diseases-The-Facts.htm (accessed March 16, 2011).

SUGGESTED READINGS

Bickley, L.S. (2008). *Bates' Guide to Physical Examination and History Taking,* 10th ed. Philadelphia: Lippincott, Williams, and Wilkins.

Centers for Disease Control and Prevention, National Center for Immunization and Respiratory Diseases. (2010). "Norovirus: Technical Fact Sheet." http://www.cdc.gov/ncidod/dvrd/revb/gastro/norovirus-factsheet.htm (accessed March 16, 2011).

Dillon, P.M. (2007). *Nursing Health Assessment: A Critical Thinking, Case Studies Approach.* Philadelphia: F.A. Davis.

Friedman, S.L., McQuaid, K.R., & Grendell, J.H. (2003). *Current Diagnosis and Treatment in Gastroenterology.* New York: Lange.

Houdart, R., Perniceni, T., Dame, B., et al. (1995). Predicting common bile duct lithiasis: determination and prospective validation of a model predicting low risk. *American Journal of Surgery, 170,* 38–43.

Powell, D.W. (2007). Approach to the patient with gastrointestinal disease. In Goldman, L., Ausiello, D., Arend, W., & Armitage, J.O. (Eds.), *Cecil Textbook of Medicine.* Philadelphia: Saunders.

Rodney, W.M. (2007). Gastroenterology. In Rakel, R.E. (Ed.), *Textbook of Family Medicine.* Philadelphia: Saunders.

Swartz, M.H. (2009). *Textbook of Physical Diagnosis: History and Examination.* Philadelphia: Saunders.

Chapter 11

GENITOURINARY SYSTEM

S.A. Quallich • M. Lajiness

The assessment of a genitourinary (GU) complaint should lead the practitioner to a differential diagnosis narrowed through further evaluation. Symptom analysis of lower urinary tract complaints can be aided by objective instruments, which can reliably reflect a change (improvement or worsening of the condition) in symptoms over time. Many of the disease entities can significantly affect a patient's quality of life and overall social functioning. Genitourinary conditions can impact a variety of patient behaviors, including travel, social functions, entertainment pursuits, sexual activity, sleep, and activities around the home. This chapter focuses on groups of complaints that are unique to the GU system, and it presents the most common differential diagnoses in each category.

Throughout life, hormonal influences and age-related structural changes in anatomy and tissue consistency cause variances in voiding function that affect the quality of life. In infancy, the emptying of the bladder is reflexive. As we age into puberty and adulthood, unless there is a congenital anomaly, trauma, or an intervening illness or surgery that directly affects our ability to maintain urinary control, voiding function is taken for granted. Middle adulthood and later adulthood for both men and women are the times when hormonal influences and anatomical changes are noted by their effect on quality of life. At this time, the degree to which one is able to remain continent of urine and to comfortably empty the bladder begins to affect quality of life.

In men, the prostate is under the influence of the testosterone over the entire life span. The prostate gradually undergoes hypertrophy, causing obstructive symptoms, as though liquid flowing through a tube were being slowly held back. An assessment of urinary function for men should include the International Prostate Symptom Score (IPSS), a validated, reliable instrument designed to objectively measure the amount of bother that urinary symptoms play in the overall quality of life for men (Barry et al., 1992).

In women, estrogen influences tissue elasticity and bacterial populations. Birth trauma and female surgery with the resulting scar tissue may change the anatomic relationships and musculature of the pelvis and therefore have a role in future urinary function.

Although lower urinary tract symptoms arise from different causes in men and women, the signs and symptoms can be very similar. Over the life span, storage function and bladder outlet obstruction for both genders varies more than bladder contractility. The discussion of presentation, symptoms, and diagnostic workup are directed at the evaluation of these clinical entities in the adult or geriatric patient. See the number of red flags relative to the assessment of the adult GU system. Evaluation of the pediatric patient with GU complaints, although similar, does vary and is not addressed in this chapter.

RED Flag ◀ Red Flags in the Assessment of the Genitourinary System

- Gross hematuria must be referred urgently to a urologist with accompanying studies arranged and, if possible, completed before the appointment.
- Abrupt onset or worsening testicular pain, regardless of patient age (see Chapter 12).
- Anuria and oliguria require aggressive evaluation and/or admission for management.
- Acute urinary retention must be referred to the nearest emergency department immediately.
- Large kidney masses—particularly when accompanied by the classic triad of gross hematuria, flank pain, and a palpable mass—must be referred emergently to a urologist.
- Pain associated with any GU structure that awakes the patient or prevents sleep.
- A toxic-appearing patient with poor urine output.

History

■ General History

The general history for a patient who presents with genitourinary complaints should begin with questions regarding a previous history of any similar complaints. A sexual history is appropriate, including recent changes in partners and an assessment of general sexual habits. The history should include a discussion of any recent (within the last 6 months) systemic illness; recent weight gain or loss; smoking, alcohol consumption, and illicit drug use history; a history of recent nausea, vomiting, fever, or chills; a history of other constitutional symptoms; and a history of exposure to chemicals or dyes as part of the occupational and/or social history. A general history of the genitourinary tract must also include a list of current prescription and over-the-counter, homeopathic, or naturopathic medications. Ask what remedies have been tried prior to presentation. As each presenting complaint is listed, additional specific history-taking points are discussed.

■ Patterns of Pain

Knowledge of the potential sources of GU pain and a range of pain syndromes is important to accurately assess complaints of pains. These are reviewed in Tables 11.1 and 11.2.

■ Past Medical and Surgical History

The GU-related past medical and surgical history should include any surgeries to the GU tract or reproductive structures, prostate surgery, bladder reconstructions, and previous treatment for reproductive or GU malignancies. It is vital to elicit an accurate history of any surgery that may affect the vascular or nerve supply to the urinary tract or bladder, including pelvic surgery, retroperitoneal surgery, or back surgery. Obtain a previous history of stone disease or treatment for other GU conditions, including urinary tract infections (UTIs). For women, previous pregnancies, live births, birth trauma, and manner of delivery should be assessed.

Table 11.1

Sources of Pain

Source of Pain	Spinal Level	Presentation
Kidney/renal pain	T10–12, L1	Dull, constant ache to the CVA, lateral to sacrospinalis muscle and just below 12th rib Can spread to subcostal area toward umbilicus or LLQ Results from distention of renal capsule
Pseudorenal pain	T10–12	Caused by mechanical derangement of costovertebral or costotransverse joints, resulting in pressure on costal nerves Mimics renal pain or ureteral colic Can cause costovertebral pain May radiate to ipsilateral LQ Pain is positional, acute, absent on arising, and increases during the day Pain exacerbated with heavy work
Ureteral pain	*Upper ureter:* T11–12	Due to acute obstruction
	Mid-left ureter: T12, L1	Pain due to hyperperistalsis and smooth muscle spasm as ureter tries to overcome obstruction

Continued

Table 11.1

Sources of Pain—cont'd

Source of Pain	Spinal Level	Presentation
		Back pain from renal capsular distention and colicky pain (from ureteral muscle and renal pelvic spasm): • Radiates to CVA, toward LQ, along the course of the ureter • In men, also pain to bladder, scrotum, testicle • In women, also pain to vulva *Upper ureter stone:* pain radiates to testicle (nerve supply similar to kidney and upper ureter) *Mid-right ureter stone:* pain referred from McBurney's point and can present like appendicitis *Mid-left ureter stone:* mimics pain to descending and/or sigmoid colon *Stone close to bladder:* edema and inflammation to ureteral outlet with resulting vesical (bladder) irritability
Vesical (bladder) pain	No corresponding level	*Overdistention:* suprapubic pain; other suprapubic pain is likely not bladder in origin *Pain with UTI:* usually referred to distal urethra (terminal dysuria)
Prostatic pain	S2–4	Pain directly from prostate is uncommon *Acute inflammation:* may have discomfort or fullness to perineal and/or rectal area Possible lumbosacral backache Can cause dysuria, frequency, urgency
Epididymal pain	No corresponding level	Due to acute infection Pain in scrotum Begins as pain in groin or LQ abdomen Can reach costal angle and mimic stone pain Inflammation of testicle possible
Testicular pain	No corresponding level	Very severe, felt locally Can radiate along spermatic cord to lower abdomen and/or CVA Varicocele can cause dull ache that worsens after heavy exercise (see Chapter 12)

CVA = costovertebral angle; LLQ = left lower quadrant; LQ = lower quadrant; UTI = urinary tract infection.

Table 11.2

Pain Syndromes

Genitourinary Pain Syndromes	Description
Painful bladder syndrome	Complaint of suprapubic pain related to bladder filling. May be associated with other symptoms. Increased daytime and nighttime frequency in the absence of proven urinary infection or other pathology
Pelvic pain syndrome	Persistent or recurrent episodic pain associated with symptoms similar to UTI. May include complaints of sexual dysfunction, bowel function, or gynecological function in the absence of proven pathology
Perineal pain syndrome	Persistent or recurrent episodic perineal pain related to urinary voiding or with symptoms similar to UTI. Possible sexual dysfunction (male or female)
Scrotal pain syndrome	Persistent or episodic scrotal pain of varying degree. May be associated with symptoms similar to UTI. Possible sexual dysfunction
Urethral pain syndrome	Recurrent episodic urethral pain, usually while voiding, in the absence of proven infection or other disease process
Vulvar pain syndrome	Persistent or recurrent episodic vaginal pain associated with symptoms similar to those of UTI. Possible complaints of sexual dysfunction

UTI = urinary tract infection.

■ Family History

Family history is important because it can help establish a patient's risk for various GU conditions. Include a history of GU malignancies, prostate or bladder problems, family history (particularly first-degree relatives) of stone disease, incontinence (particularly female relatives), or complaints similar to the patient's. It is recommended that the family history be as specific as possible, noting the relationship to the patient, to provide further insight into congenital or hereditary risk factors.

■ Sexual History

The degree of detail regarding sexual history is guided by the patient's presenting complaints. Sexual history should include activity from adolescence through adulthood and include the patient's sexual orientation (hetero/homo/bisexual). The number of current and lifetime sexual partners should be discussed along with any history of sexually transmitted diseases (STDs), including gonorrhea, chlamydia, herpes simplex, condyloma, HIV, or syphilis and the treatment received. A history of intravenous drug use and the date and results of the patient's last HIV test should also be noted.

Questions regarding safe sex and condom use (serial monogamy risk) and specifics about sexual practices are also relevant. The patient's preferred method of birth control should be noted. Questions regarding erectile dysfunction, premature ejaculation, change in libido, pelvic pain, or incontinence during sexual activity can also provide insight into disease pathology (see Chapters 12 and 13 for details on these topics).

Physical Examination

■ General History

Inspection

Look for suprapubic fullness, and fullness at the costovertebral angle (CVA). Examine for any visible striae or truncal obesity. Refer to male and female reproductive chapters for the specifics of genital inspection. The male patient should be standing and facing the examiner; the patient may develop an erection during the examination.

Auscultation

The examiner can auscultate the scrotum to distinguish loops of bowel from scrotal mass if a hernia is suspected. Listen over the renal artery to rule out renal artery aneurysm; otherwise, perform the usual auscultation of the abdomen as described in Chapter 10.

Percussion

Perform percussion at the CVA and flank to elicit and identify pain that may be associated with hydronephrosis or pyelonephritis. This can also help to localize or outline a suspected renal mass and to determine whether tender. The percussion of the abdomen is as indicated in Chapter 10.

Palpation

The specifics of palpation relative to the GU system pertain to the palpation of the kidneys and the inguinal regions for hernia or adenopathy as well as digital rectal examination (DRE). Palpation of the GU system is described in Table 11.3.

Diagnostic Studies

■ Laboratory Evaluation

Urinalysis

Significant urinalysis findings are described in Table 11.4.

Table 11.3

Palpation of GU System

Procedure	Technique
Digital rectal examination (DRE)	Gloved, lubricated finger is inserted into anus. Sweep back and forth across the surface of the prostate. Sweep the anal ring and the rectal walls 360 degrees. The examination can result in a sensation of pressure and possibly an urge to urinate. The prostate should be symmetric (but asymmetry is a normal variant); nontender; free of nodules; approximately the size of a walnut; and have a smooth, rubbery consistency. The examination also involves an assessment of anal sphincter tone and an estimate of prostate size in grams. This examination can be done with the patient standing and bent over, side lying, or in dorsal lithotomy position
Examination for inguinal hernia	The index finger is inserted into the scrotum and invaginates the scrotum into the external inguinal ring (scrotum should be invaginated in front of testicle); fingertips of other hand should then be placed over internal inguinal canal and patient should be asked to cough. If present, a hernia will be felt as a bulge that descends against the index finger with Valsalva maneuver
Palpation of kidneys	With the patient lying supine, for the right kidney, the examiner should place the left hand, palm up, under the 10th to 12th ribs and place the right hand on top of the abdomen, just below the right costal margin. For the left side, the examiner should reverse the hands so the right hand is under the patient's left costovertebral angle. Ask the patient to take a deep breath. When the breath is fully drawn, ask the patient to exhale. As the diaphragm moves into the thoracic cavity, the lower pole of the kidney may be felt slipping across the fingertips of the hand beneath the 10th and 12th ribs

Urine Cultures

Laboratory cultures of the urine are indicated with suspected UTI and are particularly important for recurrent UTIs or a UTI that seems refractory to treatment. Urine dipstick will show positive leukocyte esterase, positive nitrite, and greater than 3 to 5 white blood cells per high-power field.

Cytology

Urine cytology is part of a routine microscopic or gross hematuria work-up, and a positive cytology may indicate bladder, ureteral, or renal pelvic malignancy. This test should be sent from a patient's first voided morning urine on three separate days, if possible, for the greatest degree of accuracy. Urine cytology is an

Table 11.4

Urinalysis Findings

Urinalysis Component	Interpretation
Color	Bright red if urologic or anatomic cause Tea-colored or brown urine may be due to old clots, glomerulonephritis, or other medical cause
Specific gravity	May see low specific gravity with hydronephrosis, intrinsic renal disease
Protein	3–4 or higher may indicate glomerulonephritis or other decline in kidney function
Leukocyte esterase	If positive, suggests UTI (does not localize source of infection); 80%–90% sensitive; approximately 95% specific
Erythrocyte casts	Indicates glomerular source for hematuria (medical hematuria)
Crystalluria	May indicate stone disease
Nitrite	If positive, suggests UTI (does not localize source of infection); 50% sensitive; approximately 95% specific

UTI = urinary tract infection.

inexpensive means of screening for cancer in a patient with irritative lower urinary tract complaints.

Serum Creatinine and Blood Urea Nitrogen

Serum creatinine and blood urea nitrogen (BUN) provide information regarding kidney function. They are useful with suspected disease and possible obstruction due to benign prostatic hypertrophy (BPH; also called benign prostatic hyperplasia), kidney stones, or ureteral stones. Other laboratory tests are ordered at the clinician's discretion to evaluate the suspected cause of disease; they are discussed in the diagnosis sections of specific conditions.

PSA Testing

Prostate-specific antigen (PSA) is a measurable protein produced by the prostate gland. It is commonly used as a marker for the presence of prostate cancer, but it is not specific to that condition. The PSA can be elevated by infection, ejaculation within the 48 hours prior to testing, GU instrumentation, or increased volume. Guidelines for normal range (Table 11.5) are based on both age and ethnicity. Recent attempts have been made to make this test more specific to prostate cancer by establishing additional variables such as PSA velocity: If the PSA rises more than 0.75 ng/mL per year, the risk for prostate cancer is increased. Pharmacotherapy with finesteride is associated with a 50% decrease in PSA, which must be considered when evaluating results on men so treated.

Table 11.5			

Age-Specific PSA Reference Ranges

Age Range	African Americans	Asians	Whites
40–49 yr	0–2.0 ng/mL	0–2.0 ng/mL	0–2.5 ng/mL
50–59 yr	0–4.0 ng/mL	0–3.0 ng/mL	0–3.5 ng/mL
60–69 yr	0–4.5 ng/mL	0–4.0 ng/mL	0–4.5 ng/mL
70–79 yr	0–5.5 ng/mL	0–5.0 ng/mL	0–6.5 ng/mL

Adapted with permission from Richardson, T.D., & Oesterling, J.E. (1997).

■ Radiologic Evaluation

Uroradiologic Study

The simplest uroradiologic study is the KUB (kidney, ureters, bladder). It can be helpful as a screening or preliminary test, especially if clinical suspicion points to possible renal or ureteral lithiasis. A KUB study often shows calcified abnormalities in both the urinary tract and the skeletal system, and it may also demonstrate large soft tissue masses. A KUB is routinely used to track the progress of ureteral stones as they are passed and to provide a rapid method for evaluating the asymptomatic stone patient for recurrence.

Intravenous Pyelography, Intravenous Urography, and Excretory Urography

Intravenous pyelography (IVP), also known as intravenous urography or excretory urography, remains the initial and preferred study for evaluation of the renal pelvis and ureter owing in part to its moderate cost and ease of administration. It remains the gold standard for noninvasive visualization of ureteral intraluminal filling defects and urothelial abnormalities.

This test demonstrates a wide variety of upper tract lesions and is well tolerated by most patients, although it is recommended that a patient have a serum creatinine of 1.6 or less. Most commonly used to screen for filling defects, IVP may miss small filling defects (such as small ureteral tumors) as a result of the bolus of dye. Because plain abdominal films are taken after the dye injection, this test requires bowel preparation to help ensure the production of high-quality images. The number of films, volume of dye injection, and speed of the injection depend on the institution as well as on the patient's age, comorbidities, and physical condition.

IVP also provides a crude estimation of renal function. Its use is complicated by possible allergy to the dye (which can be treated with preprocedure steroids), modest soft tissue–contrast resolution, possible contrast-induced renal toxicity, and potential cardiovascular issues related to the osmotic load. No special training is required for its administration, and thus IVP is widely available. Its utility, however, is coming into question with the advent of ultrasound, computerized tomographic (CT) scanning, and CT urography because it has a lower specificity, and patients who are found to have abnormalities on an IVP often proceed to a CT or ultrasound study.

Ultrasonography

Ultrasound is a noninvasive, relatively inexpensive, and widely available procedure that avoids radiation exposure and the risk of intravenous contrast. It is widely used to image all parts of the GU system. Ultrasound is superior to IVP for the evaluation of small lesions, and it is more sensitive than IVP in the evaluation of renal masses. It has limited utility for upper tract filling defects but can be useful for differentiating between medical and urologic renal disease. Ultrasound is also limited by the patient's body habitus and the skill of the operator.

Ultrasound is excellent for examination of the scrotum and its contents and can definitively distinguish between extra- and intratesticular pathologies.

Computerized Tomography

CT can also demonstrate filling defects, but it is not cost effective as a screening tool or as an initial step in the evaluation of most GU complaints unless stone disease is highly suspected. Its main role remains in staging malignancies of the GU tract. The CT scan is a superior imaging method for the evaluation of renal and retroperitoneal pathology and is indicated when bladder or renal malignancy is suspected or when an IVP or ultrasound indicates a mass. Unenhanced helical CT scanning is also superior for the evaluation of suspected or actual stone disease because slices 3 mm thin are used. CT scans can be combined with angiography.

The advantages of CT include a quick scanning time, wide field of view, good cross-sectional views, and the ability to detect subtle differences in tissues. The disadvantages of CT include the radiation dose, low soft tissue resolution, the need for contrast media, and images limited to the transaxial plane.

Magnetic Resonance Imaging

Magnetic resonance imaging (MRI) has wide application in the evaluation of GU patients; it provides excellent images of the retroperitoneum, bladder, prostate, testes, and even the penis. The use of gadolinium as a contrast media has broadened the use of MRI further because it is well tolerated even by patients with compromised renal function. An MRI with contrast can provide increased characterization of renal masses. The MRI is clearly superior to CT in imaging the pelvis. When MRI is combined with angiography, renal vessels, renal vein thrombosis, and congenital abnormalities can be demonstrated.

The advantages of MRI include imaging in any plane, excellent soft tissue characterization, and the lack of exposure to radiation. Its disadvantages include slow scanning time, decreased imaging clarity compared with CT, heat generation, and claustrophobia for the patient.

Computerized Tomographic Urogram

A CT urogram (CT urography) is a CT test done with the addition of radiopaque dye, and it can image both the renal parenchyma and urothelium (the lining of the ureters, bladder, and urethra) with a single examination. It combines the sensitivity and specificity of a CT scan for urinary calculi and small renal masses with the sensitivity and specificity of intravenous urography for urothelial abnormalities (Kawashima, Glockner, & King, 2003). Some authors (Perlman et al., 1996) report that CT urography further characterizes masses seen on IVP and better detects small renal cell carcinomas. Its sensitivity and specificity are superior to the IVP, and it can provide a safe and more precise evaluation. It is not widely available, but it is becoming the preferred initial study in the evaluation of hematuria (Kawashima, Glockner, & King, 2003).

Magnetic Resonance Urography

Magnetic resonance urography (MR urography) is another emerging technology in the evaluation of GU pathologies. Similar to MR cholangiopancreatography, images are taken after the administration of intravenous gadolinium contrast. It is especially helpful in imaging patients with dilated tracts (Kawashima, Glockner, & King, 2003). This study is currently limited by the poor spatial resolution of the resulting images and its poor record with calculi detection. However, it provides another method for detecting urinary tract dilatation, ureteric obstruction, duplicated renal collecting systems, and urothelial tumors. The sensitivity of MR urography is currently considered to be similar to that of the CT urogram (Kawashima, Glockner, & King, 2003), but it is not yet widely available.

Differential Diagnosis of Chief Complaints

GENERAL COMPLAINTS

■ Flank Pain and Renal Colic

The kidney and ureters are described as the upper tracts. Symptoms in this anatomic area are a subjective indicator of change in the urinary outflow system. Upper tract symptoms arise from irritation in the kidney and/or blockage of urinary outflow (see Table 11.2). Causes of upper tract symptoms (UTS) include kidney stones, rarely renal cell carcinoma, and urothelial cell carcinoma.

History

Presentation can vary widely—the onset of complaints may be acute or insidious. A description of the pain is critical. Complaints can include a dull renal pain or a constant ache in the CVA area that can radiate laterally to the sacrospinalis muscle and just below 12th rib. Pain can spread to the subcostal area toward the umbilicus or left lower quadrant. The patient may describe only back pain, which is the result of renal capsular distension, and/or colicky pain from ureteral muscle and renal pelvic spasm. Associated symptoms should be explored. There may also be concurrent constitutional symptoms (nausea, vomiting, fever) and associated weight loss or gross hematuria. Determine history of self-treatment, prior episodes of similar or other GU conditions, and most recent health status. Family history should be established.

Physical Examination

General appearance should be noted, as patients with complaints of flank pain may have widely varying presentations ranging from toxic and/or cachectic to only mild discomfort. A thorough GU examination and a general abdominal examination should be completed. Presence of CVA tenderness should be elicited. Palpation may reveal a palpable renal mass if the patient is thin and/or the mass is large enough. A pelvic examination should be completed as complaints warrant, for instance in females who also have complaint of lower abdominal pain.

RENAL MASS

Renal cell carcinomas (RCCs) have been referred to as the "internist's tumor" and as one of the great masqueraders in medicine. A patient with RCC presents with extraordinary variation, from a small asymptomatic lesion found on a CT or MRI scan during an evaluation for another complaint to a full-blown paraneoplastic syndrome with liver function derangements and hypercalcemia. RCCs can secrete biologically active substances, such as gonadotropins and adrenocorticotrophic hormone (ACTH). Laboratory findings can include normochromic anemia, an elevated erythrocyte sedimentation rate, and hematuria on urinalysis. Risk factors for RCC include smoking, environmental exposure to heavy metals, and hereditary conditions such as von Hippel-Lindau disease.

Signs and Symptoms

The signs and symptoms are described as in the preceding history subsection. The patient may present with obvious symptoms or vague constitutional complaints.

Diagnostic Studies

The workup is dictated by the patient's presentation and complaints. Initial laboratory work can include a urinalysis, urine cytology, complete blood count (CBC), liver function tests, and serum electrolytes. Imaging studies can include an IVP or renal ultrasound, CT scan, or MRI; the CT scan remains the gold standard for detection of RCC. Referral to a urologist is indicated; the more symptomatic the patient, the more urgent the referral.

NEPHROLITHIASIS

Kidney stones are more common in men and rank as the third-most common condition of the urinary tract. Several varieties of stones can be formed, the majority of which are radiopaque, and after an initial episode, the recurrence rate can be up to 50%. Most stones present with acute-onset pain due to the obstruction of the upper urinary tract. The symptoms associated with a kidney stone are due to the inflammation, edema, and hyperperistalsis of the GU tract, particularly the ureter (see Table 11.2, particularly in regard to ureteral pain). The number or size of the stone(s) correlates poorly with the degree of pain. Risk factors include a history of crystalluria, low fluid intake or dehydration (such as living in a hot, dry climate), socioeconomic factors (industrialized countries), and a family history of stones. Ninety percent of stones measuring 4 mm or less will pass spontaneously, 50% of stones of 4 to 6 mm are likely to pass spontaneously, but only 10% of stones larger than 6 mm will pass spontaneously.

Signs and Symptoms

Patients will appear uncomfortable as they try to find a resting position that is not painful. They may also experience nausea and vomiting; other systemic indicators of renal colic may be noted, such as tachycardia. If a patient appears septic, referral to the nearest emergency room is mandatory.

Diagnostic Studies

The initial study can be a KUB or IVP; however, many facilities can perform a stone protocol spiral CT, a much more definitive test for the evaluation of kidney stones. Urinalysis usually shows some degree of hematuria, may indicate infection, and may also show crystals that can be a clue to the diagnosis of stone type. Referral to a urologist for management is indicated. Recurrent stone formers should also undergo a 24-hour urine collection for electrolytes (calcium, uric acid, phosphate, oxalate, phosphate uric acid) to evaluate for a metabolic condition that may be amenable to medical management.

UPPER URINARY TRACT OBSTRUCTION OR HYDRONEPHROSIS

This condition could be caused by either an obstructing stone, ureteral stricture, prostatic hyperplasia, or renal or abdominal tumor that prevents the kidney from draining. The obstruction can be unilateral or bilateral, symptoms can be sudden or gradual in onset, and progressive renal damage will occur with time.

Signs and Symptoms

Flank pain may radiate along the course of the ureter and may be accompanied by a variety of constitutional symptoms. More severe or bilateral obstruction may cause weight loss and eventual uremia. A distended kidney may be noted on palpation, and CVA pain may be present if there is infection. Genitourinary, abdominal, pelvic, and rectal examinations are indicated.

Diagnostic Studies

The workup is the same as for the evaluation of kidney stone or renal tumor. Imaging studies are the key to determining the etiology.

PYELONEPHRITIS

Pyelonephritis is a bacterial infection of the renal pelvis and parenchyma, typically caused by *Escherichia coli* ascending from the lower urinary tract. Risk factors include vesicoureteral reflux, neurogenic bladder, stone disease of any part of the GU tract, immunosuppression, and diabetes mellitus.

Signs and Symptoms

The patient will have bilateral or unilateral flank pain, fever, chills, nausea, and vomiting. Lower urinary tract symptoms, such as dysuria, may also be present. The patient will appear ill on presentation, with fever and tachycardia commonly noted. Palpation and/or percussion over the infected side is painful. There may be accompanying abdominal discomfort or abdominal distention.

Diagnostic Studies

A CBC will show leukocytosis, often with a shift to the left. Urinalysis will also demonstrate leukocytosis, RBCs, protein, and bacteria. Urine culture will be positive with heavy growth. Blood cultures may be necessary. Imaging studies should be considered if the patient appears ill or does not respond to initial outpatient management (CT scan or renal ultrasound to assess for urinary obstruction). Assessment must include the determination of whether or not the patient requires inpatient management.

AUTOSOMAL DOMINANT POLYCYSTIC KIDNEY DISEASE

A family history of autosomal dominant polycystic kidney disease (ADPCKD) should raise the level of suspicion if a renal mass is palpated. Adult-onset ADPCKD is uncommon under the age of 40.

Signs and Symptoms

Back or flank pain (60%), gross hematuria (30%), and renal stones (20%) are the most common symptoms. There may be infections in the cysts, hypertension, and decreasing renal function associated with the initial presentation. A CT scan may also reveal liver cysts concurrent with renal cysts and may begin to appear at age 30. During palpation of the abdomen, cysts on either or both kidneys may be evident.

Diagnostic Studies

A family history of liver or renal cysts will aid in diagnosis even in the absence of palpable masses. A renal ultrasound may reveal cystic lesions; a CT examination is more sensitive in the evaluation of cysts but also more costly. Once the diagnosis is established, imaging studies need not be routinely performed unless new symptoms require evaluation. Patients with an established diagnosis of ADPCKD should be followed by a urologist or nephrologist for monitoring pyelonephritis, nephrolithiasis, and renal function.

BLUNT RENAL TRAUMA

Blunt trauma typically causes damage in the transverse plane of the kidney. Damage to the kidney represents the most common injury to the GU tract. Trauma can be the result of a motor vehicle accident or contact sports and is usually seen in men and boys.

Signs and Symptoms

The patient usually has evidence of abdominal trauma, such as fractured ribs, with complaints of pain that localize to the affected side. If the injury is severe, there may be signs of shock.

Diagnostic Studies

History may be sufficient to establish that renal injury is likely. Urinalysis will show some degree of hematuria. The initial imaging study is an IVP or CT urogram for evaluation if the kidney is poorly visualized on the IVP. The patient should be referred to a urologist for further evaluation and management or to the nearest emergency department if the injury appears severe.

■ Gross Hematuria

A sudden, noticeable change in the color of urine is usually quite alarming to a patient. Gross hematuria results from a sufficient number of erythrocytes in the urine for the patient or clinician to perceive a color change in the urine. Painless, gross hematuria may be ignored by some patients, resulting in a significant delay before presentation for evaluation. Gross hematuria is often the only indication of a urologic malignancy; a malignancy is found in up to 40% of gross hematuria cases.

Therapeutic anticoagulation should not lead to either gross or microscopic hematuria. Hematuria may result if a patient becomes excessively anticoagulated. However, patients who are anticoagulated may also have coexisting urologic malignancies, and an episode of gross hematuria in an anticoagulated patient warrants an evaluation.

History

Obtain a history of the hematuria, including the urine color and any accompanying symptoms. The urine color may range from pink to red or simply look like blood is being urinated. The episode is usually painless, but it can be associated with flank pain, nausea, vomiting, or generalized dysuria with or without other LUTS. Ask about prior GU conditions, related family history, and habits. There may be an extensive smoking history or history of exposure to chemicals through the patient's job. It is vital to try to establish the timing of blood in the urinary stream, which can help predict the source of bleeding (see Table 11.6).

Physical Examination

A routine GU examination and a pelvic examination for female patients (see Chapter 13 for pelvic examination methodology) is mandatory. The physical

Table 11.6		

Possible Significance of Timing of Blood in the Urinary Stream

Description of Hematuria	Possible Site	Possible Cause
Microscopic hematuria	Any site within upper or lower urinary tract	UTI, prostatitis, urethritis, medical renal disease, bladder/ureteral/renal malignancy, stone disease
Initial gross hematuria	Anterior urethra	Stricture, meatal stenosis, urethritis, urethral cancer
Total gross hematuria	Source above bladder neck: bladder, kidney, ureter	Renal/ureteral/bladder stone or tumor; trauma; vigorous exercise; renal tuberculosis, hemorrhagic cystitis; interstitial cystitis; sickle cell disease; nephritis; ADPCKD; poststreptococcal glomerulonephritis
Terminal gross hematuria	Bladder neck, prostate, posterior urethra	BPH, regrowth BPH post-transurethral resection, bladder neck polyps, posterior urethritis, tuberculosis

ADPCKD = autosomal dominant polycystic kidney disease; BPH = benign prostatic hyperplasia; UTI = urinary tract infection.

examination is often unremarkable except in the case of a kidney stone or ADPCKD, in which case a large, boggy kidney may be palpated.

Selected Causes

Box 11.1 lists many of the most common causes of gross hematuria; it is commonly due to anatomic causes (nonglomerular bleeding).

Diagnostic Studies

Laboratory studies can include CBC, urinalysis, serum electrolytes, urine electrolytes, and urine cytology; studies are guided by the patient's presentation, risk factors for such GU diseases as bladder cancer, and comorbidities. Urine cultures are indicated with suspected UTI. Coagulation studies are performed as appropriate in anticoagulated patients. An imaging study (IVP, CT, or ultrasound) will aid in evaluating an anatomic cause for the microscopic hematuria. The patient should be referred urgently to a urologist with the following studies completed before the visit: IVP, CT, or ultrasound; BUN and creatinine; urinalysis; and at least one urine cytology.

■ Suprapubic Pain

The differential for complaints of midline lower quadrant pain includes many conditions that are not specific to the GU system. The key in evaluation of this

Box 11.1

Selected Causes of Gross Hematuria

- Arteriovenous malformation
- Autosomal dominant polycystic kidney disease (ADPCKD)
- Benign prostatic hypertrophy (BPH)
- Bladder neck polyps
- BPH regrowth post-transurethral resection
- Contamination from menstruation
- Hemorrhagic cystitis
- Interstitial cystitis
- Meatal stenosis
- Nephritis
- Posterior urethritis
- Poststreptococcal glomerulonephritis
- Renal tuberculosis
- Renal/ureteral/bladder stone
- Renal/ureteral/bladder tumor
- Sickle cell disease
- Trauma
- Tuberculosis
- Urethritis
- Urethral cancer
- Urethral stricture
- Vigorous exercise

complaint is a careful history and physical examination to localize the complaints to the actual structures involved.

History

A thorough history is indicated. Complaints on presentation may include pain to the midline lower abdomen that is constant or intermittent. The onset of the discomfort may have been acute or gradual. There may be associated complaints of perineal fullness, irritative voiding symptoms, or urinary retention. There may also be a variety of constitutional symptoms, including fever, chills, nausea, or vomiting.

Physical Examination

A routine GU examination is mandatory, including a DRE. An abdominal examination and in women, a pelvic examination (see Chapter 13 for pelvic examination methodology) are also suggested. Physical examination may demonstrate pain on palpation of the suprapubic region, and the bladder may be palpable. There may be global abdominal discomfort if gastrointestinal structures are involved. The patient may have CVA tenderness.

Selected Causes

Localization of the source of pain after physical examination, coupled with the history, aids in diagnosis of the potential cause. See Table 11.7 for examples.

Diagnostic Studies

The suspected cause guides the diagnostic workup. Laboratory studies can include CBC, urinalysis and culture, and urine cytology. The initial imaging study, if indicated, could be either a KUB or CT scan, with any further workup dictated by initial findings of the laboratory studies and imaging. The patient may require urgent referral to a urologist, general surgeon, or gynecologist.

■ Anuria, Oliguria, and Renal Failure

Although anuria and oliguria are unusual as acute complaints, the course toward renal failure can be predicted in many patients, and patients should be questioned to elicit report of decreasing urine. It remains important to establish the causes contributing to the renal dysfunction because many patients with severe kidney dysfunction will need a variety of support services, including dietitian consultations and dialysis, and select patients may be candidates for a renal transplant.

History

The history is the key to evaluating the suspected cause. The patient may report decreasing urine output over time or a recent change in medications. This can be complicated if the patient has a solitary kidney or previous renal transplant. Associated symptoms (flank pain, nausea, vomiting) must be noted; also note a history of recent IV dye administration. A thorough GU history as well as general history and review of systems should be obtained.

Physical Examination

A complete physical including routine GU examination is required. The signs and symptoms depend on the cause and are not restricted to the GU system: flank pain if stone obstruction, murmur if endocarditis, palpable bladder if BPH, generalized edema if myocardial failure.

Selected Causes

Table 11.8 lists many common causes, categorized as prerenal and postrenal.

Diagnostic Studies

The suspected cause and physical presentation guide the diagnostic workup. Laboratory studies can include CBC, urinalysis, serum electrolytes, and urine electrolytes. Initial imaging studies can include a renal or bladder ultrasound, and further workup is dictated by initial findings of the laboratory studies and imaging. A patient presenting acutely with anuria, oliguria, or renal failure requires an emergent referral for further evaluation and appropriate management based on the suspected cause.

Table 11.7

Selected Causes of Suprapubic Pain

Urethral	Prostate	Vesical	Distal Ureteral	Large or Small Bowel (See Chapter 10)	Gynecologic (See Chapter 13)
• Urethral syndrome • Urethral stenosis	• Acute or chronic bacterial prostatitis • Nonbacterial prostatitis • Prostatodynia	• Bladder cancer • Bladder stone • Interstitial cystitis • Urinary retention • Urinary tract infection	• Ascending infection • Foreign body • Stone	• Appendicitis • Diverticulitis • Inflammatory bowel disease • Malignancy	• Ectopic pregnancy • Endometriosis • Pelvic inflammatory disease • Uterine fibroids

315

Table 11.8

Selected Causes of Renal Failure, Anuria, and Oliguria

Prerenal	Postrenal
Decreased vascular volume	**Upper urinary tract obstruction**
• 3rd spacing	• Kidney stone (unilateral vs. bilateral)
• Gastrointestinal losses	• Obstructing retroperitoneal mass
• Hemorrhage	• Pregnancy
• Reduced cardiac output	**Lower urinary tract obstruction**
• Septic shock	
• Severe dehydration	• Benign prostatic hypertrophy
• Spinal shock	• Carcinoma (bladder, prostate)
	• Neuropathic bladder
Myocardial failure	• Prostatitis
	• Urethral stricture
• Cardiomyopathy	
• Ischemic heart disease	
• Tamponade	
• Valvular heart disease	
Renal/glomerular causes	
• Acute glomerulonephritis	
• Vasculitis	
Vascular	
• Renal vein thrombosis	
• Renal artery occlusion	
Medication-related	
• Anticonvulsants	
• Antihypertensives	
• Chemotherapeutic agents	
• Diuretics	
• Radiographic contrast media	

■ Microscopic Hematuria

Microscopic hematuria is rarely a patient complaint; it is usually found on evaluation, such as during a routine medical examination or monitoring of a patient's kidney function. Opinions differ as to the appropriate long-term follow-up of the patient with persistent microscopic hematuria, and ultimately the follow-up is guided by the patient's overall medical conditions and medication profile.

History

A GU history should be obtained, as described earlier in this chapter. Usually there is no history of an associated complaint; the patient may give a history of recurrent stones, recent UTI, longstanding diabetes, or other medical renal disease. The patient may be taking prescription medication that can cause renal damage when used long term, and all over-the-counter and prescribed agents should be identified.

Physical Examination

A routine GU examination is required, including pelvic examination for female patients (see Chapter 13 for pelvic examination methodology). Microscopic hematuria is often found incidentally on routine screening urinalysis, and there are no related signs.

Selected Causes

A detailed discussion of each potential differential diagnosis is beyond the scope of this chapter, and in many cases, a referral for further urologic and/or nephrology evaluation is warranted. Box 11.2 lists many common causes; microscopic hematuria is due to a physiologic process (glomerular bleeding). Small, asymptomatic stones within the GU tract can cause intermittent microscopic hematuria. Excessive anticoagulation has been known to lead to microscopic hematuria.

Diagnostic Studies

Laboratory studies can include CBC, urinalysis, serum electrolytes, urine electrolytes, and urine cytology. Hemoglobin and hematocrit are not routinely indicated except as part of the CBC: Microscopic hematuria rarely causes significant

---

Box 11.2

Selected Causes of Medical/Renal Hematuria

- Arteriovenous fistula
- Benign familial hematuria
- Berger's disease (IgA nephropathy)
- Bleeding disorder
- Bleeding dyscrasias/sickle cell disease
- Diabetes mellitus
- Drug-induced interstitial disease
- End-stage renal disease
- Exercise (marathon running)
- Familial glomerulonephritis
- History of analgesic abuse
- HIV
- Infections (e.g., hepatitis)
- Mesangioproliferative glomerulonephritis
- Postinfectious glomerulonephritis
- Systemic lupus erythematosus
- Vascular disease (e.g., renal artery embolism)

blood loss. Urine cultures are indicated with suspected UTI. Order coagulation studies as appropriate in anticoagulated patients. An imaging study (IVP, CT, or ultrasound) will aid in ruling out an anatomic cause for the microscopic hematuria.

■ Prostate Nodule, Elevated PSA, and Asymmetric Prostate

An asymmetric prostate is typically asymptomatic and not necessarily diagnostic of prostate cancer; asymmetry can be a normal finding on DRE but should be followed periodically to monitor for changes. A second opinion of a questionable finding on DRE is always a wise idea, whether from another practitioner in the clinic or by referral to a urology specialist.

An elevated PSA is relative to an individual's baseline PSA value or is a value that lies outside the established norms for race and age (see Table 11.5). PSA velocity is also a valuable way to gauge the significance of the PSA value; it describes the rapidity of increase in PSA over time. Generally, an increase in the PSA value of 0.75 ng/mL or more over 12 months should trigger referral for a transrectal ultrasound–guided prostate biopsy for a histological evaluation for prostatic carcinoma.

Age-specific reference ranges for PSA (see Table 11.5) should be used as a guide when there is no previous PSA for comparison. A prostatic nodule found on DRE necessitates a referral to a urologist or radiologist for transrectal ultrasound–guided prostate biopsy and may well be the first indication of the presence of a cancer.

History

History should include analysis of any recent voiding symptoms, discomfort, or other GU symptoms. Family history of prostate or other malignancies should be determined. Usually there is no history of related symptoms unless BPH is present, as prostatic asymmetry or enlargement may be a finding on routine physical. There may be a history of mild or moderate LUTS with obstructive features.

Physical Examination

A routine GU examination, including DRE, is required. On examination, a normal prostate is smooth with a rubbery surface (posterior surface of the gland is palpated through the rectal wall), and the lateral lobes and median sulcus, as well as the base and apex of the prostate, can usually be appreciated. The seminal vesicles should not be palpable. Documentation should reflect the gland's size (estimated in grams), consistency, symmetry, and the presence or absence of nodules. Other abnormalities found during the DRE can include hemorrhoids, condyloma, and anal fissures.

Diagnostic Studies

As noted earlier, the PSA is assessed relative to the man's age, race, and prior levels. PSA can be decreased during finesteride treatment. Recent ejaculation has no clinically significant effect on the PSA value. Men should not be asked to abstain from sexual activities before a PSA screening test (Stenner et al., 1998). Prostate biopsy is necessary and performed in urology setting.

BENIGN PROSTATIC HYPERTROPHY

BPH is a nonmalignant enlargement of the transition zone of the prostate gland; the precise etiology is unclear. Risk factors are simply advancing age and normal androgen status, although there may be an additional genetic predisposition. The terms *BPH* and *obstructive symptoms* have traditionally been used to describe a collection of complaints associated with prostate overgrowth; in 2002, the International Continence Society assigned these symptoms under the term *lower urinary tract symptoms* (detailed later in chapter). Prostate size correlates poorly with the degree of symptoms; that is, a larger size does not automatically mean worse symptoms, in part due to the subjective impressions of the patient.

Signs and Symptoms

LUTS associated with bladder outlet obstruction secondary to an enlarged prostate include urinary urgency, frequency, hesitation in getting the stream started, decreased caliber and force of stream, and nocturnal frequency of urination that is bothersome. This collection of symptoms has also been termed *prostatism*. A patient with benign prostatic hypertrophy shows symmetric or asymmetric enlargement and a firm, smooth, nontender gland.

Diagnostic Studies

If the PSA level is elevated relative to the age-specific reference, or if there has been a rise greater that 0.75 ng/mL in less than 12 months, the patient should be referred to a urologist for discussion and management, including possible prostate biopsy or surgery to improve the urinary outlet (transurethral resection of the prostate).

PROSTATE CANCER

Early-stage prostate cancer is largely asymptomatic and is found as a result of screening for prostate cancer by DRE and PSA. Histological evaluation of biopsy specimens obtained during transrectal ultrasound–guided biopsy of the prostate provides a tissue diagnosis of prostate cancer and a Gleason score, which aids in deciding treatment options. Increased risk for prostate cancer is associated with more than two first-order relatives diagnosed with prostate cancer. Family members, such as grandfathers, with prostate cancer should raise the index of suspicion.

Signs and Symptoms

An asymmetric prostate, a prostatic nodule, or an elevated PSA level may be found during a routine physical. There may be a history presented of mild or moderate LUTS with obstructive features. A prostate suspicious for malignancy will demonstrate nodular areas and/or overall hardness.

Diagnostic Studies

Definitive diagnosis is made via prostate biopsy. Routine or urgent referral to a urologist is indicated, depending on the degree of PSA elevation and/or the degree to which it has risen since the previous value in conjunction with any suspicious findings on the rectal examination.

PROSTATITIS

Prostatitis is an acute or chronic infection of the prostate gland. Acute bacterial prostatitis is usually the result of infection by aerobic gram-negative rods (coliform bacteria or *Pseudomonas*). *Enterococcus faecalis*, an aerobic gram-positive bacteria, can also cause prostatitis. Routes of infection are ascent from the urethra, reflux of infected urine into the prostatic ducts, direct extension of bacteria, and migration via the lymphatic and vascular system. It may be associated with acute cystitis and may result in urinary retention.

Signs and Symptoms

Acute symptoms commonly include fever,, low back and perineal pain, urinary urgency and frequency, nocturia, dysuria, and muscle and joint aches. Transrectal palpation of the prostate reveals a very tender, boggy, swollen prostate. Urine may smell strong and be cloudy. Gross hematuria may be present. CBC will be positive for leukocytosis and a shift to the left. Chronic prostatitis manifests as recurrent episodes of irritative symptoms of dysuria, nocturia, frequency, and urgency. Febrile episodes, gross hematuria, and hematospermia are rare. A tender, indurated epididymis is sometimes associated with chronic prostatic infection.

Diagnostic Studies

Low back pain in the sacral area differentiates prostatitis from pyelonephritis, which manifests as flank pain. A urine culture will reveal the offending pathogen. Presentation of sudden, severe onset rather than milder, recurrent episodes differentiates acute from chronic prostatitis.

CHRONIC INFLAMMATION AND PROSTATODYNIA

The etiology of male chronic pelvic pain syndrome is still not certain, although an autoimmune process is favored. Further research is required to determine the putative autoantigen, the immune responses of patients, the role of bacteria in the inflammatory process, and the patients' pain response to genitourinary insults. As yet, no diagnostic tests (other than to eliminate other pathology) and few treatments for chronic prostatodynia can be recommended on the basis of scientific evidence (Batstone, Doble, & Batstone, 2003).

Signs and Symptoms

The signs and symptoms are often similar to those of BPH or prostatitis.

Diagnostic Studies

Chronic inflammation can be diagnosed only via prostate biopsy. Routine referral to a urologist for biopsy is indicated.

■ Proteinuria

Proteinuria is another clinical entity that is discovered during an evaluation rather than presenting as GU complaint. Proteinuria is an indicator of parenchymal disease of the kidney and is commonly seen in patients with conditions such as diabetic nephropathy, nephritic syndrome, autoimmune disease, multiple myeloma, and acute inflammation of the urinary tract. It can also be the result of prolonged use or abuse of NSAIDs.

History

A thorough GU-specific and general health history should be obtained if proteinuria is present. Determine whether there is a family history of potentially contributory conditions and/or kidney disease. Proteinuria is likely to be present with no structural abnormalities found and is almost always painless. It is important to establish the timing of proteinuria (relative to the patient's medical history): transient, intermittent, persistent, or whether it is the initial episode.

Physical Examination

A routine GU examination is required. Other aspects of the examination are guided by the suspected cause (flank bruit, pericardial rub, skin lesions, edema). There are typically no signs or symptoms other than those resulting from the causative medical condition. A general physical examination should be completed.

Selected Causes

The medical/renal disease is glomerular, tubular, overflow, or tissue proteinuria.

Diagnostic Studies

Proteinuria is usually found on routine urinalysis; it may be falsely positive in the context of dilute urine. No further studies are indicated unless there are new progressive symptoms or the patient appears toxic or is manifesting other symptoms of renal or contributory conditions. Renal ultrasound or IVP studies can be considered in these cases (if the renal function can withstand contrast media). Referrals to a nephrologist for all persistent proteinuria and to an oncologist, as appropriate, are recommended.

LOWER URINARY TRACT SYMPTOMS

LUTS include a variety of complaints that help in the clinical identification of a potential diagnosis. Not all patients experience all symptoms, and the symptoms may be present in varying degrees at varying times. The symptoms are much more descriptive of lower urinary tract pathology in men and can be graded using a tool such as the American Urological Association symptom score. Box 11.3 lists the components of LUTS.

Box 11.3

LUTS

- Acute retention (suprapubic pain, severe urgency)
- Chronic retention (much hesitancy starting stream, reduced force/caliber of stream)
- Cystitis
- Hesitancy (strains to force urine)
- Interruption of stream (can be accompanied by pain radiating down urethra)
- Loss of force/decreased caliber of stream (urethral resistance increases despite increased intravesical pressure)
- Sense of residual urine
- Terminal dribbling
- Urgency (strong, sudden desire to urinate owing to hyperactivity and irritability of the bladder)

The following presenting complaints represent common manifestations of disorders of the lower urinary tract. *As part of the diagnosis, a measurement of a postvoid residual volume can be included with each differential that follows in this section if the clinical environment has the appropriate equipment. This measure will confirm that the patient is actually emptying the bladder or can provide a baseline against which to gauge interventions if the bladder is not being emptied.*

■ Dysuria

Complaints of dysuria—or burning, pain, or discomfort on urination—are more common in women than in men, largely as a result of the shorter urethral length in women. Infection is the most common cause of dysuria, and its presentation depends on which structure of the GU tract is affected. The infection can be secondary to an anatomical abnormality or abnormality of function, including postmenopausal status or prostatic hypertrophy. The patient may have undergone recent GU instrumentation or catheter placement, leading to a mechanical cause for the dysuria.

Dysuria can also be an indicator of other systemic conditions, such as diabetes mellitus, renal calculi, GU neoplasms, or depression. Debate exists over treating complaints of dysuria empirically with antibiotics, particularly when it is a recurrent complaint for a patient. The most common causes for dysuria are presented here as differentials.

History

The history should explore current voiding symptoms as well as past history of GU problems. The patient may report pain, hesitancy, urgency, frequency, and discomfort on urination and may describe bladder fullness. There is usually a negative history of fever, chills, or other constitutional symptoms. The patient may also report a color change in urine or the presence of a strong odor to the urine. The timing of pain with urination (external, initial, during, terminal) may provide clues to the cause. Female patients may have associated vaginal symptoms; both men and women should be asked about their risk for STDs. The patient should also be asked about herbal, homeopathic, or vaginal hygiene remedies that may have been tried since symptom onset. Male patients should be specifically queried about the presence of LUTS, and women should be queried about incontinence.

Physical Examination

A routine GU examination is required, including DRE and pelvic as indicated, based on the patient's gender. A CVA examination and general abdominal examination should also be performed. The patient's general appearance should be noted, including whether he or she appears toxic.

UNCOMPLICATED URINARY TRACT INFECTION

Uncomplicated UTI is one of the most common infections seen in a primary care setting and occurs among patients of all ages, but it is more commonly seen in women. The etiology of UTIs is affected by a patient's comorbidities, including age, use of catheters, or neurologic disease. The most common pathogen causing acute, uncomplicated UTIs is *E. coli*, followed by *Staphylococcus saprophyticus*, and *Klebsiella*, *Enterobacter*, and *Proteus* species. Risk factors for the development of a UTI are well established and include increasing age, recent sexual intercourse, a history of UTI, use of a diaphragm or cervical cap, and anatomic abnormalities.

Signs and Symptoms

The signs and symptoms are as described in the immediately preceding History subsection; onset is typically sudden and without other constitutional symptoms.

Diagnostic Studies

Urinalysis will confirm the presence of a UTI; hematuria, pyuria, and/or bacteriuria will be observed. However, there exists debate as to whether the specimen must be a clean-catch specimen. The leukocyte esterase test combined with the nitrite test provides a high sensitivity and specificity for infection. In women whose symptoms suggest uncomplicated UTI, a culture of greater than 10^2 CFU/mL is indicative of cystitis (Bent & Saint, 2003). Urine cultures should be considered in the patient with recurrent UTI, refractory UTI, and the patient who appears toxic. Blood for CBC and electrolyte tests should also be drawn based on the overall clinical presentation. If anatomic causes are suspected, diagnostic imaging, such as KUB or IVP, should be arranged based on the suspected cause and patient's presentation.

PAINFUL BLADDER SYNDROME/INTERSTITIAL CYSTITIS

Painful bladder syndrome (PBS)/interstitial cystitis (IC) is a poorly understood entity with a suspected cause related to a variety of factors that include autoimmune, allergic, and infectious components. Patients with IC suffer from chronic symptoms that include a combination of suprapubic pain, chronic pelvic pain, dyspareunia, and negative urine cultures in addition to dysuria. Patients may become debilitated by this disease; they may be making up to 40 trips to the bathroom in 24 hours. Interstitial cystitis is also marked by periods of remission and flare-up throughout a patient's lifetime. The prevalence of this disorder is not known. The actual diagnosis by a clinician is low, 200/100,000 population, with the estimated prevalence of symptoms at 5,000/100,000 population. Typical age at onset varies from 30 to 70, and most patients visit an average of five physicians and wait 4 years before the correct diagnosis is made.

Signs and Symptoms

Patients describe a history of irritative voiding symptoms: urinary urgency, frequency, and pain. They may also complain of suprapubic pain, dyspareunia, and chronic pelvic pain. Symptoms may worsen in the week preceding menstruation and have often been present for a period of several months or years.

Diagnostic Studies

Urinalysis will eliminate a UTI as the cause of these complaints. In order to diagnose IC, all other potential etiologies should be ruled out, including such things as carcinoma or medication-induced cystitis. Confirmation of diagnosis is via bladder appearance on cystoscopy; referral to a urologist is indicated.

SEXUALLY TRANSMITTED DISEASE–RELATED URETHRITIS

Presentation of STD-related dysuria varies by gender, with females usually more affected than males.

Signs and Symptoms

See specific signs and symptoms in male and female patients in Chapters 12 and 13 respectively. Some STDs may be accompanied by complaints of constitutional symptoms or malaise.

Diagnostic Studies

STDs can be diagnosed with the appropriate cultures, Gram stains, swabs, and serologic studies. Unless a patient appears ill and a white blood cell count seems indicated, no additional laboratory work or imaging studies are indicated. Treatment is often begun before the results of diagnostic tests are received; it is imperative to simultaneously treat the partner(s). Many STDs must be reported to the local health department.

URETHRAL SYNDROME

Urethral syndrome brings with it nonspecific complaints of frequency, urgency, and dysuria without objective clinical findings; it is more common in females during their reproductive years. Risk factors include a history of UTI, GU tract obstruction, and neurogenic bladder, and the condition is similar to prostatodynia in men.

Signs and Symptoms

The signs and symptoms are similar to those of UTI and may include complaints of back or suprapubic pain.

Diagnostic Studies

Both urinalysis and urine cultures will be negative; this is a diagnosis of exclusion. If urethral syndrome is suspected, the patient can be referred to a urologist for additional specialized testing.

COMPLICATED URINARY TRACT INFECTION

Defined as a UTI in a context that increases the likelihood of treatment failure or recurrent infection, this condition is seen in patients with abnormalities of GU anatomy (such as BPH) or functional abnormalities (such as a neurogenic bladder) and diabetes or other metabolic derangements. Other risk factors for a complicated UTI include male gender, pregnancy, extremely old or young age, or immunocompromised status. A complicated UTI can also be indicated when multiple organisms are present on culture. Complicated UTIs can evolve into more serious conditions, such as pyelonephritis.

Signs and Symptoms

Patient complaints are typically the same as for an uncomplicated UTI but often include constitutional symptoms. Symptom onset may be sudden or insidious. Prostatic symptoms may be present in men with prostate enlargement, or there may be symptoms of concurrent prostatitis (see BPH and Prostatitis sections). Complaints may also indicate upper tract involvement (see Pyelonephritis section).

Diagnostic Studies

Initially, infected urine will be noted on urinalysis. Urine culture and sensitivity are recommended, particularly if the presentation is recurrent or refractory UTI, and appropriate laboratory work (CBC, serum electrolytes, blood cultures) should be ordered according to the patient's overall presentation and other comorbidities. Imaging studies are indicated on the basis of suspicion for anatomy abnormalities or obstruction. Hospital admission may be necessary depending on the overall clinical picture, comorbidities, hydration status, and need for further evaluation.

VAGINITIS

Vaginitis can be accompanied by irritation to adjacent structures as well as vaginal discharge and vulvar irritation. See Chapter 13 for additional discussion.

POSTMENOPAUSAL STATUS

Dysuria seen in women after menopause can be accompanied by stress urinary incontinence and urinary frequency. All result from the mucosal thinning of the urethra and bladder in the absence of estrogen.

Signs and Symptoms

The signs and symptoms are similar to the complaints seen with a UTI but without constitutional symptoms. Patients may also experience vaginal dryness and related symptoms. Vaginal and urethral areas will appear pale owing to the diminished vascularity.

Diagnostic Studies

A history and physical examination are usually sufficient; a urinalysis will rule out UTI.

GENITOURINARY NEOPLASM

Bladder cancer in particular can be accompanied by complaints of bladder irritability or LUTS, along with either gross or microscopic hematuria. Symptoms of bladder irritation are also common with both BPH and prostate cancer.

Signs and Symptoms

Patients with bladder cancer may have unremarkable physical findings unless there is a large-volume invasive tumor, in which case there may be a palpable thickness to the bladder. Patients who have prostate cancer may also describe LUTS and general bladder irritability; other physical findings are typically unremarkable.

Diagnostic Studies

A urinalysis is required to confirm or investigate the presence of blood. Urine cytology is needed to evaluate for malignant cells, although this will not determine the source of the abnormal cells (bladder, ureter, renal pelvis). If malignancy is suspected or confirmed, a staging CT scan should be ordered before urgent/emergent referral to a urologist for further management.

ANATOMIC ABNORMALITY

Anatomic abnormality includes such conditions as a ureteral or urethral stricture, duplication of the collecting system, meatal stenosis, phimosis, or vesicovaginal fistula. These conditions may become apparent after surgical procedures that promote scar tissue in the urethra, prolonged catheterization, and surgeries to the pelvic region.

Signs and Symptoms

Patients may describe a gradual onset of changes to their pattern of urination, such as spraying, painful urination, frequency, and the need to push in order to urinate. Physical examination includes a pelvic examination for women and special attention to the foreskin and meatal opening in men.

Diagnostic Studies

Physical examination alone may provide the diagnosis. Urinalysis may show some degree of contamination or a UTI. Suspicion of a structural abnormality requires referral to a urologist for further evaluation; depending on the suspected location of the abnormality, a retrograde urethrogram or IVP may be considered.

■ Difficulty Urinating or the Inability to Urinate

Urinary difficulties often occur insidiously, with few complaints from the patient until the situation is advanced or has created a social difficulty. However, when a patient has difficulty urinating or emptying his or her bladder, there is a motivation to seek evaluation sooner rather than later.

History

A detailed GU history is indicated, including family history, lifestyle habits, and review of symptoms. A patient may describe recurrent or persistent UTIs, dysuria, and varying LUTS, including difficulty starting the stream or nocturia. There may be a history of recent GU instrumentation, indwelling Foley catheter, or surgery. The patient may also describe a history of declining bladder control.

Physical Examination

A routine GU examination is required, including DRE and a pelvic examination in women.

BENIGN PROSTATIC HYPERPLASIA

See p. 319.

PROSTATITIS

See p. 320.

NEUROGENIC AND NEUROPATHIC BLADDER

Neurogenic (or neuropathic) bladder is the failure of the bladder to store or to empty. There may be spontaneous and uncoordinated contractions of the bladder when it is filling, or the bladder and sphincter may not work in concert, preventing the bladder from effectively emptying. Risk factors include spinal cord injury, trauma to the central nervous system, diabetes mellitus, spina bifida, multiple sclerosis, spinal disk disease, and pelvic surgery, among many others.

Signs and Symptoms

A variety of urinary complaints may occur, including incontinence, dribbling, and retention, as well as disorders of bladder sensation. Associated complaints may reflect changes in bowel habits, sexual function, or lower extremity sensation. Physical examination involves not only a routine GU and pelvic examination but also a full neurologic examination.

Diagnostic Studies

Order a urinalysis to rule out UTI as a treatable cause that would contribute to the complaints. Conduct other laboratory studies as suspicions dictate (such as an evaluation for diabetes). Consider an evaluation of the upper tracts with IVP or renal ultrasound. Referral to a urologist is warranted for further specialized testing.

POSTOPERATIVE URINARY RETENTION

The bladder may recover sluggishly after anesthesia, requiring a patient to embark on a short-term regimen of intermittent catheterization. A history of recent surgery that required bladder catheterization should be sufficient to confirm the diagnosis. This is more commonly seen in men.

URETHRAL LESIONS

Urethral cancer is a rare condition for both men and women, but it can change the quality of the urinary stream. Some STDs can cause lesions within the urethra itself, resulting in pain and changes in the urinary stream.

Signs and Symptoms

The patient may complain of a splayed or intermittent urinary stream. The symptoms may be gradual in onset. There may be a history of STD, recent urethral trauma or instrumentation, or previous urethral stricture. Inspection may show visible lesions at the meatus.

Diagnostic Studies

Visual inspection may be sufficient to confirm the presence of lesions. Referral to urology for cystoscopic examination of the urethral tissue is recommended because lesions may indicate a urethral carcinoma.

BLADDER CALCULI

In the United States, bladder calculi are most frequently due to bladder outlet obstruction, commonly BPH. They can also be caused by an elevated bladder neck in combination with an increased postvoid residual, which results in stagnant urine.

Signs and Symptoms

The presentation may be completely asymptomatic; there may be various complaints, including urinary retention, recurrent UTI, bladder pain, microscopic or gross hematuria, dysuria, urgency, or nocturia. The bladder may be palpable due to distention. Physical examination involves palpation of the bladder and, in women, pelvic examination.

Diagnostic Studies

Urinalysis will confirm hematuria and possibly test positive for a UTI. A urine cytology and urine cultures may be considered. The initial imaging study can be a KUB, IVP, or pelvic ultrasound, all of which will demonstrate the presence of one or more stones. Referral to urology for management is indicated.

■ Decreased Force of Stream or Spraying With Urination

Any change in the pattern of urination to which a patient is accustomed can be upsetting. Some of these complaints have causes that are easily remedied and may simply be related to age and/or pelvic floor weakness.

History

The history should include prior GU conditions and procedures, and a general health history should be determined. The patient will give a history of decreased force and/or caliber of stream. Establish acute versus gradual onset, and rule out genital trauma as a contributing factor. There may be complaint of spraying with urination. Pain is not typically associated with this complaint.

Physical Examination

A routine GU examination is required, with attention to location of urethral opening, and DRE.

BENIGN PROSTATIC HYPERPLASIA

See p. 319.

EPISPADIAS AND HYPOSPADIAS

These conditions are more commonly diagnosed in infancy and have varying degrees of severity. Severe hypospadias in the infant, male or female, can be confused with an intersex condition. In a female, leaving an epispadias untreated can result in incontinence as an adult. It is not uncommon for an adult male (hypospadias occurs in one of every 300 male births) to have a slight displacement of the urethral opening that was not surgically corrected during infancy or childhood. There is also an increased incidence of undescended testes with hypospadias; other consequences include infertility and upper urinary tract damage.

Signs and Symptoms

A patient may complain of a displaced urethral opening or the inability to direct the urinary stream. Men may also complain of chordee (curvature of the penis caused by tethering of the skin and dartos fascia). A careful scrotal examination should be performed to confirm the presence of both testicles and to rule out an inguinal hernia. Rarely, the patient may present with complaints of infertility.

Diagnostic Studies

Physical examination should be sufficient to make the diagnosis. The patient should be referred to a urologist for further evaluation and management.

LESIONS RELATED TO SEXUALLY TRANSMITTED DISEASES

See discussions in Chapters 12 and 13.

DISTORTED FEMALE PELVIC ANATOMY

Cystocele, prolapse of the uterus, and failed continence surgery can all affect pelvic floor anatomy and cause urinary changes, including incontinence and changes to the quality of the urinary stream. See Chapter 13 for descriptions of these conditions.

■ Frequency, Urgency, and Hesitancy

Urinary complaints that involve frequency, urgency, or hesitancy can be seen by patient and provider alike as part of the aging process. However, in many cases, these complaints may have treatable or even reversible causes. A thorough history will sometimes uncover the cause, such as with radiation cystitis.

History

In addition to GU and general health history, it is important to explore the association with daily activities as well as the impact of the complaint on the patient's activities. All medications should be identified. These complaints may have an acute or insidious onset, particularly if irritative and obstructive symptoms are involved. The patient may provide a history of some degree of incontinence or dysuria.

Physical Examination

A routine GU examination is needed; other system examinations are dictated by history and accompanying complaints. Patients may have a palpable bladder on examination.

INTERSTITIAL CYSTITIS

See pp. 323–324.

URINARY TRACT INFECTION

See pp. 323, 325.

BENIGN PROSTATIC HYPERPLASIA

See p. 319.

NEUROGENIC OR NEUROPATHIC BLADDER

See pp. 327–328.

VOLUME- OR METABOLIC-RELATED CAUSE

The kidneys receive roughly 20% of cardiac output and have a major role in the volume and electrolyte homeostasis of the body. Changes to the fluid and electrolyte balance of the body can directly affect urinary output, such as in the osmotic diuresis seen with poorly controlled or undiagnosed diabetes mellitus.

Other examples include diabetes insipidus, metabolic acidosis and alkalosis, renal insufficiency, and congestive heart failure.

Signs and Symptoms

Volume- or metabolic-related conditions often involve varying GU complaints along with frequency, urgency, and hesitancy. Other systemic complaints representative of the particular endocrinopathy or underlying disease process will occur. The physical examination involves a routine GU examination and additional system examinations as indicated by presentation and history.

Diagnostic Studies

Urinalysis should be performed to rule out UTI as a treatable cause contributing to the complaints. Other laboratory studies can be ordered as suspicions dictate (such as evaluation for diabetes), particularly electrolytes. Referral to the appropriate subspecialty may be needed for further diagnosis and management.

DRUG-INDUCED EFFECTS

A patient may complain of frequency that she or he associates with a particular medication. Alternatively, this association may not be clear until a complete list of the patient's medications is available.

Signs and Symptoms

Signs and symptoms are primarily frequency and urgency, both of which may be complicated by coexisting GU conditions, such as BPH, some type of incontinence, or mobility issues.

Diagnostic Studies

A review of a patient's medications and administration schedule should be sufficient to determine that a diuretic is a contributing cause. Consider urinalysis to rule out a UTI.

NEOPLASTIC (BLADDER OR RENAL CANCER)

See p. 326.

■ Nocturia

As nocturia persists, patients become more likely to seek evaluation and treatment. They begin to suffer fatigue from sleep interruption and deprivation, as there may be 45 minutes or less between urges to urinate.

History

The duration of the problem may be difficult to gauge, because the onset may have occurred over several months. The patient's overall disposition and energy level should be noted. The patient should be asked to estimate the average number of episodes per night, and the presence of associated LUTS should be queried.

Physical Examination

A routine GU examination is needed; a pelvic examination and/or full physical may be indicated by history.

BENIGN PROSTATIC HYPERPLASIA

See p. 319.

INTERSTITIAL CYSTITIS

See pp. 323–324.

VOLUME- OR METABOLIC-RELATED DISORDER

See pp. 330–331.

EXCESSIVE FLUID INTAKE IN EVENING

When questioned, the patient will describe a pattern of increased fluid intake later in the day. History is usually sufficient to confirm the cause.

PHARMACOLOGICALLY INDUCED

This problem can present when a patient times the administration of a diuretic late in the afternoon or evening, with consequent complaints of urinary frequency late into the night. A review of medications and their timing should be sufficient to confirm this cause.

■ Urinary Incontinence

Urinary incontinence (UI) is a prevalent and costly public health problem. Twenty million adults have urinary incontinence or an overactive bladder, causing bothersome urinary leakage. It is estimated that 15% to 30% of the adult women in the United States experience UI. Men can experience UI after pelvic surgery and also as they age owing to prostate enlargement. The prevalence of UI increases as age increases for both genders; approximately 50% of elderly people in extended care are incontinent of urine, and 33% are incontinent all or most of the time. Given the increase in numbers of the aging population, UI will continue to affect large numbers of the population. Healthcare costs for UI exceed $20 billion annually. The lifetime medical cost of treating an older adult who has UI approaches $60,000. Added costs arise from complications of UI such as loss of wages, poor quality of life, depression, and loss of self-esteem, which increases the financial burden of UI even further (Wilson, 2006).

As a result of the constant production of urine and the bladder's finite storage capacity, incontinence will occur in anyone who does not have timely access to facilities, regardless of age, mobility, or gender. Box 11.4 lists several recognized patterns of urine loss.

The bladder has several functional features that contribute to normal continence: its normal capacity of 400 to 500 mL; the fullness sensation; the ability to accommodate various volumes without changes in intraluminal pressure; the

Box 11.4

Patterns of Incontinence

- *Stress incontinence*, or the loss of urine with activities that cause changes in intraabdominal pressure, such as sneezing, lifting, or exercise
- *Urge incontinence*, or the loss of urine that results from detrusor overactivity at unusually low volumes of urine; symptoms can include involuntary loss of urine preceded by an urgent and compelling desire to void
- *Mixed incontinence*, or a combination of both stress and urge incontinence
- *Functional incontinence*, or the inability to make it to the toilet before losing control and/or an inability to undress properly; commonly influenced by both cognitive and functional status
- *Overflow incontinence*, or a bladder that does not empty completely owing to outlet obstruction or neurogenic causes and subsequently spills urine when full

---

ability to initiate and sustain contraction until the bladder is empty; and a response to the voluntary inhibition of voiding despite the inherent involuntary nature of the organ.

The bladder receives afferent and efferent innervation from both the autonomic and somatic nervous systems. Parasympathetic innervation arises from sacral segments 2–4 and projects to the pelvic plexus, supplying both the bladder and sphincter. Sympathetic control originates at the T10–L2 level. Somatic innervation originates from S2–S3 and travels via the pudendal nerve to the external urethral sphincter and permits the sensation of fullness, inflammation, or pain depending on the specific pathway. Damage or other pathologies that affect these areas of the spine (herniated disk, spinal stenosis, degenerative changes in the vertebrae, or metastatic disease) can result in changes to bladder function and/or sensation. Diseases that result in neuropathies (such as diabetes mellitus or multiple sclerosis) can contribute to the dysfunction of bladder sensation and function.

Gender-specific anatomy may explain some of the difference in the incidence of UI. Female gender greatly increases the risk for urinary incontinence, as does childbearing. Age is a risk factor but is not causative; some age-related changes associated with the urinary tract are normal. The most significant age-related changes in women are related to decreased estrogen influence. As estrogen levels decline, the epithelium and supporting tissues of the pelvis atrophy, resulting in friable mucosa and possible prolapse of the pelvic structures. The change in relationship of the pelvic structures results in hypermobility of the bladder base, pelvic muscle weakness, and urethral weakness, resulting in stress urinary incontinence in women. The decreased glycogen content of the vaginal epithelium causes decreased lactic acid metabolism by Döderlein's bacillus, an increased pH of vaginal secretions, and therefore an increased risk for UTI.

A variety of history and assessment points aid in narrowing the etiology of a patient's specific complaints.

History

Obtain a thorough GU history, including detailed description of the type of incontinence experienced. Ask about activities that seem to trigger urine loss and any efforts the patient has taken to avoid or adapt to the incontinence. The patient will report some pattern of involuntary loss of urine; this may occur under specific circumstances or be nearly continuous. Detailing the context in which the urine loss occurs will aid with diagnosis. A general history is important, as existing comorbidities and surgical history provide additional clues to the etiology of the incontinence.

Physical Examination

A routine GU examination, including DRE, and, in women, a pelvic examination are needed.

Selected Causes

See Table 11.9.

Table 11.9

Selected Causes of Urinary Incontinence

Female	Male	Male or Female
• Childbirth • Cystocele • Estrogen deficiency (atrophic vaginitis or urethritis) • Failed previous surgery to correct incontinence • Hysterectomy • Rectocele • Vesicovaginal fistula	• Prostatic hypertrophy • Prostatitis • Postradical prostatectomy	• *Anatomic* (constipation; urinary retention; pelvic, back, or retroperitoneal surgery) • *Irritative* (interstitial cystitis, urinary tract infection) • *Metabolic* (diabetes mellitus, diabetes insipidus, aging) • *Neurologic* (dementia, peripheral or autonomic neuropathy, spinal cord trauma or lesions, multiple sclerosis, diabetes) • *Pharmacologic* (diuretics, sedatives, anticholinergics, alpha-adrenergic blockade • *Vascular* (stroke)

Diagnostic Studies

The initial evaluation should include a urinalysis to rule out reversible causes of incontinence, such as a UTI. Consider a urine culture based on urinalysis results, BUN and creatinine as history and comorbidities indicate, and measurement of a postvoid residual volume to help distinguish the type of incontinence. If an imaging study seems needed, the initial choice is renal ultrasound. Consider referral to a urologist or urogynecologist as needed for specialized testing and concerns regarding an anatomic basis for the incontinence.

REFERENCES

Barry M.J., Fowler, F.J. Jr., O'Leary, M.P., Bruskewitz, R.C., Holtgrewe, H.L., Mebust, W.K., et al. (1992). The American Urological Association symptom index for benign prostatic hyperplasia. *Journal of Urology, 148*(5), 149–157.

Batstone, G., Doble, A., & Batstone, D. (2003). Chronic prostatitis. *Current Opinions Urology, 13*(1), 23–29.

Bent, S., & Saint, S. (2003). The optimal use of diagnostic testing in women with acute uncomplicated cystitis. *Disease-A-Month, 49*(2), 83–98.

Kawashima, A., Glockner, J.F., & King, B.F. (2003). CT urography and MR urography. *Radiologic Clinics of North America, 41*(5), 945–961.

Perlman, E.S., Rosenfield, A.T., Wexler, J.S., & Glickman, M.G. (1996). CT urography in the evaluation of urinary tract disease. *Journal of Computer Assisted Tomography, 20*(4), 620–626.

Richardson, T.D., & Oesterling, J.E. (1997). Age-specific reference ranges for serum prostate specific antigen. *Urologic Clinics of North America, 24*(2), 339.

Wilson, M.G., (2006). Urinary incontinence: Selected current concepts. *Medical Clinics of North America, 90*, 825–836.

SUGGESTED READINGS

American Urological Association. (2000). "Prostate-Specific Antigen Best Practice Policy: 2009 Update." www.auanet.org/content/media/psa09.pdf?CFID=3412874&CFTOKEN=70152000&jsessionid=8430963ab8811b2477441947435f254b372e (accessed March 16, 2011).

Brownlee, N. (1999). Taking the mystery out of ureteroscopy. *Association of Operating Room Nurses (AORN), 69*(1), 162–171.

Fielding, J., Silverman, S., Samuel, S., Zou, K., & Loughlin, K. (1998). Unenhanced helical CT of ureteral stones: A replacement for excretory urography in planning treatment. *American Journal of Roentgenology, 171*(4), 1051–1053.

Grossfeld, G.D., Litwin, M.S., Wolf, J.S., Hricak, H., Shuler, C.L., Agerter, D.C., et al. (2001). Evaluation of asymptomatic microscopic hematuria in adults: The American Urological Association best practice policy—Part I: Definition, detection, prevalence, and etiology. *Urology, 57*(4), 599–603.

Grossfeld, G.D., Litwin, M.S., Wolf, J.S., Hricak, H., Shuler, C.L., Agerter, D.C., et al. (2001). Evaluation of asymptomatic microscopic hematuria in adults: The American Urological Association best practice policy—Part II: Patient evaluation, cytology, voided markers, imaging, cystoscopy, nephrology evaluation, and follow-up. *Urology, 57*(4), 604–610.

Kreder, K., & Dmochowski, R. (2007). *The Overactive Bladder Evaluation and Management.* London: Informa Healthcare.

Ouslander, J. (1997). Aging and the lower urinary tract. *American Journal of the Medical Sciences, 314*(4), 214–218.

Roehrborn, C.G., Uzzo, R.G., Burnett, A.L., Dougherty, J., Lavelle, J.P., Lofholm, P., et al. (2006). Benign prostatic hyperplasia: Applying the clinical guidelines to practice. Supplement to *Clinical Advisor* (Nov.).

Wyndaele, J. (1999). Normality in urodynamics studied in healthy adults. *Journal of Urology, 161*(3), 899–902.

Chapter 12

MALE REPRODUCTIVE SYSTEM

S.A. Quallich

Knowledge of the anatomy and the ability to focus the history on the presenting complaint are the keys to accurately assessing complaints related to the male reproductive system (see Figure 12.1). Most of the information needed to arrive at an accurate diagnosis is gained through inspection, palpation, and a precise history. Because not all assessment points are relevant to every complaint, taking a problem-focused history is vital.

History

■ General History

In order to confirm normal physiologic male development, the patient's general history relative to reproductive or genital complaints should first establish that puberty started in his early or middle teens. The history should include any past reproductive complaints; a discussion of any recent (within the last 6 months) systemic illness; recent weight gain or loss; and a smoking, alcohol consumption, and illicit drug use history. It must also include a listing of current prescription and over-the-counter medications. As each complaint is discussed in this chapter, additional general and specific history-taking points are discussed.

■ Past Medical History

The evaluation should proceed to a history of any condition that would affect the penis, testes, or hormones (including cryptorchidism, hypothyroidism, pituitary malfunction); any history of genitourinary surgeries (such as orchidopexy; YV plasty to bladder neck; inguinal hernia repair as infant, small child, or adult; epispadias or hypospadias repair; prostate surgery; bladder reconstructions; bladder surgeries; testicular surgeries); previous treatment for testicular or genitourinary malignancies; and a history of vasectomy and when it was performed.

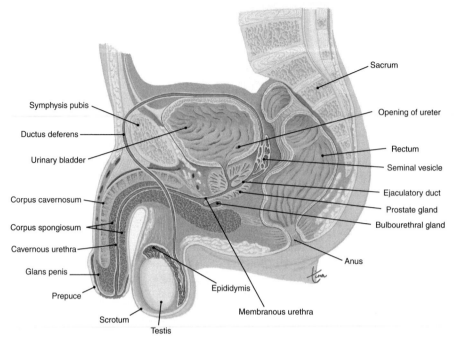

Figure 12.1 Anatomical structure of the male reproductive system. (From Scanlon, V.C., & Sanders, T. *Essentials of Anatomy and Physiology*, 4th ed. Philadelphia: F.A. Davis, 2003, p. 438. Reprinted with permission.)

■ Family History

The family history should include a discussion of testicular or other genitourinary (GU) malignancies, prostate or bladder problems in other family members (including female relatives with bladder conditions), other members of the family with complaints similar to the patient's presenting complaint, and a history of maternal medication or drug use while pregnant if known.

■ Sexual History

A sexual history is particularly relevant when the main complaint involves the GU system. The history should include recent changes in sexual partners and sexual orientation, the overall pattern of sexual activity, history of having previously fathered any children, libido, erectile function, and evaluation and treatment of a partner that may have preceded the patient's current visit.

■ Habits

This discussion will include any activity that would put the groin area at risk for trauma (such as football, hockey, marathon cycling, motocross, or riding three- or four-wheeled vehicles). It also includes any potential exposure to environmental toxins.

Physical Examination

Examination of the male patient is best done in a warm room in order to avoid exaggeration of the cremaster reflex. A routine *genital* examination, for the purposes of this chapter, involves inspection and palpation of the male genitalia. A routine *GU* examination, for the purposes of this chapter, involves the routine genital examination and digital rectal examination (DRE). Specialized examination maneuvers are indicated as needed.

■ Order of the Examination

Inspection

Look for age-appropriate development of male secondary sex characteristics; lesions or scarring of the penis, scrotum, or groin; discoloration of the penis, scrotum, or groin; asymmetry of testicles; gynecomastia; hirsutism; location and size of the opening of the meatus; and presence of scars in the abdomen, groin, or inguinal areas. The tone of the dartos muscle governs the size of the scrotum; in a cool environment, it causes the scrotum to contract.

Auscultation

Auscultate the abdomen as indicated; refer to Chapter 10. Auscultation is rarely indicated in the evaluation of male reproductive complaints except with a suspected herniation of bowel into the scrotum or as part of a complete physical.

Percussion

Percuss the abdomen as indicated; refer to Chapter 10. Percussion is rarely indicated in the evaluation of male reproductive complaints except as part of a complete physical. See box for red flag presentations.

RED Flag | **Red Flags in the Assessment of the Male Reproductive System**

- Sudden onset of acute testicular pain
- Cellulitic or necrotic changes to the skin of the scrotum, penis, perineal region
- Erection lasting more than 60 minutes after cessation of sexual activity
- Inability to urinate
- New mass, painful mass, or previously identified mass that is newly painful in the scrotum

---

Palpation

Palpation is the most important part of the physical examination. The examination requires palpation of all suspected intrascrotal masses—that is, masses that may arise from the surface of the testicle or adjacent to or separate from the testes. Table 12.1 reviews the palpation of the male reproductive structures.

Table 12.1

Palpation of Male Reproductive Structures

Male Reproductive Structure	Normal Findings on Palpation	Abnormalities and Possible Significance
Penis	• Soft and pliable along length of shaft • Meatus midline and central to glans • Foreskin should retract and draw forward easily	• Areas of fibrous plaque along shaft—Peyronie's disease • Tenderness—possibly secondary to a urethral stricture • Difficulty with foreskin retraction—phimosis, edema, balanitis, balanoposthitis • Difficulty moving foreskin forward—paraphimosis, edema • Entire shaft of penis fibrous and with reduced pliability—previous priapism • Meatus not midline or central to glans—hypospadias, epispadias
Scrotum	Loose sac of skin partially covered with hair	• Areas of erythema or nodularity—infected sebaceous glands or hair follicles • Unilateral, uncomfortable swelling of the scrotum—hydrocele, hematoma, varicocele
Testes	• Two testes, freely movable within the scrotum • Palpate between thumb and first two fingers of the hand • Firm, smooth, rubbery consistency • Average 6 cm × 4 cm in size • Symmetrical • Right testicle may be slightly anterior to left • Separate from epididymis	• Mass associated with testicle—tumor, hydrocele, spermatocele • Solitary testes—nondescent of testicle or previous surgical removal • Small, soft testicle(s)—Klinefelter's disease, history of infection, late orchidopexy

Table 12.1

Palpation of Male Reproductive Structures—cont'd

Male Reproductive Structure	Normal Findings on Palpation	Abnormalities and Possible Significance
Epididymis	• Soft ridge of tissue longitudinally posterior to the testicle • Separate from testicle	• Cystic or nodular—spermatocele, previous or current infection, history of vasectomy • Large and fluctuant—spermatocele • Localized pain—epididymitis, postvasectomy pain syndrome
Vas deferens and spermatic cord	• Soft, rubbery consistency • Smooth along its length • Able to trace vas deferens from epididymis to inguinal canal	• Absence of vas bilaterally or unilaterally—cystic fibrosis or a variant • Sperm granuloma—post vasectomy • Congested veins unilaterally or bilaterally—varicocele • Beading/nodularity of the cord—obstruction of epididymis, tubercular infection of the epididymis

■ Special Maneuvers

Table 12.2 outlines several physical examination points specific to the assessment of male reproductive complaints.

Differential Diagnosis of Chief Complaints

GENERAL COMPLAINTS

■ Testicular or Scrotal Pain

Pain in the testicles or scrotum can take many forms, including an acute, nauseating pain after trauma to the area; a dull ache with a progressive onset; and the sharp, focused pain associated with an infection. A focused history and targeted examination often provide the necessary clues to diagnosis.

Table 12.2

Physical Examination Maneuvers for Assessment of Male Reproductive Complaints

Maneuver	Description
Cremasteric reflex	Brushing or touching the skin of the scrotum in a downward direction will result in the prompt elevation of the testicle on the same side. This reaction can be aggravated by a cool room—the reflex may have engaged before any contact with the examiner
Digital rectal examination (DRE)	Gloved, lubricated finger is inserted into the anus and swept across the surface of the prostate; prostate should be symmetrical, nontender, free of nodules, approximately the size of a walnut, and have a smooth, rubbery consistency. Examination also involves estimation of anal sphincter tone
Examination for hernia	Index finger is inserted into the scrotum and invaginated into the external inguinal ring (scrotum should be invaginated in front of the testicle); fingertips of other hand should then be placed over the internal inguinal canal and patient should be asked to Valsalva. A hernia will be felt as a bulge that descends against index finger with Valsalva maneuver
Neurologic examination	Testing of superficial anal reflex (perianal sensation)—stroking the anus with a cotton swab will result in reflexive contraction of the external anal sphincter ("anal wink"). Testing of bulbocavernosus reflex—inserting a gloved finger into the anus and squeezing the glans penis will result in contraction of the anal sphincter and bulbocavernosus muscles. (These tests are most helpful when evaluating complaints of erectile and ejaculatory dysfunction)
Transillumination of hydrocele	Light source shined through mass; hydrocele will glow reddish; may feel as though it surrounds testicle; may feel turbid or tense
Transillumination of spermatocele	Light source shined through mass; should palpate testicle as separate from the spermatocele; note that the epididymis may not be palpated separately from the spermatocele; the mass feels connected to testicle at testicle's superior aspect
Valsalva maneuver to evaluate for varicocele	Performed with patient standing and in a warm room; having patient perform Valsalva will reverse the flow into the pampiniform plexus and result in palpable distention of the vessels ("bag of worms" if varicocele is of sufficient size)

History

Trauma may precede the complaint of pain in the testes or scrotum; it is important to establish the mechanism of injury if possible. The patient may report acute pain or progressive pain and tenderness after the insult. There may be a history of a sudden onset of acute pain and elevation of the affected testicle. The onset of the discomfort also may have occurred over time and could be associated with lesions or drainage from the scrotum; in such a case, the patient may also provide a history of recurrent scrotal infections and current constitutional symptoms, such as fever, chills, malaise, and nausea.

Physical Examination

A thorough examination of the genitals is vital despite that it may cause additional discomfort to the patient. Examination may reveal generalized tenderness of the scrotum and its contents, unilateral scrotal swelling, localized tenderness to one or more of the scrotal structures, or painful and edematous genitalia. If mild or moderate trauma is involved, ecchymotic areas or abrasions may be observed.

TESTICULAR TORSION

Testicular torsion is most commonly seen in early puberty and results in the loss of blood flow to the affected testicle. Compromised blood flow results in swelling and tissue necrosis after 6 to 8 hours. There are no established risk factors, but it is more common during adolescence due to the rapid growth of the testes.

Signs and Symptoms

Patients experience an acute and sudden onset of pain that localizes in the affected testicle, but it may also radiate to the inguinal areas or abdomen. This pain is often accompanied by abdominal discomfort, nausea, and vomiting. Asymmetric scrotal swelling is apparent on physical examination, with the affected testicle being somewhat elevated. The affected testicle may also have a somewhat horizontal lie. Traditional landmarks within the scrotum may be difficult to assess because of edema, and the cremaster reflex may be absent on the affected side.

Diagnostic Studies

Testicular torsion is a true urologic emergency that must be identified quickly. If it is suspected, the patient must be immediately referred to the closest emergency department for evaluation and probable surgery to try to preserve the testicle.

FOURNIER'S GANGRENE

Fournier's gangrene is a progressive necrotizing fasciitis of the genitals and perineum most commonly seen in males in their sixth decade and usually caused by a combination of aerobic and anaerobic organisms. It can progress to involve the entire perineal area, abdominal wall, and buttocks. Risk factors for its development include poor personal hygiene, phimosis, diabetes, alcoholism, malnutrition, chemotherapy or radiation treatment, perirectal or perianal infections, and local trauma to the genitals or perineal area (such as surgery).

Signs and Symptoms

There may be a prodromal period of generalized discomfort followed by erythema and edema in the affected areas. Cellulitic changes are apparent on physical examination and may be accompanied by crepitus, dark purple coloration, necrosis, eschar, and a foul odor. Often there are constitutional complaints of fever, chills, nausea, and vomiting, and the patient may progress to frank sepsis. Specific urologic complaints may be noted as well: dysuria, urethral discharge, or urethral obstruction.

Diagnostic Studies

A scrotal ultrasound can be helpful in defining areas of crepitus, but this should not delay referral. If Fournier's gangrene is suspected, the patient must be immediately referred to the closest emergency department for evaluation and probable admission: This is a true urologic emergency that must be identified quickly.

INCARCERATED INGUINAL HERNIA
See Chapters 10 and 11.

TESTICULAR MASS OR TUMOR
Malignant tumors of the testes are uncommon, usually present between the ages of 15 and 35, are slightly more common on the right side, and arise from germ cells. The greatest risk factor for the development of a testicular tumor is cryptorchidism, with an overall incidence of 7% to 10% in the patient with a history of unilateral or bilateral undescended testes. Increased screening and early detection have significantly decreased the mortality from this malignancy, but up to 10% of patients present with pain and/or constitutional or pulmonary complaints that indicate metastasis.

Signs and Symptoms

A patient may have noticed a painless swelling of the testicle or a distinct nodule on self-examination. Minor trauma may have occurred to the affected side and initiated the onset of pain and/or swelling. The testicle gradually enlarges over time with some associated heaviness. Patients rarely complain of acute pain as their presenting symptom but rather of a dull ache or heaviness that localizes to the affected side. Physical examination reveals a distinct mass or diffuse enlargement of the affected testicle; the mass may be firm, smooth, nodular, or fixed. Palpation of the inguinal, supraclavicular, and axillary areas may show evidence of enlarged lymph nodes; examination of the abdomen may also demonstrate bulky retroperitoneal disease. In advanced disease, gynecomastia resulting from hormonal changes and wheezing due to lung metastasis may be observed.

Diagnostic Studies

The ultrasound is considered an extension of the physical examination in the case of a suspected testicular mass; a scrotal ultrasound can quickly and accurately distinguish a tumor from other intrascrotal pathologies. The biochemical markers that are helpful in the diagnosis and classification of testicular masses, in addition to routine chemistries and white blood cell (WBC) count, are α-fetoprotein (AFP) and beta human chorionic gonadotropin (β-hCG). A chest x-ray and CT scan of the chest, abdomen, and pelvis complete the metastatic workup. Removal of the testicle is necessary for an accurate pathologic diagnosis. The patient should be referred urgently to a urologist; in many cases, the removal of the testicle and prompt treatment of the associated adenopathy can be curative, depending on the stage of the disease.

EPIDIDYMITIS

This inflammation of the epididymis is caused by the spread of an infection from the bladder or urethra owing to an alteration in the urethral closure mechanism. Uncircumcised men and men with indwelling catheters, benign prostatic hypertrophy (BPH), recent GU instrumentation, or prostatic surgery are at risk for epididymitis. In heterosexual men younger than 35, the causative organisms are likely to be *Neisseria gonorrhoeae* and *Chlamydia trachomatis.* In homosexual men, the causative organism is usually *Escherichia coli.* In cases in which an organism associated with a sexually transmitted disease (STD) is suspected, the exposure to the organism can significantly predate the development of epididymitis. If epididymitis is left unrecognized and untreated, it can progress to an abscess or chronic infection with resulting fibrosis, chronic scrotal pain, and infertility.

Signs and Symptoms

Complaints usually involve a sudden onset (over 24–48 hours) of painful swelling in the scrotum, which can be unilateral or bilateral. Pain may decrease with elevation of the scrotum (Prehn's sign), although this is an unreliable indicator. There may be an associated urethral discharge and/or fever, and complaints of urethritis, cystitis, or prostatitis are possible. On physical examination, the pain will localize to the affected epididymis with palpation, which will be swollen and indurated. The spermatic cord is usually tender and swollen, and pain may radiate to the inguinal canal and/or flank. Examination can be difficult, as inflammation can distort the anatomy, and manipulation is likely to increase the patient's complaints of pain.

Diagnostic Studies

An ultrasound will differentiate between testicular torsion and epididymitis, and can be helpful in establishing the correct diagnosis in cases of the acute onset of pain. Laboratory tests are not usually necessary, although the patient may exhibit an elevated white count with a fever. If an STD is suspected on the basis of history, a Gram stain of a urethral smear can be ordered, and the partner must also be treated to prevent recurrent episodes.

ORCHITIS

Orchitis is usually caused by the extension of an infection from the epididymis to the testicle and rarely exists independent of epididymitis. The risks and causative organisms are the same as for epididymitis. Orchitis may also occur as a sequela of mumps and occurs in up to 30% of prepubertal male patients with mumps.

Signs and Symptoms

The signs and symptoms are the same as those for epididymitis. On physical examination, the pain localizes to the affected testicle, and it may not be possible to distinguish the separation between the epididymis and testicle owing to inflammation. A reactive hydrocele may form.

Diagnostic Studies

The diagnostics are the same as those for epididymitis, although an ultrasound is not typically needed.

HYDROCELE

A hydrocele is a collection of fluid between the layers of the tunica vaginalis, which surrounds the testicle, or fluid along the spermatic cord. The fluid is primarily water with some albumin. It often occurs unilaterally, and its origin is idiopathic in adult males, although there appears to be some decreased absorption of this fluid by the tunica itself. The fluid collection may be large enough to completely encompass the testicle.

Signs and Symptoms

Hydroceles are not usually painful, and they frequently present as a unilateral swelling of the scrotum that may extend into the inguinal canal. There may be associated heaviness or discomfort during specific activities, such as prolonged standing, prolonged sitting, or bicycling. If the hydrocele is large enough, it is possible for the scrotal skin to suffer excoriation and erythema. It may not be possible to feel the testicle during a physical examination if the hydrocele is large enough. A hydrocele can be confirmed with transillumination. A large hydrocele can distort the position of the other scrotal structures, particularly the epididymis, and make their identification challenging.

Diagnostic Studies

A scrotal ultrasound is not necessary but will definitively confirm a hydrocele and rule out any testicular pathology, if the testicle cannot be palpated.

VARICOCELE

A varicocele is a palpable or visible dilation of the vessels of the pampiniform plexus in the scrotum; retrograde reflux of venous blood in the internal spermatic vein dilates the pampiniform plexus. Varicoceles are more common on the left, owing to the greater distance the internal spermatic vein must traverse to the left renal vein when compared with the right. The etiology of varicoceles remains unclear, and there are no specific risk factors. It is unusual for males to exhibit a varicocele before adolescence, and most varicoceles are asymptomatic. Varicoceles are commonly diagnosed during a male infertility evaluation (semen parameters are often decreased; varicoceles represent a common cause of secondary male infertility) or, less commonly, during an evaluation for scrotal pain or a scrotal mass. If a varicocele is painful, the pain may increase with prolonged standing, exertion, or sitting; pain is rare after prolonged recumbency or sleeping. A varicocele typically presents unilaterally on the left side. The acute onset of a painful varicocele, on the left or right, may indicate obstruction of the spermatic or renal vein.

Signs and Symptoms

Most varicoceles are asymptomatic, but the patient may complain of a dull ache, fullness, pain that does not radiate, or pulling to the affected side of the scrotum. If the varicocele is large enough, it typically results in scrotal swelling that is noticeable to the patient, along with a bluish discoloration beneath the scrotal skin. Primary or secondary male infertility may be the presenting symptom. The varicocele can be exaggerated during physical examination by asking the patient to perform Valsalva's maneuver while standing; any distention of the pampiniform plexus should disappear when the patient lies down. A longstanding varicocele may cause testicular atrophy. If the varicocele is large, it may be visible during inspection ("bag of worms").

Diagnostic Studies

A scrotal ultrasound is not necessary but will definitively confirm a varicocele and rule out any testicular or scrotal pathology. The ultrasound must be specifically ordered to "r/o varicocele" to ensure that the test is done correctly for this finding. A right-sided varicocele can be a sign of right renal vein obstruction, and an abdominal CT scan should be ordered to rule out any pathology. The patient can be routinely referred to a urologist for further assessment and management, particularly if there are fertility concerns.

SPERMATOCELE

A spermatocele is usually a painless mass in the head of the epididymis that contains fluid and sperm. Since sperm are not produced until puberty, this lesion is never seen in preadolescents. Patients may complain of a scrotal mass that feels like "a third testicle" if it is sizable. If the mass is small, it can also be termed an epididymal cyst.

Signs and Symptoms

The spermatocele usually presents as a nontender mass that is clearly distinct from and above the testicle on palpation. Larger spermatoceles may present as a turbid mass; smaller lesions may feel more nodular. A spermatocele can be transilluminated.

Diagnostic Studies

Diagnostic studies are usually not necessary. A scrotal ultrasound is not necessary but will definitively confirm a spermatocele and rule out any testicular pathology. Lesions as small as 2 mm can be detected by ultrasound.

■ Testicular Mass

Any complaint of a testicular mass is considered malignant until proven otherwise.

History

The patient may report sudden or acute onset of a painful or tender testicle. Most patients are unable to report the length of time the lesion has actually been present. If a palpable mass is present, the patient may give history of increasing size and/or tenderness over a period of weeks or months. In addition to the history of how the mass has developed and any associated changes such as pain or discomfort, explore that patient's general health and review of systems, assessing urinary symptoms and presence of any systemic symptoms.

Physical Examination

A thorough examination of the genitals is vital, despite that it may cause discomfort to the patient. Pain or tenderness may be noted on the examination and may localize to the testicle, where a palpable mass can be felt either continuous with the testicle or adjacent to it. There may or may not be inguinal adenopathy associated with the testicular pain.

TESTICULAR TUMOR
See pp. 344–345.

TESTICULAR TORSION
See p. 343.

HYDROCELE
See p. 346.

SPERMATOCELE
See pp. 347–348.

VARICOCELE
See pp. 346–347.

HEMATOMA

The patient describes a steadily enlarging, firm, and possibly painful mass located unilaterally in the scrotum. The mass can be of varying sizes. The key point is a recent history of some invasive procedure, such as a vasectomy, hydrocelectomy, spermatocelectomy, or trauma sustained during sports activities or a motor vehicle accident.

Signs and Symptoms

The patient will complain of an enlarging mass that became noticeable within a few days after his surgical procedure. Physical examination will usually show a unilateral firm mass that is nontender on palpation. Pain is caused by distortion and displacement of the surrounding structures.

Diagnostic Studies

A scrotal ultrasound is not necessary but will definitively confirm a hematoma and rule out any other pathology. Small hematomas can be expected to resolve over time as they are reabsorbed. Large hematomas may need to be drained; the patient should be referred back to the provider who performed the procedure.

■ Scrotal Mass

A scrotal mass can cause great concern for patient and clinician alike and may be detected by self-examination or during a routine physical. The key to diagnosing the mass is a thorough examination of the scrotal contents in an attempt to localize the mass and identify any associated structures.

History

The patient presents with complaints of a painful or nonpainful mass in the scrotum. He may provide a long history of its presence in the scrotum or a history of recently increasing size. There may also be discomfort associated with the mass, and it may worsen with activities such as running, weight lifting, or the Valsalva maneuver.

Physical Examination

A routine genital examination is required, with additional special maneuvers based on findings and the suspected cause.

INGUINAL HERNIA

See Table 11-1 and discussions in Chapter 11.

HYDROCELE

See p. 346.

VARICOCELE

See pp. 346–347.

SPERM GRANULOMA

After a vasectomy, sperm can leak from the testicular end of the vas, causing an inflammatory reaction and granuloma formation. This granuloma helps to vent the pressure that can build up in the epididymis after a vasectomy, as sperm production does not cease. It is commonly apparent on physical examination and can be mistaken for other scrotal pathology. It may also indicate that the patient has formed antibodies against his own sperm, which can complicate attempts at pregnancy after a vasectomy reversal.

Signs and Symptoms

Usually no signs or symptoms are evident other than a nontender, firm mass at the end of the proximal vas deferens that can range in diameter up to 1 cm. In some cases, the granuloma may be tender on palpation.

Diagnostic Studies

Diagnosis is based partly on the physical examination; a scrotal ultrasound is not necessary or indicated based on the history of a vasectomy, but it will definitively confirm a granuloma at the proximal end of the vas and rule out any other pathology.

SPERMATOCELE

See pp. 347–348.

■ Penile or Genital Lesions

Complaints of lesions on the genitals are a common presentation of otherwise healthy males. These lesions may be the result of a communicable disease or other skin condition. Any sort of genital lesion is often a cause of significant anxiety to the patient. There are many additional, albeit less common, lesions that are not discussed in this section. If there is any uncertainty about the identification of a lesion, a referral to a urologist or dermatologist is appropriate.

History

The male patient may give a history of transient, recurrent, or nonhealing lesions to the penis or scrotum; there may also be a urethral discharge. The lesions may be described as small or moderately sized or as blisters or papules. The patient may describe progressively worsening and increasingly painful lesions. There may be complaints of dysuria, urethral itching, or malaise. A history of prior STDs and other skin changes is important, as is past medical history, including conditions such as diabetes.

Physical Examination

A thorough inspection is mandatory, including examination of the scrotal contents, distal urethra, and inguinal regions for adenopathy. Note characteristics of the lesion(s). The examination may also reveal scars that indicate previous lesions from STDs. Examination and culture of lesions or discharge is necessary, but also may cause additional pain to the patient.

PENILE CANCER

Relatively rare in the United States, cancer of the penis is usually a squamous cell lesion that presents on the prepuce, glans, shaft, or base of the penis. If the lesion involves the glans, prepuce, or penile shaft, it is called erythroplasia of Queyrat; if it presents on the other aspects of the male genitalia or perineal region, it is called Bowen's disease. Risk factors include not being circumcised; a history of STDs, particularly condyloma acuminatum; or a history of balanitis xerotica obliterans (BXO), which is discussed later in the chapter.

Signs and Symptoms

Patients may complain of a nonhealing ulcer, erythema that does not resolve, induration of the skin, or a lesion with a warty appearance. Patients may also report a history of difficulty with foreskin retraction—the lesion being concealed by the foreskin.

There may be associated itching and/or burning with the lesion, and there may be visible ulceration of the penile tissue. Lesions are most common on the glans. On physical examination, the presentation of a lesion has a variety of appearances, including flat and erythematous or papillary, but is typically a well-marginated lesion. The tissue surrounding the lesion may feel less pliable than unaffected areas, and the foreskin of an uncircumcised male may be difficult to retract. The entire penis must be palpated to assess the possible extent of the lesion into the corpora and deeper tissues. There may be palpable inguinal adenopathy, and the lesion may show evidence of a secondary bacterial infection. A DRE is necessary to evaluate for prostatic or urethral involvement.

Diagnostic Studies

Definitive diagnosis is via biopsy. The patient should be referred urgently to a urologist for diagnosis and management (emergently if he has difficulty voiding due to the location of the lesion). If inguinal adenopathy is present, the patient can be started on an antibiotic in advance of the urology appointment to attempt to treat any superimposed bacterial infection. A CT scan may be required to assess the extent of any inguinal adenopathy.

SEXUALLY TRANSMITTED DISEASE–RELATED LESIONS

An STD can present in many ways in the male patient. Any complaint of lesions on the genitals should be thoroughly evaluated, including questioning the patient regarding his sexual conduct and frequency of new partners.

Signs and Symptoms

Some STDs may be accompanied by complaints of constitutional symptoms or malaise. Refer to Table 12.3 for details of the lesion presentation on physical examination.

Diagnostic Studies

STDs can be diagnosed with the appropriate cultures, Gram stains, swabs, and serologic studies. Unless a patient appears ill and a WBC seems indicated, no additional laboratory work or imaging studies are indicated. Many STDs must be reported to the local health department. For complex, extensive, or refractory cases of genital warts, the patient can be referred to a urologist or dermatologist.

Table 12.3

Sexually Transmitted Diseases and Their Presentation in the Male

Sexually Transmitted Disease	Clinical Presentation in the Male
Chancroid	Tender ulcer with deep, undermined border may be soft or indurated; friable base with ragged edges; purulent exudate possible; painful lymphadenopathy
Chlamydia	Scant mucoid or mucopurulent urethral discharge; may be accompanied by mild dysuria and urethral itching
Genital *Herpes simplex*	*First episode:* Fluid-filled painful vesicles that may coalesce, with erythema to surrounding skin, and that eventually rupture, resulting in painful ulcerative lesions with erythematous edges; tender adenopathy, fever; dysuria also common. Lesions typically last 2–3 weeks, possibly up to 6 weeks
	Recurrences: Prodromal pain, burning, tingling at site where vesicles will erupt with shorter course of constitutional symptoms; lesions usually resolve after 7–10 days
Genital warts (human papillomavirus)	Soft, fleshy, exophytic lesions with raised granular surfaces; commonly seen on glans and prepuce; also present as small papular lesions on the skin or nonhealing penile lesion(s). The majority of lesions are subclinical and can be detected by using 3%–5% acetic acid
Gonorrhea	Urethral discharge may be yellowish or gray-brown, purulent, and accompanied by itching and dysuria; may be accompanied by epididymal or testicular pain; asymptomatic in 5%–10% of cases; rare superficial lesions to the penile shaft
Nongonococcal urethritis	Mild to moderate clear or white urethral discharge or thin mucoid urethral discharge; accompanied by mild dysuria and urethral itching
Pediculosis pubis	Severe pruritus; observation of ectoparasites on hair and/or skin in the genital area
Scabies	Papular or linear burrow-like lesions
Syphilis	*Primary:* Solitary, painless, nontender, and rubbery ulcer (chancre), superficial or deep, with indurated edge and no exudate
	Secondary: Papulosquamous or maculopapular rash indicative of systemic infection
Trichomoniasis	Usually asymptomatic, may cause urethritis

BALANITIS

Generally seen only in uncircumcised males, balanitis is an inflammation of the glans, commonly caused by a *Candida albicans* infection. Men with poorly controlled diabetes mellitus are at particular risk for balanitis, as are morbidly obese patients who demonstrate a retractile penis as a result of their body habitus.

Signs and Symptoms

The patient may present with a combination of symptoms that include edema, erythema, and pain of the glans; dysuria; urethral discharge; and a history of a discharge from between the foreskin and glans. Physical examination will confirm the edema, erythema, and exudates; there may be a cracked appearance to the prepuce. Palpation should always be done to the affected area to evaluate for changes in the consistency of the tissue. The patient should also be examined for any inguinal adenopathy.

Diagnostic Studies

Any exudates should be cultured for STDs and for other viral and fungal organisms; KOH (potassium hydroxide) and Tzanck preparations should also be included.

BALANOPOSTHITIS

This condition is generally seen only in uncircumcised males and is an inflammation that involves both the glans and foreskin.

Signs and Symptoms

The presentation and physical examination are similar to those for balanitis but can include an edematous and painful foreskin that may not retract.

Diagnostic Studies

Diagnostic studies are the same as for balanitis.

BALANITIS XEROTICA OBLITERANS

BXO is a variation of lichen sclerosus et atrophicus, which is common in middle-aged men and is a painful condition associated with patches of white, thinned skin. Uncircumcised and diabetic males have an increased risk, and the patient with longstanding BXO has a higher risk for squamous cell carcinoma of the penis.

Signs and Symptoms

Patients may complain of localized penile discomfort, painful erections, or urinary obstruction. On physical examination, there can be a whitish patch or patches on the prepuce or glans, and the meatus may become involved. The meatus itself may become edematous and indurated. As the condition progresses, there can be erosions, fissures, or meatal stenosis, and the foreskin may adhere to the glans.

Diagnostic Studies

Diagnosis can be made only via biopsy. If BXO is suspected, a referral to a urologist is mandatory, particularly because meatal stenosis or urinary obstruction can occur over time.

TRAUMA

The patient may present with a history of some manner of trauma (including robust sexual activity or the use of an unlubricated condom) to the genitalia, with some resulting lesions. In the case of bruising to the genitals, the causative trauma may have happened a few days earlier. The patient may also admit to the use of some kind of penile enlargement device with resulting trauma to the penis.

Signs and Symptoms

Examination of the genitalia reveals ecchymotic areas on the penile shaft, scrotum, or glans. There may also be abraded areas on the genitalia.

Diagnostic Studies

No laboratory work or imaging studies are indicated. If the resulting lesions are severe or there is evidence of infection, a referral to a urologist is recommended.

■ The Inability to Retract or Advance the Foreskin

Complaints of difficulty manipulating the foreskin occur only in males who have not been circumcised. These complaints are often accompanied by a history of chronic irritation or poor personal hygiene.

History

The patient will report difficulty at retracting the foreskin, possibly as complicated by a history of poor personal hygiene and/or a recent groin skin infection. Alternatively, there may be a history of pain and progressive difficulty with retraction. There may be complaints of the inability to advance the foreskin over the glans, possibly after a prolonged period of retraction. Pain may also be associated with any of these complaints. In addition to investigating personal hygiene, recent infections, and history of conditions such as diabetes and cardiovascular disease, explore whether similar episodes have been experienced previously.

Physical Examination

A thorough genital inspection is required along with a gentle attempt to retract or advance the foreskin.

PHIMOSIS

This condition is seen only in males who are uncircumcised. The patient will often present with a history of progressive difficulty at retracting the foreskin and, in some cases, urinary obstruction. This is commonly preceded by poor personal hygiene, chronic balanitis or balanoposthitis, or poor control of diabetes mellitus. Longstanding phimosis will create a risk for chronic inflammation and squamous cell cancer of the penis.

Signs and Symptoms

The patient may complain of pain when retracting or attempting to retract the foreskin and possibly a "ballooning" of the foreskin when voiding. If the patient reports a complete inability to retract the foreskin, physical examination may show that the opening of the foreskin has contracted to the point at which the actual opening is quite small. There may be evidence of balanitis or balanoposthitis.

Diagnostic Studies

History and presentation are usually sufficient to confirm the diagnosis. The patient should be referred to a urologist for further evaluation and management, as a dorsal slit or circumcision may be required.

PARAPHIMOSIS

Paraphimosis is a condition in which the foreskin has been retracted and cannot be advanced forward to its normal position over the glans. It results from chronic inflammation under the foreskin and is commonly preceded by poor personal hygiene, chronic balanitis or balanoposthitis, or poor control of diabetes mellitus. Over time, a tight ring of tissue forms when the foreskin is retracted, resulting in additional edema to the glans with retraction of the foreskin.

Signs and Symptoms

The patient may present with complaints of pain, swelling, and possible discoloration of the glans. Physical examination will reveal a foreskin that cannot be reduced or can be reduced with some difficulty; the shaft of the penis and glans may be tender/painful on palpation. There may be evidence of balanitis or balanoposthitis.

Diagnostic Studies

Although history and presentation are usually sufficient to confirm the diagnosis, paraphimosis is a urologic emergency; the patient should be referred to a urologist for further evaluation and management because arterial occlusion and necrosis of the glans and distal urethra may result if the paraphimosis is not reduced. Any exudates should be cultured for STDs and for other viral and fungal organisms; KOH and Tzanck preparations may also be included.

BALANITIS

See p. 353.

BALANOPOSTHITIS

See p. 353.

GENERALIZED EDEMA

The patient who suffers from generalized edema, such as that seen in cardiovascular or congestive heart failure patients, may also experience difficulty with advancing or retracting the foreskin.

Signs and Symptoms

The complaints are similar to those for phimosis or paraphimosis. Physical examination shows a swollen glans; there may be discolored skin if this condition has persisted; the glans, penile shaft, and foreskin may be painful to palpation. Generalized scrotal edema may be noted. Physical examination should also yield evidence of edema of the feet, legs, and possibly trunk, along with findings consistent with the causative condition(s).

Diagnostic Studies

History and presentation are usually sufficient to confirm the diagnosis. The patient should be urgently referred to a urologist for management if paraphimosis is noted; otherwise, a routine referral to a urologist is recommended for consideration of dorsal slit or circumcision in the case of phimosis, if personal hygiene becomes an issue (although any elective surgical intervention will be delayed by persistent edema).

■ The Absence of One or Both Testes in the Scrotum

The male may present at any age with the complaint of the absence of one or both testes in the scrotum. Evaluation of the testes is a required physical assessment point in male infants. But it is not uncommon that adolescent or adult males will present with this complaint in the absence of a surgical history that indicates a testicle was removed.

History

The patient (or possibly a parent if the patient is a minor) will complain of the absence of one or both testicles in the scrotum. If the patient is an adult, he may provide a history of difficulty conceiving with his female partner or a history of semen analysis abnormalities. If there is a failure of both testicles to descend, the patient may report late, or failure of, puberty onset. There may also be a history of inguinal or lower abdominal pain.

Physical Examination

Physical examination involves a genital examination that notes the absence of one or both testicles in the scrotum. It is vital to note the stage of development of secondary male characteristics. The patient may have a testicle that is palpable in the inguinal canal that can be tender on examination. There may be age-appropriate secondary sexual characteristics, particularly with one descended testicle.

CONGENITAL CRYPTORCHIDISM OR ECTOPIC TESTICLE(S)

This is the condition in which one or both testes have failed to descend normally into the scrotum. Descent may have stopped at any point between the renal and scrotal areas, but most commonly the undescended testes are found in the inguinal canal. In male infants with undescended testes, more than half will descend into the scrotum during the first month after birth. There are no genetic abnormalities associated with this condition, and many males with a unilaterally undescended testicle do not have trouble initiating a pregnancy, despite decreased sperm counts. There is an increased risk of infertility owing to damage to the seminiferous tubules, depending on the length of time after birth the testes were brought down into the scrotal sac. The majority of patients with bilateral cryptorchidism become appropriately androgenized as adults but are at increased risk for inguinal hernias.

Signs and Symptoms

There can be complaints of pain, as the testes may be in an uncomfortable position. The patient may complain of infertility. On physical examination, the scrotum on the affected side will be atrophic. The testes may be felt in the inguinal canal or may not be palpable at all. If the testicle is palpable, it cannot be manipulated into the scrotum. An inguinal hernia may also be present on the affected side. The stage of development of secondary sexual characteristics should be noted in postpubertal males.

Diagnostic Studies

Ultrasound is usually successful if the suspected testis is in the groin; a CT scan or MRI will detect an intra-abdominal testis in a postpubertal male. Laboratory work can include testosterone, follicle-stimulating hormone (FSH), and luteinizing hormone (LH; FSH and LH may help differentiate intra-abdominal from bilateral anorchia because both are significantly elevated in anorchia). A routine referral to a urologist for further evaluation and management should also be made.

SEVERE ATROPHY OF ONE OR BOTH TESTICLES

Severe atrophy can result from a mumps infection in the prepubertal male, although it is rare in this era of a successful mumps vaccine. The patient will give a history of mumps before puberty and will often relate a history of profound swelling of one of the testicles. Orchitis will result in approximately 30% of males who contract mumps, with approximately one-third of those developing testicular atrophy.

It is also possible to encounter severe atrophy of a testicle as the result of a varicocele that has been present for many years (see earlier section on varicoceles for details).

Signs and Symptoms

Possible signs include complaints of size differential between the testicles or altered semen analysis. On physical examination, pronounced testicular atrophy compared with the unaffected side is apparent. The affected testicle is non-tender on examination and has a softer consistency.

Diagnostic Studies

History and examination are usually sufficient. A scrotal ultrasound is not necessary but will definitively confirm the size differences and rule out any additional pathology.

KLINEFELTER'S SYNDROME

Klinefelter's syndrome is the most common abnormality of sexual differentiation, occurs in approximately 1 in 500 live births, is one of the most common causes of primary hypogonadism, and is the most common sex chromosome abnormality seen in infertile men. Patients present with the typical triad of small, firm testes; gynecomastia; and elevated urine gonadotropins. Variants of Klinefelter's may also result in increased height, diabetes mellitus, obesity, and decreased intelligence. Although testicles are not absent, their small size may lead to lack of recognition as the testes.

Signs and Symptoms

Patients complain of delayed completion of puberty and delayed virilization. There are usually few physical complaints associated with Klinefelter's disease other than possible concern regarding testicle size. Physical examination reveals a lack of development of secondary sexual characteristics (small [<3.0 cm] atrophic testes, small phallus, diminished body hair, diminished muscle bulk), and a feminine, or truncal, rather than male fat distribution that often includes gynecomastia. Patients will be tall due to a delay in the fusion of the epiphyseal plates in the long bones.

Diagnostic Studies

Karyotype analysis will show 47, XXY or a mosaic 46, XY/47, XXY. Hormone studies will demonstrate decreased or normal testosterone, decreased free testosterone, elevated estradiol, normal or elevated LH, and elevated FSH. A scrotal ultrasound is unnecessary but can confirm the presence and small size of the testes. If fertility is an issue, the patient should be routinely referred to a urologist specializing in male infertility, as semen analysis will show azoospermia.

PHYSIOLOGIC RETRACTILE TESTICLES OR MIGRATORY TESTES

The rare male patient may present with a history of one or both of his testicles "climbing into his belly" or inguinal canal. This is a normal variant due to a hyperactive cremasteric reflex. Usually it can be demonstrated in children and into puberty, at which point it resolves. Occasionally it can persist into adulthood. The patient will demonstrate normal male physiologic development.

Signs and Symptoms

The patient will report that one or both testicles retract to the point that they are no longer palpable or visible in the scrotum. The important point of the physical examination is to locate the testicle(s) and gently manipulate it (them) into usual anatomic position(s). This does not usually cause the patient pain. The scrotum will also be normally developed with no sign of atrophy.

Diagnostic Studies

The history and examination is typically sufficient. A scrotal ultrasound will aid in the diagnosis. If there is any doubt or trouble locating a testicle, the patient may be referred to a urologist.

ERECTILE FUNCTION COMPLAINTS

■ Erectile Dysfunction

Male erectile dysfunction (ED) is a common clinical complaint that may have far-reaching effects on the self-esteem and relationships of those involved. Some estimates number men with complete ED at 10 to 20 million in the United States alone; this number increases to an excess of 30 million men if moderate to complete ED is also included. The worldwide incidence of ED is projected to rise to greater than 322 million men by 2025 (Ayta, McKinlay, & Krane, 1999). The actual incidence is likely to be greater because ED is an underreported condition, and questions regarding sexual function may not be asked during routine clinic visits.

Several underlying causes contribute to ED: arteriogenic, venogenic, endocrinologic, neurologic, psychologic, and medicinal. Vascular disease is one of the most common causes of organic ED. Many epidemiologic studies have shown not only that ED coexists with hypertension but also that as the severity of hypertension increases, so do reports of ED severity from patients. The incidence of ED in diabetic men has been reported at 35% (Sullivan, Keoghane, & Miller, 2001); other investigators have reported this incidence ranging from 20% to 85%, with the incidence rising with age and degree of glycemic control. But many men will complain of erectile problems in the absence of any other currently diagnosed pathologies, and ED may provide a clue to the subtle onset of many systemic diseases. This is particularly true in patients who proceed to formal diagnoses of hypercholesterolemia, hypertension, or diabetes mellitus. However, a complete discussion of ED is beyond the scope of this chapter.

ED can be successfully treated without knowing the precise nature of its cause.

History

The patient will often give a history of declining erectile function, usually insidious and progressive, that may span several years. Alternatively, he may provide a history of relatively rapid or recent onset of decline in erectile function, perhaps associated with the history of recently starting new medication. Some degree of ED is a frequent complaint after prostate, bladder, rectal, or other retroperitoneal surgery.

The history should include several points specific to the patient's sexual functioning: the precise nature of the dysfunction (i.e., whether the problem is attaining or sustaining an erection, insufficient rigidity, penetration, absence of climax or anejaculation); whether ED occurs with all sexual partners or only specific partners; psychosocial factors, including the nature of current relationship(s); the presence or absence of nocturnal and morning erections and their quality; and any treatments (pharmacologic and nonpharmacologic) the patient has tried.

An assessment of the degree to which this condition has impacted the patient's quality of life is also important. This can be assessed using the Sexual Health Inventory for Men (SHIM), a short questionnaire that has been validated for the assessment of ED.

Physical Examination

If ED is a complaint in a man with no other recognized medical conditions, a full physical examination is necessary. In the patient with recognized chronic conditions, the focus should be on the routine genital examination along with a cardiovascular examination for cardiovascular risk assessment (Kostis et al., 2005).

Diagnostic Studies

Based on the clinical suspicion for undiagnosed underlying disease, screening begins with a testosterone level, urinalysis, CBC, glucose, BUN, serum creatinine, and cholesterol profile. A free testosterone may also be considered, particularly if hypogonadism is suspected. If these tests are inconclusive, the patient can be referred to a urologist for further evaluation with specialized diagnostic testing as well as management if first-line pharmacologic management is not sufficient. If the history and physical appear to suggest a stronger psychological than organic component to the ED, a referral to a sexual counselor or therapist would be helpful.

Categories of Erectile Dysfunction

See Table 12.4, which is representative and is not all inclusive. Systemic disease–induced causes for ED are usually a combination of other etiologic categories. Medications that contribute to erectile dysfunction are listed in Table 12.5.

Table 12.4

Categories of Erectile Dysfunction and Selected Examples

Category of ED	Examples of Causes
Arteriogenic	Atherosclerosis, hypertension, hyperlipidemia, smoking, pelvic trauma, diabetes mellitus
Cavernosal (venogenic)	Vascular disease, diabetes mellitus, Peyronie's disease, insufficient trabecular smooth muscle contraction, age
Endocrinologic	Hypogonadism, hyperprolactinemia, hyperthyroidism, hypothyroidism, diabetes mellitus, orchiectomy
Medication-induced	Antihypertensives, antidepressants, antipsychotics, alcohol abuse, smoking, antiandrogens, α-adrenergic blockers, β-blockers, tranquilizers, thiazide diuretics, centrally acting sympatholytics, cimetidine, estrogens, polypharmacy, marijuana use, chemotherapy
Neurologic	Retroperitoneal surgery, SCI, MS, diabetes mellitus, pelvic trauma, spina bifida, CNS tumors, alcohol abuse, Parkinson's disease, Alzheimer's disease, CVA, pelvic irradiation
Psychologic	Performance anxiety, depression, psychological stress, relationship issues, psychotic disorders, misinformation or ignorance of normal anatomy/function
Systemic disease-induced	CRF, coronary heart disease, COPD (fear of inducing exacerbation), CHF, hepatic failure, recent MI, cirrhosis

CNS = central nervous system; COPD = chronic obstructive pulmonary disease; CRF = chronic renal failure; CVA = cardiovascular accident; ED = erectile dysfunction; MS = multiple sclerosis; SCI = spinal cord injury.

Table 12.5

Selected Medications Reported to Contribute to Erectile Dysfunction

Medication Class	Selected Examples
Antiandrogenic medications	α-5 reductase inhibitors, luteinizing hormone–releasing hormone analogues, leuprolide acetate
Anticholinergics	Diphenhydramine
Antihypertensives	Diuretics (thiazides), vasodilators, central sympatholytics (methyldopa, clonidine), β-blockers, calcium-channel blockers, angiotensin-converting enzyme inhibitors
Benzodiazepines	Diazepam, clonazepam
Lipid-lowering agents	Lovastatin, pravastatin sodium
Miscellaneous medications	Cimetidine, lithium, baclofen
Monoamine oxidase inhibitors	Phenelzine, procarbazine

Continued

Table 12.5	

Selected Medications Reported to Contribute to Erectile Dysfunction—cont'd

Medication Class	Selected Examples
Recreational drugs	Alcohol, marijuana, barbiturates, opiates, nicotine
Tranquilizers	Haldol
Tricyclic antidepressants	Nortriptyline hydrochloride, amitriptyline hydrochloride

■ Prolonged Erection/Priapism

Priapism is the presence of a prolonged erection that occurs in the absence of sexual stimulation or that remains after orgasm. This condition usually affects only the corpora cavernosa of the penis. It is uncommon, and although it can occur in any age group, it is more common from ages 20 to 50. Priapism is usually painful, and it is a urologic emergency. Failure to reverse the erection can result in scarring of the penile corpora and permanent erectile dysfunction owing to tissue ischemia. Unfortunately, there can be a significant time delay between the onset of priapism and the patient's presentation for evaluation and treatment.

History

The patient will complain of a persistent erection that did not resolve with cessation of sexual activity or after climax. There does not have to be 100% erection to be considered priapism. The erection may have occurred spontaneously. He may complain of pain, depending on length of time the penis has remained erect (pain does not usually occur until after 6–8 hours). He may also provide a history of the use of injectable erectogenic agents, sickle-cell disease, or a history of similar episodes that resolved painlessly after a couple of hours. It is vital to establish as accurately as possible the duration of the erection.

Physical Examination

A routine genital examination will establish the presence of an erection; the corpora will be partially to fully rigid, depending on the etiology of the priapism. The penis may be tender on examination. The penis feels somewhat tense and congested, but the corpus spongiosum and glans are of normal consistency. There may be skin discoloration. A DRE, abdominal examination, and neurologic examination should also be performed.

Selected Causes

See Table 12.6.

Table 12.6	

Selected Causes of Priapism

Causes of Priapism	Explanation
Idiopathic (primary) priapism	Accounts for up to 60% of cases
Medication-induced priapism	Resulting after penile injection treatment for erectile dysfunction, some recreational or psychotropic drugs (cocaine, alcohol)
Priapism caused by other medical condition	Sickle cell disease, leukemia, pelvic tumor, spinal cord trauma, thromboembolic event, neoplastic causes due to metastases
Priapism due to trauma	Perineal or penile trauma can lead to high-flow (arterial) priapism

Diagnostic Studies

None are necessary. Priapism requires immediate referral to the nearest emergency department and often requires evaluation by a urologist.

■ Curvature of the Penis

Male patients of any age may present with curvature of the penis, which is usually noticeable only when the penis is erect. As men present at older ages, the likelihood that the curvature is congenital decreases, especially if they report that the erection was previously straight. The proper course of care for these patients is referral to a urologist for further examination and treatment, particularly in a case such as congenital penile corporal disproportion. Most complaints of curvature (in the absence of a clinically apparent plaque) are amenable to some type of surgical correction.

History

The patient will report a progressive curvature of the shaft of the penis with erection; the curve can occur at any site along the shaft of the penis. There may be a concurrent history of a decline in erectile function with the onset of curvature as well as pain with erections. Some patients report a history of some sort of trauma to the shaft of the penis with resulting bruising and pain that preceded the onset of the curvature. Alternatively, the patient may give a history that curvature has "always" been present, with no pain associated with erections, no impact to erectile function, and merely cosmetic concerns.

Physical Examination

A routine genital examination is necessary, and a palpable plaque may be felt anywhere along the shaft of the penis. Plaque can also be absent, particularly if the history indicates that the curvature may be congenital.

PEYRONIE'S DISEASE

Although the precise cause of Peyronie's disease is not known, current belief regarding its etiology is that the plaque formation results after disordered wound healing, often with calcium deposition in the plaque (Greenfield & Levine, 2005). During regular sexual activity, susceptible patients may suffer nonpainful minor trauma to the penis that leads to a decrease in the elasticity of the tissue and fibroblast formation, eventually resulting in plaque. The plaque is present in the tunica albuginea of the corpora cavernosa, which leads to shortening and curvature of the shaft of the penis. The resulting curvature can be in any direction: lateral, ventral, or dorsal. Often the quality of erection distal to the plaque is poor and prevents adequate penetration during sexual activity. Peyronie's disease is most commonly seen between the ages of 45 and 60, and complaints of ED may predate the curvature. Peyronie's disease can go into spontaneous remission, and there is a 30% association with Dupuytren's contracture of the tendons of the hand.

Signs and Symptoms

The patient complains of curvature of the penis, noticeable with erections. The curve may be progressive or may have stopped curving. If it is painful, it is only while the penis is erect. Physical examination may yield evidence of a palpable plaque that involves the tunica albuginea; the plaque is commonly located at or near the dorsal midline of the shaft.

Diagnostic Studies

History and physical examination are usually sufficient to confirm the diagnosis. A routine referral to a urologist can be considered for further treatment and possible surgical intervention.

PENILE CORPORAL DISPROPORTION

This is a relatively rare congenital condition in which the corpora cavernosa of the penis are not of identical length. This leads to painless curvature with erection; there are no associated erectile function complaints. The curvature will cause some distress to the patient, and he will seek evaluation to correct the curvature. The patient may have also (incorrectly) self-diagnosed Peyronies' disease.

Signs and Symptoms

The patient will describe curved erections without a history of having previously had straight erections. On physical examination, the difference between the corpora may be palpable. The patient will demonstrate age-appropriate development of secondary sexual characteristics.

Diagnostic Studies

Diagnosis is typically through history and physical. Routine referral to a urologist is recommended; this condition can be corrected with surgery.

PENILE FRACTURE

Penile fracture results in an acquired curvature of the penis and is the result of trauma during intercourse that causes a rupture to the tunica albuginea of one of the corpora cavernosa of the penis. The patient will present with a history of a lateral buckling of the penis and a "snap" heard during intercourse, typically when the woman is in the superior position. This is followed by possible bleeding from the urethra, loss of penile rigidity, and eventual ecchymosis of the penis. The trauma may also be less severe and result in a gradual curvature over time. Often there is an accompanying loss of rigidity or pain with subsequent erections. There may also be some disruption of the urethra.

Signs and Symptoms

The patient will complain of decreased and/or painful erections. On physical examination (including GU, rectal, and lower abdominal examinations), there may be a palpable indentation or scar at the site of the corporal rupture and possibly ecchymosis of the scrotum if the presentation is shortly after injury. If the patient presents acutely, there may be blood at the meatus. Physical findings depend on the length of time since the injury.

Diagnostic Studies

History and physical examination are usually sufficient to confirm the diagnosis. An urgent consult to a urologist should be made if the patient presents acutely. A routine referral to a urologist can be considered for further evaluation, treatment, and possible surgical intervention if the patient presents after the acute period.

■ Low Testosterone

Low testosterone is less a direct patient complaint than representative of a combination of symptoms. There may be moodiness, loss of interest in usual activities, loss of libido, fatigue, and even diminished muscle bulk. The key in its evaluation is establishing the cause of the low level of testosterone.

History

There is likely to be an insidious onset of some degree of ED, loss of libido, depressed mood, and fatigue. If this has been progressing over a significant length of time, decreased muscle mass and strength and loss of facial and body hair may occur. A thorough history is essential, including past and current conditions, prescribed treatments and other agents taken, and broad review of systems. Explore emotional status, as well.

Physical Examination

A complete physical is necessary, including routine genital examination and DRE. Attention should focus on the development of secondary sexual characteristics and testicular size. The physical examination is unrevealing in the majority of cases.

HYPOGONADISM

Hypogonadism is failure of the testes to produce normal levels of testosterone (and/or sperm). It primarily results from testicular failure; secondarily, it results from pituitary or hypothalamic causes. Combined hypogonadism is due to the decreased pulsatility of gonadotropins plus decreased testicular Leydig cell response. Hypogonadism is estimated to affect 4 to 5 million men in the United States alone; in aging males, the causes are more likely to be secondary. Hypogonadism represents the only cause of male infertility that can successfully be treated with hormone therapy, although the response is largely dependent on the length of time of the hypogonadism. A complete discussion is beyond the scope of this chapter. Table 12.7 summarizes several causes of hypogonadism.

Signs and Symptoms

In the adult male, hypogonadism is manifested by changes in sexual function, behavior, muscle mass, and some loss of secondary sexual characteristics. The patient may report mood and behavioral symptoms (depression, irritability, loss of motivation) in addition to lethargy or loss of energy. Physical examination may demonstrate some regression of secondary sexual characteristics such as hair loss and possible loss of muscle bulk. There is no change to penis or prostate size.

Diagnostic Studies

Hypogonadism can be confirmed by checking a testosterone level; morning values (ideally between 800 and 1,000) are superior to afternoon blood

---

Table 12.7

Selected Causes of Hypogonadism

Primary Hypogonadism	Secondary Hypogonadism	Combined Hypogonadism
• Aging • Chemotherapy/irradiation • Cryptorchidism • Chromosome abnormalities (e.g., Klinefelter's syndrome) • Myotonic dystrophy • Orchitis (e.g., mumps) • Testicular loss from trauma, tumor	• Aging • Hemochromatosis • Hypertrophic hypogonadism Kallmann's syndrome • Medication-induced (e.g., antiestrogens for treatment of prostate cancer) • Obesity • Pituitary mass lesions • Prolactinoma • Psychological stress • Uremia	• Aging • Cirrhosis • Sickle cell disease

samples because testosterone is secreted in the morning. If the patient is not available for morning laboratory draws, at least three afternoon values at close to the same time of day can provide an average testosterone value. If the total testosterone is low, obtain a free testosterone level, the most accurate measurement of a significant deficiency. Additional hormones can also be evaluated (LH, FSH, estradiol, prolactin, thyroid profile) if secondary causes are suspected. An MRI is necessary if pituitary lesions are suspected. A semen analysis will show oligospermia or azoospermia in the patient with hypogonadism.

CONGENITAL HYPOGONADISM

The most common variant of congenital hypogonadism is Klinefelter's syndrome. See p. 358.

OBESITY

Obesity can lead to the aromatization of testosterone in fatty tissue to estradiol, leaving lowered amounts of testosterone available for maintenance and virilization functions.

Signs and Symptoms

The patient is a clinically obese male, with possible evidence of feminization or regression of secondary male sex characteristics found on physical examination.

Diagnostic Studies

Testosterone and free testosterone levels, along with estradiol, LH, and FSH levels, should be done. Routine referral to an endocrinologist or urologist, preferably one with expertise in male infertility (if this is an issue) and andrology, is recommended.

ANDROPAUSE

Andropause is a symptom complex in the presence of low levels of testosterone that can include a decline in libido and erectile function as well as irritability and loss of ability to concentrate. As males age, there is both decreased production of testosterone and decreased clearance beginning at age 40, but it is not analogous to menopause in women because men retain reproductive capacity, and not all men decline below the normal limits for serum testosterone. Many of the complaints that accompany the aging male have shown a weak correlation with plasma testosterone levels (Bhasin et al., 2006). There is much criticism related to labeling andropause as a disease that requires treatment rather than as a natural, age-related decline.

Signs and Symptoms

The patient may have a variety of complaints, including fatigue, truncal obesity, atrophic testes, loss of facial and pubic hair, and decreased muscle bulk. Additional complaints are similar to those for hypogonadism. Physical examination supports these complaints.

Diagnostic Studies

Testosterone and free testosterone will confirm lowered levels but should be drawn as early in the morning as possible. Androgen replacement is not without risk of reproductive malignancies; referral to a urologist or endocrinologist for management can be considered.

COMPLAINTS RELATED TO MALE
FERTILITY AND SEXUAL FUNCTION

■ Infertility

In 30% of all couples being evaluated for infertility, there is a clear, significant male factor alone involved; both male and female factors are present in approximately 20% of couples seeking an infertility evaluation (Sigman, Lipshultz, & Howards, 1997). Many of these male factors can be corrected, or improved, sufficiently that the couple can conceive naturally or can take advantage of less-expensive assisted reproductive technologies. An infertility evaluation is usually initiated after a 1-year history of unprotected intercourse that fails to achieve a pregnancy, although this length of time can be shortened as the female partner's age increases.

History

The patient may give a history of trying to achieve pregnancy for a lengthy period of time. It is vital to carefully detail the duration of the couple's infertility, previous pregnancies for either partner, the regularity of the female partner's menstrual cycle, the timing of intercourse in relation to ovulation, and the use of lubricants. Inquire about any established abnormal semen analysis that may have been ordered by the female partner's clinician. There may also be a history of male or female siblings (or members of extended family) who have had trouble conceiving. Several aspects of the male's medical history are particularly important: any specific childhood illnesses (e.g., mumps, orchitis), a history of cryptorchidism, the timing of puberty, and any GU or abdominal surgeries as an infant or child.

It is possible for a couple to present with a history of little difficulty achieving a first pregnancy and yet be unsuccessful in establishing a second pregnancy (secondary infertility).

Physical Examination

A complete physical examination may demonstrate that the male has failed to attain secondary male sex characteristics, lacks the vas deferens, or is obese. A careful GU examination is required. The physical examination may be completely normal. A semen analysis should be performed, with attention to sperm concentration, morphology, and motility.

VARICOCELE

See pp. 346–347.

HYPOGONADISM

See pp. 366–367. See also sections on cryptorchidism, testicular atrophy, and Klinefelter's disease.

CONGENITAL BILATERAL ABSENCE OF THE VAS DEFERENS

Congenital bilateral absence of the vas deferens is a genetic abnormality seen with cystic fibrosis (CF) and its variants. If not previously diagnosed with cystic fibrosis, the patient may present with a history of chronic bronchitis requiring hospitalization, recurrent respiratory infections as a child and adolescent, or asthma or an asthmalike condition. There are usually no other physical complaints. There may be a family history of infertility or persistent respiratory illnesses.

Male patients with CF frequently demonstrate malformation of the epididymis; the vas deferens, seminal vesicles, and ejaculatory ducts are atrophic or absent. However, spermatogenesis is usually normal. It is possible that the patient has a much more rare unilateral absence of the vas deferens.

Signs and Symptoms

Usually there are no signs and symptoms other than infertility if the patient has not been previously diagnosed with CF. Physical examination may show complete absence of the vas deferens unilaterally or bilaterally or a palpable gap in the vas deferens. Testes are usually of normal size and consistency, and the patient will demonstrate normal libido and age-appropriate secondary sexual characteristics.

Diagnostic Studies

Physical examination is usually sufficient to confirm the absence of the vas deferens. Testosterone levels will be normal. Because this is a genetic abnormality, referrals to a urologist with expertise in male infertility, a reproductive endocrinologist, and a medical genetics consultation to discuss genetic analysis of the couple should be encouraged, as establishing a pregnancy will require high-level assisted reproductive technologies.

EXOGENOUS TESTOSTERONE SUPPLEMENTATION OR ANABOLIC STEROID USE

Supplementation with testosterone or with testosterone-like substances can result in decreased endogenous testosterone and LH, hypogonadotropic hypogonadism, and suppressed spermatogenesis. Hypogonadism induced by exogenous steroid use is usually temporary, and endogenous hormone production and spermatogenesis rebounds after approximately 4 months.

Signs and Symptoms

The patient may complain of increased or decreased libido and possible erectile dysfunction. Patients using anabolic steroids may also have skeletal muscle hypertrophy, acne, gynecomastia, and striae. There may be some noticeable testicular atrophy on examination.

Diagnostic Studies

Semen analysis will show oligospermia or azoospermia, and total testosterone will be above the normal range (or supraphysiologic with anabolic use) . Levels of LH and FSH will be decreased. Routine referral to a urologist, preferably one with expertise in male infertility and andrology, is recommended.

■ Ejaculatory Dysfunction

In some cases of ejaculatory dysfunction, the cause is idiopathic and may be due to a failure of bladder neck closure. Men with diabetes can develop retrograde ejaculation. Neurologic disease, such as multiple sclerosis and spinal cord injury, can lead to retrograde ejaculation or anejaculation. Genitourinary infections can also contribute to ejaculatory dysfunction, commonly owing to obstruction of the vas deferens or ejaculatory ducts.

History

The patient may present with complaints of cloudy urine after ejaculation, hematospermia, possible recent-onset anejaculation, oligospermia or azoospermia with a low-volume ejaculate on semen analysis, and a history of retroperitoneal or bladder neck surgery or neurologic disease. There may also be complaints related to a decreased amount of ejaculate, a decreased volume of ejaculate, or the inability to ejaculate. It is possible that ejaculatory dysfunction will present during a male infertility evaluation.

Physical Examination

A routine GU examination, which is usually benign, is needed, as is a careful inspection of the abdomen to examine for surgical scars.

Selected Causes

Refer to Table 12.8.

Diagnostic Studies

Order a semen analysis—antegrade and retrograde semen analysis if retrograde ejaculation suspected. The evaluation of the semen sample will show a fructose-negative, acidic pH, azoospermic sample if obstructed. Routine referral to a urologist for further evaluation and treatment is necessary.

■ Painful Ejaculation

Male patients may occasionally complain that they experience pain with or following ejaculation. This can be distressing and, over time, may cause avoidance of sexual activity, which in turn can affect the quality of the relationship with the partner.

History

The patient will describe pain on ejaculation, usually of relatively recent onset. The pain may localize to a specific scrotal structure or radiate into the testes.

Table 12.8	

Selected Causes of Ejaculatory Dysfunction

Selected Causes	Example
Anatomic	Congenital bilateral absence of the vas deferens, obstruction of seminal vesicles, bladder neck abnormalities, retrograde ejaculation
Functional	Premature ejaculation
Medical	selective serotonin reuptake inhibitors, monoamine oxidase inhibitors, α-blockers, antipsychotics, benzodiazepines, alcohol, methadone
Neurologic	Diabetes mellitus, spinal cord injury, multiple sclerosis
Surgical	Bladder reconstructive surgery, retroperitoneal lymph node dissection, radical prostatectomy, transurethral resection of the prostate, cystoprostatectomy

There also may be decreased volume of ejaculate, hematospermia, or difficulty with bowel movements.

Physical Examination

The examination will include a careful inspection and palpation of the scrotal contents and a DRE.

EJACULATORY DUCT OBSTRUCTION

In this condition, one or both of the ducts leading from the seminal vesicles into the prostate become partially or completely blocked. This causes only prostatic fluids to contribute to the ejaculate volume, resulting in decreased volume, possible hematospermia, and possible azoospermia if both ducts are blocked. An increased risk of obstruction is associated with recent GU instrumentation or repeated urinary tract infections.

Signs and Symptoms

Testes are usually normally sized. If the obstruction is longstanding, there may be evidence of epididymal induration on physical examination. A DRE may demonstrate distended seminal vesicles, but this condition is often difficult to distinguish.

Diagnostic Studies

The ejaculate will be of low volume, acidic, and with no sperm, fructose, or coagulation factors on a semen analysis. Routine referral to a urologist is indicated, particularly if fertility is an issue.

EPIDIDYMITIS/ORCHITIS

See pp. 345 and 346.

PROSTATITIS

See Chapter 11, p. 320.

■ Hematospermia

Blood in the ejaculate, or hematospermia, like other changes to the ejaculate, can cause concern for the male patient. Although this is a relatively uncommon complaint, it does have some common causes.

History

If the patient or patient's partner complains of blood in the ejaculate, it may have been present intermittently for several months preceding the patient's presentation. The ejaculate will be pink, reddish (new blood), or brownish tinged (old blood). The presence of blood may be intermittent or occur with each ejaculate, there may be a history of recent GU instrumentation, or the patient may describe some sense of pressure with ejaculation.

Physical Examination

A routine GU examination is necessary, including DRE.

EJACULATORY DUCT OBSTRUCTION

See p. 371.

PROSTATITIS

See Chapter 11, p. 320.

BENIGN PROSTATIC HYPERPLASIA

See Chapter 11, p. 319.

RECENT GU PROCEDURE

It is possible to have several episodes of hematospermia after a prostate biopsy, resection of the prostate, incision, or other procedure that involves trauma to the prostate. In this case, the hematospermia will be transient and self-limited and is usually not associated with pain.

Signs and Symptoms

The patient will complain of blood in the ejaculate and provide history of prior procedure.

Diagnostic Studies

History of recent procedure involving the prostate will confirm the diagnosis.

REFERENCES

Ayta, I.A., McKinlay, J.B., & Krane, R.J. (1999). The likely worldwide increase in erectile dysfunction between 1995 and 2025 and some possible policy consequences. *BJU International, 84*(1), 50–56.

Bhasin, S., Cunningham, G.R., Hayes, F.J., Matsumoto, A.M., Snyder, P.J., Swerdloff, R.S., et al. (2006). Testosterone therapy in adult men with androgen deficiency syndromes: An Endocrine Society clinical practice guideline. *Journal of Clinical Endocrinology & Metabolism, 91*(6), 1995–2010.

Centers for Disease Control and Prevention. (2010). "Sexually Transmitted Diseases Treatment Guidelines 2006." www.cdc.gov/std/treatment/2010/default.htm (accessed March 16, 2011).

Greenfield, J.M., & Levine, L.A. (2005). Peyronie's disease: Etiology, epidemiology and medical treatment. *Urologic Clinics of North America, 32*, 469–478.

Kapur, V., & Schwarz, E.R. (2007). The relationship between erectile dysfunction and cardiovascular disease. Part I: Pathophysiology and mechanisms. *Reviews in Cardiovascular Medicine, 8*(4), 214–219.

Kostis, J.B., Jackson, G., Rosen, R., Barrett-Connor, E., Billups, K., Burnett, A.L., et al. (2005). Sexual dysfunction and cardiac risk (the Second Princeton Consensus Conference). *American Journal of Cardiology, 96*(2), 313–321.

Lewis, J.H. (2000). The role of the NP in the diagnosis and management of erectile dysfunction. Supplement to *Nurse Practitioner, 25*(6), 14–18.

Rowe, P.J., Comhaire, F.H., Hargreave, T.B., & Mahmoud, A.M.A. (2000). *WHO Manual for the Standardized Investigation, Diagnosis and Management of the Infertile Male.* Cambridge: Cambridge University Press.

Seftel, A.D., Miner, M.M., Kloner, R.A., & Althof, S.E. (2007). Office evaluation of male sexual dysfunction. *Urologic Clinics of North America, 34*(4), 463–482.

Sigman, M., Lipshultz, L.I., & Howards, S.S. (1997). Evaluation of the subfertile male. In Lipshultz, L.I., & Howards, S.S. (Eds.), *Infertility in the Male*, 3rd ed. St. Louis: Mosby.

Sullivan, M.E., Keoghane, S.R., & Miller, M.A.W. (2001). Vascular risk factors and erectile dysfunction. *BJU International, 87*, 838–845.

Chapter 13

FEMALE REPRODUCTIVE SYSTEM

Laurie Grubbs

Gynecological complaints account for more than 65,000 visits annually and more than 8% of the total yearly office visits (Center for Health Statistics, 2008). Endometrial cancer is the most common genital cancer in women and occurs most frequently between 55 and 65 years. For the year 2010, there are an estimated 43,470 new cases with more than 7,900 deaths (CDC, 2010). Ovarian cancer is the leading cause of death, with the highest incidence in postmenopausal women (CDC, 2010). Approximately 12,000 women develop cervical cancer annually with over 4,000 deaths (National Cancer Institute, 2010).

Anatomy and Physiology

Figures 13.1 and 13.2 show the major structures of the female reproductive system. Figure 13.3 depicts the menstrual cycle.

■ Reproductive Hormones

- Estrogen—a group of estrogenic hormones, termed the female hormones, produced by the ovary. Estrogens are responsible for the development of secondary sexual characteristics in the female and for cyclic changes in the vaginal epithelium and uterine endometrium.
- Progesterone—a steroid hormone secreted by the corpus luteum and placenta that is responsible for changes in the endometrium in the luteal phase of the menstrual cycle making implantation possible. It is used in combination with estrogen in oral contraceptives.
- Follicle-stimulating hormone (FSH)—a hormone produced by the anterior pituitary that stimulates the graafian follicles of the ovary for follicular maturation and secretion of estradiol.
- Luteinizing hormone (LH)—a hormone produced by the anterior pituitary that stimulates ovulation, which involves rupture of the mature ovarian follicle, transformation of the follicle into the corpus luteum, and secretion of progesterone and estrogen by the corpus luteum.
- Prolactin level (PRL)—a hormone produced by the pituitary gland that, in conjunction with estrogen and progesterone, stimulates breast development

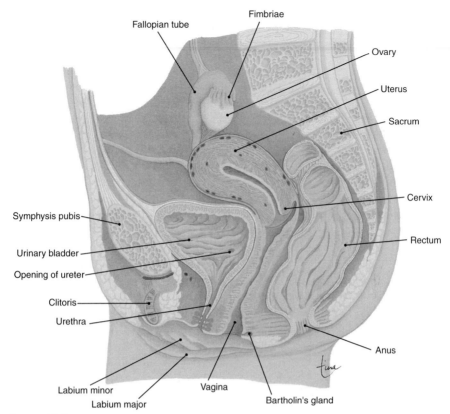

Figure 13.1 Internal female genitalia. (From Scanlon, V.C., and Sanders, T. *Essentials of Anatomy and Physiology*, 4th ed. Philadelphia: F.A. Davis, 2003, p. 441. Reprinted with permission.)

and lactation during pregnancy. In the postpartum period, sucking by the infant stimulates prolactin so milk continues to be produced. Elevations in prolactin in the female can cause amenorrhea, galactorrhea, and infertility, and in the male, impotence. These symptoms in a patient should alert the examiner to the possibility of a pituitary tumor.

- Estradiol—a steroid produced by the ovary that is a component of estrogen. It is found in large quantities in pregnant women. In the body, it is converted to estrone, another of the estrogenic hormones.
- Testosterone—an androgen and principal hormone produced by the testicle. Some testosterone is also produced by the adrenal cortex in both males and females. It is responsible for the development of secondary sexual characteristics and for sexual function in the male. It also accounts for the larger muscle mass in men compared with women and for distribution of fat in the male. It affects blood flow and other metabolic activities.
- Thyroid-stimulating hormone (TSH)—a hormone produced by the anterior pituitary that stimulates the thyroid gland to secrete thyroxine and triiodothyronine.

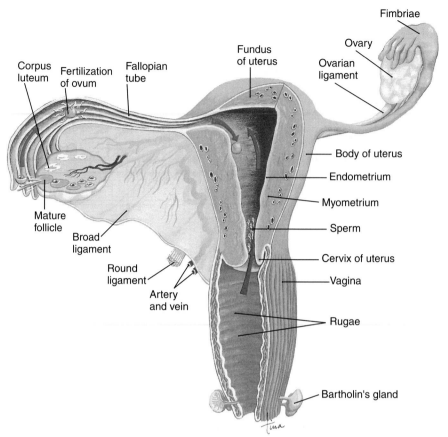

Figure 13.2 Internal structures of adnexa. (From Scanlon, V.C., and Sanders, T. *Essentials of Anatomy and Physiology*, 4th ed. Philadelphia: F.A. Davis, 2003, p. 442. Reprinted with permission.)

History

■ General Female Reproductive History

The gynecological history is complex, and complaints should not be treated lightly. Gynecological cancers may present with vague, nonspecific complaints, and an index of suspicion is necessary for early diagnosis and treatment. Last menstrual period is one of the most important questions to ask, particularly when prescribing medications, because many are contraindicated in pregnancy. If menstrual cycles are not regular, pregnancy should be ruled out first, and then other diagnoses can be considered. The menstrual history includes any episodes of amenorrhea, menorrhagia (excessive bleeding at the time of the menstrual cycle), metrorrhagia (bleeding at irregular noncyclic intervals), dysmenorrhea, and postmenopausal bleeding. Amenorrhea has many causes, including pregnancy; anorexia nervosa; excessive exercise; low body fat; and disorders or tumors of the

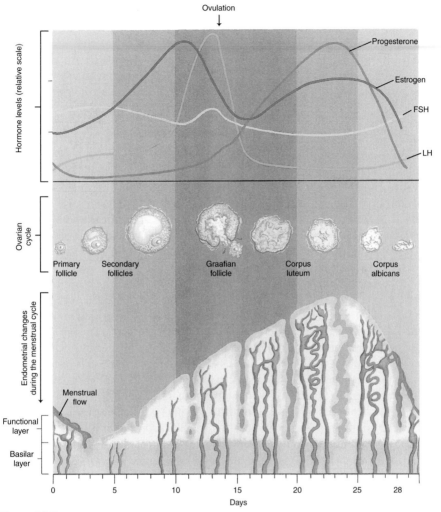

Figure 13.3 The menstrual cycle. (From Scanlon, V.C., and Sanders, T. *Essentials of Anatomy and Physiology*, 4th ed. Philadelphia: F.A. Davis, 2003, p. 447. Reprinted with permission.)

hypothalamus, pituitary gland, ovary, uterus, and thyroid gland. Menorrhagia is most commonly caused by uterine fibroids, but hematologic disorders should be considered. Metrorrhagia can be caused by anovulation, intrauterine devices (IUDs), and ovarian and uterine tumors. Primary dysmenorrhea is common and generally does not indicate pathology, particularly in the young population. It is most severe in the first few days of the menstrual cycle. Secondary amenorrhea can occur with fibroids, IUDs, cervical stenosis, and pelvic inflammatory disease (PID). The pain is more persistent with menstrual flow, and nausea, vomiting, or fever occasionally accompanies the pain. Bleeding that occurs after menopause has been established is cause for concern. It may indicate endometrial cancer, and referral for endometrial biopsy or D&C is warranted. If the patient is menopausal, ask about age of menopause, symptoms of menopause, and past or current use of hormone replacement therapy (HRT).

Ask the patient about the type of birth control being used, if any. If the patient is not in a monogamous relationship, ask about condom use. Be sure to inquire about the consistency with which the patient uses birth control methods. Often patients deny the use of birth control, deny the desire for pregnancy, and yet admit to being sexually active. This definitely indicates the need for health teaching and counseling.

Inquire about any masses or lesions that the patient may feel on the external genitalia, which could indicate infection, sexually transmitted disease (STD), vulvar malignancy, Bartholin's or Skene's gland infection/inflammation, uterine prolapse, cystocele, or rectocele.

If the patient complains about vaginal discharge, ask about the amount, color, consistency, odor, itching, burning, inflammation, lesions, and history of STDs.

Dyspareunia is one symptom that patients may be reluctant to mention or discuss, so specific inquiries should be made by the practitioner. Dyspareunia may accompany infections caused by inflammation of the vaginal mucosa, uterus, or pelvic structures; vaginal dryness or atrophy usually seen in post-menopausal women; fibroids; endometriosis; sexual difficulties; or psychosomatic illnesses.

Infertility may be caused by anovulation, decreased function of the corpus luteum, or blocked or scarred fallopian tubes. Any of these can occur despite that the patient may be having menstrual cycles. A history of menstrual irregularities may suggest anovulation or thyroid disease, either of which can cause infertility. A history of STDs could lead to scarring of the tubes. If the patient has not already done so, ask her to chart her menstrual cycles and basal body temperatures for 3 months to determine if and when ovulation is occurring.

■ Past Medical History

Past medical history includes age at menarche, menstrual irregularities, gynecological surgeries or procedures, history of ovarian cysts or uterine fibroids, endometriosis, infertility, STDs, and chronic diseases that might impact hormonal or menstrual function—the most common one being thyroid disease. Ask the patient about past or present use of medications such as oral contraceptives, HRT, fertility drugs, or thyroid medicine. An obstetrical history should include pregnancies, live births, miscarriages, and abortions.

■ Family History

Family history includes gynecological malignancies in the patient's mother or female siblings or the use of diethylstilbestrol (DES) by the patient's mother during pregnancy. Before the 1970s, DES was widely used in pregnant women with threatened abortion. Subsequently, it was found to cause abnormalities and malignancies of the reproductive tract in the children of those mothers. Its use was banned in the United States in 1971 and in Europe in 1978.

■ Habits

The matter of sexual activity and sexual partners is one of the more important areas to inquire about, especially with the high risk of HIV and other STDs. Multiple sexual partners, even in the absence of STDs, puts women at risk for infection with human papilloma virus (HPV). Smoking may also contribute to the development of HPV infection. Exercise habits, if extremely rigorous or excessive, can contribute to menstrual irregularities. Stress, if significant and prolonged, can cause menstrual irregularities. The use of drugs or alcohol may put women at risk for promiscuous behavior, unsafe sexual practices, or even date rape.

Physical Examination

■ Order of the Examination

Patients are often uncomfortable with the gynecological examination, so it is important to spend a sufficient amount of time taking the history and establishing a rapport before beginning the examination. A thorough explanation of the examination both before and as you perform it will help allay the patient's fears. Be sure to have the patient empty her bladder before beginning. The examination should start with an abdominal examination, proceed to external genitalia examination, and end with the speculum and bimanual examination.

Inspection

Inspect the abdomen for signs of masses, visible pulsations, peristaltic waves, or swelling, which might indicate ascites. Inspect the lower extremities for edema, which can be attributed to many things, one of which is lymphedema secondary to a malignancy. Inspect the external genitalia for lesions, ulcerations, inflammation, warts, swelling, discharge, or nodules. Inspect the perineum and anal areas for fissures, hemorrhoids, inflammation, lesions, ulcers, warts, or nodules. Assess the support of the vaginal outlet by asking the patient to bear down while you look for bulging at the introitus, suggesting a cystocele, rectocele, or prolapsed uterus. Observe the Bartholin's and Skene's glands for inflammation or swelling.

Auscultation

Auscultate the abdomen before beginning the gynecological examination. Listen for bowel sounds and bruits. Note any abnormalities in the bowel sounds. Gynecological malignancies can cause abnormalities of bowel sounds owing to peritoneal inflammation, infection, ascites, or gastrointestinal obstruction.

Percussion

Percuss the abdomen, paying particular attention to the suprapubic area and the right and left lower quadrants. An enlarged uterus will percuss dull in the suprapubic region. Other masses or inflammation will cause dullness or rebound tenderness as a result of peritoneal irritation. Percuss for shifting dullness in the abdomen, indicating ascites, which may be the first sign of ovarian cancer.

Palpation

Palpate the abdomen for rebound tenderness, ascites, or masses. Palpate the inguinal lymph nodes for swelling or tenderness. STDs often cause inguinal lymphadenopathy with tenderness. Ovarian cancer that has metastasized to the lymph system will cause inflammation and swelling of the lymph nodes in the inguinal area.

Speculum Examination

In addition to Pap smear samples, the standard of practice generally includes cervical samples for gonorrhea and chlamydia, and these should be taken first. Next obtain the Pap smear samples from the endocervix, cervix, and vaginal pool. If the patient has had a hysterectomy, obtain samples from the vaginal cuff, and be sure to mark the cytology slip accordingly.

Observe the cervix for inflammation, lesions, growths, nodules, discharge, or bleeding. A parous cervix is more open and may show healed lacerations. The cervix of a pregnant woman is purplish in color. Cervical polyps are common and appear as pedunculated, teardrop growths from the cervical os.

Observe the vaginal walls for inflammation, discharge, color changes, or ulcers. Infection can cause discharge and redness of the vaginal walls. Menopause causes the vaginal walls to be pale and smooth as opposed to the normal pink and rugose. Varicose veins may be seen on the sides of the vaginal walls mostly in pregnant and obese women.

Bimanual Examination

The bimanual examination is performed to determine the position, size, shape, consistency, and mobility of the uterus and ovaries. It is also used to assess tenderness that might be associated with inflammation, infection, or cysts.

The uterus should be pear-shaped, smooth, mobile, nontender, and firm but not hard. Malignancies may occur causing the uterus to be hard and fixed. Fibroids present as firm, nodular growths. Ultrasound or a computerized tomographic (CT) scan is needed to determine whether the growths are benign fibroids or malignant growths. Tenderness with movement of the cervix and uterus occurs in PID, termed cervical motion tenderness.

Variations in the position of the uterus are not considered abnormal, but significant variations may be related to back pain, especially during menses or childbirth, and occasionally to infertility. Figure 13.4 shows the common uterine positions (normal, retroverted, retroflexed, anteverted, anteflexed). The uterus can be situated in the midline, posteriorly toward the sacrum, or anteriorly toward the abdominal wall, termed normal, retroverted, or anteverted respectively. The long axis of the uterus can also be bent over on itself either backward or forward, termed retroflexed or anteflexed. A digital rectal examination is useful for indirect palpation of the uterus. It is particularly helpful if the uterus is retroverted or retroflexed.

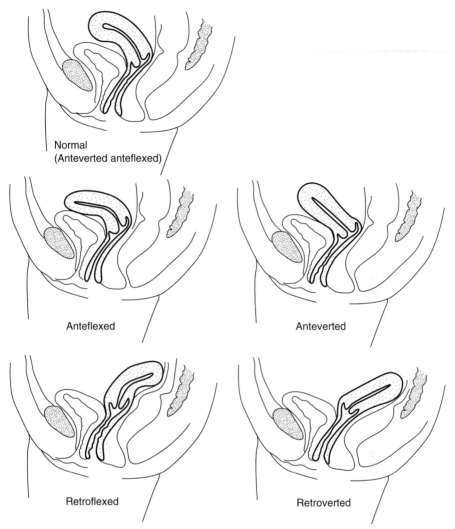

Figure 13.4 Common uterine positions. (From Swartz, M. *Textbook of Physical Diagnosis*, 3rd ed. Philadelphia: W.B. Saunders, 1998, p. 442. Reprinted with permission.)

The ovaries are small and almond-shaped, smooth, mobile, nontender, and firm. Ovaries are more difficult to palpate because of their small size and anatomical location. Ovaries are normally slightly tender on palpation. Ovarian cysts or inflammation cause a significant increase in tenderness that is easy to diagnose. Unilateral adnexal pain and tenderness in an early pregnant woman should alert you to the possibility of a tubal pregnancy, considered a surgical emergency. Malignancies may result in nodular, enlarged, hard, and fixed ovaries, but the cancer may have been present for some period of time before the physical examination signs are detected. Any masses or abnormalities on palpation of the uterus or ovaries warrant prompt ultrasound or CT.

Differential Diagnosis of Chief Complaints

■ Mass and/or Swelling at the Introitus

Vaginal infections or malignancies may lead to irritation and swelling of the external genitalia. Swelling and/or infection of a Bartholin's gland is common and presents as a very painful, inflamed, tender cyst on either side of the introitus. Nontender masses include uterine prolapse, cystocele, and rectocele. Occasionally, pregnant women develop painful varicose veins in the vagina that appear swollen and purplish in color. Inspection and palpation are most helpful in the diagnosis. Laboratory and diagnostics are usually not necessary for initial diagnosis. Referral to a surgeon or gynecologist is necessary for treatment in most cases.

History

A childbirth history is important in patients with this complaint because difficult or numerous childbirths may lead to problems with the pelvic support structures or damage to the bladder or rectal wall. Any change in elimination patterns is one of the most important questions to ask this group of patients. Ask about urinary incontinence or more frequent urinary tract infections. Uterine prolapse and cystocele can cause frequency, incontinence, and residual urine, increasing the risk for urinary tract infections. Ask about changes in bowel movements, such as constipation, difficulty with evacuation, and rectal fullness, which could be symptoms of a rectocele. Ask about recurrent infections in the Bartholin's gland, which are sometimes, but not always, related to STDs.

RED Flag ◄ **Red Flags for Examination of the Female Reproductive System**

- Significant unilateral adnexal pain in an early pregnant female
- Frank uterine bleeding in a pregnant female
- Frank uterine bleeding in a postpartum or postabortion patient for more than 7 days
- Fever or significant abdominal pain in a postpartum or postabortion patient
- Free fluid in the peritoneal cavity (ascites)
- Uterine bleeding in a postmenopausal patient
- A uterus or ovaries that are fixed, hard, or nodular on palpation

---

Physical Examination

A thorough pelvic examination including a speculum and bimanual examination are necessary. Assess for support of the vaginal outlet. It may be possible to visualize a mass or swelling in the vaginal area on inspection. If not, ask the patient to strain down while you insert your finger into the vaginal opening.

Feel for the mass to come to meet your finger when the patient bears down. Palpate superiorly, inferiorly, and on the sides over the Bartholin's glands for swelling and tenderness.

UTERINE PROLAPSE

Uterine prolapse is a downward placement of the uterus into the vaginal canal. It occurs more often in older, multiparous women as a result of injury, weakening, and stretching of the pelvic musculature and ligaments. Prolapse can be due to traumatic vaginal delivery, multiple births, chronic straining, pelvic tumors, and obesity. It may take years for the prolapse to develop, which partly explains why it is seen more often in older women. Prolapse of the uterus is often accompanied by cystocele and rectocele.

Signs and Symptoms

Early on, the patient may complain of a full feeling in the vaginal area or may be unaware that the uterus is prolapsed until it is discovered on physical examination. As the uterus prolapses further, the patient will feel a mass at the introitus or even protruding from the vagina. The patient may also have complaints of urinary frequency or incontinence owing to pressure on the bladder from the uterus. Kegel exercises and estrogen therapy, either oral or vaginal, can be used as prevention or treatment of mild prolapse. The use of a pessary will hold the uterus in place and lessen symptoms. Surgical intervention may be required, particularly when cystocele and rectocele are present.

Diagnostic Studies

The diagnosis is made by physical examination, although pelvic ultrasound may help to rule out other conditions. The degree of prolapse depends on the degree of weakness of pelvic support.

- In first-degree uterine prolapse, the uterus partially descends into the vagina.
- In second-degree uterine prolapse, the uterus descends into the introitus.
- In third-degree uterine prolapse, the uterus can be visualized outside of the vagina, and often the vagina becomes inverted.

CYSTOCELE

A cystocele occurs when a portion of the bladder herniates into the vagina. Similar to uterine prolapse, it is the result of weakness of the supporting muscles and ligaments, and cystocele often accompanies uterine prolapse.

Signs and Symptoms

Although a cystocele can contribute to urinary frequency, urgency, and infection, it is not the only cause of stress incontinence, and surgical repair of the cystocele may not resolve the incontinence. The bimanual examination reveals a smooth, soft bulge of the anterior vaginal wall that may be more pronounced with straining. Kegel exercises may be helpful, but surgical repair may be needed.

Diagnostic Studies

Pelvic ultrasound, CT scan, magnetic resonance imaging (MRI) of the abdomen and pelvis, and videocystourethrography are all useful tools for the diagnosis of cystocele.

RECTOCELE

A rectocele occurs when a portion of the connective tissue of the rectal wall herniates into the vagina. As in uterine prolapse and cystocele, rectocele occurs more often in multiparous women as they age. Breech deliveries and episiotomies also may contribute to the development of a rectocele.

Signs and Symptoms

Patients are often asymptomatic but may complain of difficulty defecating, constipation, incomplete evacuation, or a feeling of rectal fullness. Rectovaginal examination reveals a soft bulge in the posterior vaginal wall.

Diagnostic Studies

Along with the history, MRI and cystoproctography can aid in the diagnosis of rectocele. Tumors often give rise to symptoms similar to those of rectocele and must be ruled out. Surgical repair is indicated when it obstructs and impairs fecal evacuation.

BARTHOLIN'S CYSTS

The two Bartholin's glands are mucus-secreting glands located one in each lateral wall of the vagina at the introitus. They can become abscessed in acute or chronic inflammatory processes, usually as a result of STD infection or from other bacteria that are prevalent in the vaginal and perineal area but also by thickened mucus or congenital narrowing of the duct. In postmenopausal women, a malignant cause should be considered in the differential diagnosis.

Signs and Symptoms

Acutely, Bartholin's abscesses are extremely painful, in part due to their anatomical location, which makes sitting difficult. The area becomes swollen with the presence of a tender, inflamed, fluctuant cyst that is easily visualized. Systemic symptoms are usually absent. The cysts often become chronically inflamed, in which case surgery may be indicated. Occasionally, solid malignant tumors can occur in the Bartholin's glands and need prompt referral. Other considerations include vaginal wall cysts (Gartner's duct cysts), Skene's gland cysts, and urethral diverticulum, although the latter two are located superiorly to the Bartholin's gland. As previously mentioned, malignancy should always be considered in the postmenopausal woman.

Diagnostic Studies

The diagnosis is made by physical examination. A culture and sensitivity (C & S) of the fluid drained from the cyst will identify the causative organism so that proper antibiotic therapy can be instituted. If malignancy is suspected, prompt referral and biopsy are necessary.

■ Vaginal Discharge

Vaginal discharge is one of the more common complaints in both primary care and women's health. The history and physical examination are often sufficient to give a diagnosis, but in some cases, further laboratory testing may be necessary for a definitive diagnosis. If the history, physical examination, and vaginal smears or cultures lead to a diagnosis of an STD, further serology is indicated, and patient education is of utmost importance in treatment and future prevention. Where there's smoke, there's fire: When a patient presents with a complaint of vaginal discharge, several diagnoses should be considered, including yeast infection, trichomoniasis, chlamydia, gonorrhea, bacterial vaginosis, cervicitis, gynecological cancer, PID, and pregnancy.

History

The history includes the length of time the patient has had the discharge, the color and consistency of the discharge, presence of itching or odor, unusual bleeding, abdominal pain, or fever. Abdominal pain or fever suggests inflammation in the fallopian tubes and ovaries rather than just being confined to the vaginal area. It is imperative to obtain a menstrual and sexual history as well as method of birth control and history of STDs. Many health-care agencies require a pregnancy test on all patients presenting with a complaint of vaginal discharge to aid in diagnosis but also to be sure that prescribed medication is not contraindicated.

Physical Examination

A thorough gynecological examination is necessary, including a speculum examination to observe the discharge and presence of inflammation of the vaginal mucosa or cervix, a wet prep to examine the discharge microscopically, cervical cultures if necessary to rule out STDs, and a bimanual examination to rule out tenderness or enlargement of the uterus or ovaries. See Table 13.1 for differentiation of vaginal discharge.

MONILIA (CANDIDIASIS)

Monilia, otherwise known as yeast vaginitis, is one of the more common vaginal infections in young women and is caused by the fungus *Candida albicans*. It is not considered an STD, and transmission to or from sexual partners is unlikely. Since the advent of over-the-counter (OTC) preparations to treat yeast vaginitis, it is not seen in office practice as frequently. There should be a high index of suspicion in patients who complain of failure with OTC preparations because they have most likely misdiagnosed their problem or perhaps have more than one infection occurring. Patients who have documented recurrent yeast vaginitis should be screened for diabetes because this type of infection is common in the diabetic population. The high concentration of glucose in the blood offers a favorable medium for yeast to flourish. In addition, HIV is a concern

Table 13.1

Differentiation of Vaginal Discharge

Characteristic	Yeast	Trichomonas	Bacterial vaginosis	Chlamydia	Gonorrhea
Color	White	Grayish	White/yellow	Yellowish	Yellowish
Odor	Absent	Foul	Fishy	Absent	Absent
Consistency	Thick, curdy	Frothy	Creamy	Purulent	Purulent
Location	Adheres to vagina, walls	Pooled in vagina	Introitus, vagina	Introitus, vagina cervical os	Introitus, vagina, cervical os
Vulva	Erythematous and pruritic	Edematous	Normal	Normal	Normal
Vaginal	Erythematous	"Strawberry spots"	Normal	Normal	Normal mucosa
Cervix	No discharge	"Strawberry spots"	Normal	Purulent discharge	Purulent discharge
Wet Prep	Hyphae, yeast buds	Motile protozoa	Clue cells and whiff test	Numerous white cells	Numerous white cells

because yeast is more prevalent in immunocompromised individuals. Other causes include medications, particularly antibiotics but also oral contraceptives and corticosteroids.

Signs and Symptoms

The discharge associated with yeast vaginitis can be differentiated from other infections by symptomatology and wet prep examination. The discharge is very thick, curdlike, and adheres to the vaginal walls. Intense vulvar itching accompanies the discharge. Because the discharge is thick, patients often give a history of only itching and no discharge, since it adheres to the vaginal walls and may not be seen by the patient. In most cases, inflammation and swelling around the labia and introitus occur. This inflammation causes dyspareunia and burning of the labia with urination. Partners generally do not have any related complaints.

Diagnostic Studies

A high suspicion of yeast can be made on physical examination with a wet prep to confirm the diagnosis of *C. albicans*. A 10% KOH (potassium hydroxide) prep is most helpful for visualizing budding yeast and hyphae microscopically.

A saline prep should also be done in looking for alternative causes of the discharge. The presence of *C. albicans* may be reported on a Pap smear.

BACTERIAL VAGINOSIS

Although it is believed that the Gardnerella bacteria can be transmitted through sexual contact, it is not strictly considered an STD. A change in the vaginal pH to a value greater than 4.5 and a change in the bacterial flora with a decrease in lactobacilli gives rise to increases in aerobic and anaerobic bacteria. *Gardnerella vaginalis* is the most prevalent vaginal infection, although many women with this infection are asymptomatic. It is considered a risk factor for preterm labor, and pregnant women should always be treated aggressively. Also, women who are undergoing pelvic surgery are believed to benefit from treatment before surgery.

Signs and Symptoms

Of those women who are symptomatic, the overwhelming complaint is of a malodorous discharge. The odor of *G. vaginalis* is a distinct, fishy odor. The odor is usually noticeable during the pelvic examination, but a few drops of 10% KOH solution on the wet prep slide augments the odor. The discharge is fairly thick and white. Patients do not complain of itching, and the vaginal mucosa generally is not inflamed. Male partners do not complain of discharge, odor, or dysuria, although it is believed they may harbor the bacteria without being symptomatic. The higher pH of semen may be related to the higher vaginal pH that triggers the overgrowth of anaerobes and aerobes.

Diagnostic Studies

The diagnosis is made on symptomatology and wet prep. Microscopically, the wet prep shows the characteristic clue cells (epithelial cells embedded with bacteria), and the odor of *G. vaginalis* is unmistakable.

TRICHOMONAS

A sexually transmitted disease, *Trichomonas vaginalis* is a unicellular, flagellate protozoan. It is associated with an increased incidence in the transmission of HIV; therefore, women with trichomoniasis should be screened for other STDs, including HIV, gonorrhea, chlamydia, and syphilis. *T. vaginalis* has also been associated with perinatal complications.

Signs and Symptoms

The presenting complaints with trichomoniasis are discharge and itching. It can be differentiated from yeast by the discharge, which is thin and frothy rather than the thick, curdlike discharge of yeast. It can also be differentiated from *G. vaginalis* by the presence of vulvar itching and inflammation with trichomoniasis but no complaint of odor, as there is with *G. vaginalis*. Inflammation with petechiae of the vaginal walls, known as "strawberry spots," is diagnostic of *T. vaginalis*. Male partners are usually asymptomatic but harbor the organism, and they must be treated along with the patient; intercourse should be avoided or condoms used until treatment is completed.

Diagnostic Studies

T. vaginalis is easily seen on a wet prep in the majority of cases as a flagellate protozoan. If they are present, it is diagnostic. If protozoa are not seen on wet prep and trichomoniasis is suspected, a culture is recommended. Pap smears may also show the presence of *T. vaginalis* but are only 60% to 70% accurate for diagnosis.

CHLAMYDIA

Chlamydia is an STD caused by the bacteria *Chlamydia trachomatis*. It is thought to be the main cause of salpingitis and scarring of the fallopian tubes, leading to ectopic pregnancy or infertility. It can also cause conjunctivitis in the neonate if present during delivery.

Signs and Symptoms

Patients are often asymptomatic with chlamydia infections but may present with mucopurulent discharge, dysuria, abdominal pain, fever, and abnormal vaginal bleeding. Cervicitis and cervical motion tenderness on physical examination indicate PID. It is the causative organism in the majority of nongonococcal urethritis in both women and men and in most cases of cervicitis. Reiter's syndrome, a serious systemic complication of chlamydia infection that occurs more commonly in men, is characterized by urethritis, arthritis, and conjunctivitis or uveitis.

Diagnostic Studies

Chlamydia is often accompanied by gonorrhea; a Gynprobe cervical culture screens for both. A PCR (polymerase chain reaction) nucleic acid amplification is more sensitive than a cervical culture but is currently not routinely done except in cases of recurrent salpingitis or cervicitis with a negative culture. Because it is an STD, both the patient and partner should be screened and treated. Patients should abstain from intercourse during treatment, and repeat cultures should be performed at 3 weeks and 3 months.

GONORRHEA

Gonorrhea is an STD caused by *Neisseria gonorrhoeae* that can present in any degree ranging from asymptomatic to severe infection. Initially, symptoms are mild and usually begin within 7 to 21 days after exposure, although women may remain asymptomatic for weeks or months after infection. In addition to cervical or higher reproductive organ infection, *N. gonorrhoeae* can affect the urethra, rectum, and Skene's and Bartholin's glands. In spite of continued public education on STDs, the incidence of gonorrhea is increasing.

Signs and Symptoms

Patients may be asymptomatic or present with complaints of mucopurulent discharge, fever, abdominal pain, lymphadenopathy, and joint pain. Be suspicious of infection with *N. gonorrhoeae* in a young patient who complains of abrupt onset of polyarthritis. Clinically evident vaginal infection is only transitory, but infection with *N. gonorrhoeae* can persist, leading to salpingitis, abscess, and peritonitis. As with chlamydia, long-term complications include scarring of the fallopian tubes, ectopic pregnancy, and infertility. In addition, *N. gonorrhoeae* can cause conjunctivitis in the newborn in infected mothers.

Two more serious complications of gonorrhea are disseminated gonococcal infection (DGI) with bacteremia and gonococcal arthritis. In DGI, symptoms of genital infection may be absent. The patient presents instead with systemic complaints, such as fever, malaise, migratory polyarthralgias, and pustular skin lesions on the limbs. The bacteremia occasionally can lead to pericarditis, endocarditis, and meningitis; therefore, prompt diagnosis and treatment are necessary. Gonococcal arthritis presents with more severe and localized joint symptoms. The patient is usually febrile with severe joint pain, limited range of motion, redness, tenderness, and effusion of a few joints rather than disseminated as seen in DGI. Prompt treatment is required to avoid articular destruction.

Diagnostic Studies

A cervical culture, Gynprobe, is the standard diagnostic tool. It detects the presence of both *N. gonorrhoeae* and *C. trachomatis*. As with chlamydia, a PCR nucleic acid amplification can be performed and is more accurate but also more expensive and usually not necessary. A repeat culture for cure should be done in 2 to 3 months. If DGI is suspected, blood cultures or synovial fluid cultures should be drawn. In gonococcal arthritis, joint aspirate will show pus and the presence of gonococci.

PELVIC INFLAMMATORY DISEASE AND SALPINGITIS

PID is an infection of the uterus, fallopian tubes, and adjacent pelvic structures. It is often secondary to an STD or other infection of the lower reproductive tract that migrates upward into the uterus and tubes. *N. gonorrhea* and *C. trachomatis* are two of the commonly offending organisms. Pelvic infections can also occur postsurgery, postpartum, or postabortion but are generally caused from other organisms, such as staphylococcus or streptococcus.

Signs and Symptoms

Abdominal pain, mucopurulent cervical discharge, and often fever are the more common presenting symptoms. Rebound tenderness indicates peritoneal irritation. Dysuria, nausea, and vomiting may also be present. The abdominal pain is midline and often accompanied by right and left lower quadrant pain, particularly when accompanied by salpingitis. During the pelvic examination, there is pain with cervical motion and with palpation of the uterus and ovaries. Risk factors include a history of PID or STDs, multiple sexual partners, douching, and IUDs. Infertility may occur as a complication owing to scarring and occlusion of the fallopian tubes.

Diagnostic Studies

The diagnosis is based mostly on history and physical examination. A positive culture of the cervical discharge identifying a bacterial organism is helpful. An elevated white blood cell count will be present. Surgical emergencies, such as ectopic pregnancy or appendicitis, must be ruled out. Culdocentesis, endometrial biopsy, and laparoscopy can be performed if the diagnosis is unclear or to isolate the causative organism.

ATROPHIC VAGINITIS

Although atrophic vaginitis is not an infection and does not cause a discharge, its signs and symptoms can mimic the *C. albicans* yeast vaginitis. It occurs in postmenopausal women as a result of a lack of estrogen. It can occur with surgical or natural menopause and occasionally in lactating women.

Signs and Symptoms

The vaginal mucosa thins and becomes smooth and pale. The complaint most often heard from patients is itching owing to dryness and atrophy of the vaginal tissue. It is often mistaken for *C. albicans* by patients because of the pruritus, but the physical examination shows no similarity.

Diagnostic Studies

The diagnosis is made by pelvic examination. A vaginal scraping can be obtained and placed on a slide for cytological evaluation, and a maturation index can be ordered for confirmation.

■ Labial Lesions

The common causes of labial lesions include the herpes simplex virus (HSV); condyloma acuminatum; cancer of the vulva; syphilitic chancre; and, just inferior to the labia, a Bartholin's cyst. Although HSV is the most common cause of this complaint, it depends somewhat on the age and sexual history of the patient.

History

As with most gynecological complaints, a thorough sexual history is imperative. Include the number of partners, type of birth control, condom use, history of STDs, length of time in current relationship, perceived monogamy of the relationship, last Pap smear, and history of abnormal Pap smears. Ask the patient to describe the location and characteristics of the lesion and whether it is a single lesion or multiple lesions. Inquire about accompanying symptoms, such as pain, tenderness, burning, itching, excoriation, redness, swelling, or discharge. Herpetic lesions usually burn or itch in the prodromal stage and then become painful and tender, condyloma often itch but are not painful, syphilitic chancres are usually not tender, labial lesions are neither tender nor pruritic, and Bartholin's cysts present with severe discomfort and tenderness especially with sitting. The age of the patient can play a part in prioritizing differential diagnosis because labial cancer rarely occurs in women under 50 years of age.

Physical Examination

The physical examination includes a thorough visualization of the skin over the entire body to look for other lesions or skin changes, particularly in the anal area, mouth, palms of the hands, and soles of the feet. Labial lesions caused by STDs may also be present in the mouth or anus depending on sexual practices. Syphilis may manifest itself with pigmented or light-red macules or papules on the soles or palms.

Examine the abdomen for tenderness, and perform a lymph node examination, especially in the inguinal area. A thorough gynecological examination is necessary, including a speculum examination, wet prep, viral and/or bacterial cultures, and Pap smear. A scraping or biopsy of the lesion may be necessary if cancer is suspected. A blood sample for the Venereal Disease Research Laboratory (VDRL) is needed if syphilis is suspected.

HERPES SIMPLEX VIRUS

The majority of labial herpes infections are due to HSV2, and approximately 10% are due to the HSV1 that has been transferred to the labial area either by genital or oral contact. Although blood tests can be done to determine the presence or absence of antibodies to HSV1 and HSV2, it is mostly academic because the symptoms, transmission, and treatment are the same regardless of type.

Signs and Symptoms

Although antibodies to the herpes virus can be found in the majority of patients 3 weeks after exposure, the symptoms may be absent or mild enough to go unnoticed by the patient. Approximately 10% to 15% of persons who carry the virus are asymptomatic, but they can still shed the virus—they are referred to as "asymptomatic shedders." This, among other things, contributes to the spread of the herpes virus. The lesions begin with a slightly reddened area on the labia that is pruritic and tingling. There may be systemic symptoms, such as fever, headache, malaise, lymphadenopathy, and urinary frequency/dysuria. After a few days, a patchy lesion appears containing several small vesicles. The vesicles rupture, and a painful, tender, ulcerated area remains for 10 to 14 days. Lesions may be single or multiple. They may also occur on the cervix, perianal area, and mouth depending on contact area. Lesions can reoccur as frequently as once a month, often with menstruation, or as infrequently as once a year or longer. The virus may remain dormant for years until a stress or illness causes a recurrence. Treatment with antiviral medication can lessen and sometimes prevent recurrence.

Diagnostic Studies

A viral culture of the active lesion will yield positive results in the acute phase. Additionally, about 85% of patients will develop antibodies within 21 days of exposure, and a blood test will be positive for IgM antibodies. Type-specific assay tests are available to distinguish HSV1 from HSV2.

CONDYLOMA ACUMINATUM

Condyloma is one of the manifestations of the HPV, which is the most common STD. Approximately 30% to 60% of the American population has had HPV infection, and it is estimated that 50% of college women have the disease.

The peak age range for HPV is 20 to 24 years. It is diagnosed more often in women not necessarily because they have a greater incidence but because they are more likely to get regular checkups. There are over 70 types of HPV, 20 of which commonly affect the anogenital region. The virus is categorized by DNA pattern (genotype) rather than by host antibodies to the virus (serotype). Types 6 and 11 are most commonly associated with condyloma. There is an increased incidence of cervical cancer in women infected with HPV; types 16 and 18 present the highest risk for cervical neoplasias. Previous chlamydia infection was shown to be an independent and cofactor with HPV for cervical cancer risk. The incubation time is 1 to 6 months. It is highly contagious and can be transmitted through intercourse, oral/anal sex, and mother to infant. HPV can affect the respiratory tract of newborns, termed *respiratory papillomatosis*. Condyloma grow more rapidly in pregnancy; therefore, early treatment is recommended so healing can occur before delivery. However, the presence of lesions during delivery is not always a contraindication to a vaginal delivery. Those who are immunocompromised are also at greater risk for infection or proliferation of condyloma.

Signs and Symptoms

The incubation period for appearance of clinical disease is at least 3 months. Visible manifestations of HPV occur in less than a dozen genotypes, estimated at only 1% of those infected. Of those who develop condyloma, the presentation is variable. The patient may complain of itching in the area, or the condylomas may be only an incidental finding during a routine gynecological examination. Lesions are white with a rough, granular appearance with fingerlike projections often containing capillaries or a mosaic pattern. Condyloma may be single or multiple and can occur on the vagina, cervix, vulva, perineum, and perianal areas.

Diagnostic Studies

In women, diagnosing condyloma through physical examination can be a challenge. Lesions are often very small, even microscopic, and the rugae of the vaginal mucosa may mask the lesion. Applying white vinegar to a suspected lesion helps to distinguish it from normal tissue. Condyloma will turn white against the surrounding tissue when the vinegar is applied. Many of the small lesions can be seen only on colposcopy. Although there are many topical preparations for treatment, patients should be referred for colposcopy because of the microscopic condyloma that may be present. If dysplasia is seen on the Pap smear, biopsies should be taken to rule out intraepithelial neoplasia because more than 90% of the cervical neoplasias are caused by HPV. Unfortunately, barrier contraceptives offer only limited protection against the spread of HPV infection.

SYPHILIS

Syphilis is an STD caused by the spirochete *Treponema pallidum*. It is transmitted through intact or abraded mucous membranes and rapidly spreads to the lymph nodes and throughout the body. The incidence of syphilis has risen dramatically in the last 30 years with the increase in HIV and other STDs. In response, state and federal agencies put forth massive campaigns for prevention of all STDs and, in the last few years, have been able to show a decrease in newly reported cases of syphilis.

Signs and Symptoms

The primary chancre lesion occurs anywhere from 10 to 90 days after exposure. It appears as a firm, indurated, painless papule that erodes into an ulcer with raised or reddened borders. Chancres are usually single lesions and can occur on any mucous membrane or skin area. Nontender lymphadenopathy is present in the regional nodes. Genital lesions are most commonly seen in women on the external genitalia. Symptoms may be mild enough to go unnoticed, especially when they are in areas other than the genitalia, and they heal without treatment in 4 to 8 weeks.

If the primary infection is not treated, secondary syphilis develops and is characterized by more systemic symptoms, such as diffuse lymphadenopathy, malaise, fever, headache, anorexia, joint pain, and rash, which appears most commonly on the soles and palms but can also be present on the trunk. The rash can be macular, papular, or pustular, making the differential diagnosis variable. Erosion of the mucous membranes occurs, mostly in the mouth, forming grayish-white patches. Alopecia also may occur in patches. In secondary syphilis, anemia, jaundice, albuminuria, neck stiffness, and syphilitic meningitis may develop, causing cranial nerve lesions and deafness. If secondary syphilis is untreated, a latent stage develops. Approximately one-third go on to develop tertiary syphilis, although it may not manifest for many years. Tertiary syphilis affects the skin, bones, cardiovascular and neurological systems.

Diagnostic Studies

Serum for VDRL is the necessary laboratory test for diagnosis, and it will generally convert to positive 3 to 6 weeks after infection or 3 to 4 weeks after appearance of the primary lesion. False-positive serologic reactions are common, transient, and usually with a low titer. The fluorescent treponemal antibody absorption test (FTA-ABS) and the microhemagglutination assay for *T. pallidum* are more specific and assist in differentiating true from false positives. These tests remain positive regardless of treatment. *T. pallidum* can be detected by dark-field examination of specimens from skin and mucous membrane lesions, but serologic testing is more reliable. PCR is very specific for detecting *T. pallidum* in serum, spinal fluid, and amniotic fluid.

CANCER OF THE VULVA

Vulvar carcinoma accounts for less than 5% of gynecologic cancers. It occurs more commonly in women over 50 years of age. Over 90% of these cancers are squamous cell carcinomas; about 4% are basal cell; and the remaining are melanomas, Paget's disease, and Bartholin's adenocarcinoma.

Signs and Symptoms

The lesions of vulvar carcinoma are easily seen and palpated by the patient but are not recognized as serious and often do not bring the patient into the office for many months. They are often pruritic, white, macerated lesions initially on the vulva that may extend to the vagina, urethra, and anal area. They begin superficially but can become quite extensive in depth and breadth if left untreated. They may become infected, ulcerated, and necrotic.

Diagnostic Studies

Biopsy is the definitive diagnostic procedure, and for squamous cell carcinoma, radical vulvectomy with inguinal and femoral lymph node dissection is the definitive treatment. Patients should be followed closely for at least 5 years for early detection of recurrences. Prognosis depends on the depth of the lesion.

■ Abnormal Pap Smear

The Pap smear is designed to detect cancer cells in the cervix and vagina. It was developed in the 1940s, and since then, the incidence of cervical cancer has declined more than 70%. The technology for the interpretation of Pap smears has improved greatly over the years; computer-generated procedures are now being used. The recommendations vary some, but for most women, a Pap smear is recommended by age 18 or sooner if the woman is sexually active. Pap smears should be repeated every 1 to 3 years depending on the age and history of the patient.

History

Ask the patient about a history of abnormal Pap smears, cryosurgery, colposcopy, or cervical/endometrial biopsy. Ask about any history of STDs, especially HSV and HPV, both of which can cause an abnormal Pap smear. Ask about the use of DES by the patient's mother during pregnancy, since it can cause abnormalities and malignancies of the reproductive tract in the children of those mothers.

Physical Examination

While obtaining the Pap smear, a thorough gynecological examination should be performed and notations made of any cervical inflammation (cervicitis), discharge, STDs, or other reproductive abnormalities. It is important to continue Pap smears in postmenopausal women for cervical and endometrial cancer screening. Surprisingly, 25% of cervical cancers occur in women older than 65 years of age, and the peak incidence of endometrial cancer occurs in postmenopausal women between 50 and 60 years. In patients who have had hysterectomies, a smear of the vaginal cuff is still suggested as well as inspection of the vaginal mucosa and external genitalia looking for signs of malignancy.

Signs and Symptoms

Patients rarely exhibit symptoms of an abnormal Pap smear unless it is due to infection or inflammation, in which case vaginal discharge is commonly present.

Diagnostic Studies

Diagnosis is made solely through the Pap smear cytology report from the sample taken of the endocervix, cervix, and vaginal pool, or the vaginal cuff in the case of hysterectomy. The Bethesda system is the standard for reporting cervical cytology (Solomon et al, 2002). See Table 13.2 for an outline of the Bethesda System. If the Pap smear changes are due to infection or a reparative process, appropriate treatment should be instituted and the Pap smear repeated in 3 to 6 months. For other abnormalities, referral should be made to a specialist for colposcopy and/or biopsy.

■ Dysfunctional Uterine Bleeding

Abnormal uterine bleeding is much more common in the younger population, especially during the teen years when menstrual patterns are becoming established. Also, during the early reproductive years, malignancies are much less

---

Table 13.2

Bethesda System for Reporting Abnormal Pap Smears

Negative for Intraepithelial Lesion or Malignancy	Epithelial Cell Abnormalities	Other
Organisms	*Squamous cell*	
• Trichomonas • Fungal • Bacterial • Herpes simplex virus	• Atypical squamous cells of undetermined significance (ASCUS) • Low-grade intraepithelial lesion (LSIL); includes HPV/mild dysplasia/CIN 1 • High-grade intraepithelial lesion (HSIL); includes moderate to severe dysplasia, CIS/CIN 2 and CIN 3 • Squamous cell carcinoma	Other malignant neoplasms
Other Nonneoplastic Findings	*Glandular Cell*	
• Reactive cellular changes, such as inflammation, radiation, intrauterine device • Glandular cells S/P hysterectomy • Atrophy	• Atypical glandular cells of undetermined significance (AGCUS); includes endocervical, endometrial, glandular • Endocervical adenocarcinoma in situ • Adenocarcinoma, includes endocervical endometrial, extrauterine, NOS	
Other		
Endometrial cells in a woman 40 years or older		

likely to be the cause. Most cases of dysfunctional uterine bleeding are due to organic causes and to dysfunction of the hypothalamic-pituitary-ovarian axis. Bleeding after menopause has been established is cause for concern, and referral for endometrial biopsy is a must.

History

Start with the date of the last menstrual period and reconstruct as much of the menstrual history as possible, including age at menarche, menstrual patterns, and episodes of amenorrhea or abnormal bleeding in the past. Ask for a complete description of the current problem with abnormal bleeding. Important things to know include the time of onset; the pattern of bleeding (intermittent or constant); the amount and frequency of bleeding; the color of the blood (bright red or dark); and any history of trauma, vaginal discharge, recent STDs, abdominal pain, fever, or missed periods. Inquire about type of birth control and sexual activity. Determine whether there is a history of abnormal Pap smears. In postmenopausal women, ask about the use of unopposed estrogen replacement, which is a risk factor for endometrial cancer. Bleeding disorders can arise, so it is important to ask the patient about easy bruising or any recent gum or nosebleeds.

Physical Examination

Both an abdominal and a pelvic examination should be done to assess for masses or tenderness and the size, consistency, and mobility of the uterus and ovaries. During the pelvic examination, a Pap smear should be obtained to rule out cervical cancer. An endometrial biopsy might be needed to rule out endometrial cancer, especially in middle-aged and older women, but it is wise to wait for the results of the Pap smear before proceeding with a biopsy. A pelvic ultrasound or MRI should be considered to rule out pelvic mass. An hCG measurement should be performed to rule out pregnancy, and a complete blood count (CBC) and platelet count done to rule out hematologic causes.

ENDOMETRIAL CARCINOMA

Endometrial cancer can follow atypical hyperplasia or can arise de novo. It occurs twice as much in white as in black women. The peak incidence is between 60 and 70 years but has been reported in patients as young as 20 years old. Although it is the most common pelvic genital cancer in women, a complaint of dysfunctional uterine bleeding assists in early detection. Patients with hyperestrogenism due to either altered estrogen metabolism or the use of unopposed estrogen are at increased risk. Patients taking tamoxifen for breast cancer are also at increased risk.

Signs and Symptoms

Abnormal bleeding occurs in the majority of women with endometrial cancers. Spotting or bleeding of any kind in a postmenopausal woman is a red flag, and endometrial biopsy is warranted. A small number of women complain of lower abdominal pain or cramping. Physical examination is usually not helpful in the early stages but, in later stages, may reveal an enlarged, fixed uterus. It is necessary to refer the patient to a gynecological surgeon for hysterectomy.

Diagnostic Studies

A Pap smear should be part of the routine examination and may show abnormal cytology indicative of endometrial carcinoma. For definitive diagnosis and histological typing, an endometrial biopsy or D&C is necessary. The three histological types are adenocarcinoma (most common), adenocarcinoma with squamous differentiation, and adenosquamous carcinoma. Serum Ca-125, a tumor marker for ovarian cancer, is also elevated in endometrial cancer, with the more advanced stages more likely to have elevations. A complete metabolic profile, CBC, urinalysis, and chest x-ray should be performed at the time of diagnosis to identify or rule out metastases.

HORMONAL IMBALANCES

Irregular bleeding occurs more frequently early in menarche, before the body establishes a regular pattern, as well as during the perimenopausal period, when hormones are changing. Other causes of hormonal imbalances are discussed throughout this chapter.

ORAL CONTRACEPTIVES

If the progesterone component of the pill is not sufficient to maintain the lining of the uterus, metrorrhagia may occur in the luteal phase of the cycle. If a patient complains of spotting or bleeding during this time, a different pill with a stronger or different type of progesterone should be prescribed. If the bleeding continues, consider stopping the pill temporarily to determine whether that is the aggravating factor. There are enough choices of pills available to find one that most all patients can take without unwanted side effects.

FIBROIDS

Uterine leiomyomas, more commonly known as uterine fibroids, are benign growths consisting mostly of smooth muscle. The etiology is unknown, but their growth is hormone dependent; therefore, they are seen in approximately 25% of women during their reproductive years. They generally do not originate after menopause and, if present, will decrease in size after menopause. A tumor that arises in a postmenopausal woman should always have a high suspicion for malignancy rather than benign leiomyoma. Leiomyomas are more common in black women, occurring in as many as 50%. They can be single or multiple, usually measuring less than 15 cm. A very small percentage (0.1%–0.5%) may undergo malignant transformation to become a leiomyosarcoma requiring prompt surgical intervention.

Signs and Symptoms

Heavy menstrual bleeding (menorrhagia) and irregular bleeding (metrorrhagia) are the most common presenting symptoms, although a large percentage of patients are asymptomatic. Other symptoms include heaviness or fullness in the lower abdomen, pelvic pain, backache, dysmenorrhea, and urinary complaints. The pain can be severe if caused by torsion of a pedunculated fibroid. Fibroids are thought to contribute to infertility, spontaneous abortion, preterm labor, and problems with labor and delivery. Most leiomyomas can be palpated on bimanual examination, and some larger fibroids can be palpated through the abdomen. The uterus may feel enlarged, irregular, or nodular; pedunculated fibroids can be difficult to differentiate from other pelvic or abdominal masses. A retroverted uterus may obscure palpation.

Diagnostic Studies

A pregnancy test should be performed to rule that out as a cause of the symptoms. A CBC is needed in cases of heavy bleeding to determine whether anemia or platelet disorder is present. Pelvic ultrasound or MRI should be performed if symptoms of leiomyoma are present or for any palpable pelvic mass detected on physical examination. Imaging assists in differentiating ovarian cancer, leiomyosarcoma, endometrial cancer, or other neoplasms. An endometrial biopsy, D&C, laparoscopy, or laparotomy may be necessary to rule out malignancies.

VON WILLEBRAND DISEASE

Von Willebrand disease (VWD) is an inherited bleeding disorder. VWD is caused by a deficiency in or dysfunction of von Willebrand factor (VWF) and affects three to six million in the United States. VWF is further affected by factors such as race, blood type, inflammatory mediators, and hormonal status. While the condition affects both males and females and may be diagnosed at any age, it is often identified during evaluation of menstrual bleeding disorder. Bleeding can be life-threatening.

Signs and Symptoms

The severity of signs and symptoms is dependent on the severity of the condition. The patient often has experienced easy bruising, nosebleeds, and abnormal bleeding following dental procedures, surgeries, or other procedures, in addition to heavy or prolonged menses. If the patient has given birth, there is often a history of prolonged bleeding following delivery. There may be a positive family history of diagnosed bleeding disorder or of abnormal bleeding. Physical findings may not be present at the time of evaluation.

Diagnostic Studies

Complete blood count (CBC), partial thromboplastin time (PTT), prothrombin time (PT), and either a fibrinogen level of a thrombin time (TT) should be ordered to guide subsequent evaluation. These studies will not provide definitive diagnosis of VWD or rule the condition out. They will provide indication of a coagulation disorder. If VWD or another bleeding disorder is suspected, the patient should be referred to a hematologist.

ANOVULATION

The causes of chronic anovulation are numerous, with some resulting in dysfunctional uterine bleeding and some resulting in amenorrhea. The main categories for causes are as follows.

- Inappropriate feedback, including polycystic ovary syndrome; neoplasms that produce excess androgens, estrogens, or human chorionic gonadotropin; excess estrogen production associated with obesity or liver disease.
- Pituitary dysfunction related to tumors or hypopituitarism.
- Hypothalamic dysfunction associated with stress, exercise, malnutrition, or anorexia nervosa.
- Endocrine or metabolic dysfunction, including thyroid disease, adrenal hyperfunction as seen in Cushing's disease, and prolactin or growth hormone excess.

Signs and Symptoms

Anovulation may present with amenorrhea but also may present with dysfunctional uterine bleeding, polymenorrhea, or menorrhagia. The symptoms vary with the cause. Overweight may be seen with several of the causes, including hypothyroidism, polycystic ovary syndrome, and pituitary and adrenal dysfunction. Underweight is seen in anorexia nervosa, excessive exercise, hyperthyroidism, or stress-induced anovulation. Hirsutism, acne, and other skin changes can be seen with imbalances in LH, FSH, and androgens, as seen in polycystic ovary disease. Delayed puberty or regression of sexual characteristics is seen in hypopituitarism; galactorrhea can be the presenting symptom in pituitary tumors.

Diagnostic Studies

Appropriate laboratory and diagnostic testing depends on the history and physical examination and on the preliminary differential diagnosis. TSH, LH, FSH, estradiol, and testosterone levels will give information about sex and thyroid hormone levels and ovarian function. If polycystic ovary disease is suspected, a pelvic ultrasound is necessary, although it may be normal even with the disease. If pituitary or adrenal dysfunction is suspected, tests include glucose, cortisol, growth hormone, TSH, adrenocorticotropic hormone (ACTH), prolactin, LH, and FSH. Abnormalities in any of these studies may warrant MRI or CT scanning of the head.

PERIMENOPAUSE

Generally, there is no objective way to determine when the perimenopausal period begins, but from subjective data gathered from patients, menstrual changes begin to take place in the fourth decade of life.

Signs and Symptoms

FSH and LH remain normal, but patients who had regular menstrual cycles all of their lives begin to complain of more frequent periods with more dysmenorrhea or, conversely, missed periods. Patients may also begin to have sleep disturbances, decreased energy, increased weight, urinary frequency, and other complaints usually associated with menopause.

Diagnostic Studies

Pregnancy and pathology must be ruled out. The following laboratory studies and diagnostics are recommended: hCG; urinalysis; Pap smear with bimanual examination to rule out fibroids or a malignancy; CBC to rule out anemia, which can cause menorrhagia; and FSH and LH to ensure that the patient is not menopausal. A pelvic ultrasound is indicated if fibroids or malignancy is suspected. If the symptoms are established to be benign perimenopausal symptoms, then no treatment is really necessary because the symptoms are bothersome but not dangerous. However, they can be managed with low-strength birth control pills as long as there are no contraindications.

■ Amenorrhea

The four main causes of primary amenorrhea are disorders of the outflow tract, disorders of the ovary, disorders of the anterior pituitary, and disorders of the hypothalamus. Secondary amenorrhea can occur for many reasons: pregnancy, oral contraceptives, high prolactin due to a pituitary microadenoma, stress, rapid weight change, anorexia nervosa, menopause, vigorous exercise, hypothyroidism, chronic disease, and polycystic ovary disease.

History

It is necessary to determine whether the amenorrhea is primary or secondary. Primary amenorrhea is the absence of menarche by age 16. Secondary amenorrhea is the absence of menstruation for more than 3 months in a woman with past menses. If there is no past history of menses, consider the age and Tanner stage of the patient. Constitutional delay occurs in teenagers whose family has a history of late growth. These teens can experience late but normal sexual maturation. In the case of no menstrual cycle, consider also the disorders of the outflow tract and hypoestrogenic amenorrhea. If the patient has had menstrual cycles in the past, inquire as to age of onset, duration, amount of flow, regularity, and date of last menstrual period. Irregular menses is very common in adolescents and does not necessarily indicate pathology. Ask the patient about lifestyle, exercise and eating habits, and weight gain or loss that might indicate thyroid disease, polycystic ovary disease, or an eating disorder. It is necessary to know about prescription or OTC medication; use of oral contraceptives; birth control method, if any; and sexual activity that might indicate pregnancy or oral contraceptive–induced amenorrhea. Major stresses or life-changing events and/or chronic illness that can cause physical and emotional stress have been shown to cause amenorrhea. Ask the patient about the presence of galactorrhea, indicating the possibility of a pituitary tumor.

Physical Examination

A height and weight are a good start and give you an idea about several possible explanations for the amenorrhea. Short stature, obesity, or underweight are associated with both primary and secondary causes of amenorrhea. Inspect for webbing of the hands and neck that accompany the short stature of Turner's syndrome. Assess the skin for dryness and the hair for signs of dryness, thinning, or brittleness indicating hypothyroidism or altered nutritional state. Inspect the patient for hirsutism, which can occur in pituitary and hormonal abnormalities. The gynecological examination includes inspection for patency of the introitus and cervix; inspection of the vaginal mucosa for dryness or atrophy, which accompanies a lack of estrogen; a bimanual examination to determine uterine size, which can be enlarged in pregnancy or tumors; and palpation of the ovaries for cysts.

Diagnostic testing is necessary in most cases because a cessation of menses may be the only symptom, and physical examination findings may be absent. The initial step should be to rule out pregnancy with a urine or serum hCG analysis. If negative, a TSH and prolactin level should be drawn to rule out thyroid disease or pituitary tumor. A decreased TSH, indicating hyperthyroidism, can result in hypomenorrhea or amenorrhea. Hyperprolactinemia can lead to lower FSH and LH levels and hypogonadism. If the prolactin is normal and galactorrhea is absent, a pituitary tumor can be ruled out; likewise, a normal TSH rules out thyroid disease. Before ordering other expensive or extensive laboratory studies, a progesterone challenge should be given. If the patient experiences menstrual bleeding after 7 days of oral progesterone, it can be assumed that the endometrium is sufficiently prepared by endogenous estrogen and that there is at least minimal function of the ovary, pituitary, and central nervous system. This rules out primary ovarian failure and tells you that the patient has circulating estrogen. In this case, the patient is likely not ovulating and therefore is not getting the postovulatory rise in progesterone needed for menses. Polycystic ovary disease is the most common cause of anovulation, and an increase in LH, estrogen, and androgen levels along with a decreased FSH can help to confirm this. Although in polycystic ovary syndrome (PCOS) the ovaries are not always enlarged or cystic, a pelvic ultrasound may assist in the diagnosis. Adrenal dysfunction plays a part in ovarian and menstrual function, although in the case of adrenal dysfunction, menstrual irregularities are only one of many other more serious symptoms related to the action of adrenocortical hormones.

If bleeding does not occur with the progesterone challenge, estrogen should be added to the progesterone challenge to differentiate a disorder of the outflow tract from hypoestrogenic amenorrhea. An ultrasound will also assist in the diagnosis of an outflow tract disorder. In the case of no menses with the combination estrogen and progesterone challenge, an FSH and LH test as well as an MRI of the sella turcica are needed to determine gonadal failure versus hypothalamic amenorrhea caused by pituitary adenoma or other hypothalamic/pituitary abnormalities.

Figure 13.5 provides a flowchart for the evaluation of amenorrhea.

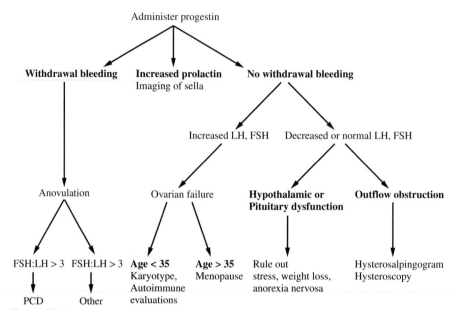

Figure 13.5 Evaluation of amenorrhea. (From Kiningham, R.B., Apgar, B.S., & Schwenk, T.L. Evaluation of amenorrhea. *American Family Physician, 53*(4), 1185–1194, 1996. Reprinted with permission.)

POLYCYSTIC OVARY SYNDROME

Formerly called Stein-Leventhal syndrome, PCOS is a hypothalamic-pituitary-ovarian axis disorder resulting in high levels of LH; low levels of FSH; a high, nonfluctuating level of estrogen; and an overproduction of androgens. It occurs in 5% to 10% of the female population.

Signs and Symptoms

PCOS is characterized by anovulation, amenorrhea, and hirsutism, although some women with PCOS have menorrhagia or dysfunctional uterine bleeding rather than amenorrhea. It also has been associated with infertility, insulin resistance, truncal obesity, and dyslipidemia. Enlarged ovaries are usually present but are not required for diagnosis. Other physical findings associated with PCOS include acne, alopecia, and acanthosis nigricans.

Diagnostic Studies

No one test can give a definitive diagnosis of PCOS: several tests assist in the diagnosis. Elevated androgen values (free testosterone, dehydroepiandrosterone sulfate [DHEAS], total testosterone) are seen in many women, most commonly free testosterone. If elevated androgen levels are present, adrenal tumors need to be ruled out. Elevated levels of LH and an elevated LH-to-FSH ratio may be present, although results vary widely depending on the timing of the laboratory testing. Prolactin and TSH levels are normal but assist in ruling out pituitary tumors or thyroid disease as a cause of the amenorrhea. Cushing's disease should be ruled out because PCOS has many similar signs and symptoms. Ultrasound of the ovaries may assist in the diagnosis, but many women who have cystic ovaries do not have PCOS. If PCOS is suspected, a glucose tolerance test, insulin levels, and a lipid profile should be done to monitor other health problems associated with PCOS. Management includes hormone therapy, insulin-sensitizing drugs, and weight loss. Weight loss will help to prevent diabetes, dyslipidemia, and cardiovascular disease and will also reduce circulating testosterone.

MENOPAUSE

Menopause is the absence of menses for at least 6 months. See Box 13.1 for physiological changes that occur with menopause.

Signs and Symptoms

In addition to inquiring about the typical menopausal symptoms, ask the patient about recent major life changes, as stress has been shown to affect menstrual regularity. Age of menopause varies greatly, although age 50 to 55 is the typical range of onset.

Diagnostic Studies

Although the absence of menses in a woman around the age of 50 years is diagnostic for menopause, measurement of FSH, LH, and estradiol levels are helpful in confirming the diagnosis. In menopause, first FSH and then LH rises, both greater than 100 mU/mL. A fall in estradiol is the last hormonal change that occurs with the decline of ovarian function. An estradiol level of less than 30 pg/mL indicates loss of ovarian function.

■ Dysmenorrhea

Dysmenorrhea is the most common gynecological complaint, particularly in the adolescent and young adult population. Primary dysmenorrhea is due to a rise in prostaglandins that occurs at the onset of menses, and it has been found that

---

Box 13.1

Physiological Changes With Menopause

- Hot flashes, fatigue, insomnia, urinary frequency and incontinence, nervousness, decreased libido, and depression
- Increased bone resorption, especially in the first 5 years of menopause leading to osteopenia and osteoporosis
- Increased incidence of atherosclerosis
- Vaginal and urethral dryness and decreased integrity
- Decreased skin turgor

prostaglandins are higher in women with dysmenorrhea. Recently, increased leukotriene levels have been found to contribute to dysmenorrhea. Other psychosocial variables may contribute, such as response to pain, anxiety, stress, and attitudes about menstruation.

Secondary dysmenorrhea is most often caused by endometriosis. Other causes include chronic PID, adhesions, IUDs, cervical stenosis, and uterine fibroids.

History

Take a menstrual history including age at menarche, menstrual patterns, and the qualitative and quantitative factors of the dysmenorrhea. Important things to know include the time of onset in the menstrual cycle, pattern (intermittent or constant), regularity of the cycles, severity and duration of the pain, amount of lost work or school time, and medications taken for relief. Also ask about any history of trauma, vaginal discharge, recent STDs, fever, history of endometriosis, infertility, or missed periods. Inquire about the type of birth control and sexual activity. Determine whether there is a history of abnormal Pap smears.

Physical Examination

Both an abdominal and a pelvic examination should be done to assess for masses or tenderness. During the pelvic examination, a Pap smear should be obtained along with cultures for chlamydia and gonorrhea. Assess for size, consistency, mobility, and tenderness of the uterus and ovaries.

PRIMARY DYSMENORRHEA

Primary dysmenorrhea is often used to describe menstrual cramping, but strictly speaking, the term should be used only to describe pain with menses that interferes with normal daily living and requires pain medicine, either narcotic or nonnarcotic.

Signs and Symptoms

The pain is in the pelvic area and begins with the onset of menses or shortly thereafter. The pain can be so severe as to be accompanied by nausea, vomiting, and diarrhea. It is short in duration, usually lasting only the first day or two of the menstrual cycle. If pain worsens over time or occurs between cycles, secondary causes should be suspected.

Diagnostic Studies

In primary dysmenorrhea, diagnosis is by history because menstrual pain is a subjective complaint and cannot be measured objectively. However, if a secondary cause is suspected, an examination should be done to inspect for vaginal discharge that might indicate infection, and cervical cultures are needed to test for gonorrhea and chlamydia. A bimanual examination should be done to palpate for tenderness that might indicate infection or fibroids. Laboratory tests and diagnostics to consider include a serum hCG for pregnancy, a pelvic ultrasound to rule out fibroids or endometriosis, an endometrial biopsy, and possibly laparoscopy if endometriosis is suspected in order to determine the extent of disease. Oral contraceptives will diminish the severity of the dysmenorrhea along with NSAIDs or other pain medication.

ENDOMETRIOSIS

Endometriosis is characterized by a proliferation of endometrial tissue in sites other than the lining of the uterus. It typically grows on the outside of the uterus, tubes and ovaries, broad ligament, uterosacral ligaments, large and small bowel, bladder, ureters, vagina, and cul-de-sac. It is almost exclusively found in premenopausal women and is estimated to cause as much as 50% of infertility in women. Several theories exist, but the exact cause is unknown. Theories include retrograde menstruation with transport of endometrial cells, lymphatic transport of endometrial cells, metaplasia of coelomic epithelium, or immune response resulting in endometrial hyperplasia. In addition, there seems to be a genetic predisposition, with a 6% to 10% increase in patients with first-degree relatives who have endometriosis.

Signs and Symptoms

The main symptom of endometriosis is dysmenorrhea, which sometimes makes it difficult to differentiate from primary dysmenorrhea. Other presenting symptoms include dyspareunia, infertility, and constant pelvic and low back pain that occurs before menses. Adhesions may cause chronic pelvic pain unrelated to menstrual cycle. The physical examination may reveal a fixed uterus as a result of adhesions, causing pain on uterine movement; nodules on the posterior vaginal fornix; and tenderness in the adnexal area. In many patients, the physical examination is unremarkable.

Diagnostic Studies

The history and physical examination generally lead you to suspect endometriosis, but the definitive diagnosis is made through laparoscopic surgery and biopsy. The lesions seen in endometriosis, termed *endometrial implants*, appear as dark red to dark brown lesions that give the appearance of a powder burn from a gunshot. They appear on the peritoneal, bladder, uterine, and ovarian surfaces. Over time they become thickened and produce scar tissue. Ultrasound may give information about the extent of the disease but should not be used as the sole diagnostic tool. Various hormonal treatments are helpful, as are laparoscopic ablation of extrauterine endometrial tissue and lysing of adhesions with the goal of restoring pelvic anatomy.

UTERINE FIBROIDS

Along with dysfunctional uterine bleeding, leiomyomas can cause dysmenorrhea, which is often one of the presenting complaints. See the section on fibroids under dysfunctional uterine bleeding, pp. 397–398.

■ Ovarian Cancer

Although patients do not come in with a chief complaint of ovarian cancer, the symptoms and physical findings are usually vague or nonexistent, making it a differential diagnosis or a diagnosis of suspicion rather than one based on history or physical examination. Ovarian cancer has the highest mortality of the gynecological malignancies because as much as 85% of cases have metastases outside the ovaries at the time of diagnosis, and the cancer is usually widespread before the patient has signs or symptoms. It occurs most often in postmenopausal women and in women with a positive family history.

History

The history should include both abdominal and gynecological complaints, as many patients with ovarian cancer present with vague gastrointestinal complaints. A menstrual history is necessary because some of the patients have dysfunctional uterine bleeding. A positive family history of ovarian cancer is a red flag, as is a patient history of other gynecological or breast malignancies.

Physical Examination

In the premenopausal female, 95% of ovarian masses are small (less than 8 cm), cystic, and benign, although ovarian malignancies do occur in this population. In the postmenopausal female, there should be a high index of suspicion for ovarian cancer. Early symptoms are vague and include mild lower abdominal discomfort, feelings of fullness, bloating, distention, nausea, dyspepsia, constipation, and urinary frequency if the tumor is large. Abnormal uterine bleeding is uncommon. Pelvic pain, anemia, ascites, and cachexia are seen in late disease.

The characteristics typical of a malignant ovarian mass include solid, fixed, nodular, nontender, and bilateral. The abdominal examination is essential, looking for distention, changes in percussion, or ascites. As the cancer metastasizes, lymphadenopathy occurs, especially in the inguinal and supraclavicular areas. The cancer spreads by direct extension to the abdominal and pelvic peritoneum and through lymph nodes. Laboratory and other diagnostics are needed for a definitive diagnosis.

Pelvic examination has been shown to have a low sensitivity and specificity for ovarian cancer, with many tumors smaller than 10 cm being missed. Several diagnostic studies are useful for detecting ovarian cancer. The Ca-125 blood test by immunoassay is used as a tumor marker for treatment decisions but can also be used as a diagnostic tool. False-positive elevations do occur with endometriosis and pelvic surgeries; therefore, tests should be interpreted with caution and followed up with an ultrasound. Transvaginal ultrasound will show a solid, irregular mass that may be adhered to adjoining structures. A Pap smear may contain malignant cells. X-rays may show metastatic lung or bone lesions. Prognosis is poor, with a mean survival of 18 months. Surgery is necessary for staging and also as the mainstay of treatment, along with chemotherapy and possibly radiation.

OVARIAN CYSTS

Several factors differentiate ovarian cysts from ovarian cancer. The primary factor is that cysts are fluid-filled sacs, and cancer is a solid tumor. Ovarian cancer is much more prevalent in women over 50 years of age, although it can occur in younger women. Ovarian cysts are common in the younger population and tend to occur in the latter half of the menstrual cycle. Many spontaneously resolve. Others may need surgical intervention, if they become twisted, owing to the risk of gangrene.

Signs and Symptoms

Right or left lower quadrant pain is usually the presenting complaint. Pelvic examination reveals significant tenderness in the affected adnexal area. Rebound tenderness may be present. Follicular cysts are most common, and the pain typically occurs in the second half of the menstrual cycle. These cysts usually resolve with menses and require no further treatment. Other cysts—including corpus luteum cysts, inflammatory cysts occurring with tubo-ovarian abscess, and endometriotic cysts—may require surgical intervention.

Diagnostic Studies

Tubal pregnancy must be ruled out immediately with a urine and/or serum hCG. Transvaginal ultrasound will give the best information for differentiating a blood- or fluid-filled cyst from a solid mass.

HYDATIDIFORM MOLE AND CHORIOCARCINOMA

These solid tumors are part of a category of gestational trophoblastic neoplasias. In the United States, the incidence is 1 in 1,500 pregnancies. Risk factors include low socioeconomic status and age under 18 or over 40 years (Crombleholme, 2009).

Signs and Symptoms

Clinical signs are those of a missed abortion: uterine bleeding, nausea, vomiting, and enlarged and/or tender uterus and ovaries. Collapsed vesicles from the mole may pass through the vagina.

Diagnostic Studies

A quantitative hCG should be done because these values may differ from those of a normal pregnancy. Grapelike clusters within an enlarged uterus in the absence of a fetus and placenta are diagnostic for hydatidiform mole. In partial hydatidiform mole, pelvic ultrasound may show an embryo or gestational sac. These partial moles are slow growing but are more likely to become choriocarcinomas. A solid mass on ultrasound is suspicious for choriocarcinoma and requires biopsy for diagnosis.

UTERINE FIBROIDS

See Dysfunctional Uterine Bleeding, p. 395.

GASTROINTESTINAL, LIVER, AND PANCREATIC CANCERS

See Chapter 10, pp. 262, 290.

IRRITABLE BOWEL SYNDROME

See Chapter 10, p. 282.

■ Sexual Dysfunction

There are many causes of sexual dysfunction that may have a physical or psychological origin or a combination of both. Dysfunction generally stems from decreased desire, decreased arousal, orgasmic dysfunction, and physical discomfort.

History

A sexual history should be part of the gynecological review of systems, although it is often omitted as a result of examiner discomfort or a failure to view it as an integral part of the examination. If problems exist, the examiner should explore with the patient her relationships, life circumstances and changes, medical conditions, surgeries, sexual activity and behaviors, sexual development, and fertility issues.

Physical Examination

There are no special examinations to be done for sexual dysfunction, although hormonal assessment may be helpful. A thorough gynecological examination is adequate to determine whether there is a physical cause for the problem. If dyspareunia is part of the complaint, a pelvic ultrasound may assist in the diagnosis of structural pathology.

LOSS OF LIBIDO AND DECREASED SEXUAL RESPONSE

Decreases in libido and sexual response are not uncommon with aging, although it is an erroneous stereotype to assume that sexual desire or functioning automatically declines with age. Inhibited or decreased sexual desire has many causes, including aging, marital discord, drug or alcohol abuse, pregnancy, physical illness or discomfort, depression, history of sexual abuse, sexual phobias, and anxiety.

Signs and Symptoms

The diagnosis of inhibited sexual desire is primarily a subjective one based on patient history. If organic causes such as illness and physical discomfort are ruled out, a thorough psychological evaluation is recommended. As previously mentioned, desire and response may slow with aging, but a good history should be able to discern when a psychological evaluation is warranted. In the aging client, lubricating agents may be helpful to deal with decreased or uncomfortable stimulation due to loss of lubrication.

Diagnostic Studies

Although a thorough history is most helpful, serum for free testosterone will show an androgen deficiency, which has been blamed for decreased libido, particularly in the postmenopausal woman.

DYSPAREUNIA

The causes of dyspareunia are numerous and include vaginal infection or irritation, PID, endometriosis, pregnancy, atrophic vaginitis, decreased lubrication, episiotomy, labial lesions, Bartholin's cysts, adhesions from previous gynecological or abdominal surgeries, and psychological causes.

Signs and Symptoms

The age of the patient should be considered because decreased estrogen can cause atrophic vaginitis and thus decreased lubrication leading to dyspareunia. The history can give information about pregnancy or delivery difficulties, past surgeries, and the possibility of adhesions. The history should include a thorough sexual history to uncover any psychological issues. A pelvic examination should be done looking for vaginal discharge, inflammation, or lesions.

Diagnostic Studies

Structural abnormalities should be ruled out, and transvaginal ultrasound may be helpful. If vaginal discharge is present, wet prep and cultures should be obtained to rule out infection. Blood samples for hormonal testing may be necessary, particularly if mucosal atrophy is evident on physical examination.

VAGINISMUS

Vaginismus is a painful contraction of the lower vaginal and thigh adductor muscles that occurs unconsciously in a woman who does not desire penetration. It most often occurs in young women who have been molested, sexually abused, or raped, or it is secondary to gynecological trauma or medical procedures.

Signs and Symptoms

The physical or psychological causes can be uncovered during history and physical examination. A good history, inquiring specifically about sexual abuse, is necessary. Involuntary vaginal spasm can be observed during the pelvic examination, and the patient often exhibits avoidance behavior in response to the examiner and the pelvic examination.

Diagnostic Studies

Once structural and other physical causes have been eliminated, vaginismus can be treated with gradual dilation techniques. In many instances, psychotherapy is necessary.

■ Infertility

The workup for infertility is complex and must be referred to a gynecologist specializing in infertility. The causes are numerous but generally fall into the categories of anovulation, implantation failure, hormonal failure, chromosomal abnormalities, or low sperm count in the male partner. Preliminary tests that can be initiated by the nurse practitioner include the following.

- Pelvic examination to ensure that the cervix is open and that there are no uterine abnormalities.
- Basal body temperature charts to plot monthly ovulation and menstrual patterns.
- Laboratory testing including TSH, FSH, LH, and estradiol.
- Ultrasound—shows the position of the uterus, the presence of fibroids or other growths, and the thickening of the endometrium that may occur in endometriosis, all of which can affect fertility.
- Hysterosalpingography—radiography of the uterus and fallopian tubes to assess patency and the presence of any structural abnormalities.
- Sperm count for the male partner—this is one of the first things that should be done in an infertility workup.

REFERENCES

Center for Disease Control and Prevention (2010). *Cancer topics: Ovarian Cancer* http://www.cdc.gov/cancer/ovarian/index.htm (accessed March 17, 2011).

Center for Health Statistics. (2008). Centers for Disease Control and Prevention: Gynecologic Cancers. http://www.cdc.gov/cancer/gynecologic/basic_info/ (accessed March 17, 2011).

Crombleholme, W.R. (2009). Obstetrics. In McPhee, S.J., & Papadakis, M.A. (Eds.), *CURRENT: Medical Diagnosis & Treatment 2008*, 48th ed. Stamford, CT: Appleton & Lange Medical Books.

Holschneider, C.H. (2006). Premalignant and malignant disorders of the uterine cervix. In DeCherney, A.H., Nathan, L., & Goodwin, T.M. (Eds.), *CURRENT: Obstetric and Gynecological Diagnosis & Treatment*, 10th ed. New York: Appleton & Lange Medical Books.

Kiningham, R.B., Apgar, B.S., & Schwenk, T.L. (1996). Evaluation of amenorrhea. *American Family Physician, 53*(4), 1185–1194.

National Cancer Institute. (2010). *Cancer topics: Endometrial cancer.* Available at: http://www.cancer.gov/cancertopics/types/endometrial (accessed March 17, 2011).

National Cancer Institute. (2010). *Cancer topics: Cervical cancer.* Available at: http://www.cancer.gov/cancertopics/types/cervical (accessed March 17, 2011).

Solomon, D., Davey, D., Kurman, R., Moriarty, A., O'Connor, D., Prey, M., et al. (2002). The 2001 Bethesda System: Terminology for reporting results of cervical cytology. *Journal of the American Medical Association, 287*(16), 2114–2119.

United States Cancer Statistics: 1999–2006 Incidence and Mortality Web-based Report. (2010). Atlanta, GA: Department of Health and Human Services, Centers for Disease Control and Prevention, and National Cancer Institute. Available at: www.cdc.gov/cancer/cervical/index.htm

Chapter 14

MUSCULOSKELETAL SYSTEM

Mary Jo Goolsby

The bones and muscles provide the infrastructure for the stability and movement of the body. Individual abilities and limitations in strength, movement, ease, and grace are defined by the abilities of this system to respond to stimuli. Limitations are a result of disease, injury, metabolic disorders, and lack of conditioning, which can lead to temporary or permanent disability. Complaints related to the musculoskeletal system are common across the lifespan. The types of problems vary among age groups.

Over 100 rheumatologic problems can cause musculoskeletal pain, swelling, and/or stiffness. There are over 33 million persons in the United States with arthritis; the majority are women. In fact, arthritis is the leading cause of disability in the United States. Even though the incidence of several of the chronic joint disorders increases with age, approximately two-thirds of patients with arthritis are under 65 years old.

As with all systems in the body, the musculoskeletal system is closely linked with other systems. The neurological and circulatory systems and the skin are most often associated with problems that also affect the musculoskeletal system. Problems affecting one system often produce associated problems in others. Problems with the musculoskeletal system most often relate to the joints, but the examination must also include the bone and associated muscles and joints to obtain a complete picture of the problem.

Assessment of Musculoskeletal Complaints

Patients who have musculoskeletal problems usually present with pain, deformity, or weakness. Joint pain, in general, is the most common problem, and backache, specifically, is the most common disorder for which patients seek health care. The examination is often centered on the joints where the pain is focused, but frequently muscles and nerves are also a focal point of the examination. Conditions associated with joint pain can be categorized into four major groups: mechanical problems, soft tissue conditions, inflammatory diseases, and noninflammatory diseases. Conditions frequently associated with joint pain include osteoarthritis, tendonitis, infection, gout/pseudogout, and rheumatoid arthritis. A number of presentations are indications of urgent problems, requiring immediate recognition and definitive treatment. It is essential that the history and physical be directed to identify any of the symptoms or signs noted in the Red Flag box.

RED Flag ◀ **Red Flags in the Assessment of the Musculoskeletal System**

- History of major trauma
- Hot and/or swollen joint(s)
- Systemic/constitutional symptoms
- Focal or diffuse weakness
- Neurogenic pain
- Claudication
- Unrelenting nighttime pain
- Poorly localized pain

History

■ General Musculoskeletal History

It is important to complete a thorough symptom analysis for any musculoskeletal complaint. When a musculoskeletal disorder is suspected, the review of that system should include a history of associated pain, discomfort, swelling, redness, stiffness, crepitus, limitation, and weakness. The onset and progression of symptoms are important to help differentiate among traumatic or acute problems and chronic conditions. The musculoskeletal history should be appropriate to the patient's age because many problems occur among certain age groups more often than others.

■ Past Medical History

Identify any history of musculoskeletal disorders, and procedures. The history of both remote and recent trauma and/or other injuries, and how they occurred, should be determined. Disorders to ask about include recent infections, which could explain symptoms such as polyarthritis, monoarthritis, or generalized aches, as well as the history of rheumatoid arthritis, osteoarthritis, osteoporosis, gout, or other musculoskeletal problems. The treatment and response related to any identified musculoskeletal problem(s) should be noted. Obtain a list all current and recent prescribed and over-the-counter medications. The medication list may shed light on disorders previously omitted from the overall medical history and may also provide clues to the etiology of complaints. Table 14.1 lists some medications that are commonly associated with musculoskeletal effects. Ask about previous treatments from physical therapists, chiropractors, and practitioners of other disciplines relative to musculoskeletal complaints.

Table 14.1	
Medications With Musculoskeletal Effects	
Medications	**Possible Musculoskeletal Side Effects**
Diuretics	Secondary hyperuricemia
Chemotherapies for malignancies	May increase hyperuricemia
Hydralazine, procainamide, chlorpromazine, methyldopa, isoniazid, and oral contraceptives	Triggers for systemic lupus erythematosus
Anti-inflammatories, statins, fibrates, erythromycins	May cause rhabdomyolysis

In addition to specific musculoskeletal disorders, determine whether the patient has a history of skin disorders that might suggest a cause for the musculoskeletal complaint, such as gonococcal arthritis, Lyme disease, or systemic lupus erythematosus. Several endocrine disorders may result in musculoskeletal symptoms, including hyperparathyroidism, hyper- and hypothyroidism, and diabetes. History of any neurological problems should be established.

■ Family History

Identify the family history of various types of arthritis, osteoporosis, gout, and other musculoskeletal disorders. Also determine the history of related systems.

■ Habits

Identify all drugs and herbal remedies used. Ask about use of devices such as crutches, cane, walker, splint, or sling. Obtain a history of normal daily activity and any limitations realized since the presenting complaint was first noticed. Have the patient identify all occupational, social, and recreational physical activities, particularly those that require repetitive motions and/or stressors to the musculoskeletal system. Environmental issues associated with where the patient works, lives, and spends recreational time should be explored.

Physical Examination

■ Order of the Examination

The musculoskeletal examination is primarily limited to inspection and palpation. After an initial observation of the patient's general appearance, gait, and gross range of motion (ROM), the remainder of the examination is usually performed in a head-to-toe sequence. However, depending on the presentation, the general survey may be followed by a more focused examination of the affected area, with comparison to the opposite side/structures. Although assessment involves both inspection and palpation, there are specific procedures used to assess individual joints that combine inspection with palpation to determine muscle tone, muscle strength, ROM, and joint stability. As specific complaints are assessed, the problem can be further identified by having the patient point to the specific region or site that is most painful and by more carefully assessing that area.

General Survey

As the history is obtained, observe the patient's general appearance, including body build, posture, obvious deformities, general gait, movement, and any assistive aids used (crutches, walker, cane, bracing, etc.). A limp, guarding, or obvious weakness can provide a valuable indication of a musculoskeletal or neurological problem and how the patient is compensating. Notice whether the patient appears comfortable in the current position, guards a particular extremity or region during the initial portion of the visit, and so on. Observe the patient's general skin condition. Note the vital signs.

Inspection

The focused musculoskeletal examination begins with inspection. For overall assessment, it is essential that the patient disrobe, usually to his or her underwear. When examination is limited to a specific region, it is essential that the region be completely free of clothing to allow adequate observation. Once the patient is disrobed, the general posture should again be noted, as well as any deformities, limited motion, and asymmetry of bony pairs or muscle groups. Identify any skin lesions, scars, bulges, and areas of redness or swelling. Direct the patient through a variety of maneuvers intended to demonstrate ROM and general ability to control movement. These include a variety of gaits (normal, heel-toe, on-toes, on-heels, etc.), as well as full ROM of all joints without resistance. In addition to general inspection, more focused attention should be paid to any area of complaint. If an effusion, bulging, and/or redness are detected, the cause is more likely an inflammatory condition.

Palpation

For complete musculoskeletal examination, palpation involves assessment of each joint, as well as the major muscle groups and accessory structures, such as ligaments and tendons. Joint assessments are complex. During palpation, note any palpable deformities, nodularities, tenderness, swelling, or warmth. Palpate muscles for tone, size, and tenderness. Note any palpable crepitus. Areas of warmth suggest inflammatory or infectious cause of pain. Point tenderness is important as a potential indicator of bursitis or tendinitis as well as a defining feature of fibromyalgia.

■ Range of Motion

Active motion of the major joint groups is determined prior to assessing passive and/or assisted motion. In each case, note any limitations or complaints. The patient's response to active motion provides clues to how the examiner should best support the limb through passive motion. A goniometer provides an objective measure of ROM. Although a loss of motion occurs to some degree with age, it is usually minimal. Substantial loss is an abnormal finding except in the distal finger joints. An injured or diseased joint will likely be painful on motion, and active ROM may be limited to a greater degree than passive ROM. Motion in an abnormal plane may indicate looseness in ligaments. Crepitus and grating on movement indicates roughness in the surfaces of articulating bones. Clicks can occur from previous injuries to the joints, abnormalities of a meniscus, or merely from soft tissue sliding over bone.

■ Ligamentous Tests

When a patient complains of pain or injury to a joint, the stability of the joint should be determined. Ligamentous tests involve applying stress to the ligaments by a variety of maneuvers that typically involve the examiner flexing or extending the joint while applying pressure in a particular direction and determining the "feel" of the resulting movement, including any laxity, crepitus, or pain. Ligamentous stressing of a joint should start with only gentle pressure and then be repeated with increasing amounts of pressure/stress so that the test remains within the patient's pain tolerance yet provides information on the degree of laxity in a joint with any particular amount of stress.

■ Muscle Strength and Tone

Muscle strength is determined by asking the patient either to resist the examiner's attempt to flex or extend a muscle group or to flex or extend the muscles against the examiner's resistance. Muscle strength is graded 0 (no evidence of strength) to 5 (complete or full resistance). Pain, contracture, and disease can all affect muscle strength. Table 14.2 depicts a rating scheme for muscle strength.

Table 14.2		

Muscle Strength Assessment

Muscle Strength Assessment	Grade Notation	% Normal
No muscle contraction noted when resistance applied	M0	0
A slight muscle contraction seen or palpated but insufficient for joint movement	M1	10
Weak contraction when the joint is held in position. Full passive range of motion	M2	25
Contraction weak but there is full active movement against resistance	M3	50
Some muscle strength against resistance	M4	75
Normal strength is present	M5	100

Joint and muscle pain typically increase when the muscle is stretched and the joint is extended. For instance, an injured hamstring muscle is more painful when the leg is straightened/extended and the muscle pulled tight. Joint and tendon pain also increase when the area of injury is stressed.

Assessment of the muscle tone helps to determine nerve supply. A relaxed muscle should retain a slight residual tension, or tone. To assess muscle tone, passively stretch the muscle, ask the patient to relax, and then palpate the muscle, comparing side to side. It takes practice on the part of the examiner to develop a smooth motion when performing passive stretching. Alternatively, assessment of muscle tone can be combined with a determination of the patient's resistance to passive movement. Tense patients, those with increased muscle tone, will have increased resistance to passive movements. Flaccid or hypotonic muscles may indicate peripheral nervous system disease, cerebellar disease, or spinal cord problems. A spastic muscle has increased resistance, which may vary as the limb is moved, as in "cogwheeling," such as that found in patients with parkinsonism. Resistance with both flexion and extension is called lead-pipe rigidity, as is sometimes seen in parkinsonism.

■ Special Maneuvers

A variety of special maneuvers are indicated during the assessment of specific muscle, ligament, and/or joint groups. Some of the major maneuvers are described in subsequent sections on specific complaints.

Diagnostic Studies

The range of diagnostic studies relevant to musculoskeletal assessment is immense. Plain radiographs provide the appropriate first image for most musculoskeletal complaints. However, a number of other imaging studies are available, depending on the presentation and suspected condition. These include computed tomograph (CT scans), magnetic resonance images (MRIs), myelograms, ultrasound, nuclear scans, and others. Arthroscopic procedures provide an invasive means to visualize the internal joint structures. Arthrocentesis allows for aspiration of fluid to determine pyogenic or gouty arthritis. Doppler studies may be helpful in determining problems with blood flow, clotting, and inflammation in the veins. Blood work to determine the presence of infectious, metabolic, rheumatologic, or other disorders may also be needed.

Differential Diagnosis of Chief Complaints

Pain is a common complaint associated with musculoskeletal disorders. Any complaint of musculoskeletal pain requires further symptom analysis. The analysis is very similar regardless of the specific joint or region involved. Box 14.1 identifies the basic symptom analysis for musculoskeletal pain. The subsequent sections of this chapter refer to this box.

Box 14.1	

Musculoskeletal Symptom Analysis

Questions to determine what causes and/or relieves the pain:

- What, if anything, has been done to relieve the pain, and what was the response?
- Is there any situation or activity that relieves or diminishes the pain?
- Does anything seem to trigger the pain or make it worse?
- Is the pain worse or better at any particular time of day?

Questions to identify the type or quality of the pain:

- How can the pain be described?
- Is it burning, cramping, aching, sharp?
- Is it constant, throbbing, shooting?
- How bad is the pain on a scale?

Questions to determine the location and radiation of the pain:

- Where exactly does it hurt the most? (Ask the patient to point to the area where the pain is the worst.)
- Where does the pain radiate? Where else has there been pain?

Questions about associated symptoms:

- What other symptoms have been noticed since the pain first occurred?
- Have any other sensations, such as tingling or numbness, been noticed?
- Has there been any weakness, swelling, redness, limited motion, or popping?
- Have there been any other generalized symptoms, such as fever, malaise, or decreased energy?

Questions about the temporal sequence of the symptoms:

- When was the pain first noticed? What was the patient doing at the time?
- Since the pain was noticed, has it been persistent or intermittent?
- Since its onset, has the pain gotten worse or stayed the same?

■ Polyarthralgia

Polyarthralgia usually refers to arthralgia, or pain, in five or more joints, as opposed to monoarthralgia involving only one joint or oligoarthralgia involving two to four joints. Arthralgia is differentiated from arthritis in that arthralgia simply indicates joint pain/discomfort, whereas arthritis indicates associated joint inflammation. Therefore, one can have arthralgia with or without accompanying signs of arthritis.

The differential diagnosis for polyarthralgia is broad and includes infections, rheumatic conditions, noninflammatory degenerative disorders, malignancies, and endocrine disorders, for example. For this reason, it is critical that the history and physical examination obtain the necessary information to narrow the differential diagnosis.

History

Essential components of the history include a description of the nature of symptom onset and progression as well as the presence of extra-articular symptoms. Establish whether the pain and any other symptoms have been constant, progressive, and/or intermittent and whether the same joints are consistently involved or the pain migrates among differing joints. Family history is important, particularly for autoimmune disorders, rheumatoid arthritis, and osteoarthritis.

Physical Examination

When examining a patient who complains of pain in multiple joints, it is important to determine the distribution of the involved joints, noting the degree of symmetry and the types of joints (large weight-bearing versus small joints) affected. The presence of inflammatory signs helps to differentiate arthritic conditions from noninflammatory arthralgias. Other important signs include the presence or absence of nonarticular signs, including abnormalities of the integumentary, cardiac, gastrointestinal, genitourinary, neurologic, and/or lymphatic system.

Diagnostic Studies

Many diagnostic studies can be used to evaluate musculoskeletal complaints. Imaging studies are commonly used to evaluate the structure and integrity of affected joints. The range of relevant imaging studies is broad, although plain films are generally the first images indicated. Depending on the presentation, appropriate laboratory studies include a complete blood count, a metabolic profile, a urinalysis, and a variety of rheumatologic tests. Analysis of synovial fluid is often warranted to differentiate among potential etiologies.

RHEUMATOID ARTHRITIS

Rheumatoid arthritis (RA) is a progressive, inflammatory, and erosive condition that usually affects multiple joints. In addition to the articular changes associated with RA, there is a range of systemic effects. RA is an autoimmune condition.

Signs and Symptoms

RA typically affects the joints symmetrically. Symptoms may wax and wane, but the effects are cumulative and progressive. Although RA can affect any joint, it commonly affects the small joints of the hands and feet, and this is often helpful in diagnosis. Affected joints are often tender, swollen with effusions, warm, and inflamed. Nodules and deformities are common to RA. The disease most commonly affects metacarpophalangeal and proximal interphalangeal joints. Over time, a variety of typical RA deformities develop, including subluxation of the metacarpophalangeal joints and ulnar deviation and hyperextensions of the proximal interphalangeal (swan neck) joints.

Diagnostic Studies

A variety of laboratory tests are used to diagnose RA, including the rheumatoid factor, which is positive in up to 80% of persons with RA, but not specific to this disorder. It is often falsely positive in patients with other diseases, including lupus, sarcoidosis, and syphilis. RA is often associated with normocytic, hypochromic anemia as well as elevations in sedimentation rate and C-reactive protein. Other laboratory tests that may be positive at diagnosis include antinuclear antibody (ANA) and anticitrullinated protein (anti-CP) autoantibodies. The anti-CP autoantibodies are more specific to RA than the rheumatoid factor.

OSTEOARTHRITIS

Osteoarthritis (OA) is another common cause of polyarthralgia. This progressive disorder is associated with age and with wear and tear. Osteoarthritis causes a loss of cartilage and progressive erosion of bone.

Signs and Symptoms

Compared with RA, OA has a higher likelihood of affecting larger joints, such as the hips and knees. Like RA, OA also frequently involves the small joints of the hands, although it tends to occur at the distal interphalangeal joints (Heberden's nodes) and proximal interphalangeal joints (Bouchard's nodes). Most frequently, the second and/or third digits and the base of the thumb are involved. The distribution is asymmetrical. The pain and stiffness associated with OA often improve with moderate use and are worse after extended periods of rest. If three or more metacarpophalangeal joints are swollen, the differential should include rheumatoid arthritis.

Diagnostic Studies

Plain films reveal progressive changes, including diminishing joint space, sclerosis, and osteophyte formation. The sedimentation rate is negative, and the rheumatoid factor is negative.

FIBROMYALGIA

The etiology of fibromyalgia is not known. This complex, multifactorial disorder affects approximately 2% of the population and occurs primarily in females. Although patients may present with complaints of multiple joint pain, the disorder does not actually involve joints. Instead, it is a noninflammatory soft tissue disorder.

Signs and Symptoms

The most common symptoms are generalized pain, stiffness, and decreased ROM, with multiple-point tenderness. The diagnostic criteria currently rest on a patient reporting point tenderness in at least 11 of 18 specified sites (Fig. 14.1) in addition to the presence of widespread pain for at least 3 months. The most common tender sites are in the neck, shoulders, spine, and hips. Other common symptoms include morning stiffness, anxiety, depression, sleep disturbances, "brain fog," and irritable bowel syndrome.

Diagnostic Studies

There are no definitive diagnostic biomarker studies for fibromyalgia.

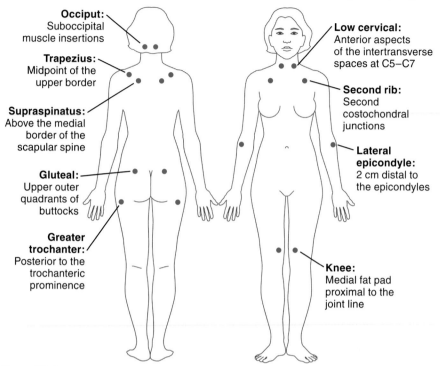

Figure 14.1 The 18 pressure points must be accurately located and tested by applying just enough pressure with one finger to barely blanch the nailbed.

SYSTEMIC LUPUS ERYTHEMATOSUS

Systemic lupus erythematosus (SLE) is a chronic autoimmune disorder that has widespread effects. The prevalence is much higher in women, particularly in the childbearing years, than in men.

Signs and Symptoms

SLE has many potential symptoms. The classic findings include a malar rash. Patients often have arthralgias, myalgias, fever, fatigue, Raynaud's syndrome, and neuropathy. SLE effects depend on the organs involved. Cardiovascular, renal, pulmonary, hematologic, neurological, ophthalmic, gastrointestinal, dermatologic, and musculoskeletal symptoms are possible.

Diagnostic Studies

The diagnostic findings depend on the organs involved, and diagnosis can be difficult. A positive ANA (antinuclear antibody) occurs at some point in the condition in the majority of patients but is neither consistent nor specific for SLE. Positive anti-DNA and lupus erythematosus prep are also common to SLE. The sedimentation rate and C-reactive protein level are increased. Other helpful laboratory studies include complete blood count with differential, creatinine, albumin, and urinalysis. Imaging study selection depends on the presentation.

SARCOIDOSIS

Sarcoidosis is an inflammatory disorder in which patients develop granulomas and a wide range of symptoms, including arthritis. It is most commonly diagnosed in persons between ages 20 and 40.

Signs and Symptoms

Although the disorder may be asymptomatic, it often is accompanied by multiple symptoms, including joint pain. Arthralgias occur in approximately 3% of patients with sarcoidosis, and the most commonly affected joints include the ankles, feet, and hands. The patient may complain of constitutional symptoms, including fatigue, fever, and altered appetite. Respiratory symptoms, including cough, wheezing, and shortness of breath are primary symptoms. Others include lymphadenopathy, rash, eye changes, and palpitations.

Diagnostic Studies

Appropriate diagnostic studies depend on the symptoms and involved organs. However, definitive diagnosis involves biopsy of involved organs. Other laboratory abnormalities depend on involved organs. There is often an elevated sedimentation rate and normocytic, normochromic anemia. Chest films should be ordered when sarcoidosis is suspected.

REACTIVE ARTHRITIS

This syndrome is described by several terms, including Reiter's syndrome and seronegative arthritis, and is the most common cause of migratory arthritis in young males. The complex of symptoms develops following an infection, usually chlamydia. However, other associated causes include shigella, salmonella, and clostridia.

Signs and Symptoms

Multiple joints are involved, primarily those of the lower extremities, as well as the vertebrae. The distribution of affected joints is asymmetrical, and the arthritis is migratory. In addition to the arthritis pain, often present are urethritis, conjunctivitis, and/or iritis, as well as diarrhea and fever.

Diagnostic Studies

There are no studies specific to Reiter's syndrome, although the sedimentation rate and C-reactive protein are often elevated, and studies may identify the offending infectious agent.

GONOCOCCAL ARTHRITIS

This polyarthritis is also common in young men and follows infection with gonorrhea. Gonococcal arthritis occurs as part of disseminated infection.

Signs and Symptoms

The polyarthritis is often migratory and affects lower extremities as well as the hands. In addition to the arthritis, the syndrome usually includes a nonpruritic dermatitis and tenosynovitis. Generalized muscle aches and fever are also common.

Diagnostic Studies

The sedimentation rate and C-reactive protein are often elevated. Plain films will reveal joint distention, which can later progress to joint destruction. Synovial fluid with increased polymorphonuclear leukocytes and positive culture occur in fewer than 50%.

GOUTY ARTHRITIS

Gout is a form of arthritis that results from the deposition/collection of microcrystals within a joint space. The offending agents are usually urate crystals. The condition usually occurs after middle age and is associated with an elevated uric acid level.

Signs and Symptoms

Gout is a classic cause of monoarthritis but more rarely affects multiple joints. It should be considered when polyarthritis recurs over a long period of time. Even though most cases involve a joint in the lower extremities, other joints may be affected. Acute pain usually develops in one joint, with swelling, redness, and warmth, and the severity of the pain increases rapidly. ROM of the affected joint(s) is limited by pain, and there is significant tenderness to the site. Patients who have had gout for an extended time often have gouty tophi, which are soft tissue nodules containing urate crystals. The olecranon bursa is a common site for tophi development, and the tophi are often painful.

Diagnostic Studies

Plain films are generally negative unless the condition has persisted for a long period of time. In this case, films may reveal "punched-out" lesions of the bone. The uric acid level is elevated. Joint aspirate will reveal crystals. There may be a mild increase in white blood cells, and sedimentation rate is increased.

LYME DISEASE

Lyme disease is caused by the bacterium *Borrelia burgdorferi,* and is transmitted by a bite from a deer tick. Whereas the incubation period ranges from 3 to 30 days, the onset of symptoms typically appears in 7 to 14 days.

Signs and Symptoms

Although the disorder can be asymptomatic, the patient generally develops migratory polyarthralgia, myalgia, and neurological findings, including meningitis and/or neuropathy. An early finding is a solitary target lesion that may be followed by multiple lesions.

Diagnostic Studies

The diagnosis is often based on the physical findings. Definitive diagnosis is based on laboratory studies. Initially, an enzyme-linked immunosorbent assay

(ELISA) or indirect immunofluorescent immunoglobulin G (IgG) antibody is obtained; if the initial test is positive, it is followed by Western blot.

ACUTE RHEUMATIC FEVER

Acute rheumatic fever is becoming more rare in the United States. However, this disease should be considered when children and young adults develop polyarthralgia. This complex of symptoms occurs following an infection with streptococci, typically streptococcal pharyngitis.

Signs and Symptoms

There is typically a history of recent sore throat preceding development of pain in the larger joints. The pain is often migratory. Cardiac symptoms may be present, including heart failure, murmur, or pericarditis. Other signs include fever, rash, and subcutaneous nodules. The rash is usually a faint pink and nonpruritic.

Diagnostic Studies

There may be elevations of sedimentation rate and C-reactive protein as well as a prolonged PR interval on electrocardiogram. Throat culture is positive in approximately 25% of patients.

■ Neck Pain

Neck pain is a common complaint and may originate from the neck structures or radiate from another region. Many of the potential causes are benign and self-limiting. Neck pain may also be an indication of a rheumatologic disorder, traumatic injury, or neurological disorder. Signs and symptoms associated with neck pain are listed in the Red Flag box.

RED Flag Red Flags in the Assessment of the Patient with Neck Pain

- History of injury/trauma preceding onset of pain
- Associated neck stiffness (nuchal rigidity) with fever
- Neck pain in a child
- Pain that is unrelenting and/or worsening in patients who have tried and failed conservative treatment
- Acute, severe pain, with or without radicular symptoms, upon awakening in the morning
- Pain relieved by elevating the arm above the head on the side of the pain
- Severe pain, with or without radicular symptoms, on flexion or extension of the neck
- Chronic neck pain with weakness of upper or lower extremity(ies), stumbling, muscle atrophy, bowel or bladder incontinence
- Pain with a history of malignancies

History

When a patient presents neck pain, it is important to obtain a thorough history of the complaint as well as any associated symptoms. An analysis of the pain should be completed (see Box 14.1). Determine whether there is any accompanying pain in other areas, including the head, shoulders, back, and upper extremities. Ask about stiffness or decreased ability of motion as well as whether certain motions or positions increase the discomfort. Identify the patient's normal occupational and recreational activities as well as any unusual exertion/activities. Always determine whether recent injury or trauma has occurred.

Physical Examination

The examination relevant to neck pain varies depending on the presentation. For recent trauma, a brief examination to determine stability may be performed and then radiographs obtained before proceeding with further examination. Otherwise, the examination should be thorough and performed with the patient undressed from the waist up. It can be helpful to observe the patient as he undresses, noting movement and any apparent discomfort or weakness. Observe the patient's general posture, head placement, cervical curve, and symmetry of movement. The neck structures should be observed and palpated, noting any deformity, tenderness, muscle spasms, or other abnormalities. Active ROM of the neck should be performed in all planes (flexion, extension, rotation, lateral flexion) within the patient's tolerance, followed by passive movement if any limitation are identified. Pain associated with movement is noted. Assess the range of motion of the upper extremities. The strength and tone of the neck and upper extremities should be determined, as should reflexes.

Diagnostic Studies

The history and clinical findings should guide the determination of when to order diagnostic studies. Patients with a recent onset of neck pain but no neurological symptoms and no history of trauma do not necessarily require imaging, and the selection of diagnostic studies is guided by clinical judgment. However, any patient with a history of trauma and neck discomfort should have a minimum of a three-view radiograph ordered: anteroposterior, lateral, and open mouth views. Similarly, patients presenting with a history of chronic pain should have plain cervical films, consisting of anteroposterior, lateral, and open mouth views. Oblique views are often included. A CT scan should be obtained for patients who have a history of trauma and who present with neurological signs, altered sensorium, or abnormal radiographic findings. When patients have neurological symptoms, an MRI should be ordered as well. When the patient cannot tolerate or has other contraindications to the use of an MRI, the CT scan should be obtained and followed by a myelogram, as necessary. Electromyography and nerve conduction studies are helpful in identifying level of involvement.

CERVICAL DISK DISEASE

Cervical disk disease results from compression associated with herniated cervical disks. When cervical disk disease is identified or strongly suspected, the patient should be referred for specialist evaluation and definitive treatment.

Signs and Symptoms

Cervical disk disease is frequently manifested by morning tightness, stiffness, and/or pain. Coughing and straining can increase the pain, which may radiate to the shoulder and arm. Elevating the arm may provide relief. Numbness along the medial border of the scapula is a common finding. There may be radicular sensations, including paresthesias or pain that is sharp or burning in the shoulders, arms, or back. The actual distribution of radiating symptoms depends on the affected nerve root. Neurological findings include altered upper extremity deep tendon reflexes, weakness, and sensation. If disk rupture is due to trauma, the onset of symptoms will typically be acute.

A positive Spurling's sign is noted if this maneuver reproduces neck and radicular pain, suggesting herniated disk. Spurling's sign is tested for by lightly pressing downward on the top of the patient's head while tilting back and toward the side of pain. Lhermitte's sign may support suspicion of a herniated disk. This test is conducted by having the patient flex the neck in a chin-to-chest motion and is positive if an electric shock–like sensation down the spine results. The sign may also be positive in a number of other conditions, including spondylosis and Chiari I malformation.

Diagnostic Studies

Plain films often identify the diminished disk space. An MRI is indicated for chronic neck pain with diminished disk space and/or neurological findings.

CERVICAL SPONDYLOSIS/STENOSIS

Cervical spondylosis results from bone spur development associated with degenerative arthritis. The term *cervical stenosis* is used when the degenerative changes are more focal than diffuse. In both instances, the bony osteophytes compress the spinal cord so that both motor and sensory neurological symptoms may result. Patients in whom cervical spondylosis is identified should also be referred to specialty evaluation and treatment.

Signs and Symptoms

Neck tenderness is a common finding of cervical spondylitis. The neurological symptoms and clinical findings are specific to the affected nerve root. These can include radicular pain and dysesthesias, abnormal deep tendon reflexes, and weakness.

Diagnostic Studies

Plain radiographs identify osteophyte formation and may suggest narrowing of spaces. An MRI will identify the site(s) and degree of compression.

NECK STRAIN

Neck strain is a common problem, which can be caused by positioning or overuse/repetitive use of the neck and related structures. Acceleration injury, or whiplash (typically seen following a car accident), is also a form of neck strain.

Signs and Symptoms

The most common symptom of neck strain, regardless of the cause, is neck pain. However, there is often associated occipital, shoulder, and/or upper back pain. The history usually identifies the source of the strain. With more severe strain, such as is seen with acceleration injuries, other common complaints include paresthesias of the upper extremities. The general strength and reflexes of the upper extremities should be within normal limits, and the patient should be neurologically intact.

Diagnostic Studies

Radiographs should exclude cervical fractures and subluxation if trauma has occurred or any neurological findings are present. If spasm is present, the only radiologic finding may be loss of the lordotic curve.

SYRINGOMYELIA (SYRINX, HYDROSYRINGOMYELIA)

Syringomyelia is a fluid cavity in the spinal cord that can occur in the cervical and/or thoracic areas. The most common cause of syringomyelia is Chiari malformation (see Chiari Malformation in the Headache or Cephalalgia section of Chapter 15). Less common causes include spinal tumor, arachnoiditis, trauma, or idiopathology.

Signs and Symptoms

The patient often describes burning pain in the neck or thoracic area and paresthesias or numbness in the neck or thoracic areas as well as in the extremities. Progressive weakness of the extremities and limited ROM of the neck and/or back may occur. Other possible symptoms include bladder retention or incontinence and diminished sensation, strength, and reflexes. The gait may be altered.

Diagnostic Studies

The test of choice for diagnosis of syringomyelia is an MRI of the cervical, thoracic, and lumbar spine with and without contrast. The area of the spine that is imaged is determined by the area of symptoms reported by the patient.

PATHOLOGIC FRACTURE AND METASTATIC TUMOR

Any spontaneous fracture should be explored for possible relation to carcinoma, either metastatic or multiple myeloma, in an older adult.

FIBROMYALGIA

See p. 419.

■ Low Back Pain

Low back pain (LBP) is extremely common. Nearly three-fourths of the world's population will have at least one disabling episode of LBP in their lives. It is the most common cause of limited activity and most common reason for office visits for patients under 45 years of age in the United States. Most episodes are self-limited and resolve in less than 3 weeks. However, the longer an employee is absent from work owing to LBP, the lower the chance the employee has of returning to the workplace. The cause of LBP can be difficult to differentiate/diagnose, and the condition may be poorly treated. Many patients forgo standard medical assessment and treatment in favor of chiropractic care.

History

As with all pain syndromes, it is important to obtain a detailed history of the onset and progression of the pain. A thorough pain history should be completed, noting its quality, location, radiation, and intensity, as well as any exacerbating and relieving factors. A thorough review of systems is necessary to identify any associated symptoms that may indicate an urgent problem. These include altered bowel and/or bladder function, fever, weight loss, and/or weakness. The medical history should identify previous episodes of back pain and other musculoskeletal disorders and should include the treatment and responses for them. Specifically ask about a history of malignancy, arthritis, recent infection, and neurological disorders. Family history should be obtained. The patient's recreational and occupational activity patterns should be determined. A history of all medications, both over the counter and prescription, should be identified. See the Red Flag box for signs and symptoms associated with low back pain.

RED Flag ◀ **Red Flags in the Assessment of the Patient with Low Back Pain**

- Pain is associated with neurologic deficits (weakness, altered sensation, bowel/bladder changes)
- Pain in a child
- Pain is associated with fever and/or stiff neck
- Pain is associated with unexplained weight loss with or without a previous history of malignancy
- Pain is worse at rest
- Pain is associated with radiation to the abdomen or stomach area
- Pain is related to history of urinary tract infections, drug use, or other infections (including AIDS)
- Pain increases with coughing/sneezing or straining

Physical Examination

The physical examination should begin by noting the patient's posture and apparent level of comfort. The standing patient should be directed through a series of maneuvers to assess the back motion, including flexion, hyperextension, lateral flexion, and rotation, as the smoothness of motion, range of motion, and any obvious signs of discomfort are noted. Next, palpate along the spinal column with the patient standing and then bending forward. Note the presence or absence of the natural curvature. Observe the patient walking on heels and on toes, noting any signs of weakness.

Next, with the patient resting supine on the examination table, the straight leg maneuver should be performed. This test is often misinterpreted. However, as the patient rests supine with both legs extended, the examiner should passively elevate one leg at a time. A positive test is indicated if the patient experiences discomfort with the initial elevation rather than once the hip has been hyperflexed beyond 50 degrees. Note whether any pain is experienced on the side of the raised leg or contralaterally. Consider the results of the straight leg test in combination with the rest of the physical examination, including neurosensory and reflex testing. If the results indicate nerve impingement or disk injury, further radiographic testing is then indicated.

Throughout the assessment, be attentive for signs of serious diseases associated with low back pain, including malignancy, abdominal aortic aneurysm, fracture, and bone infection.

Diagnostic Studies

The following diagnostic tests should be considered on the basis of history and presentation.

- Lumbar x-rays with anteroposterior/lateral and flexion/extension views provide information about bony abnormalities. Acute fractures and subluxation are often discernable on plain x-rays.
- An MRI of the lumbar spine with and without contrast is the test of choice for diagnosis of herniated disks, intra- or extradural mass lesions, spina bifida occulta, and cauda equina syndrome.
- A CT scan with myelogram is not commonly used because MRI is a more sensitive test for determining tissue abnormalities. However, for those in whom MRI is contraindicated, a CT myelogram is useful. This is an invasive test, and the patient should understand the risks and benefits before proceeding.
- Electromyography and nerve conduction tests may help to determine the exact nerve root involved in the setting of radiculopathy associated with low back pain.

MECHANICAL LOW BACK PAIN

Mechanical low back pain is extremely common, and most individuals experience some type of mechanical back pain at least once in their life. The causes are varied.

Signs and Symptoms

Pain in the back, buttocks, and thigh may be severe. The onset occurs after new or unusual exertion. There is no history of major trauma, systemic infection, or malignancy. Pain relief is achieved when lying down. Physical examination reveals paravertebral tenderness/spasm, scoliosis, or loss of natural lumbar lordosis with no neurological signs or radiculopathy.

Diagnostic Studies

None are needed.

HERNIATED INTERVERTEBRAL DISC

Herniated disks are most common after age 30. Symptoms are dependent on the degree of disk protrusion and are often referred to as sciatica.

Signs and Symptoms

A flexion injury or trauma may precede the onset of symptoms. Lying with hips flexed provides pain relief. Associated paravertebral tenderness and spasm often result in awkward posture. The acute phase is associated with radicular irritation and symptoms, including diminished reflexes and strength. Major prolapse may be associated with bilateral weakness and bowel and bladder dysfunction. Pain associated with chronic irritation is usually dull and unilateral.

Diagnostic Studies

The diagnostics include MRI, CT, or myelogram. Electromyography (EMG) may give supporting documentation regarding the nerve damage.

SPINAL STENOSIS

Caused by progressive degenerative spine changes, spinal stenosis is most common at middle age or later.

Signs and Symptoms

Spinal stenosis pain is usually worse during the day. It is aggravated by standing and relieved by rest. The pain varies from severe to mild. The level of neurological findings varies and can include weakness and bowel or bladder dysfunction. OA signs may be present.

Diagnostic Studies

Radiological findings may indicate extensive vertebral osteophytes and degenerative disk disease. An MRI or CT scan can be helpful if initial x-rays are inconclusive.

OSTEOARTHRITIS

See p. 419.

MALIGNANCY

When assessing back pain, it is important to consider that the complaints and findings may suggest a malignancy. Back pain in a patient with cancer is an indication of metastasis.

Signs and Symptoms

The patient is often over 50 years of age and presents with dull pain that has gradually increased in intensity. Neurological findings vary by the level of involvement. A fever may be associated. The potential increases with a history of another malignancy.

Diagnostic Studies

When malignancy is suspected, plain films should be ordered, followed by CT, MRI, and/or bone scan.

SPINAL INFECTION

Vertebral osteomyelitis is rare, but it should be considered, particularly with at-risk patients. These include persons with advancing age, history of IV drug use, and compromised immune systems.

Signs and Symptoms

The history includes fever and chills with possible weight loss. The pain is often worse at night. There is point percussive tenderness and elevated temperature. There are usually no neurological complaints; this is dependent on the degree and level of involvement.

Diagnostic Studies

In advanced infections, plain films reveal vertebral destruction. An MRI with enhancement is more diagnostic. While a bone scan could be used for patients who cannot tolerate MRI, they are not specific. Blood cultures should be obtained. The sedimentation rate and C-reactive protein are elevated.

COMPRESSION FRACTURE

Compression fractures are most commonly associated with osteoporosis and have a higher incidence with age.

Signs and Symptoms

The patient complains of back pain that may range from mild to severe. Onset can be gradual or acute. With acute onset, the patient can often describe a precipitating injury. There is a loss of height. Kyphosis results from thoracic fracture and lordosis from lumbar fracture. Depending on the degree of deformity associated with the fracture(s), pulmonary symptoms may be present.

Diagnostic Studies

Plain films reveal compression deformity with loss of vertebral height and/or wedge deformity.

ANKYLOSING SPONDYLITIS

Ankylosing spondylitis is one of the spondyloarthropathies, which have genetic predispositions and are inflammatory disorders. The incidence is higher in men than in women, and onset is generally in young adulthood. Neck pain is a late symptom and often occurs some time after the development of low back pain.

Signs and Symptoms

Early symptoms include low back pain and stiffness, which gradually become persistent and increase in severity. Later, the pain may again become intermittent. Other symptoms can include bony tenderness, malaise, loss of appetite, fever, and fatigue. There is loss of spine mobility, and posture gradually changes with flexion of the neck, increased kyphosis of the thoracic region, and loss of the lumbar curve. Although chest expansion is affected, respiratory function usually remains intact.

Diagnostic Studies

The gene *HLA-B27* is present in most patients. Most have elevations of erythrocyte sedimentation rate and C-reactive protein as well as some degree of anemia. Radiographs show abnormality of the sacroiliac joint with progressive erosion. A CT scan is useful to identify sacroiliitis.

■ Shoulder Pain

Shoulder pain arises both from disorders affecting the shoulder structures and conditions involving other structures, such as the neck. The shoulder includes complex structures, and many of the conditions have very similar symptoms and physical findings. Shoulder pain in young patients (under 45 years old) is often related to trauma. Shoulder pain in older patients (over 45) is more often related to degenerative disease. Biomechanical trauma to the shoulder accentuates degenerative changes and symptoms. Shoulder syndromes frequently arise from inflammation. Most frequently, the capsule of the glenohumeral joint, supraspinatus tendon, and the subacromial bursa are involved. When patients present with shoulder pain, always consider the possibility of cardiac, cervical neck, or gastrointestinal cause.

The history should be directed to identify any potential injuries from trauma or overuse as well as any previous experience of shoulder pain. Determine whether the onset was acute or gradual. Ask about any activities or positions that are associated with diminished or increased pain. Details on self-treatment and response are important to elicit. Personal and family history of autoimmune and inflammatory disorders should be investigated.

The physical examination for shoulder pain starts with observations of the patient's poster and how the arm is "carried." General ROM, palpation, and testing of strength and sensation are important. A number of maneuvers are helpful in differentiating the source of shoulder pain; they are depicted in Figures 14.2 through 14.6 and are referred to in the following sections, as appropriate.

TRAUMA

Trauma to the shoulder can result in a range of injuries, including brachial plexus injury, acute rotator cuff tear, acromioclavicular injury, and fractured clavicle.

Signs and Symptoms

The history includes the traumatic event, such as direct blow, fall on the shoulder, or twisting injury. Physical findings will be consistent with the degree of trauma and involvement of the shoulder and other structures. Rotator cuff injuries (see next subsection) typically result from chronic impingement, but they can result from acute trauma. A fall or blow to the shoulder area may result in a fractured clavicle, which is often associated with an obvious deformity at the site of the fracture and significant pain when pressure is applied over the fracture site. Acromioclavicular separation or strain typically results in an obvious deformity as well as pain, which increases as the arm is elevated. The presence of deformity depends on the severity of separation/displacement. A brachial plexus injury with trauma to C5–7 is indicated by paresthesia and/or sharp pain that radiates to the arm, paired with significant weakness and decreased sensation.

Diagnostic Studies

An x-ray should be ordered for any complaint of shoulder pain following an acute trauma.

ROTATOR CUFF SYNDROME AND IMPINGEMENT SYNDROME

The rotator cuff consists of the supraspinatus, infraspinatus, subscapularis, and teres minor. Injury to the rotator cuff is typically due to chronic impingement with degenerative changes over time. It is most common in persons over 40 years of age. Impingement results in rotator cuff tendinitis and/or bursitis of the subacromial bursa. As the structures thicken, increased mechanical injury occurs.

Signs and Symptoms

The patient typically complains of anterior and lateral shoulder pain that increases with arm elevation and reaching overhead. The pain is usually progressive and may be associated with repetitive activities. Pain at night may cause sleep disturbance. ROM is typically preserved. Apley's (see Fig. 14.2) and Hawkins' (see Fig. 14.3) tests may reproduce the pain, depending on the component of the rotator cuff involved. There may be point or diffuse tenderness to the shoulder area. Crepitus and/or arm weakness suggest an acute tear.

Diagnostic Studies

Plain films are often normal but may show subacromial spurs.

ROTATOR CUFF TEAR

Injury to the rotator cuff usually follows chronic impingement and degenerative changes over time. Injury to the structures may also result from trauma.

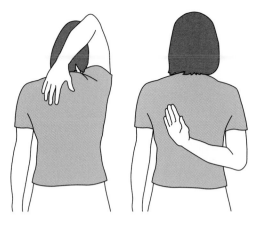

Figure 14.2 Apley's test involves range of motion as the patient reaches overhead and behind the lower back to touch the scapula.

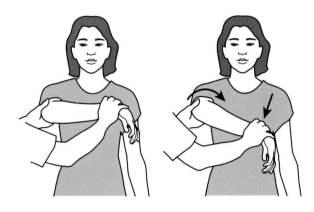

Figure 14.3 Hawkins' test involves internally rotating the patient's arm as it is elevated to 90 degrees.

Signs and Symptoms

Pain associated with a tear of the rotator cuff is sudden in onset and may be worse at night. Associated weakness and atrophy of surrounding structures occurs, and ROM is limited. The limitation is sometimes connected with the pain, as it is painful for the patient to lift the arm; however, weakness of the periarticular structures also contributes to weakness. With a large tear, the patient will be able only to shrug the shoulder but not lift the arm. Tenderness is greatest at the supraspinatus insertion, and pain may radiate to the deltoid region. Crepitus is often noted with rotation at 60 to 120 degrees of abduction, as this maneuver compresses the injured tissue. To compensate, the patient may rotate the palm up (supination) during abduction, which rotates the shoulder and widens the rotator cuff, decreasing the pain on movement. Apley's (see Fig. 14.2), Hawkins' (see Fig. 14.3), and the empty can (Fig. 14.4) tests may be positive, depending on the location of the tear.

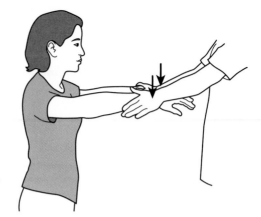

Figure 14.4 The empty can test involves the patient's arms held anteriorly with thumbs down (as if holding an empty can) while resisting downward pressure applied by the examiner.

Diagnostic Studies

Plain films are usually not helpful unless the injury has been longstanding, in which case some sclerosis may be noted. Diagnosis can be confirmed by arthrogram, which should be considered if shoulder pain persists or the onset of pain was preceded by trauma.

BICEPS TENOSYNOVITIS

Inflammation of the biceps tendon is another frequent cause of shoulder pain. The patient is usually middle aged or is an athlete with repeated injuries related to the throwing motion.

Signs and Symptoms

Tenderness is noted with active and passive motion as well as with palpation of the tendon sheath. The tendon becomes inflamed in the bicipital groove that can be felt on palpation. A positive Yergason test (Fig. 14.5) suggests biceps

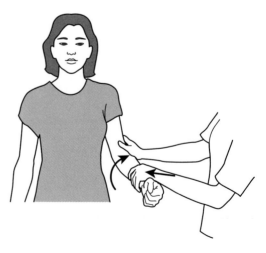

Figure 14.5 Yergason's test involves the patient holding the arm with elbow flexed 90 degrees, in thumb-up position, and then attempting to further flex and supinate the arm as the examiner offers resistance.

tendon instability or tendonitis. The test is positive if pain is produced at the bicipital groove.

Diagnostic Studies

No radiological testing is indicated.

ADHESIVE CAPSULITIS ("FROZEN SHOULDER")

Frozen shoulder encompasses a variety of conditions associated with shoulder stiffness and limitation of motion. Although many other terms are used to refer to this condition, the most commonly accepted term is *adhesive capsulitis*. There is controversy regarding the etiology.

Signs and Symptoms

The patient is unable to abduct the affected arm beyond 90 degrees with the scapula on that side stabilized/immobilized. A period of pain without limited motion often precedes the loss of motion. Then, progressive stiffness associated with the pain may occur until the patient recognizes inability to perform certain tasks requiring elevation of the arm or reaching behind the head/back. At the point that passive and active ROM are affected, there is generally diffuse tenderness.

Diagnostic Studies

Plain films may be helpful in identifying other disorders that cause secondary adhesive capsulitis, such as osteoarthritis, fracture, avascular necrosis, and calcific tendinitis.

GLENOHUMERAL INSTABILITY

Unlike the other conditions affecting the shoulder, glenohumeral instability is most common in young patients who are physically active. The instability can result in displacement of the humeral head in various directions.

Signs and Symptoms

The patient will experience sudden onset of pain and be unwilling to move the arm. The displacement may follow an acute injury/trauma or may be associated with specific movements or overuse. A positive apprehension test suggests glenohumeral instability. This can be somewhat validated by performing the relocation test, in which the apprehension test is immediately followed by placing mild anterior pressure on the arm paired with external rotation. With glenohumeral instability, the pain produced with the apprehension test (Fig. 14.6) is typically diminished.

Diagnostic Studies

Plain film will identify the direction of instability and may show a defect of the humeral head that is associated with the instability.

CARDIAC PAIN

When patients present with complaints of exertional pain in the shoulder region, it is important to maintain a level of suspicion for referred cardiac pain.

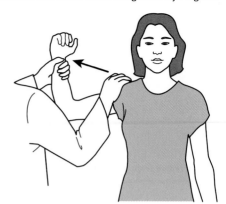

Figure 14.6 The apprehension test involves the patient holding the arm in a neutral position, elevated to 90 degrees. Then the examiner places mild pressure on the anterior aspect of the arm while externally rotating the arm.

The presentation would likely include pain relieved with rest, and the patient would likely have a history of cardiac risk factors. See Chapter 7.

PULMONARY PAIN

Pulmonary disorders can be associated with pain that is referred to the shoulder region. See Chapter 8.

REFERRED ABDOMINAL PAIN

Certain abdominal conditions, such as gallbladder disease, may result in pain that refers to the shoulder. See Chapter 10.

■ Elbow Pain

Pain related to the elbow is commonly mechanical in origin. The elbow is a very complex joint, with articulations between the humerus and radius, the humerus and ulna, and the ulna and radius. The innervation is also complex, with risk for entrapment between the various soft tissue and bony structures. Overuse and repetitive movement is responsible for many causes of elbow pain. However, rheumatoid, gouty, and septic arthritis can also affect the elbow.

TRAUMA

As with other joints, the elbow is at risk for acute trauma, which can result in fracture or dislocation or can trigger reactive tendinitis. The presentation will be specific to the trauma experienced.

EPICONDYLITIS

Epicondylitis involves inflammation of the tendon/tendon insertion of the forearms. This tendinitis results in either lateral elbow pain associated with overuse of the wrist extensors (tennis elbow) or in medial elbow pain associated with overuse of involving wrist flexion and rotation (golfer's elbow).

Signs and Symptoms

Point tenderness is noted at the medial or lateral epicondyle. The onset and severity of pain is usually gradual and progressive but may have relatively acute onset following an activity involving significant repetitive use. The pain may be referred to the forearm and is increased by the offending motion (wrist flexion, extension, or rotation). Pain is usually greater when the motion is made against resistance. There may be a locking sensation with motion and the area of point tenderness may be swollen.

Diagnostic Studies

Plain films are often normal but may reveal spurs, loose bodies, and/or loss of joint space. Imaging is indicated particularly if there is a history of trauma.

OLECRANON BURSITIS

The olecranon bursa is superficial and at risk for repeated trauma. Olecranon bursitis can result from repetitive overuse, trauma, and infection.

Signs and Symptoms

The patient complains of swelling and tenderness at the "tip" of the elbow over the olecranon. Point tenderness is common, although it is found most frequently in patients with septic bursitis. Septic bursitis is also often associated with a skin lesion either over the bursa or distal to the elbow and/or an elevated body temperature.

Diagnostic Studies

Plain film will be negative. An aspiration of the bursa should be performed for culture (septic bursitis) as well as determination of whether there is a collection of crystals (gouty bursitis) and/or elevated white cell count (greatest in septic bursitis).

NURSEMAID ELBOW

Also known as pulled elbow or toddler's elbow, nursemaid's elbow involves the head of the radius slipping under the annular ligament in children, usually between 1 and 4 years of age. The condition occurs when traction is applied to the young child's hand or wrist.

Signs and Symptoms

There is a history of sudden onset of pain associated with sudden immobility of the affected arm as the child protects the elbow. The parent may be able to identify a situation in which the child's hand was held and traction applied: The child may have moved in an opposite direction or injury could occur while pulling the arm through clothing. There is no associated swelling or inflammation. Examination is otherwise normal with the exception of resistance to attempts to move the arm, elbow, and, possibly, wrist. There may be tenderness along the upper margin of the radius.

Diagnostic Studies

None are usually indicated unless history suggests need to rule out fracture.

GOUT

Whereas gout typically involves a lower extremity joint, it is a frequent cause of elbow inflammation.

RHEUMATOID ARTHRITIS

Rheumatoid arthritis is a systemic condition but may affect individual joints. See pp. 418–419.

OSTEOARTHRITIS

See p. 419.

■ Wrist and Hand Pain

Pain and numbness of the hand and wrist may be unilateral or bilateral, but they are usually associated with injuries related to overuse. The hands are common sites of both osteoarthritis and rheumatoid arthritis.

The history should include a thorough description of the pain and its impact on activities as well as personal and family history of inflammatory or autoimmune conditions. Ask about occupational and recreational routines to identify potential overuse, ergonomic, or traumatic etiologies.

The examination includes careful inspection and palpation of the structures of the wrists, hands, and fingers with side-to-side comparisons. ROM and strength are tested.

CARPAL TUNNEL SYNDROME

The carpal tunnel is a space located on the anterior aspect of the wrist between the carpal bones and a ligamentous band through which the median nerve and several tendons traverse. With overuse and repetitive movements, the various tissues may hypertrophy, causing a loss of space and impingement on the median nerve. The types of activities associated with carpal tunnel syndrome include computer use and painting.

Signs and Symptoms

Carpal tunnel syndrome causes a range of neurological symptoms, including pain, paresthesia, and weakness. Frequently, nighttime pain is an early symptom. There may be a swelling at the wrist related to inactivity or flexion at night. The pain and/or paresthesias typically involve the anterior aspects of wrist, medial palm, and first three digits on the affected hand. However, pain may radiate up the forearm to the shoulder with numbness and tingling along the median nerve. Over time, hand weakness often develops. Pain and paresthesia are often relieved by the patient "shaking" the affected hand in a downward fashion; this is called the flicking sign. A positive Tinel's sign is elicited by tapping on the median nerve at the carpal tunnel, causing pain and tingling along the median nerve. Phalen's maneuver reproduces the pain after 1 minute of wrist flexion against resistance.

Diagnostic Studies

Nerve testing, including nerve conduction studies, is indicated to determine the location and extent of the compression. An ultrasound may depict synovitis.

DE QUERVAIN'S TENDONITIS/TENOSYNOVITIS

De Quervain's tenosynovitis involves irritation of a tendon located on the radial side of the wrist, near the thumb. With overuse, the tissues surrounding the tendon sheath hypertrophy, causing pressure on the tendon and making it difficult to move.

Signs and Symptoms

The pain is usually limited to the radial aspect of the wrist and area immediately around the base of the thumb. Pain increases with use of the hand, such as with gripping maneuvers. Other symptoms include swelling, decreased sensation, and limited ROM with a locking sensation with thumb motion. The Finkelstein maneuver (Fig. 14.7) is used to diagnose De Quervain's disease. A positive test results in pain, which is often severe. Patients who can repeatedly open and close the fist with smooth thumb motion are unlikely to have De Quervain's.

Diagnostic Studies

Plain films of the wrist are normal.

GANGLION CYSTS

Ganglion cysts are common soft tissue abnormalities involving the wrist and/or hand. The fluid-filled cyst typically develops adjacent to a tendon sheath. The etiology is not clear, but ganglia are believed to be associated with some degenerative or traumatic damage to tendon sheaths.

Signs and Symptoms

There is an obvious swollen defect over the fluid-filled ganglion cyst, and the area often becomes inflamed and painful. The presence and severity of discomfort is variable and may be mild and/or limited to hand motion. The size of the ganglion cyst may vary over time. The cyst should transilluminate.

Diagnostic Studies

Plain films will be negative. Ultrasound will reveal the cystic structure.

OSTEOARTHRITIS

See p. 419.

RHEUMATOID ARTHRITIS

See pp. 418–419.

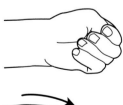

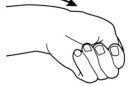

Figure 14.7 Finkelstein's maneuver involves the patient making a fist, with the fingers flexed over the thumb, which is flexed against the palm of the hand, and then holding the fist closed while flexing the wrist toward the ulnar surface.

■ Hip Pain

There are many potential causes of hip pain. Among adults, the most common cause is OA with degenerative changes. In younger patients, the cause is often strain of the muscles or tendons. In comparison to other joints, the hip is often difficult to assess, in part because much of the joint and its periarticular structures lie deeper than those of other joints.

As with other joint-specific pain, it is critical to obtain a history of the pain's onset, progression, and nature, starting with the questions in Box 14.1. Previous experience with hip pain as well as inflammatory or degenerative conditions must be explored. History of recent activities and trauma is important.

The examination begins with noting the patient's posture and apparent limitations or discomfort with walking, sitting, rising, and so forth. The ROM should be thoroughly tested, actively, passively, and against resistance. Note pain, crepitus, clicking, and limitations.

OSTEOARTHRITIS

OA causes degenerative hip changes and is a frequent cause of hip pain in adults, becoming more prevalent after age 50. In younger patients, it may be secondary to trauma or congenital problems, such as a congenital hip dislocation or slipped capital femoral epiphysis. See p. 419.

TROCHANTERIC BURSITIS

Trochanteric bursitis involves a presumed inflammation or irritation of the gluteus maximus bursa, which surrounds the greater trochanter. Other problems that result in changes in the patient's gait tend to increase the stress on the joint.

Signs and Symptoms

The patient presents with pain from the lateral hip and thigh to the knee or numbness. Pain is precipitated by walking, climbing, or prolonged standing. There is point tenderness at the greater trochanter, with increased pain on resisted abduction and external rotation.

Diagnostic Studies

X-rays are usually not helpful and may show no abnormalities.

ASEPTIC/AVASCULAR NECROSIS OF THE FEMORAL HEAD

This condition involves bone deterioration associated with diminished circulation stemming from trauma or other disorders, such as malignancy, sickle cell disease, lupus, infections, or Legg-Calvé-Perthes disease. It is also associated with the use of corticosteroids and radiation treatment. Avascular necrosis can also affect other structures, such as the humeral head and knee.

Signs and Symptoms

The patient presents with complaints of hip pain and difficulty bearing weight. There is a history of an offending medication, trauma, or condition. Actual onset of pain can be very sudden or gradually recognized. In addition to weight bearing, other activities, such as coughing and other non-weight-bearing movements, often increase pain, and the pain often persists at rest and occurs at night. ROM is significantly limited. Pain often radiates down the thigh.

Diagnostic Studies

Early in the progression, plain films may be normal or reveal increased bone density. As collapse of the affected bone occurs, the density increases. However, these changes may not be evident until the disorder is very advanced. For this reason, definitive diagnosis is made with MRI, which is more sensitive than plain films. Bone scan will show increased uptake in the region surrounding the necrotic bone.

TENDONITIS

This inflammation of the iliopsoas tendon typically follows overuse activities, with strain and/or inflammatory changes. The condition can be acute or chronic.

Signs and Symptoms

The patient usually can identify recent activities that included repetitive motions and/or risk for straining tendon structures related to hip. The onset of pain is delayed until some time following the repetitive activity. The pain is localized and increases with further activity. There is often a snapping or catching sensation. Point tenderness and swelling may be present.

Diagnostic Studies

The diagnosis is typically made on physical findings and history alone. Plain films will be normal. While an MRI or ultrasound may reveal the injury to tendon, these studies are not usually indicated or ordered.

INFLAMMATORY ARTHRITIS

RA and other forms of inflammatory arthritis, such as gout and Reiter's syndrome, should be considered in assessment of hip pain. See elsewhere in this chapter.

SLIPPED FEMORAL CAPITAL EPIPHYSIS

This condition causes hip pain in adolescents. Slipped femoral capital epiphysis involves slippage of the femoral epiphysis on the femoral neck. It is more common in overweight male adolescents during a time of rapid growth. Because the patient often presents with referred pain to the groin, thigh, or knee, diagnosis and treatment are frequently delayed.

Signs and Symptoms

Progression of symptoms is usually gradual, with stiffness progressing to pain and subsequent development of a limp. There is usually no history of preceding activity or trauma. Pain often involves the buttocks and/or groin and can radiate to the medial knee. The presentation may be knee pain, with normal knee examination. Comfort is increased with external rotation of the hip;

passive internal rotation of flexed hip increases pain. If advanced, avascular necrosis may occur, resulting in collapse of the femoral head. The condition is often bilateral, although the complaint may be limited to one hip.

Diagnostic Studies

Plain films with anteroposterior and lateral frog leg views reveal widening of the epiphyseal line and/or femoral displacement.

■ Knee Pain

The knee is vulnerable to injury from recreational and occupational activities and a variety of conditions. Assessment of the knee requires skill and practice in performing special maneuvers, such as McMurray's test and tests of ligament integrity, including the drawer test and Lachman's test.

This section does not address knee fractures. However, the Ottawa knee rules provide a set of evidence-based criteria by which to determine when radiographs of the knee are warranted following trauma. The criteria have been shown to have 100% sensitivity and 49% specificity for fracture of the knee. According to the findings, films should be ordered only if at least one of the following criteria are met: the patient is at least 55 years of age, tenderness is present at the tibial head, isolated tenderness is present at the patella (i.e., no other knee tenderness), the patient cannot flex the knee to 90 degrees, or the patient cannot bear weight for four steps (i.e., two steps on each foot) even with limping.

A number of special maneuvers are useful in differentiating the cause of knee pain. These are shown in Figures 14.8, 14.9, and 14.10 and referred to in subsequent sections, as appropriate.

MENISCUS (LATERAL, MEDIAL) TEAR

Tears or disruptions of the meniscus sheath of cartilage are associated with osteoarthritis in older persons and with athletic activities in younger persons.

Signs and Symptoms

There is typically a sudden onset of pain and swelling over the lateral or medial joint line as well as locking and painful popping. Onset often follows a twisting injury. Point tenderness is present over the joint line, with mild effusion. A positive McMurray's test is often present (see Fig. 14.8).

Diagnostic Studies

If meniscal tear is suspected, plain films are of little use, as they are usually negative. An MRI will reveal the defect in most cases. Arthroscopy can be performed alternatively or as a follow-up to the MRI.

LIGAMENTOUS INJURIES

The anterior, medial, and lateral knee ligaments are vulnerable to injury in athletic activities. The mechanism through which the anterior cruciate ligament (ACL) is typically injured involves deceleration combined with sudden turning or pivoting. The medial collateral ligament (MCL) is most prone to injury

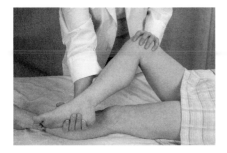

Figure 14.8 McMurray's test assesses the menisci. The medial meniscus is tested with the hip flexed and the knee externally rotated as the examiner moves the knee from full flexion to extension. To test the lateral meniscus, the knee is internally rotated during the procedure. A snap heard or felt during this maneuver suggests a tear of the tested meniscus.

through motions that place valgus stress on the knee. Compared with ACL and MCL injury, damage to the lateral collateral ligament (LCL) is much rarer but typically occurs when sudden varus stress is placed on the knee.

Signs and Symptoms

The patient often relates history of an acute trauma followed by onset of pain, swelling, and limited mobility. Often patients recall hearing or feeling a "pop" at the moment of injury. ACL injury is identified through a positive drawer (see Fig. 14.9) and/or Lachman's test (see Fig. 14.10). Laxity of the LCL is assessed by placing varus stress on the knee with the leg both extended and flexed.

Diagnostic Studies

Radiographs are generally not indicated. If there is an ACL injury, plain film may reveal the presence of a tibial avulsion fracture. Tears are revealed with MRI.

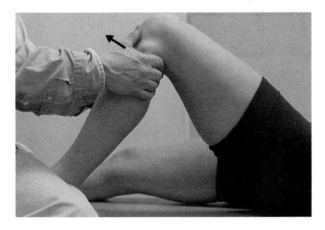

Figure 14.9 The drawer sign is elicited by the examiner holding the patient's leg at the level of the tibial tubercle and pulling anteriorly on the lower leg as the patient's knee is flexed at 90 degrees. The test is positive for anterior cruciate ligament injury when there is laxity and forward motion and for posterior cruciate ligament injury if there is laxity in posterior movement.

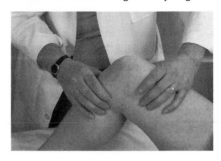

Figure 14.10 Lachman's test is performed with the patient's knee flexed to 30 degrees, noting laxity in anterior and posterior movement of the lower leg with the maneuver. Laxity of the medial collateral ligament is assessed by placing valgus stress on the knee first with the leg extended and next with it flexed at 30 degrees.

CHONDROMALACIA PATELLA

Chondromalacia patella is seen in young active persons of either gender. The condition is also commonly called patella-femoral syndrome and runner's knee. In some cases, this condition is associated with other problems, such as congenitally high-riding patellae and tight hamstrings.

Signs and Symptoms

The pain involves the anterior knee, often develops gradually, and is moderate in intensity. For some, there is sudden onset of patellar pain. The pain is often noticed when rising to stand after sitting for a prolonged time. Runners sometimes indicate that their discomfort was first noticed when running downhill or walking up and down stairs. The pain is relieved during rest. Pain can be reproduced by pressing the patella against the femoral condyles, and there is tenderness around the patella. Other maneuvers that reproduce the pain include applying pressure against the patella as the patient extends the lower leg, flexing the quadriceps, and moving the patella from side to side. Crepitus and effusion are often present.

Diagnostic Studies

Diagnostic studies are not necessarily warranted. However, sunrise x-rays may reveal irregular surfaces of the patella.

PATELLAR TENDONITIS

Tendonitis can develop in any of the knee tendons but is most common with the patellar tendon. It most commonly affects boys during their teens and is also referred to as jumper's knee.

Signs and Symptoms

The patient complains of pain inferior to the patella, at the site of the patellar tendon. The pain is often vague and increases with walking, climbing stairs, or jumping. There is point tenderness over the tendon, and pain can be reproduced by having the patient extend the knee against resistance. There is usually no effusion or crepitus.

Diagnostic Studies

None are indicated.

PREPATELLAR BURSITIS

Bursitis often accompanies tendinitis and is also associated with mild trauma. Prepatellar bursitis is also called *housemaid's knee,* which is common to persons whose occupation requires extended periods of kneeling, such as plumbers and carpet layers. This bursitis can also be caused by an infection.

Signs and Symptoms

The patient complains of pain in the area inferior to and over the patella, and there is swelling and inflammation of the bursa. The swelling and pain can occur suddenly, and there is point tenderness over the affected area. The pain is worse with activity and does not bother the patient at night. The problem can become chronic.

Diagnostic Studies

No diagnostic studies are generally performed. However, aspiration of the bursa can be performed to assess for crystalline deposits (gout) or signs of infection.

OSGOOD-SCHLATTER DISEASE

This self-limited condition occurs in adolescents and involves inflammation of the site where the patellar tendon inserts on the tibia.

Signs and Symptoms

The patient complains of pain centered 2 to 3 inches inferior to the patella. The pain ranges from mild to severe. Pain may occur primarily only with extensive activity or persist regardless of activity level. Point tenderness and swelling are often present.

Diagnostic Studies

Images are not necessary, as the diagnosis is made on history and physical findings. However, if plain films are ordered, they often reveal an area of ossification over the tibial tubercle.

BAKER'S CYST

This is a popliteal cyst that often arises secondary to some other knee condition or injury. This synovial cyst develops from fluid of the gastrocnemio-semimembranous bursa.

Signs and Symptoms

Baker's cysts can cause mild to moderate discomfort in the posterior knee/popliteal space. The cyst is palpable as an area of fullness. Other physical findings depend on associated knee problems, such as meniscal tear.

Diagnostic Studies

Diagnosis is typically based on physical findings of the palpable cyst. However, an ultrasound of the popliteal space will provide definitive diagnosis.

OSTEOARTHRITIS

See p. 419.

INFLAMMATORY ARTHRITIS

See p. 418.

■ Ankle and Foot Pain

Although this section does not address fractures, the Ottawa ankle and Ottawa foot rules provide evidence-based criteria to determine when, following acute trauma/injury, radiographs are warranted. These are summarized in Table 14.3. The identified specificity and sensitivity are based on adequate training in application of the rules.

SPRAINS

Sprains are the most common of all ankle injuries. Most ankle sprains involve the lateral ligament complex and are caused by forceful inversion and plantar flexion.

Signs and Symptoms

The patient relates the history of an injury followed by sudden onset of pain. Pain is noted in the region of the strained muscles or ligaments with local tenderness on palpation. Ankle stability is assessed in a manner similar to that used to test the ligaments of the knee. By immobilizing the lower leg, grasping the foot while applying anterior and posterior stress, a drawer test is achieved. Valgus and varus pressure can also be applied, with inversion and eversion of the foot. Sprains can be classified using the Ottawa guidelines to provide information concerning the degree of disability and requirements for treatment. Table 14.4 lists the classifications for strains.

Diagnostic Studies

Unless indicated by the presence of one of the findings described by the Ottawa ankle rule, no diagnostic imaging is warranted.

Table 14.3	
Ottawa Ankle and Foot Rules	
Ankle Rule: Order Film If One of the Following Is Met	**Foot Rule: Order Film If One of the Following Is Met**
Inability to bear weight for four steps (both immediately and in emergency department)	Inability to bear weight for four steps (both immediately and in emergency department)
Bone tenderness at posterior edge or tip of either malleolus	Bone tenderness at navicular or base of fifth metatarsal
Sensitivity = 100%	Sensitivity = 100%
Specificity = 79%	Specificity = 79%

Table 14.4	

Classification of Strains

Grade	Degree of Injury
I	Partial tear but no instability or opening of the joint on stress maneuvers
II	Partial tear with some instability indicated by partial opening of joint on stress maneuvers
III	Complete tear with complete opening of joint on stress

PLANTAR FASCIITIS

Plantar fasciitis is often incorrectly referred to as heel spur pain. In fact, this condition can occur in the absence of a calcaneal spur. It involves inflammation of the plantar fascia associated with biomechanical tension on the fascia, most commonly involving the site of insertion at the calcaneal tubercle.

Signs and Symptoms

The history includes pain on the undersurface of the heel, worse upon weight bearing after periods of rest or dorsiflexion of the toes. It can be present in one or both feet, but bilateral problems may represent an early symptom of gout, RA, or ankylosing spondylitis. There is point tenderness at the fascia insertion site.

Diagnostic Studies

Images are not warranted. The absence of a calcaneal spur does not rule out the condition. However, plain films can rule out stress fracture.

ACHILLES TENDINITIS

Chronic overuse of the muscles of the calf or extreme stress on the Achilles tendon from activities such as jumping can lead to inflammation.

Signs and Symptoms

Passive stretching of the tendon by dorsiflexion of the ankle reproduces this pain. Tendon ruptures may occur. The patient cannot stand on the ball of the foot and has tenderness and hemorrhage at the site of rupture. The ankle ROM is usually diminished. Thompson's test is positive if a rupture has occurred. Thompson's test involves squeezing the calf, a maneuver that causes plantar flexion in a normal foot. With Achilles tendon rupture, there is a loss of movement in the foot when the calf is squeezed.

Diagnostic Studies

X-ray can be helpful to rule out fracture. Ultrasound identifies the degree of tendon thickening.

HALLUX VALGUS, OR BUNION

This is an enlargement of the metatarsophalangeal joint of the great toe resulting in lateral deviation.

Signs and Symptoms

Pain and deformity are the initial complaints with soft tissue tenderness and redness.

Diagnostic Studies

X-rays will rule out degenerative changes and differentiate soft tissue injuries from deformity.

GOUT

The great toe is the most common site of gouty arthritis, which can also affect other areas of the foot or ankle. See p. 437.

OSTEOARTHRITIS

See p. 419.

RHEUMATOID ARTHRITIS AND OTHER FORMS OF INFLAMMATORY ARTHRITIS

See p. 419.

■ Myalgia

Myalgia, or muscle pain, is a nonspecific complaint accompanying many conditions. The history and physical examination are essential in arriving at a definitive diagnosis. Whereas myalgia is a finding in many conditions, it is the central complaint in others, which are described in the following sections.

FIBROMYALGIA

Myalgia is often the primary complaint in fibromyalgia. See p. 419.

POLYMYALGIA RHEUMATICA

Polymyalgia rheumatica is usually identified in adults aged 60 or older. The actual etiology of this condition is unknown. Giant cell arteritis occurs in about 15% of those with polymyalgia rheumatica, and the two conditions may be different expressions of the same etiology.

Signs and Symptoms

The patient typically complains of sudden onset of widespread pain. Commonly affected sites include the neck, shoulders, and pelvis. Pain is accompanied by fatigue and stiffness. The stiffness is most profound in the morning. There is no actual muscle weakness. Unlike RA, there is no small joint inflammation and effusion.

Diagnostic Studies

The C-reactive protein and sedimentation rate are often elevated. Biopsy and EMG are normal.

RHEUMATOID ARTHRITIS

Although RA typically affects multiple joints, it is not unusual for patients to present with complaints of muscle aches. See pp. 418–419.

INFECTION

A variety of infections cause varying degrees of myalgia. Myalgia is a common component of viral syndrome.

Signs and Symptoms

The patient describes acute onset of symptoms, which often includes complaints more specific to the infectious agent. There is often an elevated temperature and signs of infection.

DRUG-INDUCED MYALGIA

Myalgia is associated with several medications, including diuretics, anticonvulsants, lipid-lowering agents, hydralazine, chloroquine, and procainamide.

Signs and Symptoms

The signs and symptoms are dependent on the medication taken. If the myalgia is related to rhabdomyolysis, the urine is often reddish-brown.

Diagnostic Studies

In general, no diagnostic studies are ordered. However, when drug-induced myalgia is present, there is often eosinophilia. For drug-induced SLE, ANA is positive. For rhabdomyolysis myalgia, the serum creatine kinase is significantly elevated.

Conclusion

All evaluations of muscle and joint problems should be made with concern for the patient's optimal function and pain reduction. The possibility of systemic disease should be ruled out, and x-rays should accompany the examination. Injury may result in an insurance claim that requires clear and concise documentation, which should always be a result of detailed and follow-up examinations.

SUGGESTED READINGS

Bickley, L.S., & Szilagyi, P.G. (2003). *Bates' Guide to Physical Examination and History Taking.* Philadelphia: Lippincott, Williams, and Wilkins.

Dillon, P.M. (2003). *Nursing Health Assessment: A Critical Thinking, Case Studies Approach.* Philadelphia: F.A. Davis.

Greene, W.B. (2005). *Essentials of Musculoskeletal Care*, 2nd ed. Rosemont, IL: American Academy of Orthopaedic Surgeons.

Mercier, L.R. (2008). *Practical Orthopedics*, 6th ed. St. Louis: Mosby.

Swartz, M.H. (2005). *Textbook of Physical Diagnosis: History and Examination.* Philadelphia: Saunders.

Chapter 15

NEUROLOGICAL SYSTEM

Mary Jo Goolsby • Laurie Grubbs

Neurological conditions are commonly encountered in primary care settings. Often neurological problems result in nonspecific symptoms that require careful investigation for timely diagnosis. Some of the content described in this chapter overlaps that in others. For instance, dementia and delirium are described here in detail but are also addressed in the chapters addressing mental health (Chapter 17) and elderly patients (Chapter 20). Hearing changes and sensory vision are addressed in Chapters 4 and 5, respectively.

History

■ Chief Complaint and the History of Present Illness

The history of present illness should include the primary symptom or constellation of symptoms, the associated factors, and the onset and duration of the symptoms. Ask the patient to describe the chief complaint in his or her own words. Ask whether the primary symptom began acutely or gradually and whether an injury or traumatic event precipitated the onset of symptoms. If an injury was involved, explore the mechanism of injury, any associated loss of consciousness, and emergent treatments at the time of injury. Ask whether there has been any change in the character, severity, location, or duration of the symptoms. Identify measures that make the symptom better or worse (e.g., lying down, movements, Valsalva, medications).

■ General History and the Review of Systems

The general history should include a review of all body systems because symptoms of neurological diseases often overlap with other systems. For example, endocrine disorders may manifest themselves with symptoms of lethargy, fatigue, dizziness, or paresthesias; musculoskeletal disorders may manifest as weakness, muscle atrophy, and balance or gait problems; and psychiatric disorders may mimic signs of neurological dysfunction. Therefore, a thorough review of systems is recommended.

Specific to the neurological system, the review should include questions to determine whether the patient has experienced headaches or other pain, sensory changes, motor disturbances, confusion or other altered thought processes, dizziness, syncope, or altered speech.

■ Past Medical and Surgical History

The past medical history should include all disorders for which the patient has been treated in the past. This includes both recent and remote history. If the patient is a child or adolescent, inquire about common childhood illnesses and immunizations. Ask whether the patient has ever been treated for the same or a similar complaint. If so, identify what diagnosis was made at that time, what treatments were rendered, and the response. The history should include conditions that have potential neurological effects, including cardiovascular disorders, such as atherosclerosis or hypertension; endocrine disorders, such as diabetes or hypothyroidism; and malignancies. Include any history of blood transfusions and allergy or adverse reaction to medications or treatments. Explore the history of surgery or interventional procedures and experience with anesthesia. Identify history of any serious injuries. Document all medications, including over-the-counter and herbal agents, as well as the patient's understanding of their indication.

The specific neurologic history should include any past neurological disorders, excluding the presenting chief complaint. This includes stroke, carotid artery disease, head or spine trauma, altered level of consciousness, exposure to toxins or infectious diseases (such as tick bites, spider bites, mononucleosis, insecticides), seizures, or psychiatric disorders.

■ Social History

Ask about the current and past use of tobacco (cigarette, cigar, pipe, smokeless), alcohol, or drugs, including the quantity and duration of each. Document the amount of caffeine the patient consumes per day (include coffee, tea, caffeinated beverages, chocolate). Identify the type and frequency of activity performed and any recreational risks. Document the patient's highest level of education and current and former occupations, including any possible occupational hazards.

■ Family History

Inquire about the immediate family history, including parents, siblings, and children. Family history of neurological diseases, including familial tremor, stroke, cerebrovascular disease, and neuromuscular disorders are particularly important. Establish whether there is a family history of cardiovascular, endocrine, or other conditions with neurological effects. Also include any family history of substance abuse or mental illness.

Physical Examination

The neurological examination should start with a review of the patient's vital signs and general survey. The breadth of the actual examination will depend on the patient's presentation. However, familiarity with each aspect is important, and these are described next.

■ General Appearance and Affect

Observe the patient while entering the room and during the interview. Note general appearance as it relates to nutrition, body habitus, cleanliness, attention to grooming, and affect. Observe physical appearance of the skull, identifying any asymmetry or gross lesions. Note fluidity of movements, gait, and facial expressions. Abnormalities that may be detected during the assessment of general appearance include obesity, cachexia, poor grooming, sullen or flat affect, involuntary movements, hyperactivity, jocularity, and obvious craniofacial deformities.

■ Mental Status

A good screening tool for use in the outpatient setting is the Mini-Mental Status Exam described in detail in Chapter 20. Ask the family or significant other whether the patient's behavior patterns have changed. If the patient does not speak or write English, have an interpreter available during examination. Box 15.1 describes the components of the mental status examination. Mental status abnormalities include confusion, inability to recall recent or remote events, inability to concentrate on conversation or examination, confabulation,

---

Box 15.1

Mental Status Components

Orientation—the patient should normally be aware of person, date, and place. Ask the patient his or her full name, current date, and place in which the examination is being done.

Memory—recent and remote memory should normally be intact. Ask what the patient had for lunch yesterday (recent) and where he or she graduated from elementary school (remote).

Fund of knowledge (take into consideration the patient's level of education)— ask about any recent news events or significant upcoming or past holiday.

Attention span—ability to focus on the interviewer without being easily distracted. Ask the patient to repeat a short list of numbers (e.g., 7-8-9-3-0-2). Inability to repeat six or more numbers indicates attention deficit.

Concentration—ability to concentrate on a question or task. Ask the patient to remember three unrelated words (*red, happy,* and *five*) and then to repeat them in 5 minutes, or ask the patient to count backward from 100 by 7.

Language—use and understanding of language. Ask the patient to write a full sentence or to spell *world* backward. Distinguish between dysphonias and dysarthrias, as these indicate mechanical disturbances often due to cranial nerve dysfunction. Assess fluency of speech by asking the patient to repeat "no ifs, ands, or buts about it." Dysfluent speech is Broca's aphasia. Speech that is devoid of content indicates Wernicke's aphasia.

Abstract thoughts—ask the patient to interpret a common proverb (e.g., a stitch in time saves nine), or ask the patient to answer an abstract question (e.g., "Is my sister's brother a man or a woman?").

inappropriate crying or laughter, slurred speech, word-finding difficulty, jocularity, or difficulty with abstract reasoning.

■ Cranial Nerve Examination

Examination of the cranial nerves (CNs) offers information about localization of the abnormality. Table 15.1 summarizes the CN examination.

Table 15.1	

Cranial Nerve Examination

Cranial Nerve	Technique
CN I, olfactory	After establishing patency of nostrils, assess ability to recognize smell such as alcohol swab, soap, or coffee (never ammonia); test one side at a time. (Abnormalities: inability to discriminate between odors, asymmetric sense of smell)
CN II, optic	Check visual acuity, visual fields; observe optic disk. (Abnormalities: diminished vision, optic disk pallor, papilledema; see Chapter 5)
CN II, optic	Test pupil responses to light and accommodation. (Abnormalities: asymmetry of pupil size or reaction, ptosis; see Chapter 4)
CN III, oculomotor CN IV, trochlear CN VI, abducens	Observe relative position of each eye and eye movements. (Abnormalities: asymmetrical gaze, nystagmus, limited movement of either eye or both eyes)
CN V, trigeminal	Assess facial and corneal sensation and masseter muscles tone/strength. (Abnormalities: asymmetric facial sensation, inability to blink upon threat, inability to clench jaw, jaw pain)
CN VII, facial	Observe facial symmetry during conversation, at rest, during exaggerated expressions, assess strength of eyelids, taste on the anterior two-thirds of the tongue, sensation and elevation of the palate. (Abnormalities: decreased or absent taste, palate numbness, facial asymmetry or droop, asymmetric facial sensation)
CN VIII, vestibulocochlear	Assess hearing and balance. (Abnormalities: positive Romberg, poor balance, altered acuity of hearing, tinnitus)
CN IX, glossopharyngeal CN X, vagus	Assess swallowing, gag reflex, and quality of voice; observe palate elevation, taste and sensation. (Abnormalities: absent gag reflex, dysphagia, asymmetry or deviation of uvula, asymmetric decreased/absent taste or numbness of the tongue, hoarseness/altered voice quality)
CN XI, spinal accessory	Assess head movement, strength of sternocleidomastoid (SCM) and trapezius muscles. (Abnormalities: asymmetric movements or weakness.) *Note:* Both central and peripheral lesions cause ipsilateral SCM weakness: central lesions cause ipsilateral trapezius weakness, whereas peripheral lesions cause contralateral trapezius weakness.

Continued

Table 15.1

Cranial Nerve Examination—cont'd

Cranial Nerve	Technique
CN XII, hypoglossal	Observe tongue position and movement. (Abnormalities: fasciculations, atrophy, tongue or palate deviation) The tongue will deviate *toward* the side of the lesion.

■ Motor Function

If possible, the assessment of motor function should begin as the patient walks into the room and becomes seated. Note the strength of handshake. Observe posture, resting movements of limbs, blinking frequency, and facial movements. More detailed assessment involves attention to isolated muscle groups, noting strength, tone, bulk, and contour of muscles. Box 15.2 provides one scale for grading muscle strength. Abnormalities include a lack of muscle tone, rigidity, cogwheel rigidity, atrophy, asymmetric strength, spasticity, flaccidity, fasciculations, and tremor.

■ Reflexes

Test deep tendon reflexes in all extremities. Some patients will have diminished or absent reflexes, which is a normal variant providing that the finding is symmetrical. If necessary, reinforcement can be accomplished by having the patient clench the jaws or tighten muscles of extremities not being tested. The grading scale for reflexes is provided in Box 15.2. The nerves related to each of the reflexes are listed in Box 15.3. Special reflex maneuvers include the Babinski reflex, assessing for upper motor neuron lesions of the lower extremities, and the Hoffman response, assessing for upper motor lesions of the upper extremities. Abnormalities of the deep tendon reflexes include hyperreflexive responses, with clonus. Diminished or absent reflexes are particularly important if limited to specific sites, while others remain intact.

Box 15.2

Reflex Grades

0 = absent
1+ = hyporeflexia
2+ = normal
3+ = hyperreflexia
4+ and 5+ = abnormally strong contractions with clonus

Box 15.3

Deep Tendon Reflexes

Biceps: C5, C6
Brachioradialis: C5, C6
Triceps: C6, C7
Patellar: L3, L4
Achilles: S1

■ Coordination

Test fluidity of movements. Inability to coordinate volitional movements suggests cerebellar dysfunction. Also note any involuntary movements, such as tremors, or an inability to perform tests. Box 15.4 lists coordination tests.

■ Cerebrovascular

Auscultation of the carotid arteries is an important portion of the neurological examination, particularly for elderly patients or those with a history of tobacco abuse. The patient should be asked to hold his or her breath during auscultation. A bruit in the carotid artery may be an indicator of potential stroke or carotid artery stenosis and should be followed by further tests, such as carotid duplex and carotid ultrasound.

■ Funduscopic Examination

The funduscopic examination is fully described in Chapter 5, p. 97.

■ Sensory Examination

The sensory examination should be the final portion of the neurological examination. The sensory examination indicates the patient's ability to interpret cutaneous sensory information. The test is performed with a clean, unused safety pin, the end

---

Box 15.4

Coordination Tests

Finger to nose testing—ask the patient to touch your index finger with his or her index finger, then touch his or her nose repeatedly. Poor coordination of movement indicates dysmetria.

Rapid alternating movements—ask the patient to perform rapid pronation and supination of the hand on his or her thigh or on the examining table.

Heel-to-shin testing—ask the patient to take the heel of one side and repeatedly move up and down the shin of the opposite leg.

Romberg—ask the patient to stand with feet together, arms abducted outward with palms up, and eyes closed. Positive Romberg is observed as a swaying motion, or inability to maintain balance, and indicates cerebellar dysfunction.

of a cotton swab, and a tuning fork. Test each dermatome individually for sharp/dull and vibratory discrimination. Asymmetry of sensation implies impaired sensory distribution to the particular dermatome being tested.

Differential Diagnosis of Chief Complaints

■ Headache or Cephalalgia

Headache is one of the most prevalent presenting complaints in the outpatient clinical setting, as well as a leading cause of missed days of work. The occasional headache sufferer accounts for the expenditure of billions of dollars annually for over-the-counter symptom remedies. Those who suffer one or fewer headaches per month are unlikely to seek professional advice; however, those who suffer chronic pain of two or more episodes per month are more likely to consult their health-care provider.

The considerable frequency of headache in the general population has led to the development of the International Headache Society (IHS) classification of headaches (IHS, 2004). This classification is useful for appropriate diagnosis and treatment of headaches. Headaches are broadly categorized as primary (e.g., migraine, tension, or cluster) and secondary (associated with space-occupying masses, infection, trauma, or substances).

History

The history is critical to head pain assessment and is often more telling than the physical examination. The headache history should follow the basic history format, with an emphasis on the head pain episode(s). Key elements of the history should include full symptom analysis. Have the patient describe the pain in his or her own words (throbbing, aching, pressure, sharp, stabbing), rate the severity (on scale of 1 to 10), and point to the area of pain. An account of activities preceding the onset of the headache(s) may help to identify potential triggers, such as straining, exertion, coitus, foods, substances, and the like—although the relationship may be coincidental rather than causative. Determine whether onset of pain was acute or gradual in onset and its duration. If similar headaches have been experienced previously, ask about prior treatments and response. Identify any associated symptoms, such as fever, nausea, vomiting, confusion, stiff neck, or vision changes, as well as the history of any prodromal symptoms or aura. Determine whether the patient has recently altered any habits, such as caffeine intake. Identify all recently used over-the-counter or prescribed drugs, illicit/recreational drugs, tobacco, and alcohol. Determine whether the patient has recently experienced or been exposed to a viral or bacterial infection, traveled out of the country, or had exposures to any environmental toxins. Inquire about a history of lung disease or obstructive sleep apnea (OSA), since cerebral hypoxia can cause headache. Ask about any recent trauma, specifically a fall or blow to the head. Explore with the patient his or her occupation, habits, family stressors, marital relationship, sexual factors, social relationships, hobbies, and coping strategies. A thorough psychosocial investigation should precede additional testing. See the Red Flag box for headache presentations.

RED Flag ◀ **Red Flags in the Assessment of Patients with Headaches**

- Acute onset, severe headaches described as "the worst headache of my life" in a patient who has no history of headache
- Unrelenting headaches, unrelieved with conservative treatments or with pain that steadily worsens
- New-onset headaches in patients over 50 years of age without previous history of headache
- Lancinating, "ice-pick" head pain
- Severe headaches associated with a stiff neck and/or fever
- Persistent headaches following trauma to the head or neck
- Headaches that are significantly different in pattern or severity in a patient with a longstanding chronic headache history

---

For recurrent headaches, a headache diary is helpful in arriving at a definitive diagnosis. Although details can be simply recorded on a calendar, a number of headache diaries are available and downloadable via the Internet. Regardless of the format used, the diary should provide a space for the patient to identify daily whether a headache was experienced. When headache is experienced, the form should allow the patient to identify the type, severity, and duration of pain experienced; accompanying symptoms; treatment and response; and any suspected triggers.

Physical Examination

The neurological examination for headache should include all of the basic elements with an emphasis on the cranial nerves. Vital signs should be recorded, noting blood pressure and heart rate to assist in determining possible vascular components of the headache, and any fever, which may indicate an inflammatory or infectious process. The physical examination should include examination of the eyes/fundi, neck, throat, sinuses, and nose. Pay particular attention to the funduscopic examination, which can provide information about increased intracranial pressure. Palpate the head and temporal arteries for any gross abnormalities. The remainder of the neurological examination should be conducted to detect any sensory or motor dysfunction, difficulty with coordination, diminished reflexes, or altered mental status. Lesions/tumors of the brain, in particular, may cause subtle or insidious symptoms, requiring a thorough examination and strict attention to detail.

Patients exhibiting any of the red flags noted previously require immediate definitive diagnosis. For example, any patient with an acute, severe headache, described as "the worst headache of my life," with or without associated symptoms, should be referred immediately to the emergency department because this type of complaint may indicate an intracranial bleed. Any patient with headache associated with fever and stiff neck should be referred to the emergency department for evaluation of possible meningitis. Any patient over the age of 50 with new onset of headache that is unrelieved by medication and without previous history of headache should trigger suspicion of a space-occupying lesion, and imaging studies should be obtained to further assess the complaint.

Diagnostic Studies

Depending on the presentation and findings, further studies may be warranted. Box 15.5 provides a brief discussion of diagnostic studies relevant to the assessment of headache.

MIGRAINE HEADACHE

Migraine is one of the most common vascular headache types and accounts for a significant percentage of clinic and emergency department visits each year. They occur more frequently in women, with the typical onset at approximately age 6 through adolescence. The majority of patients report a family history of

---

Box 15.5

Diagnostic Studies for Headache

Magnetic resonance imaging (MRI) with and without contrast is the test of choice for diagnosis of occult lesions and organic disorders unless contrast is otherwise contraindicated. The MRI should be performed in the sagittal, axial, and coronal planes.

Computerized tomographic (CT) scan is a useful screening tool for emergent detection of expanding mass lesions such as subdural or epidural hematoma, hemorrhagic stroke, or large mass lesions. CT with contrast will help to visualize mass lesions, although it is less sensitive than MRI. CT of the brain also helps to determine evidence of hydrocephalus.

Plain skull films are helpful in identifying bony, extracranial abnormalities, such as skull fractures or lesions. However, they lack the sensitivity to diagnose intracranial abnormalities.

Lumbar puncture (LP) is an invasive test to be performed only when symptoms warrant and if no expanding mass lesion is found on contrast MRI of the brain. Patient must be fully informed of the risks and benefits of procedure.

Select laboratory studies such as complete blood count (CBC), erythrocyte sedimentation rate (ESR), and basic metabolic profile are used to detect infectious processes, anemia, and metabolic abnormalities. Thyroid function tests (TFTs) identify hypothyroidism.

migraine. Onset of migraine is uncommon after the age of 40 years. Thus, patients with an onset of headache beyond this age should be evaluated for other head pain etiologies. Migraines often subside or completely resolve during pregnancy and menopause. The IHS defines migraine as a recurring, idiopathic headache that generally lasts 4 to 76 hours. They generally do not occur daily and are often associated with the menstrual cycle. The frequency of episodes can be one to four times per month or only several times per year. Migraines can occur with or without aura.

Signs and Symptoms

Typical migraine pain begins unilaterally but may become generalized and may lateralize to the opposite side and/or radiate to the face or neck. The pain ranges from a dull ache to a throbbing or pulsatile pain. The pain is often severe and/or incapacitating and is often aggravated by movement, light, and noise. Accompanying symptoms may include nausea, vomiting, photophobia, phonophobia, osmophobia, dizziness, chills, and/or ataxia. There may be tenderness to palpation of the temporal arteries. Auras, if experienced, may include blurred vision and scotoma and/or other prodromal symptoms such as anorexia, irritability, restlessness, or paresthesias lasting from 30 minutes to 3 hours before the onset of migraine pain. The patient may be able to identify headache trigger(s); common migraine triggers are listed in Table 15.2.

Diagnostic Studies

Although not usually indicated, further diagnostic studies may be desired to rule out other conditions, based on the history and physical examination. These tests can include complete blood count (CBC), erythrocyte sedimentation rate (ESR), metabolic profile, computed tomography (CT) scan with contrast, and magnetic resonance imaging (MRI) of the brain with and without contrast. It is often helpful to ask the patient to keep a headache diary and record any factors precipitating the headache.

Table 15.2		
Headache Triggers: Migraine, Cluster, Tension		
Migraine	Cluster	Tension•
• Stress	• Smoking	• Stress
• Caffeine	• Alcohol	• Fatigue/lack of sleep
• Altered sleep	• Vasodilators	• Anxiety/depression
• Specific foods, missed meals	• Seasonal changes	• Caffeine/tobacco overuse
• Menses	• Altitude changes	• Latent hostility
• Alcohol		
• Hormone supplements		

CLUSTER HEADACHE

One of the most severe and incapacitating forms of headache is the cluster headache, so named because the pain occurs in episodic clusters of attacks. The pain of cluster headache can be so intense as to precipitate suicidal thoughts or actions in order to find relief. Cluster headaches are more common in men, with onset in the second to third decades of life. Rare cases have been reported in children.

Signs and Symptoms

There is usually complaint of headaches that are episodic and unpredictable in nature and that may be cyclic. Episodes often occur more frequently in spring and autumn. Cluster periods last, on average, 2 to 3 months and may remit for months to years. Remissions are typically shorter than 2 years. The pain is not preceded by aura. Cluster headaches have rapid crescendo patterns, peaking in approximately 10 to 15 minutes and often lasting 30 to 60 minutes per episode (rarely lasting over 2 hours each). Attacks occur as frequently as two to three times per day. The pain is generally in the area of the trigeminal nerve and is described as unilateral, penetrating, sharp, excruciating, and unrelenting in nature. There may be associated unilateral lacrimation, nasal congestion or rhinorrhea, pallor, flushing, conjunctival redness, ptosis—all on the *same side* as the pain. Some people may experience bradycardia during the episode. During an episode, the patient is restless, may hold the head, and is often anxious and unable to sit still. Cluster headache triggers are listed in Table 15.2.

Diagnostic Studies

Diagnostic studies and work-up are not definitive but should be selected if needed to rule out other disorders. These include MRI or CT scan of the brain with contrast, dental examination for possible trigeminal neuralgia, ESR, CBC, and basic metabolic profile. An ophthalmologic examination with dilation may help to rule out ocular causes of the pain.

TENSION HEADACHE

Tension headaches are quite common. Whereas many people with episodic tension headaches do not seek treatment, those who suffer from frequent or chronic tension headaches may enlist the help of their provider. Other terms to describe tension headache include stress headache, essential headache, idiopathic headache, and muscle contraction headache. Tension headaches can occur with equal frequency among men and women, in any age group, and within any socioeconomic group.

Signs and Symptoms

Typical symptoms of tension headache include mild to moderate, nonthrobbing, pressure, or squeezing pain that can occur anywhere in the head or neck. The pain often starts slowly as a dull and aching discomfort that progresses to holocranial pain and pressure. The pain can recur intermittently, lasting from minutes to hours, and usually remitting with rest or removal of the stressful trigger. There is usually no associated nausea and vomiting. Although patients may report photophobia and phonophobia, it is less severe than those associated with migraines. Tension headaches are not aggravated by movement or activity. The neck muscles are often tight to palpation. Tension headache triggers are listed in Table 15.2.

Diagnostic Studies

Diagnostics and further work-up should be ordered only if necessary to rule out other conditions.

SUBDURAL HEMATOMA

Subdural hematomas can be either acute or chronic. Acute subdural hematomas are usually associated with an acute head injury and can cause a range of symptoms, including headache and loss of consciousness. A chronic subdural hematoma in the elderly population may enlarge significantly before the patient begins to notice head pain.

Signs and Symptoms

The headache associated with subdural hematoma is generally dull and aching in nature and may be transient. The history often includes a blow to the head, fall, or other injury, which preceded the pain. The pain will gradually worsen over days to weeks. In older adults, the history of head trauma may be more remote than in younger patients. A change in mentation may precede pain in older patients. The physical findings vary depending on the severity of the trauma but may include progressive neurological deterioration, which may advance to include coma.

Diagnostic Studies

A CT scan of the brain is the test of choice in the acute setting and will show both acute and chronic subdural hematoma. An MRI of the brain with and without contrast will demonstrate any associated abnormalities.

SUBARACHNOID HEMORRHAGE

Head trauma is the most common cause of subarachnoid hemorrhage (SAH). However, an SAH can be spontaneous, stemming from a ruptured aneurysm, vascular malformations, uncontrolled hypertension, or hemorrhagic disease. Persons who smoke have a significantly higher risk of SAH. SAH most typically occurs in adults 50 to 60 years of age. *This type of headache represents a true medical emergency and necessitates immediate referral or transfer to a local emergency department for triage and treatment.*

Signs and Symptoms

The pain associated with SAH is generally described as severe and acute in onset. The onset is often described as a thunderbolt or lightening. The severity is described as "the worst headache of my life." It is generally made worse by lying down. There is often associated nausea and/or vomiting and possible rapid deterioration in neurological function.

Diagnostic Studies

A noncontrast CT scan of the brain is the test of choice in the acute setting. If SAH is included in the differential diagnosis, a lumbar puncture is generally not recommended in the acute phase because it may result in increased bleeding or herniation. If a vascular abnormality is found, magnetic resonance angiography or conventional angiogram is generally recommended to determine the exact etiology.

VIRAL OR BACTERIAL MENINGITIS

Meningitis involves inflammatory central nervous system (CNS) disease generally caused by either viral or bacterial infection. The etiology of meningitis includes community acquired, posttraumatic, aseptic, carcinomatous, or transferred from another bodily source. The most common organisms belong to such genera as *Streptococcus, Neisseria (meningitides), Haemophilus (influenzae), Listeria, Staphylococcus (aureus)*—as well as gram-negative bacilli and gram-positive cocci. Meningitis can affect persons of all ages, including children. Patients with meningitis represent a medical emergency and should be referred to an emergency department for treatment.

Signs and Symptoms

The headache associated with meningitis is described as diffuse and throbbing and is often severe or intense in nature. There is usually associated fever, photophobia, phonophobia, nausea/vomiting, and nuchal rigidity. Patients can rapidly decline to delirium, seizures, and, if untreated, coma. On neurological examination, the patient may be lethargic and febrile and have altered mentation along with nuchal rigidity and/or guarding, contracted and sluggish pupils, and a generally "toxic" appearance. Brudzinski's and Kernig's signs are helpful in assessing potential meningeal conditions (see Box 15.6). Delirium or acute

---

Box 15.6

Meningeal Tests

Brudzinski's test—with patient lying on examination table, gently flex the patient's neck to a chin-to-chest position. The test is positive if the patient attempts to lift legs and flex hips to relieve pain caused by the maneuver.

Kernig's test—with patient resting on examination table, hold leg with hip and knee flexed. Without moving the upper leg, slowly extend the knee, straightening the leg. The test is positive if the maneuver results in pain, with the patient flexing the neck in attempt to relieve the pain.

confusion necessitates immediate transfer to an emergency department for treatment, as the patient can rapidly deteriorate to coma.

Diagnostics Studies

Diagnostic tests should include CBC, ESR, C-reactive protein, and CT scan or MRI to rule out a mass lesion. A lumbar puncture (to obtain cerebrospinal fluid [CSF] for cell count, protein, glucose, and cultures) is generally performed only after ruling out a mass through imaging.

CHIARI MALFORMATION

Chiari malformations are brainstem malformations. There are three types of Chiari malfunction. Chiari type I is most often associated with occipital headaches and generally seen in the adult population but can be diagnosed at any age. Type I symptoms may be very vague and transient, and it is often misdiagnosed as another neurological disease. Type II is generally diagnosed in infants or children and is associated with myelomeningocele or other open neural tube defects or in adults with undiagnosed spina bifida occulta or tethered cord. Type III malformation is rare, diagnosed in infants, associated with cervical myelomeningocele or pseudomeningocele, and carries a very poor prognosis.

Signs and Symptoms

The typical presentation of Chiari malformation includes a persistent headache that occurs most often in the occipital area and may radiate diffusely or behind the eyes. The headache is triggered or worsened by the Valsalva maneuver or by flexion/extension of the neck. There is often complaint of neck or skull base pain as well as dizziness or disequilibrium, also worsened by movement or flexion/extension of the neck. Other complaints may include tinnitus and decreased hearing; weakness, numbness, paresthesias, and extremity pain; extreme fatigue, difficulty sleeping, and generalized body weakness; difficulty swallowing and voice hoarseness (often with diminished or absent gag reflex); and altered memory or concentration.

Diagnostic Studies

The test of choice for the diagnosis of Chiari malformation is an MRI of the brain and brainstem with and without contrast.

BRAIN ABSCESS

Brain abscess can be caused by an extension of an existing extracranial infection, extension of a blood-borne infection, intracranial procedures, or penetrating head injury. Infections of the lung, heart, ear, or sinus are the most common sources of abscess transference. The cause is idiopathic in approximately 25% of the cases. Inquire about recent visits to developing countries because abscess is more common and easily spread in these geographic areas, and inquire as well about recent or remote consumption of poorly cooked meats or unwashed vegetables. The most common vector is streptococcus.

The abscess generally causes head pain only after the lesion has enlarged enough to result in mass effect on the brain tissue, so timely treatment for brain abscess requires immediate transfer to an emergency department for neurosurgical and infectious disease consultation.

Signs and Symptoms

If the condition represents an extension of a preexisting problem, the history will be consistent with that condition as well as with the symptoms specifically related to the abscess. The history usually includes a gradual onset of symptoms that progress as the inflammatory process increases. These symptoms include headache, nausea (with or without vomiting), lethargy, and fever. Over time, if the lesion expands, the symptoms progress to include seizures, lethargy, hemiparesis, and altered mental status. If left untreated, the patient can rapidly decline to seizures and coma.

Diagnostic Studies

Diagnostic tests for patients suspected of brain abscess include CBC (may be normal in the early stage or in older patients), ESR, C-reactive protein, and blood cultures (may be negative). An MRI of the brain with and without contrast will show enhancing lesions, and this is the test of choice for localization. Magnetic resonance spectroscopy may also help in determining the activity of the abscess. Lumbar puncture is not recommended in the initial work-up for intracranial abscess.

TUMOR

An intracranial malignancy can result in a wide range of complaints and findings, depending on the size and location of the mass, as they commonly stem from the increased pressure on tissues, obstruction of the circulation, and/or increased intracranial pressure. Because the brain tissue does not feel pain, most patients do not present with headache until the lesion is large enough to significantly increase intracranial pressure. Meningioma is the most likely tumor to cause headache. Brain tumors include benign, primary malignant, and metastatic lesions.

Signs and Symptoms

Progressive neurological deterioration is one of the most common symptoms of an intracranial mass lesion. Many elderly patients may show slow, progressive mental decline over months to years and may be misdiagnosed as depressed or demented. Head pain generally overlies the area of the mass lesion. Tumors of the sella generally refer pain to the vertex. The pain associated with tumors is often described as dull, aching, and transitory. New-onset seizures in the adult population should be considered the result of a mass lesion until proven otherwise. Vomiting without nausea implies increased intracranial pressure. Some persons report improvement in their symptoms for a brief time after vomiting. Unilateral extremity numbness/paresthesias and weakness may be either slowly or rapidly progressive. Mass lesions of the cerebellum may cause disequilibrium or gait disturbance. Acute unilateral hearing loss or tinnitus may imply a lesion of the acoustic nerve, and unilateral visual disturbances may imply a lesion or compression on the optic nerve. The physical examination may reveal alterations in vital signs, particularly new-onset hypertension. The neurological examination may be normal until the lesion exerts enough mass effect to increase intracranial pressure or obstruct the flow of CSF. Focal neurological findings may include anisocoria, unilateral hearing loss, nystagmus, visual field defects, extremity weakness, numbness or paresthesia of the extremities, tongue deviation, and papilledema.

Diagnostic Studies

An MRI of the brain with and without contrast is the imaging study of choice for assessment of intracranial lesions. Magnetic resonance spectroscopy will help to assess cell activity within the tumor. If suspicious for metastasis, imaging of the suspected area may aid in evaluation of the tumor type. If a lesion is found in the cerebellum, an MRI of the cervical spine will help to assess for any drop lesions. Surgical biopsy of the intracranial tumor is the test of choice for definitive diagnosis of tumor type.

TEMPORAL ARTERITIS

Temporal arteritis is also referred to as giant cell arteritis or cranial arteritis. It is characterized by chronic inflammation and the presence of giant cells in large arteries, usually the temporal artery, but can occur in the cranial arteries, the aorta, and coronary and peripheral arteries. It affects the arteries containing elastic tissue, resulting in narrowing and eventual occlusion of the lumen. It occurs more among persons over 50 years of age and is slightly more common in females than in males. The cause is unknown, but there seems to be a genetic predisposition. If left untreated, arteritis can rapidly lead to blindness that is often irreversible.

Signs and Symptoms

The most common chief complaint is bitemporal, frontal, or vertex head pain that is lancinating, sharp, or "ice pick" in nature. The pain can be quite severe and debilitating. Patients often complain of visual changes, including amaurosis, diplopia, blurred vision, visual field cuts, eye pain, periorbital edema, and intermittent unilateral blindness. Other common presenting symptoms include scalp and/or jaw tenderness, facial pain, and tenderness to palpation over the affected artery. The pain is generally hemicranial but can be bilateral or diffuse. There may be eye pain, which is usually bilateral; periorbital edema may be present. Other potential associated symptoms include an intermittent fever (generally low grade), nausea, and/or weight loss.

Diagnostic Studies

In temporal arteritis, the white blood cell count may be elevated, although often it is normal in older patients. The ESR and C-reactive protein may be elevated. Definitive diagnosis of arteritis is determined by temporal artery biopsy. An MRI of the brain with and without contrast will help to rule out other structural causes; however, its use is not definitive for the diagnosis of arteritis. Patients with acute visual change should be referred immediately to a neurologist or neuroophthalmologist to prevent blindness from ischemic optic neuropathy, which occurs in approximately 20% of patients; treatment with corticosteroids should be started immediately while diagnostic studies are completed.

MEDICATION-OVERUSE HEADACHE, OR ANALGESIC REBOUND HEADACHE

Susceptible patients who take analgesic or abortive medications on a frequent basis for recurrent headaches may develop medication-overuse headaches. In addition to the susceptibility of the individual patient, the regularity with which the particular agent is taken is an important variable; overuse or rebound headache should be considered in patients who develop chronic, daily headaches during therapy for primary headaches. Although this discussion is specific to the development of chronic headaches following overuse of headache agents, chronic headaches can also be associated with overuse of or withdrawal from a variety of other agents or may be an adverse effect of a wide range of substances. Withdrawal may require detoxification.

Signs and Symptoms

The headache is usually described as migrainelike. History reveals frequent use of analgesic or abortive agents (acetaminophen, aspirin, compounds, codeine, triptans, etc.) taken, for example, 15 or more times a month, usually for a period of 3 or more months. The chronic daily headaches resolve or revert to the earlier pattern of frequency when the patient is successfully withdrawn from the associated drug for a period of 2 months.

Diagnostic Studies

None are warranted unless to exclude other potential causes. Urine and/ or serum toxicity screens may aid in determining the levels of certain medications.

TRAUMA

Blunt trauma to the head can result in acute or chronic headache, regardless of whether there was loss of consciousness or traumatic brain injury (TBI). Generally, the severity of the trauma is correlated with the duration of the headache, but that is not always the case.

Signs and Symptoms

The headache related to trauma is highly variable in frequency, intensity, and duration and can be difficult to manage. The pain may be localized to the site of the injury or generalized. The patient may be irritable and/or may complain of dizziness, difficulty with concentration, and difficulty sleeping owing to the pain. Stress and/or depression may play a role.

Diagnostic Studies

An acute head injury with complaint of severe headache warrants an emergency CT scan, MRI, and/or skull x-ray to rule out a cerebral contusion, subdural or intracerebral hematoma or hemorrhage, or skull fracture.

CEREBRAL HYPOXIA/EDEMA

Cerebral hypoxia results in edema and can occur in TBI, chronic obstructive pulmonary disease (COPD), and sleep disorders, specifically sleep apnea.

Signs and Symptoms

In TBI, the hypoxia can be severe and neurological injury significant, ranging from temporary loss of consciousness to a vegetative state. In chronic, low-level hypoxia—as seen in COPD and sleep apnea—the headache is dull and persistent. Hypertension may also be present in these individuals.

Diagnostic Studies

The diagnosis for TBI is usually obvious from the history of trauma. For chronic hypoxemia, arterial blood gases, oxygen saturation readings, pulmonary function tests, CBC results, and sleep studies can help in determining the cause.

■ Altered Mental Status

Alteration in mental status is generally a chief complaint of the elderly population. However, some unusual forms of dementia can be diagnosed as early as the second decade of life. The causes of mental status changes include, but are not limited to, Alzheimer's disease, multi-infarct state, stroke, CNS infections, neurodegenerative disorders, head injury, mass lesions, metabolic disorders, and hydrocephalus. It is estimated that approximately 10% to 20% of mental status changes are due to treatable causes, such as vitamin B deficiency, polypharmacy, intoxication or drug abuse, and infectious processes. Chapters 17 (on mental health) and 20 (on older patients) include additional content on altered thought processes. It is important to consider psychiatric conditions in the differential diagnosis for altered mental status.

History

A thorough history of the chief complaint should emphasize the mental status baseline and changes that have occurred. It is best if a family member or significant other can be present when taking the history because the patient may not have full awareness of the mental status changes. Identify when the mental status change was first noted by the patient or others. Determine whether onset was an acute change or developed over time; ask whether the changes are most notable at any particular time of day. Identify the baseline level of function and cognition. Determine the highest level of education, current or previous occupation, and daily routine, including whether ability to perform activities of daily living independently has been affected. Determine whether the patient is aware of any functional change, as patients in the early stages of dementia often have insight into their functional capacity changes. Note whether the patient is easily frustrated with level of abilities or cognition. Ask whether the patient's interpersonal relationships have been altered. Identify any history of excessive use of alcohol or drugs, any exposures to environmental toxins (lead, ammonia, carbon monoxide, heavy metals), or recent trauma. Review all current medications because polypharmacy, especially in the elderly population, can cause states of confusion. Review recent or remote exposure to any infectious disease, such as AIDS, herpes, meningitis, mononucleosis, or syphilis. Explore psychosocial factors, such as depression, anxiety, or the loss of a loved one. See the following box for red flags associated with mental status changes.

RED Flag ◀ **Red Flags in the Assessment of Patients With Mental Status Changes**

- Acute changes associated with fever, stiff neck, or headache
- Acute changes in the elderly (The patient should be worked up for a possible infectious process, particularly urinary tract infections.)
- Acute changes associated with any type of head trauma
- Progressive changes associated with gait disorder and/or incontinence
- Gradual but significant changes

Physical Examination

The neurological examination should focus on assessment of cognition and mental status by using the Mental State Examination or another validated screening instrument. Observation of the patient is a key element in the neurological examination for the patient with mental status changes and should include the patient's dress and personal grooming, affect, any obvious agitation or frustration, and reliance on a significant other for assistance during the history or examination. Note the fluidity of speech and speech content, and note whether the speech reveals a flight of ideas, confabulation, or echolalia (repeating vocalizations of others), as well as whether hallucinations are suggested. Assess orientation by asking the patient to recite his or her full name, current location/place (clinic, hospital, home, etc.), and the date (day of the week, month, or year). Knowledge of time is generally impaired first, followed by place. The inability to recite or recognize one's name implies a significant deficit in mental status. All of the areas addressed in Box 15.1 should be considered during the mental status examination.

Diagnostic Studies

The range of potential diagnostic studies for a complaint of mental status change is immense, and studies should be selected on the basis of history and physical findings. Basic metabolic profile should be considered to determine metabolic abnormalities with particular attention to electrolytes, BUN, creatinine, calcium, and liver functions. Other common studies include serum B_{12} and folic acid levels. For older patients, consider urinalysis to rule out urinary tract infection and chest x-ray and pulse oximetry for respiratory compromise. A CBC with differential can determine evidence of infectious process or anemia. HIV, fluorescent treponemal antibody absorption test (FTA-ABS) for tertiary syphilis, and Lyme serology are important to establish specific infectious condition. An ESR can be used to assess inflammatory process. Thyroid function tests should be considered to evaluate thyroid status.

A 24-hour urine for heavy metals and/or toxicology screen should be considered. An electroencephalogram can determine the presence of subtle seizure activity or localized slow wave activity; or lumbar puncture for CSF studies should be ordered if CNS infection is suspected.

DELIRIUM

Delirium can be observed in both elderly and younger patients and is generally defined as an *acute* confusional state, affecting all aspects of cognition and mentation, and is often related to a treatable disorder. These include an almost endless list of potential causes, such as, but not limited to, the following: intoxication, substance abuse, medication overdose, polypharmacy, infectious processes, mass lesion, intracranial bleed, thyroid imbalance, metabolic disturbances, encephalopathy, anemia, hypoxia, acute obstructive hydrocephalus, vitamin B deficiency, nutritional deficiency, and environmental exposures.

Signs and Symptoms

The signs and symptoms of delirium generally have a more acute or rapidly progressive onset as opposed to the slow, gradual decline noted in the organic dementias. The acute mental status change is often associated with other signs or symptoms—such as hallucinations, illusions, incoherent speech, and constant aimless activity—that help to narrow the differential diagnosis. Table 15.3 describes some of the associated findings for several of the causes of treatable delirium or confusion. The history may reveal trauma, exposure to toxins, or medications if these are responsible for the mental status changes. In spite of the confusion, the patient's sensorium is usually intact, although some conditions (such as intoxication and severe metabolic derangements) result in altered level of consciousness as well.

STROKE

Stroke is one of the leading causes of death in the United States. Patients with stroke often have a history of hypertension, diabetes, cardiac disease, hyperlipidemia, smoking, drug or alcohol abuse, and family history of stroke. Strokes are divided into two main categories: thrombotic and hemorrhagic; however, the two can be difficult to differentiate using clinical signs and symptoms.

Table 15.3	

Select Treatable Causes of Symptoms Associated With Delirium/Confusion

Condition	Findings
Vitamin B deficiencies	Depending on the particular deficiency, peripheral neuropathy, skin and/or mucous membrane changes, fatigue, constipation
Hypothyroidism	Fatigue, depression, skin/hair changes, cold intolerance, constipation, anemia
Infections	Highly dependent on the condition; for meningitis, nuchal rigidity and fever
Nutritional deficit	Weight loss, nausea/vomiting, anorexia, weakness, electrolyte imbalances

Signs and Symptoms

The onset is usually an abrupt altered level of consciousness accompanied by hemiparesis or hemiplegia. Patients may experience confusion, memory impairment, and aphasia. Signs and symptoms vary with the location and severity of the stroke. Mentation and cognitive changes may be temporary or permanent depending on the extent of injury. Communication alterations stemming from fluent or receptive aphasia may be mistaken as dementia.

Diagnostic Studies

A CT scan, without contrast, is the preferred imaging study in early stroke because hemorrhage may be difficult to determine on an MRI in the first 48 hours. In studies of ischemic stroke patients, researchers have shown the reversibility of abnormalities on CT/MRI through the use of thrombolytic therapy within a three-hour window.

PARKINSON'S DISEASE

Although altered mental status is usually not the first manifestation of Parkinson's disease (PD), mild cognitive dysfunction is often seen. Because of the flat affect and facies that patients with PD exhibit, these symptoms may be mistaken for psychosis, depression, or dementia, which can often coexist. PD occurs in all ethnic groups, with approximately equal sex distribution, and usually begins between 45 and 65 years of age. Another form of PD, known as posttraumatic parkinsonism, or dementia pugilistica, is a combination of dementia and parkinsonism that develops in boxers or persons sustaining repeated blows to the head. Parkinsonian symptoms may also occur secondary to a number of other causes, including medications, infections, and toxins. The following discussion is not inclusive of the range of secondary parkinsonism.

Signs and Symptoms

Unilateral pill-rolling tremor at rest is usually the first symptom. The tremor is maximal at rest but absent during sleep and can be differentiated from essential tremor, which is absent at rest and worsens with voluntary movement. The bradykinesia of PD affects gross and fine motor movement, speech volume, swallowing, and blinking. There is generally no muscle weakness, and deep tendon reflexes are normal. Although Alzheimer's disease can manifest with rigidity, bradykinesia, and gait disorders, no resting tremor is seen with Alzheimer's. Nonspecific secondary manifestations include cognitive dysfunction, sleep disturbances, constipation, dysphagia, blurred or double vision, nocturia, frequency, urgency, autonomic dysfunction (such as erectile dysfunction), dizziness, and drooling.

Diagnostic Studies

No diagnostic studies are specific to PD, and the patient should be referred to a neurologist for definitive diagnosis. If secondary parkinsonism is suspected, laboratory studies such as a metabolic profile or toxicology screens may be warranted.

NORMAL PRESSURE HYDROCEPHALUS

The etiology of normal pressure hydrocephalus is not fully understood. It is seen primarily in persons over 60 years of age and involves enlargement of the ventricles, often without increased CSF pressure; intraventricular pressures may be high or normal. One of the theorized causes includes intermittent pressure increases. It is slightly more common in men than in women.

Signs and Symptoms

The patient often first notices some degree of gait disorder, followed by the onset of a "clouding" of thought processes, which gradually progress. The typical picture is a patient who has a triad of gait disturbance, altered thought processes, and urinary incontinence. Strength and sensation are usually within normal limits. However, focal neurological findings are present and include increased deep tendon reflexes, the inability to tandem walk, positive Babinski, and/or positive Romberg.

Diagnostic Studies

Imaging (MRI/CT) should be completed to provide definitive diagnosis.

TUMOR

See pp. 464–465.

BRAIN ABSCESS AND CNS INFECTION

See pp. 463–464.

ORGANIC, PROGRESSIVE DEMENTIAS

Whereas dementia generally affects persons over 60 years of age, persons in the fourth and fifth decades of life can show mental status changes as a result of some offending cause. Although Alzheimer's dementia is a frequent cause of progressive organic dementia, other causes with similar findings include Pick's disease, alcoholism-related dementia, and the causes discussed separately in the previous entries. Chapters 17 and 20 also include brief discussions of progressive dementia of this type.

Signs and Symptoms

Unlike delirium, most organic dementias develop over months to years. There are typically no physical motor or sensory alterations until the condition is advanced. Memory impairment is the predominant symptom. There may be impairment in another area of cognitive functioning, such as with aphasia (producing language as well as understanding it), agnosia (perceptual impairments not due to dysfunction of the primary sensory organ), apraxia (inability to perform complex motor acts), and impairment in executive functioning (inability to plan, organize, sequence, and think abstractly). Progressive mental status changes associated with focal motor or sensory findings should not be attributed to Alzheimer's or Pick's diseases.

Diagnostic Studies

The studies are based on the history and presentation. It is crucial to rule out any correctible cause of confusion or altered mental status in a timely manner.

■ Dizziness and Vertigo

Patients interpret the subjective complaint of dizziness differently. Therefore, it is important to determine a true vertigo, during which the patient experiences a spinning sensation, from lightheadedness, which typically has a different etiology. Table 15.4 differentiates between lightheadedness and dizziness/vertigo.

Table 15.4	
Causes of Vertigo and Lightheadedness	
Symptom	Causes
Lightheadedness/presyncope (sense of faintness)	Dehydration Hypotension Hypoglycemia/hyperglycemia Heart block Infection Cardiovascular and cerebellar perfusion
Vertigo/disequilibrium (sense of motion/spinning)	Vestibular disturbances Middle ear disturbance Cerebellar

History

The typical dimensions of the symptom are important—particularly onset and duration—because many cases of dizziness are paroxysmal, short, and self-limiting. Dizziness that is not vertigo is often associated with quick movement or bending over and is often worse upon first arising in the morning or when rising from a recumbent position. Vertigo, by contrast, describes the sense of spinning. It can occur at any time of the day or night. Many people report vertigo associated with listing to one side while walking, often running into walls or door jams while walking. Nystagmus is often associated with vertigo but rarely with dizziness. Nausea and vomiting can be associated with both dizziness and vertigo.

Dizziness that becomes frequent or lasts extended periods of time deserves closer investigation. Sustained periods of dizziness with near fainting can be a precursor to syncope or stroke and may have a neurovascular or cardiac etiology. Recently, neurocardiogenic syncope, also called vasovagal syncope, has drawn attention as a common cause of dizziness and fainting. It is due to a sudden decrease in blood pressure and heart rate after prolonged standing, with stress, or from dehydration. It is due to sympathetic sensitivity causing a reflexive response that suddenly causes bradycardia and venous dilation. Hypotension and dizziness result.

Dizziness can also be a precursor (or aura) of seizures. Dizziness that leads to disequilibrium can result in inability to drive, falls, and injuries and can be quite disabling for some persons. Lightheadedness in the elderly or in persons with vascular insufficiency is not uncommon. It is crucial to identify any associated symptoms, specifically nausea, vomiting, fevers, vision changes, speech disturbances, and numbness or weakness of the face or extremities.

The history of head or ear trauma as well as exposure to infections should be determined. A thorough review of the patient's current medications must be included because polypharmacy can cause dizziness in many patients. Social and recreational history is important. Activities such as scuba diving, high-elevation hiking, or air travel can contribute to the development of dizziness, as can dehydration related to exercising in the heat. Other potential causes include alcohol or substance abuse. Because dizziness can be associated with hyperventilation or anxiety, ask about a history of anxiety or panic attacks. Review the family history of stroke, seizures, Ménière's disease, or other conditions associated with dizziness or vertigo. Refer to the Red Flag box that lists red flag presentations of dizziness.

RED Flag ◄ **Red Flags in the Assessment of Patients With Dizziness/Vertigo**

- Near fainting or fainting
- Slurred speech, numbness of the face or limbs, or loss of limb movement
- Visual changes, particularly diplopia
- Acute onset, associated with nausea/vomiting

Physical Examination

The neurological examination should focus on vital signs, gait, station, and CN function. Blood pressure should be taken both lying and standing, looking for orthostatic changes. Measure the rate and regularity of the pulse and obtain an electrocardiogram if necessary. Note fever that might indicate infection. The examination should include an assessment of gait, including tandem walking. Gait ataxia is noted when the patient is so uncoordinated that he or she cannot walk a straight line without stumbling. The Romberg test should be performed; a positive Romberg test is noted when the patient is unable to maintain an upright posture, with feet together and arms extended, and sways or falls to the side. The finger-to-nose test should be performed, observing for dysmetria, and rapid alternating movement is tested, observing the smoothness of motion.

CN testing is important, particularly CNs II, III, IV, and VI. The eye nerves are particularly sensitive to increases in intracranial pressure. Note any vision or pupillary changes. Note decreases in visual fields, and note nystagmus on upward, downward, or lateral gaze with extraocular movements. Assess any asymmetry in facial sensation or movements (CN VII), which could indicate a transient ischemic attack or cerebrovascular accident or pressure on the nerve from a tumor. Cranial nerve VIII is the most sensitive to tests for vestibulocochlear abnormalities. Always perform the Rinne and Weber tests to localize hearing loss or tinnitus.

Diagnostic Studies

The studies useful in assessing dizziness are identified in Box 15.7.

BOX 15.7

Diagnostic Studies for Dizziness

MRI of the brain with and without contrast will help to rule out evidence of a mass lesion or demyelinating process.

MRI of the internal auditory canal is sensitive for mass lesions on the inner ear and acoustic nerve.

Audiogram is useful for assessing inner ear and hearing damage. This can also be helpful in assessing inflammatory disorders.

Electronystagmogram is useful for determining eye movements in relation to a stimulus and helps with localizing the lesion to the nerve.

Carotid ultrasound or duplex will determine vascular insufficiency.

Brainstem and auditory evoked potentials help with determining whether the defect lies with the nerve or within the inner ear.

Tilt table test can be performed to rule out neurocardiogenic syncope.

Home blood pressure monitoring may be helpful for those patients with hypo- or hypertension–induced dizziness.

CENTRAL NERVOUS SYSTEM LESIONS

The causes of CNS vertigo include brainstem vascular disease or tumor, arteriovenous malformations, cerebellar tumor, multiple sclerosis, and vertebrobasilar migraine (Aminoff & Kerchner, 2011).

Signs and Symptoms

The findings depend on the location and progression of the lesion. Most patients present with disequilibrium or dizziness. Children may present with gait disorders.

Vertigo from central lesions is constant and causes difficulties with the activities of daily living. Other symptoms may be present, such as CN dysfunction, motor and sensory dysfunction, and cerebellar dysfunction.

Diagnostic Studies

An MRI of the brain with and without contrast is the test of choice for diagnosis of central lesions. An MRI of the internal auditory canal is sensitive for mass lesions on the inner ear and acoustic nerve.

MÉNIÈRE'S DISEASE

The exact cause of Ménière's disease is unknown. However, the symptoms are associated with increased fluid and pressure in the labyrinth.

Signs and Symptoms

Ménière's disease commonly involves a triad of symptoms: severe vertigo, tinnitus, and hearing loss. The vertigo is transient but recurrent. The tinnitus and hearing loss may also be intermittent and/or recurrent but often become worse over time. A sensation of ear fullness may precede an episode. During the episode, vertigo is often debilitating and is associated with nausea and vomiting. Although the tinnitus and hearing loss are usually unilateral, some patients experience bilateral symptoms. Vestibular maneuvers, including Nylen-Barany, are often positive, reproducing the patient's complaint.

Diagnostic Studies

Because the symptoms and findings of Ménière's disease and acoustic neuroma are so similar, MRI is helpful to exclude tumor. A number of other studies, including auditory evoked potentials, are typically performed by specialists.

CENTRAL AUDITORY AND VESTIBULAR SYSTEM DYSFUNCTION

Diseases in this category include acoustic neuroma, vascular compromise, and multiple sclerosis (MS). Acoustic neuromas are benign and are one of the most common intracranial tumors. Due to their location, they affect hearing and speech discrimination.

Vertebrobasilar insufficiency is seen mostly in the elderly and is exacerbated by extension of the neck or changes in head position. Migraines and vascular loops may cause vascular compromise and vertigo. Multiple sclerosis can also cause chronic imbalance and unilateral hearing loss. See under Weakness in Chapter 16, pp. 488–492.

Signs and Symptoms

The vertigo from central lesions is more likely to be persistent and chronic rather than intermittent, as is seen with other causes of vertigo. The dizziness may be described as a constant sense of disequilibrium rather than a true vertigo. Unlike benign positional vertigo, central and vestibular nystagmus is "often nonfatigable, vertical rather than horizontal in orientation, without latency, and unsuppressed by visual fixation" (Aminoff & Kerchner, 2011). Unilateral hearing loss should be suspect for acoustic neuroma or MS. A history of migraines may suggest vascular compromise.

Diagnostic Studies

An MRI with and without contrast of the internal auditory canal is necessary for a definitive diagnosis of acoustic neuroma. Magnetic resonance angiography or a cerebral angiogram is used to diagnose vascular abnormalities. A lumbar puncture and an MRI with and without contrast are necessary for a diagnosis of MS.

VIRAL (SEROUS) OR BACTERIAL (SUPPURATIVE) LABYRINTHITIS

Labyrinthitis is caused by the invasion of the ear by bacteria or a virus. The bacterial is more serious because it may lead to meningitis. Prompt treatment with antibiotics is necessary.

Signs and Symptoms

Labyrinthitis is characterized by severe vertigo, nystagmus, and hearing loss. Suppurative labyrinthitis may be secondary to bacterial otitis media or other bacterial infection. Serous labyrinthitis can be secondary to a variety of viral illnesses, including measles, mumps, chickenpox, influenza, mononucleosis, and adenovirus.

Diagnostic Studies

The diagnosis is mainly made by history and physical examination. A CBC or mono spot can assist in the diagnosis, and a culture of the fluid from the middle ear will differentiate a bacterial from a viral cause.

CHOLESTEATOMA

See Chapter 6, p. 131.

HEAD TRAUMA/PERILYMPHATIC FISTULA

A fistula may form from a blow to the head or from barotraumas significant enough to cause a rupture of the round or the oval window.

Signs and Symptoms

Vertigo, ataxia, nausea, vomiting, and hearing loss can result from this fistula. A medical history provides the necessary information for an index of suspicion for this cause of dizziness.

Diagnostic Studies

In addition to a good history, a CT or MRI of the head can assist in the diagnosis. Surgical repair is necessary.

BENIGN PAROXYSMAL POSITIONAL VERTIGO/ CUPULOLITHIASIS

Benign paroxysmal positional vertigo, or cupulolithiasis, is a common condition resulting from particles or debris into the posterior semicircular canal. It can occur spontaneously with motion or position change or as a result of vascular or labyrinth trauma.

Signs and Symptoms

Characterized by sudden-onset dizziness lasting less than 30 seconds and following a head position change, cupulolithiasis may be accompanied by nystagmus. It usually subsides but may recur at any time.

Diagnostic Studies

In addition to the history, a provocative test for positional nystagmus can be performed, although it is not always positive. The provocative test involves moving the patient quickly from a sitting position to a lying position with the head turned to the side and the head dependent over the side of the examination table. After a few seconds, vertigo and nystagmus occur. This response fatigues with immediate repetition of the test. A CT or MRI may be necessary to rule out CNS lesions; however, the vertigo associated with CNS lesions is not as severe, does not have a latency period, and does not fatigue. The Epley repositioning maneuver, also called vestibular exercises, can assist in alleviating the problem.

REFERENCES

Aminoff, M.J., & Kerchner, G.A. (2011). Nervous system disorders. In S.J. McPhee, M.A. Papdakis, & M.W. Rabow (Eds.), *Current Medical Diagnosis and Treatment* (pp. 927–994). New York: Lange Medical Books/McGraw Hill.

International Headache Society (IHS). *Classification of Headaches.* www.ihs-classification.org/en/02_klassifikation (accessed March 17, 2011).

Olesen, J. (Ed.). (2004). International classification of headache disorders, 2nd ed. *Cephalalgia 24*, Supplement 1, 9–160.

SUGGESTED READINGS

Beers, M., Porter, R., & Jones, T. (Eds.). (2006). *Merck Manual of Medical Therapeutics*, 18th ed. Rahway, NJ: Merck.

McPhee, S.J., Papadakis, M.A., & Rabow, M.W. (Eds.). (2011). *CURRENT Medical Diagnosis & Treatment.* New York: Lange Medical Books/McGraw Hill.

Weiner, W.J., & Goetz, C.G. (2004). *Neurology for the Non-Neurologist.* Philadelphia: Lippincott, Williams, & Wilkins.

Chapter 16

NONSPECIFIC COMPLAINTS

Laurie Grubbs

History and Physical Examination

Some of the more challenging chief complaints for any health-care practitioner are those "generic" complaints that have a multitude of causations: fatigue, weakness, dizziness, numbness/tingling, headache, and so on. Deciding which system to start with is often difficult. Because there are so many possibilities for the origin of these complaints, all systems should be considered, although the neurological and cardiac systems are often a good place to start. Proceed with the history in the typical format because the complaint may be related to past health problems, medications, or a familial or genetic predisposition, or it may be a new-onset problem. Be sure to include in your review of systems the questions under the general assessment, such as weight loss, changes in appetite, fevers, chills, night sweats, lethargy, weakness, inability to perform the activities of daily life, changes in mental status, and nutritional patterns. Pay attention to the general appearance and behavior of the patient, including personal hygiene, dress, grooming, speech patterns, mood, and affect. Patients who are depressed or ill may show signs of poor hygiene and flat affect.

Differential Diagnosis of Chief Complaints

■ Fatigue

A complaint of fatigue has strong psychological overtones, making it extremely important to consider a psychological as well as a physical cause. There are a multitude of possible causes of clinically significant fatigue, including hyperthyroidism, hypothyroidism, infection, diabetes, heart disease, autoimmune disorders, renal disease, hematologic disorders, cancer, sleep disturbances, lung disease, medications, nonprescription drugs, alcohol, stress, anxiety, and depression.

History

Key symptoms to inquire about include generalized weakness, easy fatigability, and mental fatigue. A thorough medication history, including over-the-counter drugs, is imperative. Ask about tobacco, alcohol, and other drug use. Investigate a past history or family history of cardiac, respiratory, endocrine, gastrointestinal (GI), or hematologic disease. A family history of type 2 diabetes mellitus (DM) presents a significant risk of the patient developing it as well. Thyroid disease seems to show a family predisposition. A history of anemia in a patient should raise the index of suspicion for chronicity. Always ask the date of the last menstrual period for young women regardless of whether she is using oral contraceptives. Other common causes, particularly in the elderly, include arrhythmias, congestive heart failure (CHF), infection, and malignancy. Two uncommon causes of fatigue could be adrenal dysfunction (Addison's and Cushing's diseases), but patients might describe weakness rather than fatigue, especially in the case of Cushing's disease in which there is muscle wasting. It is important to take a thorough psychosocial history as part of the review of systems. Ask about living arrangements, relationships with family and significant others, environment, occupational history, economic status (including job satisfaction), daily profile (rest–activity patterns, exercise habits, social activities), and patterns of health care. In today's society, it is not uncommon for a person to be working, caring for children, and caring for elderly parents, possibly as a single parent and sole family support. People are often not aware of the physical toll that long-term stress can take on the body and immune system.

Physical Examination

The physical examination should follow most closely with the system suspected as causing the fatigue, although other systems should be included. The practitioner's index of suspicion involves many variables, including the age of the patient, current health, past history, and presenting symptoms. As usual, vital signs are a good place to start. Hypotension, bradycardia, tachycardia, or fever could indicate a cardiac or infectious cause or Addison's disease. Unexplained weight loss might indicate a thyroid disease, DM, Addison's disease, malignancy, or depression. In the head, ears, eyes, nose, and throat examination, particular attention should be paid to examination of the thyroid and lymph system. Significant findings in the cardiac examination include an arrhythmia or murmur, which might be compromising cardiac output, or ventricular hypertrophy, which could indicate heart failure. Electrocardiogram (EKG) changes may demonstrate the ventricular hypertrophy seen in heart failure or the conduction delays seen in Addison's disease. Shortness of breath, tachypnea, or adventitious sounds may indicate a cardiac or respiratory cause of the fatigue. Masses in the abdomen might indicate a malignancy. Bruits, particularly over the renal arteries, could affect blood flow to the kidneys, giving rise to renal impairment and fatigue. Skin changes may be seen in thyroid disease, with dry skin seen in hypothyroidism and moist skin in hyperthyroidism, or in Addison's disease, which causes hyperpigmentation. A thorough neurological assessment is also in order, especially in the elderly because depression and dementia are more common and could present as fatigue or lethargy. The remainder of the assessment involves laboratory or other diagnostics, which are discussed under each differential diagnosis.

STRESS, ANXIETY, DEPRESSION, AND DYSTHYMIA

Psychiatric disorders may be responsible for as much as 50% of the complaints of fatigue (McPhee & Papadakis, 2010). With the increased acceptance and recognition of depression as an illness, and with the treatment choices now available, patients are much more likely to seek help for depression. Often they are not aware of being depressed, and they present with somatic symptoms such as fatigue.

Signs and Symptoms

Subjectively, patients admit to feelings of sadness, hopelessness, and worthlessness with diminished interest in both work and recreation. There may be cognitive complaints, such as difficulty thinking and concentrating, obsessive ruminations, and difficulty making decisions. There may be difficulty sleeping, appetite changes, loss of energy, and decreased libido. Often depression is accompanied by anxiety or agitation, as well as by various somatic complaints, such as fatigue, headache, nausea, and irritability.

Diagnostic Studies

There are many diagnostic tools to evaluate depression and other psychiatric problems. The Beck Inventory of Depression is widely used. In clinical family practice, abbreviated "bedside questionnaires" can be used to evaluate the patient for referral to a mental health counselor.

TYPE 2 DIABETES MELLITUS

The incidence of type 2 DM in the United States has risen dramatically in the last decade mainly owing to the rise in obesity, and it was estimated that 8.3% of the population in 2010 had diabetes (NIDDK, 2010). From 1980 through 2005, the number of Americans with diabetes increased from 5.6 million to 15.8 million (CDC, 2008). Patients who are overweight and sedentary, with a positive family history, are at high risk for developing type 2 DM.

Signs and Symptoms

Polydipsia, polyphagia, and polyuria are the hallmark signs of diabetes, but fatigue, weight loss, and blurred vision are often the symptoms that bring patients into the office.

Diagnostic Studies

A fasting glucose level higher than 110 mg/dL is considered diagnostic for diabetes. A glucose tolerance test can also be done to look for fluctuations in glucose metabolism. A test of the hemoglobin A1c level gives an estimation of blood glucose over the previous 3 months. HgbA1c levels are an excellent way to monitor long-term diabetes control.

HYPOTHYROIDISM

Primary hypothyroidism is the most common form and is thought to be autoimmune in origin. The incidence of hypothyroidism is greater in women and more common in people over 40 years of age.

Signs and Symptoms

Because the onset of hypothyroidism can be insidious, patients may not be aware that their thyroid levels have diminished. Common signs and symptoms include fatigue or lack of energy, puffy face, constipation, intolerance to cold, hypotension, bradycardia, dry skin, menorrhagia, modest weight gain, diminished deep tendon reflexes (DTRs), and dulled cognition. In the elderly, the presenting symptom may be CHF. Also see the subsection Goiter in Chapter 4, p. 82.

Diagnostic Studies

Whereas the physical examination may raise the index of suspicion, the measurement of the thyroid hormones, T_3 and T_4, and thyroid-stimulating hormone (TSH) confirms the diagnosis. Because thyroid function requires a feedback loop between the pituitary gland and the thyroid gland, in hypothyroidism, the T_3 and T_4 levels are below normal and the TSH is above normal.

MALIGNANCY

A malignancy any place in the body may cause the patient to feel fatigued. It is often an indirect cause of fatigue stemming from anemia, shortness of breath, decreased appetite, nausea and vomiting, decreased renal function, or a variety of other symptoms caused by the malignancy.

Signs and Symptoms

The signs and symptoms depend on the system where the malignancy exists. If a patient presents with a primary complaint of fatigue, an index of suspicion for a malignancy should alert you to ask about other signs or symptoms that the patient might have noticed. If malignancy is advanced enough to cause fatigue, there are usually other symptoms present.

Diagnostic Studies

The diagnostics also depend on the system thought to be involved. A complete blood count (CBC), urinalysis, and general chemistries, as well as liver functions and a chest x-ray, are helpful. Depending on the age of the patient, a mammogram and/or colonoscopy may be warranted. New-onset anemia, especially in an older person, should be thoroughly investigated, as it may be secondary to blood loss or decreased red blood cell (RBC) production as a result of colon cancer or a hematologic malignancy.

ANEMIA

The anemia may be primary or secondary to a hematologic disease or a malignancy. It is important to determine whether the anemia is due to decreased production or increased destruction of RBCs owing to diseases affecting the bone marrow, blood loss, or other hemolytic conditions. A patient with a history of anemia should alert the practitioner to start there with the differential diagnosis of fatigue. Ask about the cause or type of anemia and any past or current treatments.

Signs and Symptoms

Fatigue and decreased activity tolerance may be the symptoms that bring the patient to the clinic. The degree of fatigue is often proportional to the degree of anemia; however, patients with longstanding anemia compensate and may be asymptomatic, even with a significant anemia. Along with fatigue, the patient may appear pale with pale conjunctivae and mucous membranes. There may be neurological symptoms, such as paresthesias or decreased proprioception, as is the case in B_{12} deficiency. Cardiac functioning may be affected with severe, longstanding anemia.

Diagnostic Studies

A CBC with differential is the first laboratory test to obtain. A reticulocyte count assists in determining whether the anemia is due to increased destruction of RBCs, resulting in a high reticulocyte count, or to decreased production of RBCs, resulting in a low reticulocyte count. Bilirubin in the urine or an elevated serum bilirubin suggests RBC destruction. Serum iron, total iron-binding capacity, ferritin, and B_{12} tests give important information about the specific type of anemia. Positive hemoccult tests alert the practitioner to the need for a GI consultation to determine the source of bleeding.

CHRONIC RENAL FAILURE

The main causes of chronic renal failure are diabetes and hypertension (greater than 50%). Polycystic kidney disease and glomerulonephritis account for another 25%, and the remaining causes are unknown (McPhee & Papadakis, 2010). The three stages of chronic renal failure are diminished renal reserve, renal insufficiency in which azotemia develops and is reflected in elevations of plasma urea and creatinine, and uremia, which is accompanied by fluid and electrolyte imbalances.

Signs and Symptoms

Patients with mild renal dysfunction are generally asymptomatic, but as the disease progresses, vague symptoms appear. Fatigue and weakness as well as decreased cognitive functioning and irritability, are early signs. Patients may complain of nocturia, which is due to the kidney not concentrating the urine at night. Many of these early signs are nonspecific, and patients often pass them off as a normal part of aging. GI complaints, such as nausea, vomiting, and anorexia, are common and contribute to the muscle wasting and fatigue. Patients may complain of a metallic taste in the mouth. Hypertension may develop from fluid overload and can result in CHF. Pericarditis may develop, producing a friction rub. Neurological symptoms include muscle cramps and twitching, peripheral neuropathy, difficulty concentrating, and sleep disturbances. Pruritus is a common and very uncomfortable symptom, and as patients become more uremic, crystals called uremic frost, may appear on the skin. The skin often takes on a yellowish-brown tone and is easily bruised.

Diagnostic Studies

The abnormal laboratory values are numerous. A blood chemistry will reveal an elevated blood, urea, nitrogen (BUN) and creatinine. Metabolic acidosis, hyperphosphatemia, hypocalcemia, and hyperkalemia are present. A normocytic, normochromic anemia is present. Imaging studies of the kidney may be helpful if the chronic renal failure is due to a structural problem in the kidney; otherwise, imaging may not be helpful.

ARRHYTHMIAS

Both atrial and ventricular arrhythmias may cause fatigue. They may be secondary to age, coronary artery disease, valvular heart disease, or endocrine diseases. Atrial fibrillation is very common in the elderly, with an increased incidence due to the aging population. Other atrial and ventricular arrhythmias can occur in any age with or without the presence of other disorders. Supraventricular tachycardia is usually paroxysmal in nature and results from an abnormal pathway within or around the atrioventricular node. Intraventricular conduction delays may be seen in Addison's disease, in which fatigue is a common symptom. The only ventricular arrhythmias that might present with a complaint of fatigue are bigeminy or trigeminy. Ventricular tachycardia or ventricular fibrillation are life threatening, and the patient generally does not remain conscious after the onset of the arrhythmia.

Signs and Symptoms

In atrial fibrillation, the symptoms generally depend on the ventricular response rate. The patient may be very symptomatic, with shortness of breath, decreased exercise tolerance, and fatigue, or he or she may be completely asymptomatic. In supraventricular tachycardia, the rate is usually quite high, up to 200 beats per minute, and the patient is aware of palpitations. Shortness of breath and fatigue may accompany supraventricular tachycardia, particularly if the arrhythmia persists. With bigeminy and trigeminy, patients are usually aware of palpitations or the sensation of missed beats. They may complain of shortness of breath and probably have more of a complaint of weakness or lightheadedness rather than fatigue.

Diagnostic Symptoms

An EKG is a simple way to quickly and definitively diagnose an arrhythmia as long as it is occurring when the patient presents to the office, clinic, or emergency department.

CONGESTIVE HEART FAILURE

CHF, commonly occurring in the elderly or in patients with past myocardial infarctions or cardiomyopathy, can often present with complaints of fatigue, decreased activity tolerance, and/or shortness of breath. A detailed discussion of CHF can be found in Chapter 7 on p. 197.

CHRONIC OBSTRUCTIVE PULMONARY DISEASE

Chronic obstructive pulmonary disease such as chronic asthma/bronchitis, bronchiolitis, and emphysema may be associated with fatigue. These conditions are discussed in Chapter 8, p. 214.

PREGNANCY

Females of child-bearing age should always be asked the date of their last menstrual period, and some index of suspicion should be present for any young female who presents with a complaint of fatigue.

Signs and Symptoms

Missed menstrual cycle, fatigue, breast tenderness, and nausea are the typical pregnancy signs and symptoms.

Diagnostic Studies

A urine or serum hCG is diagnostic.

MONONUCLEOSIS

Mononucleosis is a viral infection that typically occurs in adolescence and early adulthood and is caused by the Epstein-Barr virus. Mononucleosis is described in Chapter 6, pp. 154–156.

FIBROMYALGIA

Fatigue is a common finding in fibromyalgia and is described in detail in Chapter 14, pp. 419–420.

ADDISON'S DISEASE

Addison's disease is a chronic, progressive hypofunctioning of the adrenals caused by atrophy or destruction of the adrenal cortex, usually with an autoimmune origin. Other causes include medications, tuberculosis, amyloidosis, malignancy, or inflammation. It affects both genders equally and can be seen in all ages. The main hormones produced by the adrenal gland are cortisol, aldosterone, and adrenal androgens. Addison's disease is characterized by electrolyte imbalance—there is an increase in Na^+ excretion and a decrease in K^+ excretion that lead to low blood levels of Na^+ and Cl^- and high levels of K^+. This produces volume depletion, dehydration, and hypotension. The cortisol deficiency causes alterations in carbohydrate, fat and protein metabolism, and insulin sensitivity. The metabolic changes lead to hypoglycemia, decreased liver glycogen, and thus fatigue and weakness. The decreased cortisol levels affect melanocyte-stimulating activities, producing the characteristic hyperpigmentation of the skin.

The acute form of the disease, termed adrenal crisis, is a more severe and life-threatening form and is characterized by profound weakness, severe abdominal and back pain, nausea, vomiting, diarrhea, confusion, renal shutdown, and circulatory collapse.

Signs and Symptoms

Weakness and fatigue are early signs of Addison's disease. The patient may complain of lightheadedness owing to volume depletion, and orthostatic hypotension is found on examination. In most cases, the skin and mucous membranes are hyperpigmented, especially over creases, bony prominences, and nipples. The patient may complain of anorexia, nausea, vomiting, or diarrhea, and weight loss is evident. A complaint of lightheadedness or syncope may lead the practitioner to do an EKG, which shows decreased voltage as a result of a small heart and prolonged PR and QT intervals.

Diagnostic Studies

The blood chemistry findings suggestive of Addison's disease include low serum Ca^+, high K^+, elevated BUN, decrease in plasma bicarbonate, and low fasting glucose. The CBC may show an elevated hematocrit owing to volume depletion, a low white blood cell count, lymphocytosis, and increased eosinophils. Chest x-ray shows a small heart and possibly evidence of tuberculosis. Abdominal films may show calcifications in the adrenals and renal tuberculosis. More sophisticated tests can be performed using an adrenocorticotropic hormone challenge to determine its effect on plasma cortisol levels. Other drugs can help to differentiate primary from secondary adrenal insufficiency. Replacement of adrenal hormones results in a good prognosis for these patients.

■ Sleep Disorders

Sleep disorders can obviously contribute to fatigue and affect daily performance. Common disorders associated with sleep disturbances include insomnia; obstructive sleep apnea (OSA); restless leg syndrome; pain syndromes; substance abuse; congestive heart failure; asthma; stress, anxiety, depression, and dysthmia; and fibromyalgia.

History

The history should explore the type of sleep disturbance experienced. Determine how many hours the patient sleeps each night. Ask if the patient experiences trouble falling asleep, awakens through the night, or awakens early. Determine whether the patient feels rested when he or she awakens. A sleep diary may help to determine the type of disturbance experienced. A complete medical and mental health history are necessary to explore both physical and psychological etiology because there are numerous causes of sleep disturbances. Ask about chronic and acute conditions that could interfere with sleep, including those that affect the respiratory system, cause pain, or affect emotional state. A medication history may reveal that the patient is self-medicating in order to fall sleep or may identify medications that contribute to sleep alterations. A history of illegal drug or alcohol use is significant. A family history may help to uncover hereditary or psychosocial links. Living conditions and environmental exposures are important to explore as are occupational and recreational activities. It is important to ask how, if at all, the altered sleep affects daily activities.

Physical Examination

Vital signs, body mass index, and oxygen saturation should be obtained. A thorough mental status and neurologic examination is a good place to start. An examination of the mouth, throat, and respiratory system are necessary to assess for conditions that might cause obstructive sleep apnea. Check for peripheral pulses, sensation, and edema in the lower extremities to assess for decreased circulation or neuropathy. Examine the thyroid for enlargement or nodularity as well as for systemic signs and symptoms of thyroid disease.

PRIMARY INSOMNIA

Insomnia has a multitude of causes, including age, menopause, chronic illness, pain, stress, anxiety, depression, poor sleep habits, endocrine disorders, or medications. The DSM-IV criteria for primary insomnia are as follows (American Psychiatric Association, 1994):

1. The sleep disturbance is defined as difficulty initiating or maintaining sleep, or nonrestorative sleep, for at least 1 month.
2. The sleep disturbance (or associated daytime fatigue) causes clinically significant distress or impairment in social, occupational, or other important areas of functioning.
3. The sleep disturbance does not occur exclusively during the course of narcolepsy, breathing-related sleep disorder, circadian rhythm sleep disorder, or a parasomnia.
4. The disturbance does not occur exclusively during the course of another mental disorder (e.g., major depressive disorder, generalized anxiety disorder, a delirium).
5. The disturbance is not due to the direct physiological effects of a substance (e.g., a drug of abuse, a medication) or a general medical condition.

Signs and Symptoms

Daytime sleepiness, irritability, and cognitive impairment are the most common symptoms of insomnia. Patients may also complain of weight changes, anxiety, and depression.

Diagnostic Studies

A polysomnogram can be performed but only to rule out physiologic causes. It is important to ask the patient to keep a sleep diary for at least 1 week. A sleep history is important and should include estimated time to fall asleep, awakening time and total sleep time, number of times awakening during the night and amount of time staying awake, number and length of naps, amount and time of alcohol and caffeine intake, amount of stress during the day, amount of daily exercise, appetite during the day, a rating of level of fatigue and irritability during the day, and medication use. Treatment depends on the cause, but behavioral changes and/or pharmaceutical sleep agents may be necessary.

OBSTRUCTIVE SLEEP APNEA

With obesity becoming epidemic, the incidence of OSA is also increasing. Besides obesity, other predisposing and risk factors include narrowed upper airways, macroglossia, tonsillar hypertrophy, sleep medicines, alcohol, smoking, nasal obstruction, and hypothyroidism. It occurs more in middle-aged men.

A thorough medication history, respiratory history, neurologic history, and mental health assessment should be performed.

Signs and Symptoms

One of the more common symptoms of OSA is snoring, usually reported by the spouse. The spouse may also report prolonged periods of cessation of breathing and restlessness. The patient may complain of frequent nighttime awakening, morning drowsiness, headache (caused by carbon dioxide buildup in the brain), cognitive impairment, and impotence and weight gain, which can be both a cause and an effect. Systemic hypertension is a complication of OSA but often resolves when the cause of the apnea is corrected.

Diagnostic Studies

An overnight sleep study (polysomnogram) is diagnostic for sleep apnea. It records sleep wave activity, breathing patterns, heart rate and rhythm, and oxygen saturations. Oxygen saturations drop during periods of apnea, and brady- or tachyarrhythmias may occur. A CBC may show erythrocytosis to compensate for the hypoxemia. If possible, the underlying cause should be corrected.

RESTLESS LEG SYNDROME (RLS)

Although the exact cause of RLS is unknown, it has been associated with obesity, pregnancy, smoking, iron-deficiency anemia, peripheral neuropathy, heavy metal toxicity and other toxins, endocrine disorders, renal failure, caffeine and alcohol use, and certain medications, particularly H_2 blockers and some antidepressants. A hereditary basis has also been suggested.

Signs and Symptoms

RLS is characterized by an uncontrollable need to move the limbs, especially during times of rest and relaxation.

Diagnostic Studies

RLS is diagnosed primarily through the history. Laboratory tests include CBC to check for anemia, complete metabolic panel for endocrine and renal disorders, and tests for heavy metals.

PAIN SYNDROMES

Pain should be explored as a potential cause of sleep disturbance. Pain is described in general in the following sections, and specific types of pain are described in earlier chapters.

SUBSTANCE ABUSE

See Chapter 17.

CONGESTIVE HEART FAILURE

See Chapter 7.

ASTHMA

See Chapter 8.

STRESS, ANXIETY, DEPRESSION, AND DYSTHMIA

See p. 480.

FIBROMYALGIA

See Chapter 14, pp. 419–420.

■ Weakness

Although many of the previously discussed diagnoses for fatigue could also fit into a chief complaint of weakness, this complaint connotes a lack of strength rather than a feeling of lethargy, and it is manifest in many neurological diseases as well as in adrenal dysfunction, hyperthyroidism, and malignancy.

History

The history should include the type of weakness; whether it is proximal weakness, which might alert you to thyroid disease, malignancy, or adrenal dysfunction; or distal weakness, which would raise an index of suspicion for a neurological cause especially if accompanied by paresthesias. Ask the patient when and with what types of activities the weakness is most prominent and how much it interferes with activities of daily living. Inquire about changes in speech patterns or slurring that might indicate a neurological cause. Ask whether there are any cognitive or personality changes, which are often seen with adrenal dysfunction. The review of systems should include headache, cold or heat intolerance, change in appetite, weight gain or loss, nausea, vomiting or diarrhea, changes in balance or gait, numbness or paresthesia, diplopia or other vision changes, and difficulty with speech or swallowing.

Physical Examination

The physical examination should focus on the neurological and musculoskeletal examinations because both are closely related and provide much information about the type, site, and severity of the weakness. Evaluate muscle mass, strength, and tone; the condition of the joints; and any fasciculations or spasticity. A complete neurological examination should be done, including cranial nerves, mental status, motor and sensory function, and DTRs. Assess the skin for any color or texture changes, as seen in adrenal or thyroid dysfunction. The head and neck should be assessed particularly for lymphadenopathy or enlarged or nodular thyroid.

MULTIPLE SCLEROSIS

Multiple sclerosis (MS) is a degenerative, demyelinating disease that is most often diagnosed in the second to fourth decades of life. It occurs more often in women than in men. The presentation of MS is often vague and transient, with episodic remission and exacerbation. Patients may have remitting or primary progressive MS. The etiology is unknown, but it is thought to be autoimmune. A genetic susceptibility is suspected because it is seen more in those of western European lineage who live in temperate zones.

Signs and Symptoms

Visual disturbances may be the initial presenting symptom, indicating a plaque on the optic nerve. Associated visual disturbances include diplopia, blurred vision, tunnel vision, scotoma, or amaurosis. The visual changes are usually monocular. The patient may complain of intermittent weakness, paresthesias, or numbness of the face or extremities that occurs intermittently, and that may resolve for weeks to months. Patients may report episodes of falling or stumbling with gait ataxia. Hyperreflexia may be noted, particularly in the lower extremities. Other symptoms include bladder incontinence or retention. Spastic bladder may also occur. In later stages, mental status changes may be noted. Initial symptoms are typically intermittent, and the disease may go undiagnosed for months or years.

Diagnostic Studies

MS is a clinical diagnosis and a diagnosis of exclusion. A thorough neurologic examination is essential. An MRI of the brain and/or spine with and without contrast reveals demyelination of the white matter of the brain, spinal cord, and optic nerves. Lumbar puncture for cerebrospinal fluid analysis may show oligoclonal bands (IgG) and protein less than 55 mg/dL; however, this is not a definitive test for diagnosis.

MUSCULAR DYSTROPHIES

There are seven types of muscular dystrophy, and they are subdivided by chromosomal inheritance, age of onset, and characteristic symptoms.

Signs and Symptoms

The symptoms, occurring anywhere from a year old to late adulthood, are characterized by progressive muscle weakness and wasting. There may also be mental retardation, skeletal deformities, and cardiac involvement.

Diagnostic Studies

Diagnosis is made by genetic testing. Creatine phosphokinase is increased in some types. An electromyogram (EMG) may be helpful to distinguish among various muscle diseases.

MYASTHENIA GRAVIS

Myasthenia can occur at any age and may be associated with other autoimmune diseases. Limb weakness and fatigability of the affected muscles is a diagnostic sign. Symptoms are due to a variable blocking of neuromuscular transmission by autoantibodies that bind to acetylcholine receptors. Ocular, facial, masticatory, and pharyngeal muscles are most often affected. Ocular symptoms are also discussed under Myasthenia Gravis in Chapter 5, p. 114.

Signs and Symptoms

The eye symptoms of diplopia and ptosis are common early signs. Other symptoms include dysphagia, weakness in the extremities, and respiratory difficulties. Symptoms fluctuate during the day and often relapse or remit over long periods of time, but ultimately the disease is progressive. Sustained activity of the affected muscles increases the weakness, and symptoms improve with rest. Patients may require life support if respiratory effort is significantly affected.

Diagnostic Studies

A highly sensitivity test for the diagnosis of myasthenia gravis is the measurement of serum levels of circulating acetylcholine receptor antibodies. The Tensilon test is definitive and involves blocking acetylcholine by administering edrophonium chloride. If the patient has myasthenia, the symptoms will temporarily worsen after the administration of edrophonium chloride.

POLYMYOSITIS AND DERMATOMYOSITIS

Polymyositis is a systemic disease of unknown etiology. When rash is present, it is termed dermatomyositis, and with this form, there is an increased risk of an associated malignancy, particularly ovarian cancer. It is more common in women and in those over 60 years of age.

Signs and Symptoms

Bilateral proximal muscle weakness is the main symptom and occurs in all cases. Weakness of the legs precedes weakness of the arms, and weakness of the neck flexors may be seen. Symptoms may occur suddenly or be more gradual and insidious in nature. The rash typically has a butterfly pattern on the face with reddish lesions over the eyes and periorbital edema. Redness and telangiectasias of the hands and nails is highly suggestive of dermatomyositis, and Raynaud's syndrome may be associated.

Diagnostic Studies

Diagnosis is established by EMG and confirmed by a muscle biopsy of the affected proximal muscles. Biopsy is the only definitive diagnostic test. Creatine phosphokinase is rarely normal in active disease and is a good indicator of disease activity. Other possible enzyme elevations include aldolase, serum glutamic-oxaloacetic transaminase (SGOT), serum glutamic pyruvic transaminase (SGPT), and lactate dehydrogenase (LDH), although not specific. Myositis specific antibody (MSA) and myositis associated autoantibodies (MAA) may help to differentiate from an underlying malignancy (Hashmat, Daud, & Brannagan, 2006).

AMYOTROPHIC LATERAL SCLEROSIS (LOU GEHRIG'S DISEASE)

Amyotrophic lateral sclerosis belongs to a group of motor neuron diseases and is characterized by mixed upper and lower motor neuron deficits.

Signs and Symptoms

Amyotrophic lateral sclerosis is characterized by muscle weakness and atrophy, usually starting in the hands and then progressing randomly and asymmetrically. Other common symptoms include muscle cramps, fasciculations, spasticity, dysarthria, dysphagia, and increased DTRs. Over 90% of patients are dead within 3 to 5 years.

Diagnostic Studies

An EMG is the most helpful diagnostic test. Muscle biopsy shows histological changes owing to denervation.

GUILLAIN-BARRÉ SYNDROME

Guillain-Barré is an acute, rapidly progressive polyneuropathy that is often preceded by a virus, surgical procedure, or immunization. It is thought to have an immune etiology.

Signs and Symptoms

Symmetric weakness and paresthesias are the main symptoms. The weakness usually begins in the legs and then proceeds to the arms. Over 50% of patients develop respiratory involvement, which may require mechanical ventilation. Autonomic dysfunction can occur in severe cases and can be fatal. The maximal degree of weakness usually occurs in the first 2 to 3 weeks.

Diagnostic Studies

The diagnosis can be made mainly on clinical presentation. Increased protein in the cerebrospinal fluid and EMG abnormalities assist in confirmation of the diagnosis.

HYPERTHYROIDISM

Although we think of hypothyroidism as causing fatigue, hyperthyroidism can cause symptoms of muscle weakness and lead to difficulty in performing the activities of daily living. Patients have different subjective experiences of their symptoms; therefore, some may describe weakness, whereas others may describe fatigue.

Signs and Symptoms

Common signs and symptoms include muscle weakness, nervousness, insomnia, tachycardia, increased sweating, moist skin, intolerance to heat, exophthalmos, weight loss, hypertension, and hyperreflexia. In the elderly, the presenting symptom may be atrial fibrillation.

Diagnostic Studies

Even though the physical examination may increase suspicions, measuring the thyroid hormones, T_3 and T_4, and TSH confirms the diagnosis. The T_3 and T_4 levels are above normal, and the TSH level is below normal, sometimes to the point at which it is barely measurable.

CUSHING'S DISEASE

Cushing's disease is caused by excess cortisol and corticosteroid hormones, either endogenous or exogenous. Endogenous causes of cortisol hypersecretion include pituitary adenomas; other malignancies, such as small cell lung cancer; and adrenal tumors. Exogenous causes are related to the administration of steroids for the management of other chronic diseases. A thorough medical history will alert the practitioner to chronic diseases or medications that may be causing or contributing to the cushingoid signs and symptoms.

Signs and Symptoms

Although weakness can be profound because of the muscle wasting that occurs, it is generally not the first symptom that brings the patient to the office. For women, it may be oligomenorrhea or amenorrhea and hirsutism; for men, impotence. Patients develop a "moon face" and "buffalo hump" with central obesity and thin extremities. Hypertension and osteoporosis develop over time. Purple striae around the thighs, breasts, and abdomen are characteristic of Cushing's; patients are prone to easy bruisability, acne, and skin infections with poor wound healing. Patients complain of excessive thirst and polyuria owing to glucose intolerance, and they are prone to renal calculi. Changes in mental health are common and range from mood swings to psychosis.

Diagnostic Studies

The most accurate way to diagnose Cushing's disease is to give intravenous Decadron at bedtime and then check for elevated cortisol levels 8 to 10 hours later. A 24-hour urine for cortisol and creatinine helps confirm the diagnosis. Glucose tolerance testing shows elevated glucose resulting from insulin resistance. A CBC may show leukocytosis with granulocytosis and lymphopenia.

MALIGNANCY

Weakness caused by a malignancy may be associated with the decreased functioning of the organ involved (e.g., lung), or the weakness may be due to a secondary anemia or to weight loss. See individual chapters for specific malignancies.

■ Fever of Unknown Origin

Fever of unknown origin (FUO) is defined as a temperature of at least 101°F for at least 3 weeks without discovery of the cause (Merck Manual, 2002). In children, over 50% of fevers are due to upper respiratory or viral illness; in adults, one should be more suspicious of malignancy.

History

The history should include the timing and degree of the fever. Recent travel or exposure to illnesses or certain animals is often very helpful. Travel outside the United States can be particularly problematic, and one should consider such diseases as malaria, typhoid, tuberculosis, mycobacterium avium complex, or HIV. Brucellosis and histoplasmosis should be considered if there is animal exposure. Weight loss might indicate a malignant process or might be due to anorexia caused by the fever. As usual, a thorough medicine history, past medical history, and family history might alert the practitioner to a possible cause. Any recent infection should be investigated first because it may not have been adequately treated. A history of frequent infections could raise the index of suspicion regarding an immunocompromised condition, such as HIV, leukemia, or lymphoma. It is important to inquire about sexual practices.

Physical Examination

The physical should include examination of the skin for lesions, redness, increased temperature, or edema, which might indicate infection or an inflammatory process. Examine the lymph nodes. If there is lymphadenopathy in a particular area, it might lead you to the point of infection. If it is generalized, consider lymphoma, leukemia, or HIV. A cardiac assessment is important especially listening for a murmur or friction rub. Pericarditis or endocarditis has a variety of causes and may present as unexplained fever, shortness of breath, precordial pain/tenderness, and tachycardia. The lung assessment is crucial because over 50% of FUOs in children are caused by an upper respiratory illness. Observe the skin and nail beds for cyanosis. The abdomen should be palpated for tenderness or masses; smoldering cases of appendicitis, cholecystitis, pancreatitis, or hepatitis might cause a lingering fever.

INFECTION

Any infection, viral or bacterial, can cause prolonged fever. Patients usually have some other complaint that alerts you to the cause of the fever. If bacterial, it can be treated with antibiotics, which should resolve the symptoms. Viral illnesses are more problematic because supportive measures are generally all that can be provided. Be watchful for a secondary bacterial infection to develop with some prolonged viral illnesses.

Signs and Symptoms

The signs and symptoms are highly variable depending on the source of the infection. Expected are the typical symptoms that accompany a fever, such as headache, malaise, anorexia, and possibly chills. A thorough review of systems is necessary to detect the underlying source of the fever, if not completely obvious by other complaints.

Diagnostic Studies

Although the diagnostics vary with the underlying cause, ordering a CBC with differential, urinalysis, and chest x-ray is a good place to start with any complaint of FUO. Blood cultures as well as cultures of bodily fluids may be necessary. In babies, a lumbar puncture is recommended to rule out meningitis. Rising antibody titers for or rapid tests for influenza viral infections may be helpful. Ultrasound or CT scan of the abdomen will identify abscesses or other infections in the abdomen, including diverticulitis, peritonitis, cholecystitis, possibly pancreatitis, or appendicitis. A CT scan of the chest can detect cardiac vegetation, which might suggest pericarditis or endocarditis as a cause for the fever.

MALIGNANCY

Many malignancies can cause fever, but lymphoma and leukemia should be at the top of the differential list. Acute leukemia is more common in children, and the chronic leukemias are more common in middle-aged to elderly adults.

Hodgkin's lymphoma is more prevalent in children and young adults, whereas non-Hodgkin's lymphoma is more common in middle-aged to elderly adults. Burkitt's lymphoma is more common in HIV patients.

Signs and Symptoms

With leukemia, common symptoms include unexplained fever, easy bruising or bleeding, fatigue, bone or joint pain, and enlarged liver or spleen. With lymphoma, common symptoms include fatigue, fever, night sweats, lymphadenopathy, and weight loss.

Diagnostic Studies

A CBC is the first and easiest laboratory test to perform. The abnormalities in the CBC vary some with the type of leukemia—acute or chronic, lymphocytic or myelocytic—but in general there is a proliferation of immature white cells (blasts), anemia, and low platelet count. In lymphoma, there is a leukocytosis, lymphocytopenia, and possibly thrombocytosis. A hypochromic, microcytic anemia is often present. A bone marrow biopsy confirms the diagnosis in both leukemia and lymphoma.

DIFFUSE CONNECTIVE TISSUE DISORDERS

The connective tissue disorders include rheumatoid arthritis, Sjögren's syndrome, Behçet's syndrome, vasculitis, systemic and discoid lupus erythematosus, polymyositis, polymyalgia rheumatica, temporal arteritis, and polyarteritis. Although fever can be present in any of the connective tissue disorders, muscle and joint pain are more common presenting symptoms. The specific signs, symptoms, and diagnostics for each of these diseases are beyond the scope of this text.

IMMUNODEFICIENCY DISORDERS

Immunodeficiency disorders are numerous and are characterized as primary or secondary, with the secondary being more common than the primary disorders. The primary disorders are classified into B-cell deficiencies (antibody), T-cell deficiencies (cellular), phagocytic disorders, and complement disorders. The secondary immunodeficiencies are classified by cause and include hereditary and metabolic diseases (chromosome abnormalities, uremia, DM, malnutrition, nephritic syndrome, myotonic dystrophy, and sickle cell disease), infectious diseases (rubella; cytomegalovirus; viral exanthemas; mononucleosis; and severe bacterial, viral, or fungal infections), infiltrative and hematologic diseases (histocytosis, sarcoidosis, lymphoma, leukemia, myeloma, and aplastic anemia), those caused by surgery and trauma (burns, splenectomy, and anesthesia), and those caused by immunosuppressive agents (radiation, chemotherapy, corticosteroids, and other immunosuppressive drugs). Specific signs, symptoms, and diagnostics are beyond the scope of this text. Some of these are discussed in other chapters.

DRUG REACTION

The most likely drugs to cause fever are the chemotherapeutic agents used to treat cancer, mainly as a result of leukopenia. The medical history along with a CBC should be sufficient to make this diagnosis. Allergic reactions to any drug, particularly the antibiotics, can cause fever as well as rash. The history is usually sufficient to identify the cause of the fever.

■ Unexplained Weight Loss

Unexplained weight loss is considered significant if it is greater than 5% of the usual body weight over a 6- to 12-month period and often indicates a serious medical or psychological illness.

History

Malignancy, diabetes, digestive diseases, thyroid disease, and depression should top the list of differential diagnoses for unexplained weight loss. A thorough history and review of systems will alert the practitioner to other complaints that could give clues to the cause, such as cough, hemoptysis, shortness of breath, nausea, vomiting, diarrhea, steatorrhea, hematemesis, melena, fatigue/weakness/lethargy, changing or new moles, persistent pain, enlarged lymph nodes, abnormal menstrual bleeding, breast discharge, and chronic headaches. A thorough medicine history is critical especially in the elderly or those with chronic diseases who are on a multitude of medicines. A psychosocial history is critical, especially in the elderly client who may not be eating due to the inability to shop for groceries because of financial or transportation problems, inability to prepare meals resulting from a functional limitation, poorly fitting dentures or no dentures, or loss of appetite owing to depression or medications. Inquire about smoking and alcohol intake, which can increase the risk for both weight loss and malignancies.

Physical Examination

Patients with unexplained weight loss due to malignancy may look cachectic, pale, and lethargic, or they may look well depending on the amount and cause of the weight loss. Weights over the past year should be plotted out to see how much weight has been lost over a period of time. A slow weight decrease in the elderly is not uncommon and may simply be due to a lack of appetite, to institutional food, or to disinterest in food resulting from a decreased sense of taste and/or smell. A full physical examination is necessary, paying particular attention to any masses, tenderness, swelling, or lymphadenopathy.

MALIGNANCY

Depending on the stage of the malignancy, any are capable of causing weight loss as either a primary or secondary symptom. However, the most common malignancies to cause weight loss are GI, lung, hematologic, and musculoskeletal.

Signs and Symptoms

The signs and symptoms vary with the source of the malignancy, and many are asymptomatic except for the complaint of weight loss.

Diagnostic Studies

Ordering a CBC and blood chemistries is a good place to start; a chest x-ray and hemoccult cards can also be helpful depending on the age and medical history.

The results of these and the history should assist in narrowing down the search. Other diagnostics such as CT or MRI should be ordered as needed.

STRESS, ANXIETY, DEPRESSION, AND DYSTHMIA
See Chapter 17, pp. 505–515.

EATING DISORDERS
See Chapter 17, pp. 518–522.

FUNCTIONAL AND FINANCIAL MALNUTRITION

Depending on the patient population, malnutrition may be a reason for unexplained weight loss. It is common in the very poor and in the elderly owing to the inability to purchase, prepare, and consume the proper, varied diet. Eating disorders, depending on the severity, may result in malnutrition. In developing countries, malnutrition is a huge problem, but it is not common in the United States except in the elderly and poor populations.

Signs and Symptoms

Aside from the weight loss, other signs of malnutrition include dry skin and hair, pale conjunctivae, cheilosis, glossitis, bruising, lethargy, decreased vibratory sensation, decreased DTRs, bone demineralization, liver or heart enlargement, muscle wasting, lower extremity edema, and growth failure.

Diagnostic Studies

Malnutrition has a variety of consequences that can involve several body systems. A complete metabolic profile, CBC, and thyroid studies are recommended. Electrolyte imbalance is common especially if the malnutrition is brought on by anorexia or bulimia, and it can be life threatening. Kidney and liver functions may be affected as well. Depending on the chronicity of the problem, dual energy x-ray absorptiometry should be considered because bone health may be at risk. In severe cases, heart failure may ensue, and an echocardiogram or more invasive cardiac testing may be needed to evaluate cardiac functioning.

DRUG REACTION

A few drugs actually cause weight loss (thyroid replacement in greater than therapeutic doses, SSRIs, neuroleptics), but many drugs cause anorexia with weight loss as a secondary side effect. Because drug side effects vary greatly among patients, it is not possible to supply an exhaustive list of drugs that cause anorexia. A few that seem to be most problematic are digitalis, many psychotropic medications, chemotherapeutic agents mostly as a result of nausea, stimulants such as pseudoephedrine or other drugs used to treat obesity, and drugs used to treat attention deficit/hyperactivity disorder.

A complete medication history including over-the-counter medications may allow the practitioner to identify the cause of the weight loss. If a drug is suspected, it should be changed if possible. For patients on multiple drugs, the suspected agents should be discontinued or substituted one at a time in order to determine the offending agent.

MALABSORPTION

Malabsorption falls into two main categories: impaired digestion and impaired absorption, and there are many diseases that fall into each category. Diseases that fall under impaired digestion include gastrectomy, barosurgery, chronic pancreatitis, chronic liver failure, biliary obstruction, lactose intolerance, diverticula, and Zollinger-Ellison syndrome. Diseases that fall into the impaired absorption category include intestinal infections, alcohol, celiac disease, tropical sprue, Whipple's disease, amyloidosis, ischemic or infarcted bowel, Crohn's disease, volvulus, and intussusception.

Signs and Symptoms

The signs and symptoms vary according to the underlying problem, but common symptoms include weight loss, flatulence, abdominal bloating, edema in the lower extremities resulting from protein deficiency, muscle weakness, possibly diarrhea or steatorrhea, dehydration, glossitis, and bruising. A variety of abnormal findings can be associated with malabsorption syndromes, including iron, folic acid or B_{12} deficiency anemia; calcium deficiency; vitamins A, B, C, and D deficiencies; and niacin deficiency. A combination of weight loss, diarrhea, and anemia should raise the possibility of malabsorption.

Diagnostic Studies

There are as many diagnostics as there are causes of malabsorption. Measurement of fat in the stool is the most valuable diagnostic for diagnosing malabsorption, and a 3- to 4-day stool collection is advised. Stool specimens for ova and parasites and culture and sensitivity will help to rule out infectious causes. Absorption tests, flat plate of the abdomen, upper GI with small bowel follow-through, endoscopy, and small bowel biopsy may be necessary for definitive diagnosis.

HYPERTHYROIDISM

Hyperthyroidism is covered earlier in this chapter.

Pain Assessment

In the last decade, pain assessment has become the fifth vital sign, driven by studies reporting that pain was undertreated. In 1999, the Joint Commission on Accreditation of Healthcare Organizations (JCAHO) developed pain assessment and management standards that have been incorporated into health-care facilities at all levels. The new standards call for health-care organizations to:

1. Recognize patients' rights to control pain.
2. Screen for pain.
3. Perform a complete assessment when pain is present.
4. Record the assessment in a way that facilitates regular reassessment and follow-up.
5. Set a standard for monitoring and intervention.
6. Educate providers and assure staff competency.

7. Establish policies that support appropriate prescription or ordering of pain medicines.
8. Educate patients and families.
9. Include patient needs for symptom control in discharge planning.
10. Collect data to monitor the effectiveness and appropriateness of pain management (JCAHO, 2001).

Pain is a multifactorial condition and a common reason for which patients seek health care. Pain can be classified in many ways—acute, chronic, recurrent, or transient. Alternatively, it can be classified by the quality of the pain (gnawing, burning, deep), severity (mild, moderate, severe, excruciating), impact (debilitating, disabling), or related diagnosis (cardiac, neuropathic). Regardless, when pain is a presenting condition, the symptom should always be explored. When a presenting complaint of pain does not readily respond to the initial treatment, it warrants more detailed analysis. In 2006, approximately one-third of adults aged 20 and older who reported pain indicated that their pain had lasted less than 1 month (CDC, 2006).

■ Signs and Symptoms

The PQRST pneumonic (palliative/provoking, quality, radiation, severity, timing) will guide your history for pain assessment. In assessing pain, it is critical to identify the precipitating, palliative, and provocative factors because pain is often not constant over time. Questions on precipitating and palliative factors are also helpful in identifying how the pain limits the patient's typical activities. The quality and quantity of pain may vary, and it is essential to have the patient describe what is meant by a complaint of pain. Ask the patient to describe the pain using common words as he or she would to a family member or neighbor so that you can determine whether it is deep, boring, sharp, gnawing, burning, stabbing, aching, and so forth. The region where the pain is most noted and any area of radiation or secondary pain areas are important to identify. A body diagram may be helpful in achieving this goal: The patient can mark where the pain is located and then rate the severity and quality of pain in various regions. Related symptoms should be explored as well. The severity of pain can be measured in many ways. The most commonly used are the numerical rating scales (NRS; the patient rates the pain on a 0–10-point range); the visual analog scale (VAS; the patient notes a point corresponding to the degree of pain along a 10-centimeter scale with poles of *no pain at all* to *worst possible pain*); and verbal rating scales (VRS; the patient is asked to complete scales using verbal descriptors such as *no pain, mild pain, considerable pain,* and *most severe pain*). Certainly the timing of the pain is important because it helps to identify the situation in which onset was first recognized, including any preceding physical or emotional trauma and how the pain has progressed since first noticed. For instance, it is critical to understand whether the pain has been constant, intermittent, transient, or recurrent.

A past medical history and history of all current and recently taken medications is an important component of pain assessment. Identify history of any neurological, cardiac, gastrointestinal, musculoskeletal, and emotional conditions. Ask about family history. Explore the patient's social history, including any current or recent stressors, the occupational and recreational activities, and activities of daily living. Ask the patient to describe how, if at all, normal activities have been affected by the pain.

The physical examination is guided by the history. In addition to basic vital signs, the general appearance is crucial. However, it is important to remember that patients may not always exhibit behavioral indications of their pain. The physical assessment for specific types of pain (joint, chest, throat, etc.) are described in earlier chapters.

■ Diagnostic Studies

As noted earlier, common pain scales include various forms of VRS, VAS, and NRS pain ratings. There are a number of more detailed options, such as the Pain Faces Scale for pediatric patients and the McGill Pain Questionnaire, which includes sensory and emotional aspects of pain as well as a pain diagram. Pain diaries are often helpful and should be kept for at least a week. Whichever method is used should be culturally sensitive and appropriate to the patient's age and verbal/literacy abilities.

A number of diagnostic studies may be warranted for further exploration of pain and should be selected on the basis of the history and physical findings.

REFERENCES

American Psychiatric Association. (1994). *Diagnostic and Statistical Manual of Mental Disorders*, 4th ed. Washington, DC: American Psychiatric Association.

Beers, M.H. (2006). *Merck Manual of Medical Therapeutics*, 18th ed. Rahway, NJ: Merck.

CDC Centers for Disease Control and Prevention, Health and Human Services. (2006). "Adults Reporting Pain or Stiffness in the Past 30 Days." http://www.cdc.gov/Features/dsJointPain/ (accessed March 17, 2011).

Centers for Disease Control and Prevention, Health and Human Services. (2008). "Diabetes Data and Trends." www.cdc.gov/diabetes/statistics/prev/national/figpersons.htm (accessed March 17, 2011).

Hashmat, A., Daud, Z., & Brannagan, T.H. (2006). "Dermatomyositis/Polymyositis." eMedicine from WebMD. www.emedicine.com/neuro/topic85.htm (accessed March 17, 2011).

Joint Commission on Accreditation of Healthcare Organizations. (2001). "Pain Assessment Standards." www.jointcommission.org/pain_management/ (accessed March 18, 2011).

McPhee, S.J., & Papadakis, M.A. (Eds.). (2010). *CURRENT Medical Diagnosis & Treatment*. New York: Lange Medical Books/McGraw Hill.

National Center for Health Statistics, Diabetes. http://www.cdc.gov/nchs/fastats/diabetes.htm (accessed March 17, 2011).

National Institute for Diabetes and Digestive and Kidney Diseases, NIH. National Diabetes Statistics. (2011). http://diabetes.niddk.nih.gov/dm/pubs/statistics/index.htm#allages (accessed March 17, 2011).

Chapter 17

PSYCHIATRIC MENTAL HEALTH

Valerie A. Hart • Patricia Hentz

Unlike other clinical areas discussed in this book, the differential diagnosis of psychiatric conditions can depend less on laboratory findings and physical assessment data than on patient's complaints and reports of symptoms. As a result, the art of interviewing and skills of active listening are critical when attempting to rule out conditions with similar symptoms. In addition, the clinician must grapple with the question of whether a presenting symptom is genuine or instead represents factitious behavior or malingering, is related to substance abuse, is a medical condition, or represents any of the overlapping symptoms within one of the categories covered in this chapter.

This chapter also looks at "medical mimics," or conditions that may easily be categorized as psychiatric in nature but that appear to have confusing medical presentations. The chapter focuses on common Axis I and Axis II psychiatric disorders and common symptoms or complaints. Since many disorders have overlapping symptoms, critical indicators are presented with examples of focused questions to guide practitioners in determining the differential diagnosis. Owing to practical limitations, this is not intended to be an all-inclusive review but rather a choice of diagnostic areas most likely to be encountered by advanced practice clinicians in a primary care setting.

Diagnosis of a psychiatric illness requires attention to physical and biological indicators along with a psychiatric evaluation. Psychiatric symptoms may present in response to a medical illness, may be triggered by medications, or may be a very normative response to a stressful life event, such as in the case of grieving a loss. When a psychiatric illness is believed to be the primary problem, a comprehensive psychiatric evaluation is indicated to achieve an accurate diagnosis. For example, when a client presents with complaints of feeling tired, having difficulty sleeping, and feeling agitated and anxious, the practitioner must rule out a medical illness, determine whether the symptoms are in response to medications, and explore whether they are related to a stressful life event. When these possibilities are ruled out, a psychiatric evaluation may be indicated. Conducting a psychiatric evaluation helps prevent the frequent treatment mistake of focusing on the obvious symptoms of sleeping difficulty, anxiety, or agitation and missing an underlying depression. In such situations, a minor tranquilizer might be prescribed that could actually exacerbate depression by depleting serotonin. The basic disorder may be a depression with coexisting anxiety symptoms.

Comprehensive Psychiatric Evaluation

A comprehensive psychiatric evaluation leads to a diagnosis that encompasses five major axes: clinical disorder (Axis I), personality disorder (Axis II), physical disorders/medical conditions (Axis III), psychosocial and environmental problems/stressors (Axis IV), and the degree of functional impairment (Axis V). Targeted questions in the following areas aid in determining the appropriate psychiatric diagnosis. Although it is not critical to follow this guide in a lock-step manner, attention to the major areas can help prevent an inaccurate psychiatric diagnosis. This section provides a brief overview of the psychiatric evaluation. The sections that follow highlight various psychiatric problems and offer additional guides for assessment.

■ Problem Identification and Chief Complaint

Identify the reason for seeking care at this time in the patient's own words. Because many common symptoms fall within a variety of psychiatric diagnoses, the practitioner looks for specific clusters of symptoms to determine the diagnosis. So, given the chief complaint, "I have been feeling tired recently. I have not been able to sleep well, and I have felt restless during the day and anxious," many more details are necessary to accurately diagnose.

■ History of Present Illness

A symptom analysis similar to that done for nonpsychiatric complaints is indicated to determine the history of the specific complaint and to identify any associated problems. This analysis can be integrated into the general assessment. It should explore the time line related to symptoms, the relationship of symptoms to life events, any recent conflicts or stressors, any drugs that are used, and how the current level of functioning differs from the client's previous level of functioning. If, at the initial presentation of a complaint, the patient indicates that the problem has existed for some time, the sequence of events leading up to the visit at this particular time may identify important triggers that have either exacerbated the problem or convinced the patient (or family member) that help was needed for the problem.

■ Pertinent Past Psychiatric History

It is important to determine whether the client has a history of any psychiatric disorders. If so, determine the extent of the illness and all prior and current treatments, medications, and outcomes or responses to the treatments. Ask the patient whether he or she believes that prior treatments were beneficial and how well they were tolerated.

■ Pertinent Social History

The social history is an essential part of the psychiatric history. It is important to explore questions about education, family relationships, social networks, potential abuse history, and employment. This part of the history should include information on all drug and alcohol abuse because many psychiatric disorders mimic substance abuse. Psychiatric symptoms may actually stem from adverse effects of a prescribed, over-the-counter, or recreational drug. The following sections on specific complaints and problems identify medications associated with each of the complaints discussed. Obtaining a history of occupational and recreational activities and of performance of activities of daily living provides crucial information about how problems affect an individual's overall life. Finally, the social history is important in determining the disposition of a patient following assessment and diagnosis.

■ Pertinent Family History

Obtain a family history, including questions about psychiatric history as well as medical and genetic illnesses.

■ Medical History and the Review of Symptoms

Many times, psychiatric symptoms are a result of underlying medical conditions. In such cases, the focus for treatment is the medical condition. For example, the following sections identify medical conditions that can cause or exacerbate mental health symptoms, including depression, anxiety, eating disorders, and alterations in thought processes. It is important to identify all allergies or intolerances to both psychotropic and other medications.

■ Mental Status Examination

The mental status examination comprises five major areas: (1) appearance and behavior, (2) mood and affect, (3) speech and thought processes, (4) thought content and perceptual abnormalities, and (5) sensorial, cognitive, and intellectual functioning.

Appearance and Behavior

To assess appearance and behavior, observe gait, dress, grooming, posture, gestures, and facial expressions as the history is performed. Note the patient's apparent nutritional status. Note whether the patient maintains eye contact or exhibits any unusual behaviors during the history. For example, a patient presenting with mania might exhibit psychomotor agitation, distractibility, colorful clothes or bizarre combinations of clothes, excessive makeup, and intrusiveness. The client's behavior may range from entertaining to very irritable.

Mood and Affect

Mood is the subjective experience as self-reported. Ask the client to describe how he or she feels: well, happy, depressed, anxious, and so on. In contrast, affect is the practitioner's impression. Note whether your impression is that of a happy, depressed, anxious, flat, or other type of affect.

Speech and Thought Process

The tone, quality, quantity, and rate of speech are important indications of mental status. For instance, in mania, the speech may be pressured, loud, dramatic, and exaggerated; in depression, the speech may be soft and monotone with little or no spontaneity. In addition to noting speech patterns, consider whether the client's thought processes are clear, logical, and organized. With altered thought processes, a patient's speech may indicate irrelevant information (loose associations), frequent change of topics (flight of ideas), vagueness (circumstantiality), permanent departure from the topic of conversation (tangential thought), halted speech (thought blocking), or other signs of a formal thought disorder.

Thought Content and Perceptual Abnormalities

During the mental status examination, it is important to determine whether the patient is experiencing abnormal content of thought, such as hallucinations or delusions. Ask whether the patient sees things that others cannot see or hears voices that others cannot hear. If so, it is important to explore what type of hallucination is experienced. To assess for delusions, ask the patient whether he or she has any powers or abilities that others do not have or thoughts that others would consider strange. Determine whether the patient has obsessions or compulsions or experiences feelings of hopelessness, worthlessness, or guilt.

When patients are experiencing mental health problems, it is vital to assess for suicidal ideation or intent. Sixty percent of depressed clients have suicidal ideations. Patients should be asked whether they have previously performed any acts of self-harm or have any thoughts of harming or killing themselves in the future. Positive responses require more detailed assessment of current suicidal risk.

The Sensorium and Cognitive and Intellectual Functioning

Determine each patient's general level of orientation and alertness. Alertness may be affected or blunted by mental health problems such as depression. To assess the level of intelligence, ask about common knowledge issues. Often this assessment can be incorporated into the exploration of the client's history, work, and education. Judgment can be assessed in relation to how the client has handled situations in the past as well as any current challenges. Insight may be determined by evaluating the patient's understanding of current health status or living situation.

■ Assessing for Potential Medical Mimics

Whenever faced with a mental health complaint, it is vital that the differential diagnosis initially include any medical problems that could be correctable. This category includes nonpsychiatric health problems and the myriad of medications and treatments that may result in complaints similar to those of psychiatric problems. Hedeya (1996) provides a set of rules designed to help spot medical mimics (Box 17.1). The mnemonic "THINC MED" is useful when evaluating for underlying medical conditions that present as psychiatric symptoms (see Box 17.2).

Box 17.1

Rules to Follow for Spotting Medical Mimics

1. Never assume that an emotional symptom has a psychosocial cause until physical causes are fully explored.
2. Always have your patients get a complete physical if they have not had one since the onset of symptoms.
3. Look for a history that does not fit.
4. Check personal and family history thoroughly.
5. Be suspicious when the onset comes late in life (e.g., a first psychotic break after age 40) and/or when no stressors are present.
6. Be suspicious of a recent onset of headaches, loss of function, unusual perceptions, visual disturbances, paranormal experiences, or hallucinations.
7. Ask about all drug use, including over the counter and illicit.

Box 17.2

THINC MED

The following are major categories of medical mimics.

T Tumors
H Hormones (thyroid, adrenals, gonadal, insulin)
I Infections and immune diseases (AIDS, Lyme disease, mononucleosis, lupus, syphilis)
N Nutrition (B_{12}, B_1, B_6, manganese, iron overload)
C Central nervous system (head trauma, multiple sclerosis, seizures, Parkinson's disease, Huntington's disease)
M Miscellaneous (sleep apnea, anemia, congestive heart failure)
E Electrolyte abnormalities and toxins (K^+, NA^+, chemical exposures)
D Drugs (also include nicotine and caffeine)

Differential Diagnosis of Chief Complaints

■ Anxiety

Anxiety disorders make up the most common category of psychiatric conditions and are responsible for frequent patient use of the health-care system. Anxiety disorders affect approximately 40 million American adults (National Institute of Mental Health, 2009). Both functional impairment and morbidity have been linked to anxiety disorders, and recent studies suggest that chronic anxiety disorders may increase the rate of cardiovascular-related mortality. Anxiety disorders often go unrecognized and untreated in primary care (Kroenke et al., 2007). The etiology of anxiety disorders is a complex dance of genetic predisposition and environmental factors, as in many other psychiatric conditions. It is important to distinguish between *normal* anxiety, which everyone experiences, and anxiety that reaches the level of psychopathology. Anxiety is an unpleasant feeling of apprehension, often accompanied by perspiration, palpitation, stomach discomfort, restlessness, difficulty sitting still, and even tightness in the chest. Anxiety is usually differentiated from *fear* in that when one is fearful, there is an identifiable dreaded object, as opposed to anxiety, in which there is no specific focus. Whereas anxiety is a normal response to stress, pathologic anxiety is distinguished by the intensity, duration, level of impairment to coping it renders, and whether there is an environmental trigger.

Anxiety is quite common in the general medical setting. Patients with a single anxiety disorder are 56% more likely to be frequent users of medical services (Schmitz & Kruse, 2002). More than 90% of patients with anxiety present primarily with somatic complaints in primary care and emergency department settings (Stern & Herman, 2000). Patients with anxiety often present with the following symptoms: chest pain (with negative angiogram), irritable bowel, unexplained dizziness, migraine headache, and chronic fatigue. The medical workup for this type of patient relies on both the medical and psychiatric histories, the medication and drug histories, and the physical and neurological exams.

When assessing a patient who may be anxious, the most obvious indicators are those involving the sympathetic nervous system, such as increased heart rate, blood pressure, pallor, dry mouth, increased respiration, and sweating. These familiar signs are representations of the fight-or-flight response. Patients may also exhibit behavior connected with parasympathetic activity, such as pacing, tapping toes or fingers, and adjusting clothing (displacement activities) (Shea, 1998). Children and adolescents with anxiety disorders may present with headache, stomachache, or excessive worry and fears (Connolly & Berstein, 2007).

The *Diagnostic and Statistical Manual of Mental Disorders*, Fourth Edition (Text Revision), or DSM-IV-TR, lists 12 anxiety disorders: (1) panic disorder with agoraphobia, (2) panic disorder without agoraphobia, (3) agoraphobia without history of panic disorder, (4) specific phobia, (5) social phobia, (6) obsessive-compulsive disorder, (7) posttraumatic stress disorder, (8) acute stress disorder, (9) generalized anxiety disorder, (10) anxiety disorder due to a general medical condition, (11) substance-induced anxiety disorder, and (12) not otherwise specified.

Medical Problems and Medications

As with all mental health symptoms, the first step in the differential diagnosis is to rule out any general medical condition (Box 17.3) or medication use as the physiological cause of the anxiety. After ruling out a medical condition, the answers to the initial questions determine the next steps.

 MEDICATIONS CAUSING ANXIETY

Caffeine
Thyroid medications
Theophylline
Albuterol

Panic Disorder

Panic disorder is a syndrome characterized by recurrent unexpected panic attacks about which there is persistent concern. Panic attacks are discrete episodes of intense anxiety that peak within 10 minutes and are associated with autonomic arousal (cardiac, pulmonary, gastrointestinal, and neurological symptoms) as well as feelings of depersonalization/derealization and the fear of dying, losing control, or going crazy. After an initial attack, the apprehension of a future attack often occurs and is referred to as anticipatory anxiety. The anticipation is often as distressing (if not more so) to patients as the experience of an actual episode. Questions that should be included in the history in order to assess for panic disorder and panic attack are listed in Box 17.4.

Generalized Anxiety Disorder

Patients with generalized anxiety disorder are worried most of the time about many different concerns both reasonable and unfounded. For this diagnosis, the

---

Box 17.3

Medical Conditions Associated With Anxiety

- Hyperthyroidism
- Congestive heart failure
- Asthma
- Chronic obstructive pulmonary disease
- Malignancy

- Pheochromocytoma
- Hyperadrenal
- Hypoglycemia
- Epilepsy
- Myocardial infarction

Box 17.4

Questions for Assessing Panic Disorder and Panic Attack

1. *"Have you had episodes when you felt nervous, frightened, anxious, uneasy in situations when most people did not feel that way? Did the feelings peak within 10 minutes?"* **(panic disorder)**

2. *"Do you feel nervous in places where you might have a panic attack or when escape might be difficult, such as in a crowd; standing in a line; on a bridge; in a bus, plane, or train?"* **(agoraphobia)**

Questions Related to Panic Attack

1. *"In the past, did these episodes occur unexpectedly?"*
   a. *Was your heart racing?*
   b. *Did you have difficulty breathing?*
   c. *Were your hands sweaty?*
   d. *Did you have chest pain?*
   e. *Did you fear that you were dying?*
   f. *Did you feel dizzy or think you were going to faint?*

2. *"Have you had an episode and then for a month or more feared having another episode, or attack?"*

DSM-IV-TR requires several episodes of worry to occur on most days for at least a 6-month period of time. Patients find this worry impossible to control and usually associated with somatic symptoms, often sleep complaints, muscle pain, bowel function, mood, or problems at work or in relationships. Questions for assessing generalized anxiety disorder are listed in Box 17.5.

Social Phobia

Social phobia is characterized by a marked fear of being the center of attention or behaving in a way that will result in embarrassment or humiliation; this phobia is also characterized by marked avoidance of these situations. The fears are

Box 17.5

Questions for Assessing Generalized Anxiety Disorder

1. *"Have you been worried about many things over the past 6 months?"*

2. *"Are these worries present most days?"*

3. *"Do you find it difficult to control your worries?"*

4. *"Do they interfere with your ability to concentrate on what you are doing?"*

manifested in social situations, such as eating or speaking in public or entering a social gathering, meeting, or classroom. Symptoms of anxiety, such as blushing, and/or fear of vomiting, urgency, micturition, or defecation are also often present. Social phobia can be associated with panic attacks. It must be differentiated from normal shyness and appropriate fear as well as from schizophrenia, hypochondriasis, obsessive-compulsive disorder, and paranoid personality disorder. The content of the anxiety determines the steps in a decision tree. In panic disorder, with or without agoraphobia, anxiety is related to the fear of having additional episodes and the ramifications of the episodes. Specific phobia and social phobia are related to specific fears. Specific phobias, according to the DSM-IV-TR, are divided into animal type; nature type; blood, injection, injury type; situational type (elevators, tunnels); and other.

Obsessive-Compulsive Disorder

Obsessions (recurring thoughts) and compulsions (recurring actions) over which the patient has little or no control are the hallmark of this condition. The obsessions and compulsions interfere with everyday functioning and cause embarrassment because the sufferer is well aware of the bizarre nature of the behavior. The link to anxiety is that the behavior and thinking is an attempt to control anxiety. The most common obsession is that of "contamination" and washing or avoidance of a particular object that is contaminated. Along with anxiety, patients often experience shame and self-loathing. Another common obsession is self-doubt, such as in checking to see that routine safety chores are done, then making multiple trips to recheck in order to satisfy the doubt. Guilt is a common derivative of this obsession. Intrusive thoughts are another common class of obsessions in which repetitive thoughts of either an aggressive or sexual nature haunt a patient and cause severe distress. The major differentials for obsessive-compulsive disorder include phobias, depressive disorders, schizophrenias and obsessive-compulsive personality disorder, and Tourette's disorder.

Posttraumatic Stress Disorder

Posttraumatic stress disorder is a cluster of symptoms that occur as a result of exposure to stressful or traumatic situations. The patient may experience flashbacks, memories, recurring dreams, or avoidance behavior that was not present before exposure to the stressor. The patient must exhibit either an inability to recall some important aspect of the period of exposure to the stressor (depersonalization, derealization, or dissociative amnesia) or show marked anxiety and increased arousal (difficulty sleeping, irritability, the startle response, motor restlessness, hypervigilance, poor concentration). Differential diagnosis includes head injury, substance abuse, other anxiety disorders, mood disorders, dissociative disorders, borderline personality disorder, and malingering.

■ Mood Disorders

This section examines several categories of mood disorders, discusses clusters of symptoms, and presents the process of continuing assessment. The mood disorders presented are major depressive disorder, dysthymic disorder, cyclothymic disorder, bipolar disorder, seasonal pattern depression, postpartum depression, and premenstrual dysphoric disorder.

Depression is a clinically heterogeneous disorder resulting from a combination of genetic and environmental factors. The expression of depression is quite variable (Hentz, 2005, p. 15). It can present in a variety of ways, and the cluster of symptoms can vary markedly from one individual to the next. For example, depression may cause severe sleep disturbance for one individual and hypersomnia in another. Some individuals with depression complain of weight gain, whereas others lose weight because they find it hard to eat. Avolition is a common presenting feature in depression, but some individuals experience restlessness and agitation. Symptoms of depression include changes in mood, cognition, behavior, and motor function (Box 17.6). The accurate assessment of presenting symptoms is key to treatment. Based on diagnosis and symptoms, a combination of psychotherapy with medication is often the most effective approach.

The goal in the treatment of depression is remission. The risk of recurrence of depression is 50% after one episode, 70% after two episodes, and 90% after three episodes. Early detection and treatment are critical, as is early intervention when signs and symptoms of recurrence are detected. There is a 5% to 11%

Box 17.6

Symptoms of Depression

Mood Symptoms

Depressed mood	Tears
Anhedonia	Loss of hope
Loss of reactivity	Loss of interest
Loss of self-esteem	Social withdrawal

Psychomotor Retardation Symptoms

Loss of energy	Decreased interest in activities
Cognitive symptoms	Subjective inefficient thinking
Subjective inability to concentrate	Thoughts of dying
Pessimism	Free-floating anxiety
General rating of anxiety	Phobias

Behavioral Symptoms

Psychomotor agitation	Subjectively described restlessness
Irritability	Suicidality
Guilty ideas of reference	Fatigue and exhaustion
Depressed mood worse in morning	Loss of appetite or increased
Sleep disturbances	appetite (carbohydrate craving)
Early waking	Hypersomnia

lifetime prevalence for depression; morbidity is comparable to angina and advanced coronary artery disease. The ability to accurately diagnose depression is critical. Untreated and undertreated depression significantly increases the risk of suicide: 1 out of 7 people with recurrent depressive illness commits suicide; 70% of suicides have depressive illness; and 70% of suicides see their primary care provider within 6 weeks of suicide. Suicide is the seventh leading cause of death in the United States (Stahl, 2000).

Symptoms of depression can be vague, such as fatigue, loss of appetite, and sleep disturbances. Research has shown that up to 30% of individuals who fully meet the criteria for major depression actually deny being depressed (Shea, 1998). Tools such as the Hamilton Rating Scale for Depression (HAM-D) are helpful in assessing for depression; however, they are not a replacement for skillful interviewing.

The assessment of depression includes questions designed to identify whether or not the person is experiencing a general loss of pleasure in life or in activities he or she usually enjoys. It is important to determine whether there is any sense of being sad or a general dysphoric mood and whether any neurovegetative symptoms are evident. Manic and hypomanic symptoms should always be actively sought. As with other mental health assessments, the past psychiatric history and history of alcohol and/or drug use should always be elicited; they are commonly associated with depression. What appears to be major depression may actually be a result of alcohol or street drug use (Shea, 1998).

Medical Problems and Medications

Several medical conditions (Box 17.7) and numerous medications (Box 17.8) can be associated with symptoms of depression. If medications are the contributing cause, switching medications may be advised.

Box 17.7

Medical Problems That Can Present With Symptoms of Depression

Addison's disease	infectious hepatitis
AIDS	malignancies
anemia	menopause
asthma	multiple sclerosis
chronic fatigue syndrome	postpartum hormonal changes
chronic infection	premenstrual syndrome
congestive heart failure	rheumatoid arthritis
Cushing's disease	systemic lupus
diabetes	ulcerative colitis
hyperthyroidism	uremia
hypothyroidism	

Box 17.8	

Drugs That Can Cause Depression

- Antihypertensives (reserpine, propranolol, methyldopa, guanethidine mono-sulfate, and clonidine hydrochloride)
- Corticosteroids and hormones (cortisone acetate, estrogen, and progesterone)
- Antiparkinsonian drugs (levodopa and carbidopa, amantadine hydrochloride)
- Antianxiety drugs (diazepam, chlordiazepoxide)
- Accutane
- Birth control pills

Major Depression

To meet the criteria for major depressive episode, an individual must have symptoms over a 2-week period that represent a change from previous functioning, with at least one of the symptoms being a depressed mood or a loss of interest or pleasure (APA, 2000). Five of the nine criteria for major depression must be met during a 2-week period, as well as either depressed mood or diminished interest during the 2-week period.

1. Depressed mood most of the day, nearly every day, as indicated by either subjective report (e.g., feels sad or empty) or observation made by others (e.g., appears tearful). Children and adolescents may display irritability.
2. Markedly diminished interest or pleasure in all, or almost all, activities most of the day, nearly every day (as indicated by either subjective account or observation made by others).
3. Significant weight loss when not dieting, weight gain (e.g., a change of more than 5% of body weight in a month), or a decrease or increase in appetite nearly every day. In children, consider failure to make expected weight gains.
4. Insomnia or hypersomnia nearly every day.
5. Psychomotor agitation or retardation nearly every day (observable by others, not merely subjective feelings of restlessness or being slowed down).
6. Fatigue or loss of energy nearly every day.
7. Feelings of worthlessness or excessive or inappropriate guilt (which may be delusional) nearly every day (not merely self-reproach or guilt about being sick).
8. Diminished ability to think or concentrate or indecisiveness nearly every day (either by subjective account or as observed by others).
9. Recurrent thoughts of death (not just fear of dying), recurrent suicidal ideation without a specific plan, or a suicidal attempt or a specific plan for committing suicide.

If these criteria are met, additional symptom analysis is needed to explore changes in appetite, sleep, activity, energy concentration, and thoughts of self-harm. The HAM-D is a 21-item rating tool to identify the severity of depression and evaluate the patient's response to treatment. The mnemonic "SIGECAPS" is helpful for remembering criteria for depression (see Box 17.9).

An individual with major depression may experience difficulty with routine personal care and present as unkempt, unclean, and with a slowness of movement. In contrast, an individual with agitated depression experiences "a nagging need to move" (Shea, 1998). Thought process and content may reflect an inability to plan and make life decisions, called "blocking of the future." A marked slowing in thinking often occurs and is reflected in slowness in responding to questions and in long pauses. This change in cognition can be described as the stream of thought being frozen by an unexpected drop in temperature. In contrast, individuals with agitated depression experience thought process as a stream of thought in a turbulent boil (Shea, 1998). Restricted thought content, or "ideational caging," is the experience of having thoughts trapped within a small network of themes or ruminations.

Dysthymic Disorder

Unlike major depression, individuals with dysthymic disorder are more functional. Dysthymic disorder is marked by a longstanding, pervasive mood of sadness or depression for most of the time over a 2-year period. Individuals often state, "This is just the way I always am." Along with the depressed mood, at least two of the following symptoms need to be present: poor appetite or overeating, insomnia or hypersomnia, low energy or fatigue, low self-esteem, poor concentration or difficulty making decisions, and feelings of hopelessness. In children, the mood may be irritable rather than depressed, with a minimum duration of 1 year (APA, 2000). In other words, to meet the criteria of dysthymic disorder, the patient's sad, depressed, or irritable mood must present as stable.

Dysthymic disorder can precede major depression; however, it is important to note that if dysthymic disorder is not present before a major depression, the symptoms following treatment of major depression should be viewed as a partial response rather than as dysthymic disorder. If the depression is partially relieved, individuals may meet the criteria of apathetic responder. They present with a reduction of depressed mood, continuing anhedonia, lack of motivation, decreased libido, lack of interest, cognitive slowing, and decreased concentration. Anxious responders demonstrate a reduction of depressed mood; continuing anxiety,

---

Box 17.9

SIGECAPS

S	Sleep	**C**	Concentration
I	Interest	**A**	Appetite
G	Guilt	**P**	Psychomotor
E	Energy	**S**	Suicidality

especially generalized anxiety; worry; insomnia; and somatic complaints (Stahl, 2000). Apathetic responders and anxious responders are often associated with ineffective treatment of the major depression. In such cases, medications need to be adjusted. For a diagnosis of dysthymic disorder after a major depression, the individual must first meet the criteria for a full remission or have been diagnosed with dysthymic disorder prior to the major depression.

Bipolar Disorder

Assessment of depression should always be followed by an assessment of bipolar disorder. Major depressive and bipolar disorders must be distinguished from episodes of a substance-induced mood disorder or those due to a general medical condition (e.g., multiple sclerosis, stroke, hypothyroidism).

Approximately 10% to 15% of adolescents with recurrent major depressive episodes will develop bipolar I disorder. Mixed episodes are more prevalent in adolescents and young adults than in older adults. In males, the first episode is more likely to be manic, whereas females usually present first with depression. Women with bipolar I disorder have an increased risk of developing subsequent episodes during the postpartum period (APA, 2000).

Bipolar disorder is a cluster of disorders that reflect a marked flux in mood. A manic episode is a distinct period of a persistently elevated, expansive, or irritable mood lasting at least 1 week. This mood must coexist with at least three of the following symptoms: inflated self-esteem or grandiosity, decreased need for sleep, pressure of speech, flight of ideas, distractibility, increased involvement in goal-directed activities or psychomotor agitation, and excessive involvement in pleasurable activities with a high potential for painful consequences. Hypomanic episodes differ from manic episodes in the degree of severity. Hypomanic episodes are not usually sufficiently severe to cause marked impairment in social or occupational functioning or to require hospitalization (APA, 2000). They may, however, evolve into fully manic episodes. The mnemonic "DIG FAST" is helpful for remembering the critical criteria for mania (see Box 17.10).

Bipolar I disorder is characterized by the occurrence of one or more manic episodes or mixed episodes. Mixed episodes are characterized by a period of time

---

Box 17.10

DIG FAST

D Distractibility; leaving tasks unfinished
I Insomnia; decreased need for sleep
G Grandiosity; increased self-worth
F Flight of ideas
A Activity increased; goal directed
S Speech is pressured, hyperverbal, and rapid
T Thoughtless risk (sex, money)

(lasting at least 1 week) in which the criteria are met both for manic episode and for a major depressive episode nearly every day. Social and/or occupational functioning are severely impaired as the individual experiences rapidly alternating moods (APA, 2000). To aid in the differential diagnosis for bipolar I disorder, explore whether the patient has experienced episodes of feeling "high," with noticeably increased energy and elation, requiring less sleep than normal, and/or experienced rapid thoughts. Ask about episodes of feeling unusually creative or productive that were noticeable to others. Also explore episodes of anger, irritability, and/or rage.

Completed suicides occur in 10% to 15% of individuals with bipolar I disorder. Suicide ideation and attempts are more likely in the depressive or mixed state (APA, 2000). Therefore, suicide risk should always be assessed in a psychiatric evaluation. Box 17.11 lists several questions for assessing suicide risk. If the responses identify a detailed plan for ending life, a lack of hope that things can be better in the future, or an inability to identify reasons for not dying (such as not wanting to leave loved ones), it is considered a psychiatric emergency, requiring immediate intervention.

Bipolar II disorder is determined when the clinical course includes one or more major depressive episodes and at least one hypomanic episode. The symptoms cause clinically significant distress or impairment in social, occupational, or other important areas of functioning (APA, 2000). To meet the bipolar II criteria, the individual has not experienced a manic or mixed episode.

Cyclothymic Disorder

Cyclothymic disorder is a chronic, fluctuating mood disturbance including hypomanic and depressive symptoms that do not meet the criteria for manic episode. In addition, the depressive symptoms lack the severity, pervasiveness, or duration to meet the criteria for depressive episode. To meet the criteria for cyclothymic disorder, symptoms must be present over a 2-year period without

---

Box 17.11

Questions for Assessing Suicide Risk

1. *"Have you been thinking that you would be better off dead or wishing that you were dead?"*

2. *"Do you have thoughts of harming yourself?"*

3. *"Have you being thinking about suicide?"*

4. *"If you have been thinking about suicide, do you have a plan? If so, describe the plan."*

5. *"Have you recently attempted suicide?"*

6. *"In the past, have you thought about or attempted suicide?"*

a lapse of symptoms longer than 2 months. Many individuals function with minor distress or impairment in social, occupational, or other areas. Individuals may present as temperamental, moody, unpredictable, inconsistent, or unreliable (APA, 2000).

Mood Disorders With Specifiers

Seasonal Pattern

Seasonal pattern depression is differentiated from the other mood disorders by the essential feature of onset and remission that is consistently related to specific times of the year. It may have features similar to those of bipolar or major depression. In most cases, episodes begin in the fall or winter and remit in the spring. A key factor is that the mood is not related to situational stressors or cyclical patterns of work or life demands. Assessment involves tracking symptoms to demonstrate clear evidence of a temporal/seasonal relationship.

Postpartum Onset

There is no simple cluster of symptoms to assess during the postpartum period. Onset may be immediate or as late as 6 months after delivery. Baby blues occurs in up to 70% of women postpartum. Given the social pressures to "be happy" with the birth of a new baby, women often mask their underlying depression, a phenomenon called smiling depression. Symptoms common in the postpartum onset include fluctuation in mood, mood lability, and preoccupation with the infant's well-being. Severity of symptoms is the key. On a continuum, thoughts can range from focused and realistic regarding the infant's well-being to obsessive or even delusional. At highest risk are women who have experienced a postpartum episode with psychotic features. Their risk of recurrence is 30% to 50%. Women with a history of depression are also at greater risk. The Edinburgh Postnatal Depression Scale can help identify postpartum depression. See Figure 17.1 for postpartum mood conditions.

Premenstrual Dysphoric Disorder

Premenstrual dysphoric disorder (PMDD) is characterized by recurrent symptoms that occur during the luteal phase of the menstrual cycle and remit during menstruation. Even though many women express mood changes and other symptoms during the premenstrual phase, 5% to 9% fully meet the criteria for PMDD. Differential diagnosis includes bipolar disorder, thyroid dysfunction, premenstrual syndrome, exacerbation of unipolar depression, anxiety disorder, and cyclothymic disorder. Careful tracking of symptoms for at least 2 months is advised to determine a diagnosis of PMDD (Box 17.12).

■ Substance-Related Disorders

This category includes disorders associated with alcohol and drugs, medication side effects, and toxin-induced mental states. Owing to the effect of certain substances on mood, cognition, perception, and behavior, patients may present with a confusing array of symptoms. In the DSM-IV-TR, substance-related

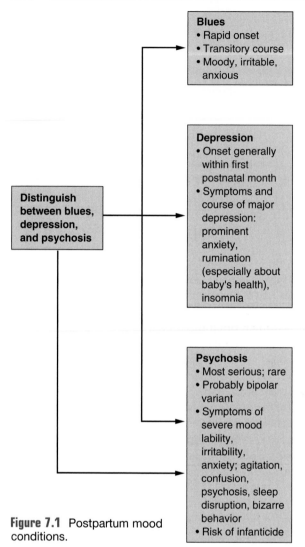

Figure 7.1 Postpartum mood conditions.

disorders are cross-referenced in the following disorders: delirium (intoxication and withdrawal), substance-induced dementia, amnesic disorder, psychotic disorder, mood disorder, anxiety disorder, sexual dysfunction, and sleep disorder.

Comorbidity with other psychiatric conditions is high in this population. Antisocial personality disorder is present in a high percentage (35%–60%) of patients presenting for treatment of substance abuse and dependence. Other psychiatric disorders associated with substance-related disorders include mood disorders and anxiety disorders.

Prioritizing the differential diagnosis demands ruling out delirium, dementia, and amnesic disorder. Initial symptoms to be alerted to include a change in

Box 17.12

Premenstrual Dysphoric Disorder

- Note recurring physical and emotional symptoms in late luteal phase, dissipating 1 or 2 days after menses.
- Encourage prospective rating of symptoms.
- Document precipitants.
- Document treatment response history.
- Rule out medical illness with symptoms that mimic premenstrual syndrome.
- Obtain family psychiatric history.
- Note use of stimulants, other mood-altering agents, water-retaining drugs.

cognition, including memory impairment, and disturbed consciousness. If no change of consciousness or memory impairment is present, then look for specific symptoms, which may indicate a substance-induced disorder.

A careful history, physical examination for signs of intoxication or withdrawal, and laboratory analysis will determine substance use. If a substance is identified, the clinician must consider whether a causal relationship exists between the substance use and the psychiatric symptom. Are the symptoms a direct effect of the substance? Is the substance abuse a means of "self-medicating" for a primary psychiatric disorder? Are the psychiatric symptoms and substance abuse independent of one another? Questions related to the timing of the development of psychiatric symptoms and substance use will help determine whether the patient has a primary psychiatric condition or a true substance-abuse disorder. Substance abuse can mimic many common psychiatric symptoms, such as depression, apathy, agitation, anxiety, panic attacks, thought disturbances, paranoia, and psychosis. Thus, during the assessment of *any* psychiatric illness, the use and possible abuse of substances must be evaluated.

Before reviewing an assessment of substance abuse, there are several terms to clarify. The first is *use* versus *abuse*. Sanctioned uses of drugs (e.g., caffeine) have been defined by a culture, vary among cultures, and can change over time. Abuse from a cultural perspective is the self-administration of any drug in a culturally disapproved manner that causes adverse consequences. From a physiologic standpoint, *use* and *abuse* take on different meanings, with a focus on the chemical neurotransmission and the degree of clinically significant impairment or distress. The terms *addiction* and *dependence* are frequently confused. Addiction is not defined as a condition in the DSM-IV. It is a behavioral pattern, as Stahl describes it, of drug abuse characterized by overwhelming involvement with use of a drug (compulsive use) and securing its supply and by a high tendency to relapse after discontinuation. Dependence is the physiological state of neuroadaptation necessitating continued administration to prevent the appearance of a withdrawal syndrome (Stahl, 2000).

Alcohol dependence can be screened for by asking the patient whether he or she has a history of taking three or more alcoholic drinks within a 3-hour period, on three or more occasions. If the answer to this screening question is affirmative, further assess by asking whether the individual has increased the amount of alcohol consumed in order to achieve the same effect, has drank alcohol to avoid hang-over, has experienced shaking, sweating, or agitation upon cutting back. Additional signs of dependence include a patient who has drunk more than intended, tried to stop or reduce drinking, and/or reduced time spent in other activities because of drinking (Sheehan et al., 1998). The criteria for alcohol abuse relate to use that causes adverse consequences. Box 17.13 presents questions used to determine alcohol abuse.

Assessment of drug use, dependence, and abuse follows the questions presented related to alcohol dependence and abuse, after determining which drugs are used. The screening question is, *In the past 12 months, did you take any of the drugs listed below* [see Table 17.1 for a list of drugs] *more than once to get high, to feel better, or to change your mood?* (Sheehan et al., 1998). Ask whether the patient has experienced withdrawal symptoms upon trying to cut back.

■ Eating Disorders

Eating disorders encompass much more than a list of symptoms. The incidence of eating disorders among young people has increased two to five times since 1955, with anorexia nervosa listed as the third-most common chronic illness of adolescence (Stashwick, 1996). According to statistics, it is estimated that 0.5% to 1% of girls 14 to 19 years of age suffer from anorexia nervosa; 1% to 5% fit the DSM-IV criteria of bulimia nervosa; and 10% to 50% fall under the eating disorder not otherwise specified (NOS). Although both men and women are affected by cultural norms of physical attractiveness, the impact on self-esteem is greater for women. Recent results from a large-scale national study suggest that binge eating disorder may occur at a rate higher than previously thought (Hudson et al., 2007).

Box 17.13

Questions to Screen for Alcohol Abuse

1. *"Have you been intoxicated, high, or hung over more than once when you had responsibilities at school, work, or home? Did this cause any problems?"*

2. *"When you were intoxicated in any situation, were you physically at risk? For example, were you driving a car?"*

3. *"Did you have any legal problems because of your drinking?"*

4. *"Did you continue to drink even though your drinking caused problems with your family or other individuals?"*

Table 17.1

Abused Substances

Group	Common Commercial or Street Names
Stimulants	Amphetamines, "speed," crystal meth, "rush," methylphenidate, diet pills, cocaine (snow, dust, flake, nose candy, crack)
Narcotics	Heroin, morphine, hydromorphone, opium, merperidine, methadone, codeine, oxycodone
Hallucinogens	Lysergic acid diethylamide (LSD, "acid"), mescaline, peyote, phencyclidine (PCP, "angel dust," "peace pill"), psilocybin, 2,5-dimethoxy-4-methyl-amphetamine (DOM, "STP"), "mushrooms," 3,4-methylenedioxyamphetamine (MDA), or 3,4-methylenedioxymethamphetamine (MDMA, "ecstasy")
Inhalants	"Glue," ethyl chloride, nitrous oxide ("laughing gas"), amyl or butyl nitrate ("poppers")
Cannabis	Marijuana ("pot," "grass," "weed," "reefer"), Hashish ("hash"), THC
Tranquilizers	Methaqualone, triazolam ("reds"), diazepam, alprazolam, lorazepam, triazolam, barbiturates, meprobomate
Miscellaneous	Steroids, nonprescription sleep or diet pills, gamma-hydroxybutyric acid (GHB, date rape drug).

Anorexia and bulimia have different profiles even though many symptoms can overlap. For example, about 50% of normal-weight individuals with bulimia have a history of anorexia, and approximately 47% with anorexia exhibit bulimic behaviors. The dominant feature of anorexia is the drive to lose weight. Common patterns include restricting food intake and exercising excessively.

Individuals with bulimia are characterized by cycles of binge eating followed by purging; the severity of the disorder determined by the frequency of the binge–purge cycles. In severe cases, the bulimia becomes the center of their life, and all other aspects of life revolve around the binge–purge cycles.

Many adolescents and young adults do not meet the full criteria for anorexia or bulimia but exhibit many of the characteristics. They may fit the diagnosis of eating disorder (NOS). As explained in Schwitzer et al. (2001, p. 158), eating disorders are driven by "(1) perfectionism regarding body image, romantic and other personal relationships, and grades; (2) a fragile sense of self, feelings of inadequacy, and a need to be bolstered by others; (3) self-doubt expressed as sexual intimacy questions and ambivalence about whether one is thin enough to attract a romantic partner and whether one should want to please a partner at all; and (4) a sense of powerlessness in intimate relationships and the world generally." There exists a "high incidence of diagnostically subthreshold problems centering around dissatisfaction with body image. Overall, 35%–45% of adolescent females report difficulties with weight control, regard themselves as too fat, or aspire to become thinner" (Schwitzer et al., 2001).

The aspects that differentiate eating disorders from the "normal" cultural obsessions with weight and thinness are the amount of time and energy involved in the thinking and behaviors associated with an eating disorder and the degree to which it interferes with social functioning. A long-term, large-scale study has found that an Internet-based intervention program may prevent some high-risk college-aged females from developing an eating disorder (Taylor et al., 2006).

Anorexia Nervosa

Individuals with anorexia are below 85% of the normal weight for their height that cannot be attributed to a medical condition. It can also be determined by a body mass index equal to or below 17.5 kg/m² (APA, 2000). Individuals with anorexia do not believe they need to gain weight and have an intense fear of becoming fat even though they are underweight. This fear is not relieved if additional weight is lost. More often, weight loss is accomplished through a reduction in total food intake, particularly high-calorie foods, leading to a diet limited to very few foods.

While the restricting pattern is more common in anorexia, binge–purge behavior may also exist. Although purging may follow a binge episode, purging may also be used even after the consumption of small amounts of food. A significant physical finding in anorexia is an irregular menstrual cycle or amenorrhea. Questions used to screen for anorexia are listed in Box 17.14.

Bulimia Nervosa

Individuals with bulimia are usually within the normal range for weight. The essential features of bulimia nervosa are binge eating and the use of inappropriate compensatory methods to prevent weight gain, such as vomiting or purging. Binge eating is the consumption of a large amount of food in a "discrete period of time" (APA, 2000). High-calorie foods are often preferred, and binging is associated with the abnormally large amounts of food consumed rather than with a craving for a specific type of food, such as carbohydrate. A feature of bulimia is an inability to control binges. Individuals with bulimia have a high degree of dissatisfaction with appearance and often have low self-esteem.

Physical findings may be a noticeable loss of dental enamel on the lingual surfaces of the front teeth as a result of recurrent vomiting. Teeth may become

---

Box 17.14

Questions to Screen for Anorexia

1. *"Do you think your current weight is normal or excessive?"*

2. *"Do you think that any part of your body is still too fat?"*

3. *"Do you have concern or fear about gaining weight even though you are underweight?"*

chipped, and there may also be an increase in dental cavities. The parotid glands may also be enlarged. Calluses or scars may be noted on the dorsal surface of the hand from inducing vomiting. If the dominant hand is used, calluses or scars may be evident on only that hand. There may be electrolyte imbalances—frequently hypokalemia, hyponatremia, and hypochloremia. Assessment for bulimia nervosa includes the questions listed in Box 17.15.

Eating Disorder Not Otherwise Specified

Many individuals present behaviors consistent with some of the features of anorexia and bulimia but do not meet the full criteria for either. The patient may exhibit the thinking patterns common to anorexia, such as an extreme fear of gaining weight or an obsessive need to control the amount or types of food eaten; however, she or he is not below the 85% mark for weight and may not experience irregular menses or amenorrhea. Individuals may also present with features of bulimia, such as binge eating and using compensatory mechanisms less than twice a week, yet not fully meet the criteria. Other abnormal patterns may include occasions of self-induced vomiting not related to binge eating or a pattern of chewing and spitting out food or not swallowing large amounts of food (APA, 2000). Because there may be no physical indicators associated with these patterns, asking directed questions about eating, weight, and body image is key.

Binge-Eating Disorder

An eating disorder in development is binge-eating disorder. The essential features include recurrent episodes of binge eating with an absence of purging behaviors. There is impaired control related to the amount of food consumed and the rate of consumption. It is characterized by the following: eating is often done alone, it is not associated with being hungry, it is done to the point of feeling uncomfortably full, and the individual feels disgust and guilt after overeating. Individuals

---

Box 17.15

Questions to Screen for Bulimia

1. *"In the past 3 months, were there times when you ate very large amounts of food, more than most people would eat, within a short period of time (2 hours)?"*

2. *"Has this occurred at least twice a week over the last 3 months?"*

3. *"Did you feel as if you could not stop eating or control what or how much you were eating?"*

4. *"Have you used any of the following methods to prevent weight gain?"*
   a. *Purging: self-induced vomiting, laxatives, diuretics, enemas, and other medications*
   b. *Nonpurging: fasting or excessive exercise*

present as overweight with marked distress during and after the binge episodes. To meet the criteria for binge-eating disorder, binges average 2 days a week for a period of at least 6 months.

■ Thought Disorders

Thought disorders are evaluated as they relate to (1) content of thought, (2) form of thought, and (3) perception. In psychiatry, thought disorders are commonly associated with schizophrenia and psychosis. However, the severity and the range of symptoms can vary significantly and often do not result from a primary psychiatric illness. Medical conditions, medications, and medical mimics often present with a clinical picture of a thought disorder.

Assessment of the *content of thought* relates to the client's ability to form an accurate assessment of reality. Major difficulties in this area may include delusions, which involve false beliefs held to be true despite proof that they are false or irrational. Examples of delusional thinking include delusions of persecution or of grandeur, somatic delusions, paranoia, and magical thinking.

The second category, *form of thought*, is assessed by listening to how the client presents his or her ideas. Does the client present with looseness of associations? In such situations, the client is unaware that the topics are unconnected. When this is extreme, the practitioner may be unable to understand what the client is talking about. Other difficulties with form of thought include circumstantiality and tangentiality. Circumstantiality is the delay in presenting a point because of numerous unnecessary and tedious details. Tangentiality is the inability to get to the point owing to the introduction of unrelated topics. The degree of circumstantiality and tangentiality can vary significantly. For example, an anxious patient might shift from topic to topic with some awareness of doing so. This would not be considered a thought disorder problem. Serious thought disorder might include neologisms (invented words), word salad (a group of words put together randomly), and clang associations (choice of words based on rhyming).

The third category, *perception*, refers to hallucinations and illusions. Hallucinations are false sensory perceptions that are not associated with external stimuli and may involve any of the five senses. Illusions are misperceptions or misinterpretations of real external stimuli.

Psychotic Disorders

In schizophrenia, psychotic features are evident with two or more of the following characteristics: delusions, hallucinations, disorganized speech, grossly disorganized or catatonic behavior, and negative symptoms. The last of these characteristics, negative symptoms, refers to affective flattening, poverty of speech, avolition, anhedonia, and social isolation. Schizophrenia subtypes include paranoid, disorganized, catatonic, undifferentiated, and residual. Differential diagnoses include schizophreniform disorder, characterized by schizophrenic symptoms of 1 to 6 months; schizoaffective disorder, characterized by a prominent mood component coexisting with the schizophrenic symptoms; delusional disorder, characterized by at least 1 month of no bizarre delusions without an active phase of symptoms of schizophrenia; brief psychotic disorder, characterized by symptoms that last more than 1 day but remit by 1 month; substance-induced psychotic disorder, characterized by symptoms directly related to an abused substance, toxin, or medication; psychotic disorder (NOS), characterized by psychotic presentations that do not meet the criteria for any specific psychotic disorder or in situations in which inadequate or contradictory information exists; and psychotic disorder due to a general medical condition (APA, 2000). Although it is difficult to absolutely differentiate psychosis associated with schizophrenia or bipolar disorder from psychosis originating from a general medical process, there are some common organic causes that should be explored. (see Box 17.16).

The assessment of psychotic disorders can be guided by the Diagnostic Questions listed in Box 17.17. If the patient answers yes to any of the questions, further probing can be accomplished by asking the patient to give an example to

---

Box 17.16

Common Causes of Delirium and Organic Psychosis

Metabolic

1. Electrolyte abnormalities (e.g., altered sodium, calcium, bicarbonate, etc.)
2. Advanced hepatic or renal disease
3. Nutritional disorders (e.g., deficits in thiamine, niacin)
4. Endocrine disorders (e.g., glucose abnormalities, disorders of the thyroid, adrenals, parathyroid)

Infections

1. Systemic (e.g., pneumonia, septicemia, malaria, and syphilis)
2. Intercranial (e.g., meningitis, encephalitis)

Neurological Disorders

1. Neurovascular (e.g., hypertensive crisis, stroke, subarachnoid hemorrhage)
2. Seizures
3. Trauma
4. Space-occupying lesions

Substances

1. Withdrawal (e.g., alcohol, stimulants, sedatives)
2. Intoxication (e.g., alcohol, stimulants, sedatives)
3. Adverse effects (e.g., digoxin, anticholinergics, levodopa, corticosteroids, barbiturates, antipsychotics, antidepressants, antidepressants)

Postoperative Sequelae

Ropper & Samuels (2009); Shea (1998); Simon, Greenberg, & Aminoff (2009).

Box 17.17

Diagnostic Questions for Psychotic Disorders

1. *"Have you ever believed people are out to get you or have been spying on you?"*
   If yes: *Do you currently believe this?* **Example:**

2. *"Have you ever thought that someone could read your mind or that you could read someone's mind?"*
   If yes: *Do you currently believe this?* **Example:**

3. *"Have you ever believed that a force outside of you had control over your thoughts or actions?"*
   If yes: *Do you currently believe this?* **Example:**

4. *"Have you ever believed you were being sent messages through the TV, radio, newspaper, or computer?"*
   If yes: *Do you currently believe this?* **Example:**

5. *"Have you ever heard voices that others around you could not hear?"*
   If yes: *Do you currently hear them?* **Example:**

---

determine the distortion of perception and thought and whether they can be considered "bizarre." In addition, check for evidence of thoughts that are based in reality. For example, if you ask, "Have you ever believed people are out to get you or have been spying on you?" and if, in reality, the person was actually being stalked, it would not be a case of delusional thinking. Delusions are considered bizarre when they are absurd, implausible, not understandable, and clearly do not relate to ordinary life experiences (Sheehan et al., 1998). Hallucinations are considered bizarre if a voice comments about the person's thoughts and behaviors or when there are two or more voices conversing with each other (Sheehan et al., 1998). The nature of hallucinations varies. Understanding the differences may help in determining whether the psychosis has medical origins, is in response to substance abuse, or is psychiatric in nature. A true visual hallucination is a perceptual image that arises from an open space and is not being triggered by an environmental stimulus. Illusions are images that *are* triggered by an actual object or stimulus. Visual hallucinations in patients whose psychosis is related to delirium differs from the classic psychosis in the following ways: the visual hallucination (1) more often occurs at night, (2) is frequently perceived as moving, (3) is briefer in duration, and (4) has no personal significance to the patient. A patient with delirium may see a snake, whereas a patient with schizophrenia may hallucinate about a deceased relative. Asking the client to state the time of day or night when he or she sees the hallucination helps in the differentiation. In medical conditions, hallucinations are often seen at night and when the patient closes his or her eyes. In schizophrenia, visual hallucinations are usually present with auditory hallucinations and occur in an otherwise normal-appearing environment and appear somewhat suddenly.

Substance abuse can produce psychotic episodes. Among the common agents are "speed," lysergic acid diethylamide (LSD), hallucinogens, marijuana, cocaine, crack, and phencyclidine (PCP). In a drug-induced psychosis, the environment appears distorted with numerous illusions and hallucinations. From a behavioral perspective, psychotic symptoms tend to be very bizarre and can be violent. On physical examination, nystagmus and hypertension may be present. Unlike schizophrenia, drug-induced psychosis usually presents with rapid-onset psychotic symptoms.

In addition to street drugs or commonly abused drugs, anticholinergic agents can precipitate delirium, especially in elderly patients. Anticholinergic medications can cause a patient to present with hyperthermia, blurred vision, dry skin, facial flushing, and delirium. The mnemonic "hot as a pepper, blind as a bat, dry as a bone, red as a beet, and mad as a hatter" can be used to describe this toxic state (Shea, 1998). It is important to note that anticholinergic syndrome may be incomplete or hidden by other medications, such as opiates, and not present as a classic anticholinergic syndrome.

Issues Related to Older Adults

The presence of coexisting medical conditions makes accurate psychiatric diagnosis and treatment a complex matter. History-taking and the mental status examination of older adults is similar to those for younger patients, but cognitive impairments make verification from a family member an important difference.

Psychiatric history includes identification (name, sex, marital status), chief complaint, history of present illness, history of previous illnesses, personal and family history, and current medication review. Past history can provide invaluable information about personality organization, coping styles, and defense mechanisms during times of stress. Family history includes adaptation to old age and the presence of Alzheimer's disease if known.

Mental disorders of old age include depressive disorders, cognitive disorders, phobias, and substance abuse, particularly alcohol. Psychosocial risk factors that predispose older adults to mental illness include social isolation and loss of friends, social roles, autonomy, and health. In 2006, there were 14.22 suicides per 100,000 adults 65 or older (Centers for Disease Control and Prevention, 2009). Studies show that up to 75% of elders who die by suicide visited a health-care provider within a month of death (Conwell, 2001), further emphasizing the importance of detection and treatment in this population.

Other common conditions related to this age group are vertigo, syncope, hearing loss, elder abuse, spousal bereavement, and sleep disorders. The very real possibility for psychiatric symptoms related to either a response to medications or a medical condition is an important concept with elderly patients.

REFERENCES

American Psychiatric Association (APA). (2000). *Diagnostic and Statistical Manual of Mental Disorder* (4th ed., Text Revision). (DSM IV-TR). Washington, DC: American Psychiatric Association.

Centers for Disease Control and Prevention, National suice statistics at a glance [online]. (2009). Available from: http://www.cdc.gov/violenceprevention/suicide/statistics/aag.html#3 [accessed October 7, 2010].

Connolly, S., & Bernstein, G. (2007). Practice parameter for the assessment and treatment of children and adolescents with anxiety disorders. *Journal of the American Academy of Child and Adolescent Psychiatry, 46*(2), 267–283.

Conwell, Y. (2001). Suicide in later life: a review and recommendations for prevention. *Suicide and Life Threatening Behavior, 31*(Suppl), 32–47.

Hedeya, R.J. (1996). *Understanding Biological Psychiatry.* New York: W.W. Norton.

Hentz, P.B. (2005). Effective management strategies. *Clinical Advisor, 6*(suppl.), 15–20.

Hudson, J., Hiripi, E., Pope, H., & Kessler, R. (2007). The prevalence and correlates of eating disorders in the national comorbidity survey replication. *Biological Psychiatry, 61,* 348–358.

Kessler, R., Chiu, W., Demler, O., & Walters, E. (2005). Prevalence, severity, and comorbidity of twelve month DSM-IV disorders in the National Comorbidity Survey Replication. *Archives of General Psychiatry, 62*(6), 617–627.

Kroenke, K., Spitzer, J., Williams, P., Monahan, P., & Lowe, B. (2007). Prevalence, impairment, comorbidity, and detection. *Annals of Internal Medicine, 146,* 317–325.

National Institute of Mental Health. (2009). *Anxiety Disorders.* Bethesda, MD: National Institute of Mental Health.

Ropper, A.H., & Samuels, M.A. (2009). *Adams and Victor's Principles of Neurology* (9th ed.). New York: McGraw Hill.

Schmitz, N., & Kruse, J. (2002). The relationship between mental disorders and medical service utilization in a representative community sample. *Social Psychiatry Psychiatry Epidemiology, 37,* 380–386.

Schwitzer, A., Rodriguez, L.E., Thomas, C., & Silimi, L. (2001). The eating disorder NOS diagnostic profile among college women. *Journal of American College Health, 49,* 157–166.

Shea, S.C. (1998). *Psychiatric Interviewing: The Art of Understanding* (2nd ed.). Philadelphia: W.B. Saunders.

Sheehan, D.V., Lecrubier, Y., Harnett-Sheehan, K., Amorim, P., et al. (1998). The Mini International Neuropsychiatric Interview (M.I.N.I.): The development and validation of a structured diagnostic psychiatric interview. *Journal of Clinical Psychiatry, 59*(suppl.), 22–33.

Simon, R.P., Greenberg, D.A,, & Aminoff, M.J. (1999). *Disorders of Cognitive Function* (7th ed.). New York: McGraw Hill.

Stahl, S.M. (2000). *Essential Psychopharmacology* (2nd ed.). New York: Cambridge University Press.

Stashwick, C. (1996). When you suspect an eating disorder, *Contemporary Pediatrics, 13,* 124.

Stern, T.A., & Herman, J.B. (2000). *Psychiatry: Update and Board Preparation.* New York: McGraw-Hill.

Taylor, C., Bryson, M., Luce, K., Cunning, et al. (2006). Prevention of eating disorders in at risk college age women. *Archives of General Psychiatry, 64,* 881–888.

SUGGESTED READINGS

First, M., Allen, F., & Pincus, H. (1995) *Handbook of Differential Diagnosis.* Washington, D.C: American Psychiatric Press.

Hollander, E. (1999). Anxiety Disturbances. In Hales, R.E., Yudofsky, S.C., & Talbott, J.A. (Eds.). *The American Psychiatric Press Textbook of Psychiatry.* Washington, DC: American Psychiatric Press.

Kessler, R.C. *National Comorbidity Survey, 1990–1992.* [Computer file]. Conducted by University of Michigan, Survey Research Center. 2nd ICPSR ed. Ann Arbor, MI: Inter-University Consortium for Political and Social Research 2002.

Othmer, E., & Othmer, S. (1994). *The Clinical Interview* (Vol. II). Washington, DC: American Psychiatric Press.

Robins, L.N., & Regier, D.A. (Eds.). (1991). *Psychiatric Disorders in America: The Epidemiologic Catchment Area Study.* New York: Free Press.

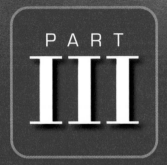

PART III

Assessments and Differential Diagnosis With Special Patient Populations

Chapter 18

PEDIATRIC PATIENTS

Sara F. Barber

Communicating With Infants and Children During the Pediatric Assessment

When assessing infants and children, it is crucial to remember that they are not merely "little adults." Obviously, infants and children have varying communication abilities and interaction skills. Pediatric assessments are more successful when providers take the time to communicate with children in an age-appropriate manner.

■ Infants

Infants are in the midst of the developmental stage of trust and mistrust, so they should be approached slowly. Be prepared for stranger anxiety in an infant of 6 to 7 months and for separation anxiety in an infant just slightly older. Owing to these normal fears, it is best to conduct most, or all, of your examination with the infant on the parent's lap. During the assessment, integrate distraction techniques, such as singing or making funny faces, and/or allow the child to hold onto a familiar security item if present. Rather than a head-to-toe approach, plan your examination in order from noninvasive to invasive (e.g., auscultate the heart and lung sounds first, and examine the ears and throat last). Remember to talk in a soothing voice and to avoid sudden movements.

■ Toddlers

Toddlers are at the height of negativism and are developmentally struggling for independence. They still have fears of parental separation, and they also fear any intrusion to their bodies. Their attention spans are short, and they can be strong-willed and uncooperative, especially when tired or ill. Allow toddlers to touch or hold some of your equipment before you begin the physical examination. Demonstrate what you are going to do on a doll or animal or parent before doing it on the child. Use distraction as much as possible, and give the child choices when they exist, such as, "Which ear should I look in first?" Be direct but friendly—tell the child what you are going to do instead of asking permission. At this age, continue to conduct as much of the examination as you can with the child on a parent's lap, working from noninvasive to invasive procedures.

■ Preschoolers

Preschoolers are magical thinkers and may have fears of pain and body mutilation. They believe that everything is "alive" and may fear unknown equipment or procedures. Involve the child in the examination by describing what you are doing and letting him practice on a doll or stuffed animal first. Move slowly and systematically, and explain in simple terms what you are doing. Choose your words carefully because preschoolers are very literal. Allow choices when possible, and praise the child frequently for helping and cooperating. A head-to-toe sequence may be possible at this age.

■ School-Age Children

School-age children generally want to be brave and cooperate, although they still fear pain and the loss of control. They often ask lots of questions and are curious about using your equipment. Allow them to examine the equipment, and provide concrete answers to their questions whenever possible because children at this age become very logical. Teach them the proper names for equipment and body parts. Modesty may begin to appear in this age group, so be sensitive to this. A head-to-toe sequence is possible for this age.

■ Adolescents

Adolescents are at the height of trying to fit in and be "normal." They worry about how they stack alongside their peers and may have concerns about their physical appearance, including their height, weight, or the presence of acne. They are striving to be independent and fear the loss of control and possibly even death. Privacy is very important at this age, so plan on examining the child without the parent unless the child prefers it otherwise. Remember to keep body parts covered when you are not examining them. Explain each step of your examination, and give the child a chance to ask questions or make choices as you progress. Be very nonjudgmental, and talk professionally but casually with them. Teach adolescents about their bodies, and stress the normalcy of their features and appearance. Reassure them that others their age feel the same way, and try to initiate discussion of sensitive subjects by utilizing this fact (e.g., "Lots of kids your age are faced with tough decisions, like whether to try drugs and alcohol. Have you been faced with any situations like that?"). Teach self-breast and testicular examinations. Give concrete information on sexually transmitted diseases, safe sex, and HIV. Give them an opportunity to ask questions.

Pediatric History and Physical Examination

Much of the content of earlier chapters regarding the assessment of specific systems is relevant to the pediatric assessment. However, the assessment of infants and children should be based on knowledge of the anticipated problems of childhood, developmental stages, and potential risks. The following section summarizes specific questions or examinations that should be considered during pediatric assessment, along with the potential findings that should be considered as red flags, warranting further assessment or consultation.

■ Head

Common Diagnoses for the Head

- Headache
- Head trauma
- Plagiocephaly

When assessing pediatric patients, remember to ask about head trauma, head growth, and the history of headaches. The head circumference should be measured at all well visits up to 2 years of age to assess for macro- or microcephaly. Assess the head symmetry and look for plagiocephaly. For the fontanel to be accurately assessed, the child should be sitting upright and not crying. Some variants that might be noted in newborns include the following.

- *Caput succedaneum*—seen at birth, usually following a traumatic vaginal delivery or vacuum-assisted delivery; edema of the soft tissue of the scalp that usually crosses the suture lines; no specific treatment; should resolve in a few days.
- *Cephalohematoma*—often appears several hours after birth and may increase for the first 24 hours; subperiosteal collection of blood that does not cross the suture lines; may take weeks to months to resolve; watch for hyperbilirubinemia.

RED Flag ◀ Red Flags for the Head Examination

- No growth in head circumference between well visits
- Enlarged head size or excessive growth between well visits

■ Eyes

Common Diagnoses for the Eye

- Conjunctivitis
- Allergies
- Corneal abrasion
- Lacrimal duct stenosis
- Strabismus

Ask about vision problems and/or history of eye drainage. The vision portion of the growth and development section of this chapter (see p. 558) provides details on specific vision and screening for children of various ages. Some variations that may be noted in newborns include the presence of "stork bites" (telangiectatic nevi) on the eyelids, nasolabial area, or nape of the neck; they appear as a purplish-red color and generally diminish and/or disappear by 12 months of age.

RED Flag | Red Flags for the Eye Examination

- Presence of white instead of red reflex may indicate retinoblastoma; an absent red reflex or opacity of the lens may indicate cataracts.
- Dilated and fixed pupils indicate severe brain damage.
- Strabismus requires referral to ophthalmology for further evaluation.

■ Ears

Common Diagnoses for the Ear

- Acute otitis media
- Middle ear effusions
- Otitis externa
- Wax impaction
- Foreign body

Ask about hearing ability and/or difficulties, ear pain, and ear drainage. The general appearance and placement of the ears is important in pediatric assessment. Ears that are set low may indicate genitourinary or chromosomal abnormalities or a multisystem syndrome such as Turner syndrome; assess for preauricular sinuses.

The otoscopic examination is described in detail in Chapter 6. The otoscopic examination should be saved for last in infants and young children because of the distress it often causes. To examine the inner ear in an infant or young child, pull the pinna down and out. For examination in an older child, pull up and back as you would with an adult. As with adults, the tympanic membranes (TM) should be mobile and intact and should appear thin, smooth, and pearly gray with bright light reflexes. The mobility of the TM should be assessed by pneumatic otoscopy if a diagnosis of acute otitis media is expected. Although crying will cause erythema of the TMs, the light reflexes and mobility should remain intact. Diagnosis of acute otitis media should not be based solely on a reddened TM. Also observe for bubbles or an obvious fluid level line behind the TM, which indicates middle ear effusion.

A young child who frequently asks for things to be repeated, seems markedly inattentive, and responds inappropriately to questions should be investigated for hearing deficit. Middle ear effusions and acute otitis media may cause hearing deficits. The Hearing portion of the growth and development section of this chapter (see p. 557) provides details on hearing screening.

RED Flag **Red Flags for the Ear Examination**

- Pain over the mastoid process, which may indicate mastoiditis
- Foreign bodies, which should be considered if the child complains of strange sounds or sensations in one ear or if there is an obvious blockage or odd color noted on otoscopic examination
- Hearing deficit

■ Nose and Sinuses

Common Diagnoses for the Nose and Sinuses

- Upper respiratory infection
- Allergic rhinitis
- Foreign body
- Sinusitis

Ask about nasal drainage, nosebleeds, and breathing interference. Note the characteristics of any drainage. Clear, watery drainage may indicate allergies, especially when coupled with pale, boggy mucosa. Persistent, copious, or purulent drainage may indicate sinusitis. Unilateral, purulent drainage is seen with foreign bodies. Bloody discharge indicates irritation that may be caused by a foreign body, infection, or excessive nose picking.

Newborns frequently have nasal congestion without other symptoms of illness ("newborn congestion"); this should resolve after 2 to 3 months. Newborns are obligate nose breathers.

RED Flag **Red Flags for the Nose and Sinus Examination**

- Reports of apnea should be investigated fully and may require hospitalization for monitoring.
- Foreign bodies should be removed as soon as possible, and referral to a specialist should be considered if removal in the office is impossible.

■ Mouth and Throat

Common Diagnoses for the Mouth and Throat

- Stomatitis
- Oral candidiasis
- Viral pharyngitis/tonsillitis
- Strep pharyngitis
- Dental caries

Ask children and/or parents about throat pain, difficulty swallowing, tooth eruption, dental trauma, and brushing habits. Table 18.13 in the growth and development section identifies the typical age of tooth eruption (see p. 565).

RED Flag Red Flags for the Mouth and Throat Examination

- An absent suck in a newborn, an obvious communication between the nose and mouth, and/or a bifid uvula should be investigated for cleft palate.
- A unilateral enlarged tonsil should be further evaluated to rule out abscess or lymphoma.

■ Lungs

Common Diagnoses for the Lung

- Asthma
- Upper respiratory infection
- Croup
- Pneumonia
- Bronchitis
- Bronchiolitis
- Gastroesophageal reflux disease (may be a cause of cough although not an obvious lung problem)
- Allergies
- Sinusitis

Ask about breathing patterns, blue spells or apnea, and cough. Children under age 7 are diaphragmatic (abdominal) breathers—this is particularly pronounced in infancy; after age 7, children become more thoracic breathers. Observe the general work of breathing, noting any use of accessory muscles, nasal flaring, and retractions. Breath sounds are heard best by having the child breathe through the mouth. Asking the child to pretend may help with breath sound auscultation; for example, to hear inspiratory sounds, have the child pretend to hold his or her breath as if preparing to go under water. Alternatively, have a child actually blow bubbles, pretend to blow bubbles, or inflate a balloon as you listen to both inspiratory and expiratory sounds.

RED Flag Red Flags for the Lung Examination

- Any abnormal breath sounds should be evaluated further with pulse oximeter monitoring and possibly a chest x-ray.
- Cough in the middle of the night or with exertion may indicate asthma, even in a child that does not wheeze.

■ Heart

Common Diagnosis for the Heart

- Innocent murmur

Ask about a history of heart murmur, cyanosis, activity intolerance, or syncope. Measure vital signs with blood pressure measurement beginning at age 3. Always assess pulse for rate and rhythm; an apical pulse should be determined in infants.

RED Flag Red Flags for the Heart Examination

- Pathological murmur
- Unequal or absent pulses
- Cyanosis

A common variation of heart rhythm is sinus arrhythmia in which the heart rate increases with inspiration and decreases with expiration. This fluctuation in rhythm will cease if the child is instructed to hold his or her breath. Assess carefully for murmurs. Up to one-half of all children have an innocent (functional) murmur. Box 18.1 includes characteristics common to innocent murmurs in general. Table 18.1 identifies characteristics of select innocent murmurs.

Box 18.1

Characteristics Common to Innocent Murmurs

- Soft, Grade III or lower
- Systolic timing
- Short duration
- Low pitched, vibratory, musical
- Rarely transmitted
- Loudest in left lower sternal border or at second/third intercostal space
- Loudest when lying down, during expiration, and/or after exercise
- Sound diminishes with position change from recumbent to sitting
- Intensity and presence may vary over time
- Child has normal growth and development, blood pressure, respiratory rate, and pulses
- No associated thrill or cyanosis

Table 18.1

Types of Innocent Murmurs

Type of Murmur	Characteristics
Still's murmur	Most common; heard most frequently from 3 to 7 years of age; described as vibratory or musical; heard best between lower left sternal border and apex with child supine; probably caused by turbulence in left ventricular outflow tract
Basal systolic ejection murmur	High-pitched, blowing sounds heard best at the pulmonic area with child supine
Physiologic peripheral pulmonic stenosis (pulmonary outflow murmur)	Short, systolic; heard best in the axillae and back; usually disappears during infancy
Venous hum	Humming, continuous murmur; heard best in the supraclavicular areas with the child sitting; can be diminished by having the child lie down, turning the head, or occluding the jugular vessels

In newborns, innocent murmurs are common and are usually systolic, grade I or II, and are not associated with other symptoms. The transition period from fetal to maternal conditions may take 48 hours. Patent ductus arteriosus is a fetal vascular connection that directs blood from the pulmonary artery to the aorta. It typically closes by day 4 following birth. However, if it remains patent, the direction of blood flow is reversed through the ductus owing to the higher pressure in the aorta. Clinical findings in a newborn with a still-patent ductus arteriosus include diaphoresis (especially during feedings) and poor feedings with easy tiring that may result in failure to thrive. Immediately postnatally, the associated murmur is soft and systolic, heard along the left lower sternal border. Soon thereafter, the sound is described as a harsh, rumbling, continuous murmur heard in the left infraclavicular and pulmonic areas. When patent ductus arteriosus is suspected, evaluation by a pediatric cardiologist is essential.

■ Breasts

Common Diagnoses for the Breast

- Normal breast bud
- Gynecomastia

Ask about tenderness, nipple discharge, and masses. Asymmetric breast development is normal in an adolescent female. Gynecomastia may be normal in males during puberty. It usually occurs during Tanner stages II and III and may last up to 2 years. Gynecomastia typically presents as a small, tender, oval mass directly under the areola that may measure up to 2 to 3 cm. If imaging of adolescent breast tissue is desired, an ultrasound should be chosen over mammogram because of the dense nature of adolescent breast tissue.

RED Flag ◄ Red Flags for the Breast Examination

- Firm, unmovable masses
- Galactorrhea—may indicate hypothyroidism or pituitary tumor

■ Abdomen

Common Diagnoses for the Abdomen

- Abdominal pain, unknown etiology (possibly related to stress or anxiety)
- Gastroenteritis
- Pyloric stenosis
- Constipation
- Lactose intolerance
- Gas
- Gastroesophageal reflux disease

Ask about diarrhea, constipation, bowel habits, reflux or spitting up, and stomachaches. A potbellied look is common in early childhood owing to poorly developed muscles. Bowel sounds should be assessed. The liver edge may be palpable 1 to 2 cm below the right costal margin with deep inspiration, and the spleen tip may be palpable 1 to 2 cm below the left costal margin with deep inspiration. Constipation may cause a palpable fecal mass in the lower left quadrant, and a rectal examination may be indicated if constipation is suspected. To aid in the abdominal assessment of a ticklish child, have the child lie with knees bent or use the child's smaller hand under your own to palpate the belly. It is also helpful to engage the child in conversation to provide distraction from what you are doing.

RED Flag | Red Flags for the Abdominal Examination

- Failure to pass first meconium stool in first 24 hours of life
- Projectile vomiting
- Blood in stool or emesis
- Chronic diarrhea or constipation
- Severe abdominal pain or guarding
- Abdominal mass

■ Genitourinary System

Common Diagnoses for the Genitourinary System

- Urinary tract infection
- Enuresis (most common is primary nocturnal enuresis—a child who has never stayed dry through the night)
- Labial adhesion
- Yeast dermatitis
- Diaper dermatitis
- Vaginitis
- Balanitis
- Retractile testes

Ask about voiding patterns (number of wet diapers in infants, frequency of urination in older children), pain, discharge, and menstrual cycle if applicable. A clean-catch urine sample should be obtained for urinalysis at all well checkups beginning at age 3, with further testing warranted with abnormal findings.

Female Genitalia

Enlarged labia or mild vaginal bleeding in a female newborn are considered a normal response to maternal hormones. Observe for labial adhesions, which occur mostly in girls 3 months to 6 years of age. No treatment is needed as long as urine and vaginal secretions are not obstructed. Observe the presence and distribution of pubic hair.

Male Genitalia

Observe the location of the urethral meatus. Hypospadias is a congenital defect that causes the meatus to be on the ventral surface of the penis, and epispadias results in dorsal placement of the meatus. Palpate the scrotum for the presence of testes; cryptorchidism is the term for an undescended testicle. If the testes are not immediately palpable in the scrotum but can be "milked" down into the scrotum, consider them descended. If one or both testes are undescended at 1 year of age, referral to a specialist is indicated. Male newborns frequently have an enlarged scrotum as a normal finding.

RED Flag ◀ Red Flags for the Genitourinary System

- Ambiguous genitalia
- Premature puberty
- Hypospadias

■ Musculoskeletal System

Common Diagnoses for the Musculoskeletal System

- Trauma or injury
- Local sprain or strain
- Torticollis
- Tibial torsion
- Osgood-Schlatter disease
- Growing pains

Ask about pain or limited movement, joint pain, and history of fractures. Although a comprehensive musculoskeletal assessment should be performed, an emphasis should be placed on specific joints.

Hips

Assessment for hip dislocation is extremely important in all infants and children under 2. Hip dislocation is most common in females and in infants delivered in a breech position (including by Cesarean section). It is more prevalent in whites, Eskimos, and Navajos. A variety of specialized maneuvers are useful in assessment for hip dislocation. Table 18.2 differentiates between the Barlow's, Ortolani's, and Galeazzi's maneuvers.

Table 18.2	

Special Maneuvers

Barlow's Maneuver

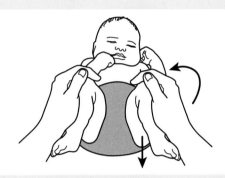

Dislocates a dislocatable hip posteriorly. With the infant supine, flex the hip, adduct the thigh, and feel for a palpable dislocation. As the thigh is adducted, the femoral head drops (or can be gently pushed) out of the acetabulum. Do the maneuver gently on an infant who is not crying.

Ortolani's Maneuver

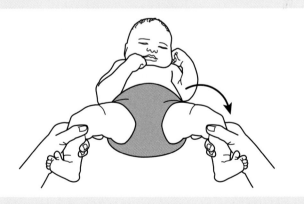

Reduces a posteriorly dislocated hip. With the infant supine, place fingers posteriorly over the greater trochanter, flex the hip 90 degrees, and abduct the thigh while pushing up with the fingers. Feel for a clunk and palpable jerk as the femur is relocated. Do the maneuver gently on an infant who is not crying.

Continued

Table 18.2	

Special Maneuvers—cont'd

Galeazzi's Maneuver

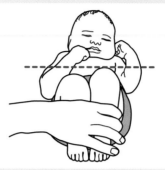

Assesses knee height for equality. With the infant supine, flex the hips and knees and place the soles of the child's feet on the table near the buttocks. Observe the knees for equal height. The sign is considered positive if the knee heights are unequal. A dislocatable hip will fall out of socket in this position and will cause the knee on the affected side to appear lower.

Although not considered definitively diagnostic of a dislocated hip, the thighs, inguinal area, and gluteal area should be assessed for asymmetric skin folds as potential indications of dislocation. When assessing for hip dislocation or dysplasia, it is essential to differentiate between normal "clicks" and the worrisome "clunk." Normal clicks may be felt when doing some hip manipulation as a result of laxity and movement of ligaments. A definitive clunk is felt when a bone (the femur) actually comes out of its socket. Even though doing these maneuvers is extremely important, it is also important to remember that as the infant ages, limited abduction becomes an increasingly definitive sign of hip dysplasia. Limited abduction (less than 60%) is also the key sign to look for in bilateral dislocation. If hip dislocation or dysplasia is suspected, radiographic studies are usually done. In an infant under 3 months of age, ultrasound is the usual choice, although this method can still give unreliable results because much of the hip joint is cartilaginous. After 3 months of age, the preferred method of radiologic evaluation is anteroposterior and frog lateral x-rays.

Gait

Observe a child's gait during well examination. Toddlers commonly walk with a wide-based gait and a bowlegged (genu varum) appearance. A knock-kneed (genu valgum) appearance is common in preschoolers.

Back

Assessment for scoliosis (a lateral curvature of the spine) should be performed at each well visit starting at age 10. If abnormal findings are present, radiographs should be obtained for confirmation and to guide possible referral. Both the age of the child and the degree of the curve will guide treatment, if any. Scoliosis is more worrisome in a child who is prepubertal because there is more growth to occur and therefore more time for a curve to worsen.

Joints

Assess joints by palpating for pain, heat, or deformity. Active range of motion gives information about how muscles and bones are working together for functional movement. Assess active range of motion by engaging a child in games in the examination room. For example, have the child perform jumping jacks, clap, pretend to be a certain animal, and/or walk heel-to-toe on a line on the floor. Passive range of motion gives information about joint mobility and stability and the limits of tendons and muscles. Excessive range of motion may indicate an unstable joint. Assess passive range of motion by flexing and extending the joints through various movements with child relaxed or lying supine.

Elbow

A child's elbow commonly and easily gets dislocated (nursemaid's elbow or toddler's elbow). Dislocation is indicated by refusal to use an arm, especially when accompanied by crying and an appropriate history.

RED Flag ◀ Red Flags for the Musculoskeletal Examination

- Refusal to bear weight or walk
- Refusal to use or bend an arm
- Heat, redness, and/or swelling of one or more joints
- Hip clunks
- Toe walking—can be a normal phase and also can be associated with cerebral palsy, tight heel cords, autism, or muscular dystrophy

---

■ Neurologic System

Common Diagnoses for the Neurologic System

- Cognitive delay
- Developmental delay
- Attention deficit-hyperactivity disorder/autism
- Neuromuscular diseases/dystrophies
- Seizure/epilepsy

Ask about episodes of seizure or loss of consciousness, tremors, or tics. A large part of the assessment of the neurological system in a child can be accomplished by observation during the visit. Watch for symmetry and quality of movement; observe gait, posture, coordination, balance, strength, and tone. Children are generally very active, and by watching the way they climb on the examination table, hop around the room, and manipulate objects and toys, you can gain a lot of information. In a newborn or small infant, observe for symmetry of movements, muscle tone, and pitch of the cry. Test deep tendon reflexes. Assess newborn reflexes—absence or persistence past expected age of disappearance may indicate severe central nervous system (CNS) dysfunction and should be investigated fully. Table 18.3 details newborn reflexes.

RED Flag ◀ **Red Flags for the Neurological Examination**

- Absence, or persistence past the expected age, of newborn reflexes
- Spasticity or poor muscle tone
- Unresponsiveness or depressed level of consciousness
- Any loss or regression of developmental milestones
- Abnormal cranial nerve responses

The pediatric assessment should integrate cranial nerve evaluation. Table 18.4 describes the pediatric assessment of cranial nerves.

During the neurological assessment, assess for developmental milestones. Although children develop at their own individual speed, any regression in developmental milestones is a major concern. The Denver II is a useful tool when evaluating developmental milestones. See information on developmental milestones elsewhere in this chapter.

Practitioners caring for children should be aware of the following two neurologic disorders and the signs and symptoms that children may exhibit, indicating the need for further evaluation.

Autism

Autism is a bioneurologic developmental disorder and generally presents before the age of 3. It is characterized by marked impairment in three general areas: social interactions, language development/communication skills, and imagination and play. Abnormal social skill development is the classic indicator of autism or autism spectrum disorders (ASDs). These social skill deficits may include abnormal eye contact, failure to respond to name, failure to use gestures or pointing, and lack of interest in other children. Language development is typically delayed in autistic children. Such children also frequently exhibit an inability to adjust to new surroundings and show an absence of imaginary play.

Ask parents if their infant studies their faces by 2 months, smiles at them by 6 months, and babbles by 1 year. Ask if their 1-year-old points to things to indicate his or her wants or just for a parent to notice the object. Does their

Table 18.3

Newborn Reflexes

	Age Appears	Age Disappears	How to Test	Response	Meaning
Rooting	Birth	3–4 mo	With head midline, stroke perioral area	Infant should open mouth and turn head toward stimulated side	Absence indicates central nervous system (CNS) disease or depression; sleepy infant may not respond
Sucking	Birth	3–4 mo	Place nipple or finger 3–4 cm into mouth; may stroke roof of mouth	Infant should have strong suck	Absence indicates CNS depression; sleepy baby may not respond
Palmar Grasp	Birth	3–6 mo	Place finger in infant's palm and press gently	Infant should flex all fingers around examiner's finger	Grasp should be strong and symmetrical
Stepping	Birth	6–8 wk	Hold infant in a standing position with feet against firm surface	Infant should "step" along, raising one foot at a time	Absence indicates paralysis or a depressed infant
Moro	Birth	4–5 mo	Make a loud noise or allow infant's head to drop down slightly	Infant's arms should spread, fingers should extend and then flex, then arms should come together; may elicit a cry	Asymmetry may indicate paralysis or a fractured clavicle; absence indicates a brain stem problem

Table 18.4	

Pediatric Assessment of the Cranial Nerves

I, Olfactory	Occlude one nostril and offer odors for identification (not frequently tested in the office unless specific concern)
II, Optic	Test visual acuity and visual fields, and examine fundi; test blink reflex in an infant
III, Oculomotor	Test extraocular movements by having child follow a light or a toy in all visual fields, and observe infants for tracking abilities; observe for asymmetry of eyelids; pupils should both constrict when light is shined in one eye
IV, Trochlear	Tested in the same way and at the same time as CN III
V, Trigeminal	For sensory, apply light touch and pressure to points across forehead, cheeks, and jaw; for motor, have child bite hard on tongue blade or observe an infant chewing on a teething toy
VI, Abducens	Tested in the same way and at the same time as CN III and CN IV
VII, Facial	For sensory, observe for eyes tearing, can offer samples for taste; for motor, have child imitate you smiling big, grimacing, puffing out cheeks, and raising eyebrows; observe for facial grimaces in an infant
VIII, Acoustic	Observe balance, do auditory testing as needed, question parents regarding hearing
IX, Glossopharyngeal	Elicit gag reflex or have child say "ah"; observe swallowing
X, Vagus	Tested along with CN IX
XI, Accessory	Have child shrug shoulders against pressure, turn head against resistance, stick tongue out
XII, Hypoglossal	Have child move tongue back and forth or push against a tongue blade; may just observe this behavior during examination of oropharynx in an infant

18-month-old imitate play with objects like a hairbrush or a phone? Does their 2-year-old put two words together meaningfully on his or her own?

If a child exhibits any of the following red flags for autism, a further and more specific evaluation is warranted.

RED Flag	Red Flags for Autism

- No big smiles or expressions of happiness by 6 months
- No back and forth sounds, gestures, or facial expressions by 9 months
- No babbling by 12 months
- No pointing, waving, or reaching by 12 months
- No words by 16 months
- No 2-word phrases by 24 months (without imitating)
- Any language regression or unusual use of language

Attention Deficit-Hyperactivity Disorder

Attention deficit-hyperactivity disorder (ADHD) is a neurobehavioral disorder that affects an estimated 5% to 10% of the school-age population. Its main symptoms are inattention with increased distractibility, poor impulse control, and motor restlessness and hyperactivity. There are three subtypes of ADHD. ADHD, predominantly inattentive type is more common in females. ADHD, predominantly hyperactive-impulsive type, and ADHD, combined type are more frequently diagnosed in males. When assessing a child for ADHD, it is important to ascertain the degree of symptoms as well as when they were first noticed and in what settings they are present. It is also important to remember that many children with ADHD have comorbid psychiatric diagnoses.

According to the DSM-IV, a child with ADHD must exhibit behavior that is developmentally inappropriate and meets the following criteria:

- has been present before the age of 7;
- has been present for at least 6 months;
- is present in at least 2 settings; and
- is not related to another disorder.

A diagnosis of ADHD should not be made quickly or without a complete evaluation. A thorough history should include any injury to the CNS, any medications the child takes, any family history of similar symptoms, and any social or family situations that might contribute to the inappropriate behaviors. Because of the importance of symptoms being present in more than one setting, it is a good idea to utilize a behavior rating scale that compares answers from both a parent and another caregiver like a teacher. The Connor Rating Scale is an example of this type of checklist.

Other diagnoses to consider when evaluating a child with ADHD-like symptoms include anxiety disorders, depression, sleep disorders, and learning disabilities.

■ Skin

Common Diagnoses for the Skin

- Viral exanthema
- Atopic dermatitis (eczema)
- Contact dermatitis
- Tinea
- Impetigo
- Cellulitis

Ask about birthmarks, lesions, and skin conditions. Common birthmarks are listed here.

- *Stork bites* commonly appear on eyelids, nasolabial area, or nape of neck; usually disappear by 12 months.
- *Nevus flammeus* (port-wine stain) is pinkish-red in color and grows as the child grows.
- *Strawberry nevus* (raised hemangioma) may not be present at birth; it usually starts out as a grayish white area and later becomes red and raised; most resolve spontaneously by age 10.
- *Mongolian spots* are usually seen in newborns of African American, Latin, or Asian descent; they are generally found in the sacral or gluteal region.

RED Flag ◀ Red Flags for the Skin Examination

- Any mole or lesion that is changing, that has irregular borders, or that is growing should be examined by a dermatologist.

Assess all skin for color, texture, and turgor; check for any rashes, lesions, pruritus, or bruising. Observe for skin conditions that may indicate underlying pathology, such as depigmented nevi, café-au-lait spots, and hemangiomas on the scalp.

Growth and Development

The growth and development of a child is one of the most important things to consider when assessing and caring for pediatric patients. Parents are very interested in how their child is growing, both physically and developmentally, and assessments of these areas by trained professionals can help indicate possible problems and the need for referral or more intensive evaluation.

■ Physical Growth

The measurement of a child's weight and height is done at every well visit. If the child is not routinely seen for well visits, this must be incorporated into visits for specific complaints/illness. The head circumference is measured at every well visit from birth to 2 years of age. Each of these measurements is plotted on a growth chart. Other charts have been developed to measure a child's body mass index and/or plot a child's weight versus height. These charts allow for a visual representation that enables practitioners to watch how a child develops in each area over time. Although parents often become interested in what percentile their child "ranks in," providers should stress the importance of watching the growth curves to compare the child against herself or himself, not against others. For example, it is much more worrisome for a child's weight or head size to drop from the 75th to the 25th percentile than it is for a child to continuously grow along the 25th percentile curve. A child whose growth is at the extremes of the growth curves but whose growth rate is normal and consistent is likely to be very healthy.

Trends

The following trends are generalizations that can be used as rules of thumb in assessing pediatric growth and development. An average American newborn weighs around 7 pounds and is 20 to 21 inches long. The average head circumference of an American newborn is 13 to 14 inches, with a chest circumference of 2 cm less than that of the head. The head circumference generally increases by a half inch per month during the first 6 months of life and a quarter inch per month during the second 6 months.

Weight

An initial 10% loss of weight occurs in the first 3 to 4 days of life. This is typically regained by 2 weeks of age. Thereafter, a child's weight typically doubles around 4 to 6 months, triples at a year, and quadruples around age 2. During the first 6 months of life, a baby gains 5 to 8 ounces a week. Between 6 and 12 months, this decreases to 3 to 5 ounces a week. During the second year of life, a child gains 8 to 9 ounces a month. Toddlers and preschoolers gain 4.5 to 6.5 pounds a year. A school-age child gains 5 to 6 pounds a year. During the pubertal growth spurt, an average American female gains 38 pounds, and an average male gains 42 pounds.

Length/Height

The length of a child typically increases by 50% at age 12 months, doubles around 4 years of age, and triples by 13 years. The average gain in length in infancy is 1 inch per month during the first 6 months, and then a half inch per month during the second 6 months. Toddlers, preschoolers, and school-age children grow 2 to 3 inches per year. During the pubertal growth spurt, American girls grow an average of 8 to 9 inches and reach 95% of their mature height by the onset of menarche or the skeletal age of 13. Boys grow an average of 9.5 to 11 inches and reach 95% of their mature height by the skeletal age of 15.

■ Development by Age

The tables in this subsection illustrate age-by-age behaviors and skills that babies and children should develop. Because every child is different, it is impossible to say that these behaviors will occur in all children at the given age. Milestones occur along a wide spectrum, and patterns considered "normal" have wide parameters. The "whole picture" of the child must be taken into consideration when comparing a child with a given standard. However, knowledge of the developmental milestones is essential when assessing infants and children. Behavioral observations and/or parents' questions can be used to determine the child's developmental progress.

Newborns/Infants

The term *newborn* is typically applied to babies from birth until 1 month of age. The period from 1 month to 12 months is infancy. The first 12 months of life represent the period of the most rapid change and maturation—both physically and emotionally. See Table 18.5 for infant developmental milestones.

Infant Developmental Red Flags

Because of the importance of early intervention in preventing and/or minimizing long-term consequences of sensory deficits, Table 18.6 is included to provide developmental red flags in infants. As always, there is some

Table 18.5

Newborn/Infant Development Milestones

Time Period	Sensory	Emotional/ Behavioral	Motor	Language
Newborn–1 mo	Sees best at 8–10 inches; cannot focus clearly; startles to loud noises	Cries a lot but responds positively to soft voice and being held	Jerky movements; grasps whatever is placed in hand; turns head	Has varying cries for different needs; may start making gurgling sounds
1–2 mo	May follow some objects with eyes (at least to midline); turns toward some sounds	May smile socially to caregiver; may quiet down in response to human face	Movements become more controlled; lifts chin for a few seconds while on tummy	Makes variety of cooing and gurgling sounds when content
2–4 mo	Focuses better but no more than 12 inches; follows objects 180 degrees by turning head side to side; prefers bright objects	Crying decreases; displays more emotions	Movements are smoother; discovers hands; may lift chest slightly while prone; may bat at dangling objects	Smiles, gurgles, and coos— especially interactively
4–6 mo	Focuses clearly; fascinated by mirror image; turns purposefully in response to voice	Very active and playful; basks in attention; acknowledges breast or bottle excitedly	Rolls from side to side; holds up chest when prone; supports head well when held in sitting position; no head lag at 6 mo	Laughs and giggles; imitates speech sounds

Table 18.5

Newborn/Infant Development Milestones—cont'd

Time Period	Sensory	Emotional/ Behavioral	Motor	Language
6–9 mo	Begins to recognize sound of own name; puts everything in mouth	May show sharp mood changes; strong attachment to mother; stranger anxiety	Rakes objects; transfers objects from hand to hand; begins to sit alone; crawling motions	Babbles and squeals; repeats sounds over and over; frequently uses syllables such as *ba, da, ka*
9–12 mo	Scrutinizes toys and objects; still puts everything in mouth	May cry when parent leaves; may resist diapering or other things he or she does not want to do; plays peek-a-boo	Refined pincer grasp; goes from sitting to lying; crawls well; may pull self to stand; cruises; may begin to walk	Imitates inflection of conversation; imitates speech sounds; says "mama" and "dada"; may say 2–3 other words; points to objects to indicate wants

Table 18.6

Infant Developmental Red Flags

Age	Social/ Emotional	Cognitive/ Visual	Language/ Hearing	Fine Motor	Gross Motor
1 mo	Excessive irritability	Doll's eyes; questionable or no red light reflex; poor alert state	No startle to sound; no quieting to voice	Absent or asymmetrical palmar grasp	Asymmetric movements; increased or decreased tone; asymmetric primitive reflexes
4 mo	Lack of social smile; depressed/ withdrawn affect	No tracking; no ability to fixate on face or object	No turning to voice or sound; no cooing or squeals	No hand-to-mouth activity	Same as above; no attempt to raise head when prone

Continued

Table 18.6

Infant Developmental Red Flags—cont'd

Age	Social/ Emotional	Cognitive/ Visual	Language/ Hearing	Fine Motor	Gross Motor
6 mo	No smiling or response to play	No looking at caregiver; no reaching for objects; no tracking	No babbling; no response to rattles, sounds, or loud noises	No grasping of objects; no holding hands together	No attempt to sit with support; head lag when pulled to a sit; persistence of primitive reflexes
9 mo	No eye contact or interactive play	No reaching for toys; no visual or oral investigation of toys	No response to name or voice; no single or double consonant sounds	No self-feeding; no solids; no picking up of toys with one hand	No sitting (including tripod sit); unequal movements or excessive one-handedness
12 mo	No response to games, books, or interactive play	No visual involvement in environment	No speech imitation	No attempt to self-feed or hold cup; no transfer of objects	No pulling self to stand; no exploring of environment

parameter for "normal," and the gestational age of the child at birth must be taken into account. However, in terms of early intervention and evaluation, it is much better to err on the side of caution and refer for further evaluation if any suspicions arise regarding the development of a child.

Toddlers

The period of toddlerhood lasts from the first birthday until age 3. During this stage, the child's rate of physical growth slows down, but the process of moving toward independence continues rapidly as toddlers acquire many new motor, cognitive, and psychosocial skills. Behavioral challenges frequently arise during this period owing to both the toddler's attempts to test limits and his or her own frustration at trying to communicate. See Table 18.7 for toddler developmental milestones.

Table 18.7

Toddler Development Milestones

Age	Cognitive	Emotional/ Behavioral	Motor	Language
18 mo	Learns cause and effect; looks for hidden objects; recognizes pictures of familiar people and objects; points to a few body parts	Likes to feed self; likes water play; prefers adults to other children	Likes to throw, roll, push, and pull toys; walks unassisted with wide stance; stoops and recovers; imitates scribbling; makes tower of 3–4 cubes	Adds gestures to speech; likes to imitate activities and speech; uses 10–20 words; may start combining two words; understands "no"
2 yr	Cannot be reasoned with; can picture objects and events mentally; concrete thinking; identifies body parts; matches some colors	"Do-it-myself" stage; may resist bedtime; gets frustrated easily; may respond with "no" constantly; learns to hold up fingers to show age; tries to get adult attention	Runs and climbs; goes up and down stairs alone; scribbling turns into more controlled movements; turns pages one at a time; builds tower of eight cubes	Uses simple sentences; seems to understand most of what is said; .uses more pronouns; learns songs/rhymes

Preschoolers

The period from age 3 to age 5 is known as the preschool stage of development. Children in this stage are usually very active, energetic, imaginative, inquisitive, and social. They also become increasingly independent with tasks such as self-care. They acquire more language skills and, as a result, can respond more verbally, which often decreases previous behavioral challenges. See Table 18.8 for preschooler developmental milestones.

School-Age Children

The school-age period of development begins with entry into school (around age 5) and lasts until adolescence. This is a period of extensive development. Children become more influenced by peers and groups outside the home, and they are expected to follow certain rules and adhere to some degree of structure in the school setting. Children often remain very imaginative as

Table 18.8

Preschooler Development Milestones

Age	Cognitive	Emotional/ Behavioral	Motor	Language
3 yr	Develops more stable sense of self; egocentric thinking; knows names of time components but does not understand sequencing; may identify some colors, letters, numbers	Learns to share and take turns; tests limits; seeks approval from adults; likes hearing stories over and over; likes imaginative and imitative play; increased curiosity about bodies	Tiptoes; rides a tricycle; kicks a ball; stands briefly on one foot; undresses self; copies a circle; can brush teeth (although not well)	Speaks about 1,000 words; tells simple stories; asks lots of questions; responds to three-part commands; may have a stuttering phase; can consistently produce *m, n, p, f, h, b,* and *w* sounds
4 yr	Uses words to solve problems; begins to understand some concepts of time; knows difference between right and wrong; begins to discern real life from make believe; identifies shapes and colors	Has penchant for silliness; shows new fears, which shows awareness of new dangers; likes to help; imitates adults; shares grudgingly; enjoys group activities and fantasy play	Runs, skips, climbs, hops with better skill; uses scissors; dresses self; holds a pencil correctly; draws recognizable shapes; draws a person with three parts; catches a large ball	Tells stories; uses four- to five-word sentences; uses prepositions; asks "how" questions; starts using past and future tenses correctly; adds approximately 50 words a month to vocabulary

they learn new things. This is the period when a child develops a sense of self and self-worth, so accomplishment and confidence become important tasks. Refer to Table 18.9 for school-age developmental milestones.

Adolescents

The period of adolescence is the transition from childhood to adulthood. Typically beginning at age 12 or 13, adolescence is a time of change and new responsibilities. With the initiation of puberty, children experience a wide array of physical, emotional, and social changes. The peer group is of utmost importance to an adolescent, and many challenges and temptations arise during this time period. During middle and late adolescence, focus on the future becomes significant, and teens gain a sense of morality as they prepare to enter the adult world. Table 18.10 lists adolescent developmental milestones.

Table 18.9

School-Age Development Milestones

Age	Cognitive	Emotional/ Behavioral	Motor	Language
5 yr	Understands time concepts; recognizes letters and some words; can learn address and phone number; begins to understand opposites; has overall image of self	Likes to please adults; enjoys family activities; embarrasses easily; submits to more rules and shows guilt over misbehavior; can participate in informal games	Displays handedness; can bathe independently; builds elaborate structures; walks downstairs alternating feet; may print name; cuts out simple shapes; copies a square	Speaks in good sentences; uses conjunctions to string thoughts together; has a vocabulary of over 2,000 words and continues to add more; masters most consonant combinations
6 yr	Loses magical thinking; starts to understand concepts of measurement (weight, length, mass); can group things into subgroups based on a common attribute; knows right from left; knows days of the week	Develops better impulse control; may enjoy and succeed at sports and arts & crafts programs; is sensitive to criticism; may resist baths; prefers socializing with same sex	Loves active play; still somewhat uncoordinated; may be reckless; can tie shoes; copies a triangle; very active	Well developed vocabulary with increasingly improved semantics; speaks with good intelligibility; may still distort some sounds/ blends *(thr, sk, st, shr, s, z, sh, ch, j)*
7 yr	Begins to use simple logic; can tell time; can group objects in ascending order; understands basic addition and subtraction principles	Less egocentric; more cooperative; usually has a best friend of same sex; seeks approval from peers; tends to be critical; tattles on others for not following rules	Has refined hand–eye coordination; rides a bike; swims; printing gets smaller; activity level decreases slightly	Produces all language sounds; uses adultlike grammar; rapid language development
8 yr	Memory span increases; understands causal relationships; can be idealistic	Adheres to simple rules; often idolizes someone; begins to show sense of loyalty; likes secrets and clubs; enjoys projects and collections	Gains better control over small muscles; writes in cursive and draws better; movements are more graceful	Articulation nears adult level; better use of pronouns; understands complex directions; better storytelling skills; likes to tell jokes and enjoys bathroom humor

Continued

Table 18.9

School-Age Development Milestones—cont'd

Age	Cognitive	Emotional/ Behavioral	Motor	Language
9–10 yr	Understands explanations; can use reference books and resources; classifies objects	Succumbs more easily to peer pressure; does not want to be different; tends to be self-critical; develops internal standards of right and wrong	Eagerly learns new skills; enjoys team competition; well coordinated with increasing dexterity and eye–hand coordination	Uses language to convey thoughts and looks at another's point of view
11–12 yr	Begins abstract thinking; increasing spans of attention and concentration	Peer acceptance is very important; critical of parents; acutely aware of opposite sex; vacillates between dependent child and independent preteen	Refines gross and fine motor skills; can do crafts and use tools well	Reading vocabulary of 50,000 words; oral vocabulary of 7,200 words; speech is grammatically correct

Table 18.10

Adolescent Development Milestones

Age	Cognitive	Emotional/ Behavioral	Motor	Language
12–15 yr	Increase in abstract thinking and decrease in concrete thinking; increased ability to relate actions to consequences	Very focused on social life, peer acceptance, physical appearance; grades may suffer; interest in sexuality increases; wide mood swings; values privacy	May enjoy and excel at a specific sport or activity; enjoys video/ computer games	Increasing ability for self-expression; may enjoy keeping a journal or diary
15–18 yr	Beginning interest in social problems; may become idealistic and altruistic; inductive and deductive reasoning; may be very introspective; increased creative ability	Risk taking is common; rejection or questioning of parental authority; may experiment with sex, alcohol, or drugs; confusion over self-image may persist	Periods of high energy alternate with periods of lethargy; may enjoy and excel at a specific sport or activity	Language skills at or near adult level

■ Hearing/Speech

Assessment of an infant's hearing is somewhat subjective (unless specific audiological testing is done), but it is essential to be aware of the signs of a hearing deficit. Hearing is critical to language development, and the failure to recognize and address a hearing deficit in infancy can be detrimental to a child's development. Basic hearing screenings should be done at each well visit. Parents should be specifically questioned regarding behaviors that indicate normal hearing. Any concerns regarding hearing should be thoroughly addressed. Part of assessing hearing is to assess for any factors that may increase the risk of a hearing deficit. See Box 18.2 regarding the risk factors for hearing deficit.

The development of language skills may provide evidence of intact hearing, and parents can be asked to identify the infant's level of interaction and language development. As long as the child is progressing (and not regressing) in language skills and there are no physical abnormalities, monitoring and intermittent assessment is acceptable during this stage. However, formal audiometry should be considered if parents express concerns about the child's hearing abilities or there are no recognizable, meaningful sounds or words at 18 months. See Box 18.3 for reasons for referral.

Box 18.2

Risk Factors for Hearing Deficit

- An affected family member
- Newborn bilirubin greater than 20 mg/dL
- Congenital cytomegalovirus, herpes, or rubella
- Defects in ear-nose-throat structures
- Birth weight less than 1,500 g
- Bacterial meningitis
- Use of ototoxic medications
- Intracranial hemorrhage
- Use of mechanical ventilation for more than 48 hr
- Head trauma or temporal bone fracture
- Infections such as mumps/measles associated with sensorineural hearing loss
- Recurrent acute otitis media or middle ear infection

Box 18.3

Reasons for Audiology Referral

- Hearing threshold levels greater than 20 dB at 500, 1,000, 2,000, or 4,000 Hz
- Presence of middle ear fluid documented for longer than 3 months
- Hearing or language skills seem to regress at any point

■ Vision

Vision is the least-developed sense in a newborn, and visual acuity is estimated to be around 20/670 at birth. However, the amazing pace at which visual acuity develops is obvious when watching the overall development of an infant's actions. At 1 month, an infant will stare at large objects. By 2 months, more detail is noticed and babies begin to enjoy gazing at a caregiver's face. As the baby reaches 3 to 4 months of age, the eyes begin to converge, and the infant starts to bring things to the mouth and develop eye–hand coordination. At this age, an infant should be able to track an object 180 degrees. Around 6 to 7 months of age, a baby can recognize different faces.

Like hearing, it is essential to assess visual acuity at all well checkups. Again, parents are the best evaluators, so they should be questioned about a baby's or child's behaviors, including tracking ability, response to new and familiar faces, the distance a child sits from a book or television, and the ability to notice details far away. Risk factors for decreased visual acuity should also be assessed (see Box 18.4).

Assessment of the red reflex should be a part of each well visit. Other things that should be assessed in a young infant include the pupillary response to light, the blink reflex, and the ability to fix and follow. An older infant or toddler should also be assessed using the corneal light reflex test and the cover/uncover test. Starting at preschool age, children should be assessed using visual acuity charts (Allen chart, illiterate E, or Sjögren hand). The school-age child and adolescent should be assessed using these measures and the Snellen chart for far vision. The Ishihara test should be used for color perception. See Box 18.5 for reasons for referral.

■ Nutrition

Assessing an infant's or child's nutrition and diet is an important part of an overall well-child evaluation and requires knowledge of anticipated intake and weight change. For infants, parents should be questioned regarding the frequency of feedings, the type and amount of formula if bottle-fed, and the baby's tolerance of feedings. Once solids are initiated, parents should be asked about what types of foods the baby is taking, how much and at what

---

Box 18.4

Risk Factors for Decreased Visual Acuity

- Prenatal infections
- Congenital cyanotic heart disease
- Structural malformation
- Family history of vision problems
- Excessive oxygenation in neonatal period
- Hearing problems

Box 18.5

Reasons for Ophthalmology Referral

- Searching nystagmus
- Strabismus (intermittent strabismus is normal until age 4–6 months)
- Absence of blinking to a threat
- Lack of vertical and horizontal following by 2 months of age
- Abnormal or asymmetric red reflex
- Asymmetric corneal light reflex
- Abnormal cover/uncover test
- Visual acuity 20/50 or worse at age 3 years
- Visual acuity of 20/30 or worse at age 5 years
- Difference in score of two lines or more between eyes on visual acuity chart
- Structural abnormality

times of the day, and how much fluid the infant is drinking now that solids have been started. As the child progresses to more table foods, part of the assessment is determining whether he or she is getting a good variety of foods, is transitioning well to table foods, and is maintaining adequate fluid intake. Table 18.11 includes information to guide the nutrition questions posed at various ages.

In addition to identifying the daily intake of meals and snacks, include questions to identify nutritional supplements and vitamins. Of particular interest is the intake of vitamin D and fluoride. Breast-fed infants who do not receive vitamin D supplementation or adequate exposure to sunlight are at risk for developing rickets. All breast-fed infants should receive a supplement of 400 IU per day of vitamin D unless they are consuming at least 500 mL a day of vitamin D–fortified formula. This practice should begin within the first 2 months of life.

Toddlers and Preschoolers

As a child reaches the toddler stage, her or his appetite naturally starts to decrease as growth starts to slow down. Toddlers are frequently easily distracted and are picky about what they eat, so mealtimes can be a challenge. Parents should be encouraged to look at their child's diet on a week-by-week rather than day-by-day basis because toddlers frequently have days when they eat very little or eat only two or three things, and then may make up for it the next day. When assessing toddlers, ask about the child's typical diet, including overall intake and any self-imposed limitations. Preschoolers frequently go on food jags, insisting on eating the same food over and over. As long as the food is not a high-sugar or empty-calorie item, parents should allow the food choice and remember that the phase usually does not last too long.

Table 18.11	

Age-Appropriate Nutritional Guidelines

Age	Intake	Anticipated Weight Change
Newborn	Requires 110–120 kcal/kg⁻¹/day⁻¹ Eats every 1.5–3 hr 20–24 oz/day	Gains 0.5–1 oz/day
2 mo	Requires 120–130 kcal/kg⁻¹/day⁻¹ Eats 6–9 times/day 20–24 oz/day	Gains 0.5–1 oz/day
4 mo	Requires 120–130 kcal/kg⁻¹/day⁻¹ Eats 24–32 oz/day	Gains 5–8 oz/week
6 mo	Requires approx. 100 kcal/kg⁻¹/day⁻¹ Eats 24–32 oz/day Solids include iron-fortified single-grain cereal mixed with water, formula, or breast milk Only one new food introduced every 3–7 days No additives, such as honey, sugar, or seasonings	Gains 3–5 oz/wk Weight usually doubles by 5–6 months
8–9 mo	Requires approx. 100 kcal/kg⁻¹/day⁻¹ Drinks 24–32 oz/day, often with sippy cup Menu slowly expanded to include tender meats and finger foods Juice limited to 6 oz/day, diluted with water	Gains 3–5 oz/wk
10–12 mo	Drinks 20–32 oz/day Menu expanded to more table and finger foods Meal pattern resembles family's (three meal/day plus snacks) Whole milk at 12 months Juice limited to 6 oz/day, diluted with water	Gains 3–5 oz/week; Weight usually triples by 12 months

School-Age Children

Energy needs for school-age children depend somewhat on the individual's body size, growth pattern, and activity level. Children aged 6 to 7 years require approximately 90 $\text{kcal/kg}^{-1}/\text{day}^{-1}$; 7 to 10 years, approximately 70 $\text{kcal/kg}^{-1}/\text{day}^{-1}$; and 10 to 12 years, 40 to 55 $\text{kcal/kg}^{-1}/\text{day}^{-1}$ depending on their size and activity. The school-age period is a time of busy schedules, and children at this age tend to skip meals and to snack more often. Also, because children spend a good part of the day away from home, parents become somewhat out of touch with what their child is eating throughout the day. Because of these habits, problems with obesity can begin at this stage.

Parents should make an effort to have easy, healthy snacks available. Healthy meals and family mealtime routines should be reinforced during this period to help prevent obesity.

Adolescents

As for school-age children, energy requirements for adolescents vary somewhat depending on body size and activity level. However, owing to the rapid growth and development during this stage, it is essential that all adolescents are consuming an adequate amount of calories, protein, vitamins, and minerals. Males typically require more kilocalories per day than females because of their larger body mass and prolonged period of growth. Teens involved in athletics also have an increased need for calories. Twelve- to 14-year-old males need approximately 60 kcal/kg^{-1}/day^{-1}, whereas females at this age need 45 to 50 kcal/kg^{-1}/day^{-1}. At age 15, daily caloric intake decreases to 40 to 45 kcal/kg^{-1}/day^{-1} for males and 35 to 40 kcal/kg^{-1}/day^{-1} for females. Daily calcium intake during adolescence should be a minimum of 1,300 mg per day.

Because of the teenage lifestyle, healthy eating habits are sometimes difficult to maintain in adolescents. The nutritional history should be considered in the context of overall lifestyle and activity. Because issues of body image and peer influence are at their peak during this age, it is essential to watch for signs of eating disorders and to caution parents on how to carefully discuss the importance of diet with their teen.

■ Anticipatory Guidance and Safety

Well checkups are not solely to examine the patient physically but also to offer advice and insight into upcoming stages and safety issues. A focus of the assessment should include identifying a child's potential risks in order to be able to appropriately counsel parents.

Create an open dialogue with parents that addresses safety topics by asking about daily practices and home environment. Table 18.12 is an age-by-age list of anticipatory guidance and safety topics, which should be covered at each well-child checkup, regarding feeding, sleeping, elimination, safety, and illness. Other issues may arise, and discussion during the visits should be based on parental concerns and questions.

■ Teething and Tooth Eruption

Assess the child's history of teething and tooth eruption. The primary teeth begin to erupt around 6 months of age. Table 18.13 identifies the typical age of tooth eruption. The eruption pattern may vary from the expected norm.

During the assessment of teething and tooth eruption, determine the level of fluoride present in the child's drinking water. It is helpful for providers to know the amount of fluoride in a community's drinking water because any recommendations for supplementation are based on those amounts. Children who do not live in a fluoridated water area but who attend school or daycare in such an area (and drink water while at school) may not need additional supplementation. The guidelines in Table 18.14 should be incorporated into the care of pediatric patients.

Table 18.12

Anticipatory Guidance

Age	Feeding	Sleeping	Elimination	Safety	Illness
Newborn–1 mo	Feed on demand; ask about duration of feeds (or amount per feeding if on formula); always hold bottle—don't prop	Back to sleep; firm mattress; avoid pillows and blankets; ask about where baby is sleeping and in what position	Breastfed stool is yellow and pasty; normal bowel frequency varies from after each feeding to every other day; ask about stool frequency and consistency	Do not leave infant alone on high surfaces; set water heater thermostat at 120 degrees; always use a proper rear-facing car seat; smoke detectors; sun protection	Call office for rectal temp higher than 100.4°F, persistent vomiting or diarrhea, refusal to feed, prolonged irritability, bulging fontanel, or yellow tinge to skin or eyes
1–2 mo	Feed on demand; may stretch out time between feeds	Same as above; some routine may slowly develop; may sleep 16–18 hr/day	Babies frequently grunt and strain while stooling; as long as stool is soft then baby is not constipated	Same as above; learn infant/child CPR	Same as above
2–4 mo	Same as above; more routine develops; may slowly increase amount of formula; no solids needed yet; avoid adding cereal to bottle	Same as above	Same as above	Same as above	Same as above
4–6 mo	Night feedings should decrease or stop; may start solids close to 6 mo	Should sleep longer stretches at night; routine nap schedule develops; if infant rolls to stomach to sleep, it is okay	Same as above	Watch for choking hazards; watch for burns from infant grabbing at hot food or liquids	Call for rectal temp over 101°F; decreased urination (no wet diaper in 8 hr); prolonged inconsolability; wheezing; cold symptoms (without fever) for over 5–7 days

562

Stage	Feeding	Sleeping	Elimination	Safety
6–9 mo	Start solids—begin with rice cereal in a soupy consistency; add foods slowly and one at a time (stick with one new food for 3–4 days); night feedings should stop	Establish consistent nighttime rituals, including reading	Stools will change in consistency with addition of solids; rice cereal can be constipating; give diluted juice if constipation is a problem	Make sure house is completely baby-proofed! Lock poisons; cover outlets; pool safety if applicable; choking hazards with new foods; sunscreen
9–12 mo	Increase table/finger foods; offer cup; offer water and diluted juice (no more than 6 oz of juice/day); establish mealtime routines	Stick with nighttime rituals; security item may help with bedtime	Same as above	Same as above
Toddler	Appetite slows; child becomes pickier; offer new foods; avoid battles	Transition to regular bed; consistent nighttime ritual; nightmares may occur; usually one nap during the day	Interest in potty training emerges; most children demonstrate readiness between 24 and 30 mo	Always use proper car seat; teach street safety; have a fire escape plan; lock guns away; lock poisons and medications; use sunscreen and bug repellent; caution about burns and falls

Continued

Table 18.12

Anticipatory Guidance—cont'd

Stage	Feeding	Sleeping	Elimination	Safety
Preschooler	Encourage balanced diet; child should use utensils correctly; pickiness may continue	Naps may decrease or stop; bedtime may be moved up when napping ceases; nightmares and terrors may occur	By age 3, 90% of children are bowel trained; 85% are dry during the day, and 60%–70% are dry at night; no interventions if still wetting at night	Same as above; water safety; begin stranger awareness and safety; continue using car or booster seat
School age	Encourage balanced diet, limiting junk foods; eat as a family; involve child in food preparation	Continue consistent nighttime ritual; average 8-year-old sleeps 9–12 hours a night	Consider interventions (pharmacologic or behavioral) if nocturnal enuresis occurs	Same as above; bike safety; fire safety; child should remain in a booster car seat until age 8 or 80 pounds
Adolescent	Encourage balanced diet and healthy food choices; limit junk and fast food	Erratic sleep patterns; napping may increase; need average of 8–9 hours of sleep per night		Seatbelts; car safety; safe sex; discourage drug and alcohol usage; reinforce sunscreen usage; keep firearms locked

Table 18.13

Patterns of Tooth Eruption

Primary Teeth	Maxillary	Mandibular
Central incisors	6–8 mo	5–7 mo
Lateral incisors	8–11 mo	7–10 mo
Cuspids/canines	16–20 mo	16–20 mo
First molars	10–16 mo	10–16 mo
Second molars	20–30 mo	20–30 mo

Permanent Teeth	Maxillary	Mandibular
Central incisors	7–8 yr	6–7 yr
Lateral incisors	8–9 yr	7–8 yr
Cuspids/canines	11–12 yr	9–11 yr
First premolars	10–11 yr	10–12 yr
Second premolars	10–12 yr	11–13 yr
First molars	6–7 yr	6–7 yr
Second molars	12–13 yr	12–13 yr
Third molars	17–22 yr	17–22 yr

Table 18.14

Fluoride Concentration in Community Drinking Water

Age	Less Than 0.3 ppm	0.3–0.6 ppm	More Than 0.6 ppm
Birth–6 mo	None	None	None
6 months–3 yr	0.25 mg/day	None	None
3–6 yr	0.50 mg/day	0.25 mg/day	None
6–16 yr	1.0 mg/day	0.5 mg/day	None

ppm = parts per million.
Data from U.S. Department of Health and Human Services, Centers for Disease Control and Prevention, http:/www.cdc.gov/mmwr/preview/mmwrhtml/rr5014a1.htm.

SUGGESTED READINGS

American Academy of Pediatrics. (2002). *Guidelines for Health Supervision*, 3rd ed., rev. Elk Grove Village, IL: American Academy of Pediatrics.

Baker, S., Cochran, W., Greer, F., Heyman, M., Jacobson, M., Jaksic, T., & Krebs, N. (2001). The use and misuse of fruit juice in pediatrics. *Pediatrics, 107*(5), 1210–1213. http://aappolicy.aappublications.org/cgi/content/full/pediatrics;107/5/1210 (accessed March 18, 2011).

Burns, C., Dunn, A., Brady, M., Starr, N., & Blosser, C. (2004). *Pediatric Primary Care: A Handbook for Nurse Practitioners.* Philadelphia: W.B. Saunders Company.

Castiglia, P., & Harbin, R. (1992). *Child Health Care: Process and Practice.* Philadelphia: J.B. Lippincott.

Ganel, A., Dudkiewicz, I., & Grogan, D. (2003). Pediatric orthopedic physical examination of the infant: A 5-minute assessment. *Journal of Pediatric Health Care, 17*(1), 39–41.

Graham, M., & Uphold, C. (2004). *Clinical Guidelines in Child Health.* Gainesville, FL: Barmarrae Books.

Greer, F., & Krebs, N. (2006) Optimizing bone health and calcium intakes of infants, children, and adolescents. *Pediatrics, 117*(2), 578–585. http://aappolicy.aappublications.org/cgi/content/abstract/pediatrics;117/2/578 (accessed March 21, 2011).

Hockenberry, M., & Wilson, D. (Eds.). (2006). *Wong's Nursing Care of Infants and Children,* 8th ed. St. Louis: Mosby.

Kleigman, R., Behrman, R., Jenson, H., & Stanton, B. (2007). *Nelson Textbook of Pediatrics,* 18th ed. Philadelphia: Saunders.

Legler, J., & Rose, L. (1998). Assessment of abnormal growth curves. *American Family Physician*, 58(1). www.aafp.org/afp/980700ap/legler.html (accessed March 18, 2011).

Millonig, V., & Mobley, C. (Eds.). (2004). *Pediatric Nurse Practitioner Certification Review Guide*, 4th ed. Potomac, MD: Health Leadership Associates.

Wagner, C., & Greer, F. (2008). Prevention of rickets and vitamin D deficiency in infants, children, and adolescents. *Pediatrics, 122*(5), 1142–1152.

Chapter 19

PREGNANT PATIENTS

Deborah Blackwell • James Blackwell

Pregnancy is considered a wellness condition and not a disease entity. The focus of care during a low-risk pregnancy is therefore on health promotion and maintenance while achieving a healthy outcome for both the woman and child. Advanced practice nurses—specifically, nurse practitioners—have a strong tradition of delivering wellness care throughout the life span in a cost-effective manner and with a high level of patient satisfaction. Caring for pregnant women is therefore congruent with the advanced practice nursing model.

Pregnancy care from nurse practitioners should ideally begin with preconception care and continue until 24 to 28 weeks of pregnancy, when the woman is usually referred to a specialty provider, which typically is either an obstetrician or certified nurse midwife, in preparation for childbirth.

The status of a woman's health directly affects the pregnancy outcome. Basic prenatal care is individualized and includes health promotion, risk assessment/screening, and the initiation of interventions (Fowler & Jack, 2008). Preconception care should be used to maximize the woman's physical and psychosocial health and allow her to make informed decisions regarding any potential health or lifestyle adjustments that may affect future pregnancies.

History

After pregnancy is confirmed, a complete medical, psychosocial (including the current living situation and social support and abuse information), family (including genetic), and reproductive history is obtained. This includes a menstrual, contraceptive, gynecologic, sexual, surgical, nutritional (including prepregnancy weight), and medication (including over-the-counter and recreational drug use) history. An estimated date of delivery (EDD) is projected at this time by using the last menstrual period (LMP). This estimation can be made either with a pregnancy wheel or by applying Naegele's rule of adding 7 days to the first day of the LMP and then subtracting 3 months (Corbett, 2007). This method of estimating the EDD depends on the woman having regular menstrual cycles of 28, plus or minus 7 days. If the EDD cannot be accurately estimated by Naegele's rule, an early ultrasound is recommended because of the linkage of specific prenatal interventions with gestational dating of the pregnancy. The EDD should be updated throughout the pregnancy for confirmation of dates by determining when quickening occurs, when fetal heart tones are first auscultated, when the fundal height is at the umbilicus, and, most accurately, through an ultrasound estimation at 16 to 20 weeks.

The reproductive history includes the contraceptive, sexual, and obstetric history. The contraceptive history elicits the last time contraceptives have been used, what types of contraceptives were used, and the dates of any unprotected intercourse. The sexual history helps identify risks for sexually transmitted diseases or ectopic pregnancies. The obstetric history consists of the number of pregnancies and their outcomes using the gravida–para–TPAL nomenclature (Table 19.1). This portion of the history also includes the year of each pregnancy, infant birth weight, gestational age at birth, type of delivery (vaginal or caesarian), length of labor, anesthesia received, and any maternal or fetal complications during the pregnancy.

Physical Examination

The initial physical examination is a systematic, complete, head-to-toe examination that is usually performed at the time of the first visit to provide baseline information. The clinical pelvimetry assessment is done at this time to ensure pelvic adequacy for vaginal delivery. Vitals signs, especially blood pressure and weight, are included with each assessment. Subsequent

Table 19.1

Pregnancy Nomenclature

Letter	Meaning	Definition
G	Gravidity	Total number of pregnancies, regardless of duration or outcome
P	Parity	Number of pregnancies after 20 weeks of gestation
T	Term	Number of pregnancies considered to be 37–40 weeks of gestation
P	Premature/preterm deliveries	Number of pregnancies between 20 and 37 weeks of gestation
A	Abortions	Number of induced or spontaneous terminations of pregnancy before 20 weeks of gestation
L	Live births	Number of living children who are alive at the time of data collection

visits are abbreviated in that they focus on the developmental stage of the pregnancy and the overall health of the mother and fetus. Components of these targeted examinations (depending on the week of gestation) include fundal height, presentation, fetal heart rate (FHR), fetal movement, the presence or absence of preterm labor signs and symptoms, cervical examination (including dilatation and effacement), urine dipstick, and timing of the next appointment.

Monitoring fetal heart rate is a vital component of fetal surveillance, providing important information on placental function, fetal hypoxia, and whether the intrauterine environment can support and sustain the fetus. The FHR can usually be auscultated at 12 weeks with an electronic Doppler and at 18 to 20 weeks with a fetoscope (Corbett, 2007). A normal fetal heart rate is 120 to 160 beats per minute. A sustained FHR of below 100 beats per minute is indicative of fetal jeopardy. If there is a question of whether the fetal heart rate is being adequately evaluated, the maternal pulse should simultaneously be assessed to ensure that the FHR and not the maternal heart rate is actually being auscultated. Leopold's maneuvers should be integrated into the prenatal assessment after 28 weeks of gestation in order to locate the most appropriate area for FHR auscultation (Figure 19.1). The provider will document the location where the fetal heart tones (FHTs) are best heard or the point of maximal intensity. This procedure can reinforce the accuracy of the fetal position as assessed by the examiner through palpation. FHTs are best auscultated through the fetal back in vertex and breech presentations and toward the mother's flank when the fetus is in a transverse lie. In vertex presentations, FHTs are usually best heard below the mother's umbilicus, in the lower abdomen, whereas for breech presentations, they are best heard at or slightly above the umbilicus, in the mother's upper abdomen.

Fundal height changes are reflective of fetal growth and correlate closely with the number of weeks of pregnancy from 18 to 32 weeks of gestation (Corbett, 2007). Assessment of fundal height provides an estimation of gestational age in relationship to uterine size. Fundal height is measured by placing the end of a tape measure at the symphysis pubis and extending it to the fundus (Figure 19.2). The uterus is usually palpable above the symphysis at 12 weeks of gestation, midway between the symphysis pubis and umbilicus at 16 weeks, and at the umbilicus at 20 weeks. Small uterine size for dates may be indicative of inaccurate pregnancy dating or intrauterine growth restriction. Large uterine size for dates may be associated with inaccurate dates, macrosomia, or multiple gestations (more than one fetus).

Laboratory Studies

Laboratory studies during the initial visit are quite extensive. These screening tests are dependent on the disease prevalence within the screened population (Table 19.2). Laboratory testing throughout the pregnancy is

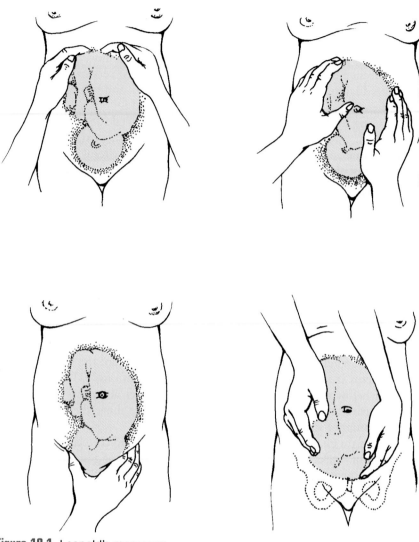

Figure 19.1 Leopold's maneuver.

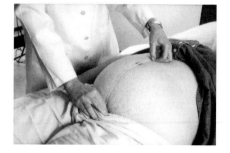

Figure 9.2 Measuring fundal heights: Fundal height in centimeters should correlate closely with number of weeks' gestation. From Dillon (2007), p. 838.

Table 19.2

Recommended Pregnancy Screening Tests

Initial Routine Tests for All Pregnant Patients	Additional Tests Depending on the Patient's History	Tests for Subsequent Pregnancy Visits
• CBC • Blood type, Rh, and antibody screen • Urine dipstick (culture and sensitivity if dipstick is positive) • Aneuploidy (quad) screen (maternal serum α-fetoprotein, hCG, unconjugated estriol [formerly known as the triple screen], and inhibin A) *(No longer dependent on maternal age)* • Rubella titer • Serology for syphilis • Hepatitis B surface antigen • Pap smear • Chlamydia/gonorrhea screening	• Sickle cell screen (Sickledex) or hemoglobin electrophoresis for African Americans • Tuberculosis screen • HIV screen • Urine toxicology screen • Diabetes screening • Herpes culture • Serum iron studies • Thyroid studies • Toxoplasmosis titer • Potassium hydroxide (KOH)/wet prep	• CBC: 28 and 36 wk • Diabetes screening: 24–26 wk • Urine culture: 12–16 wk • Repeat aneuploidy screen in second trimester • Antibody screen for Rh-negative patients: 28 wk • Retest chlamydia/gonorrhea if positive earlier: 34–36 wk • Group beta strep culture (vaginal/anorectal): 35–37 wk

dependent on presenting complaints and the developmental stage of the pregnancy. For example, a glucose screen should be done between 24 and 26 weeks of gestation, whereas an anemia screen (hemoglobin and hematocrit) should be done initially and again at 28 to 36 weeks. However, if the woman complains of a vaginal discharge later in the pregnancy, a gonorrhea and chlamydia culture could be done even if the initial screen was negative.

Prenatal Education

Prenatal education depends on when the visit occurs and any concerns uncovered during the visit, but it usually focuses on preterm labor signs and symptoms, danger signs of pregnancy, fetal movement awareness, information about prenatal classes, nutrition, exercise, weight goals, teratogens, sexuality, and infant feeding choices. The usual weight gain during pregnancy is 0.4 kg per week for a woman of normal weight, with a total of 11.5 to 18 kg for the entire pregnancy period. However, the first trimester may be only 1 to 2.5 kg (Moore, 2007). Rapid weight gain occurs during the second trimester and slows during the third trimester. The recommended weight gain for pregnancy is adjusted according to the patient's body mass index (Table 19.3).

Prenatal vitamins are started during the initial visit along with any other medications as indicated by the history or physical examination (e.g., iron or calcium supplementation). For routine pregnancies, prenatal visits are usually scheduled every month until 28 weeks of gestation. At that time, visits are scheduled every 2 weeks from 28 to 36 weeks, at which point the patient is then seen weekly until she goes into labor (Choby, 2008).

Common Chief Complaints of Pregnancy

■ Gastrointestinal Complaints

Gastrointestinal (GI) complaints are common in pregnancy, affecting 50% to 90% of pregnant women in the United States (Pandolfino & Vanagunas, 2000). These ailments can consist of mild to severe nausea, vomiting, and dyspepsia and are usually caused by increased levels of human chorionic gonadotropin (hCG) or by the effects of increased progesterone on smooth muscles in the GI tract. Evidence supporting GI ailments caused by the uterine displacement of abdominal organs is limited (Richter, 2007). The practitioner must be able to differentiate normal changes associated with pregnancy from more serious disease states and must know which diagnostic tests will not be harmful to either the mother or the fetus.

Heartburn affects 30% to 80% of pregnant women (Richter, 2007). While it may occur at anytime during the pregnancy, it usually occurs around the fifth month. Heartburn in pregnancy usually results from lower esophageal sphincter pressure, whereas hormonal changes and decreased intestinal motility is believed to cause constipation and flatulence (Christie & Rose, 2007). Causes of nausea and vomiting associated with pregnancy are unknown but believed to be related to increased levels of estrogen, human chorionic gonadotropin, estradiol, and

Table 19.3		

Recommended Weight Gain During Pregnancy

Body Mass Index	Total Weight Gain (kg)	Rate (kg/4 wk)
Less than 19.8 (underweight)	12.7–18.2	2.3
19.8–28.0 (normal weight)	11.4–15.9	1.8
28.1–29.0 (overweight)	6.8–11.4	1.2
Greater than 29.0 (obese)	6.8	0.9

From Baxley, E.G., & Brown, R.S. (2008). Patient and family education. Section A. Nutrition in pregnancy and lactation. In Ratcliffe, S.D., Baxley, E.G., Cline, M.K., & Sakornbut, E.L. (Eds.). *Family Medicine Obstetrics*, 3rd ed. Philadelphia: Mosby & Elsevier, pp. 66–73, with permission.

progesterone (Baxley, 2008; Richter, 2007). Persistent or severe nausea and vomiting, to the point of affecting the woman's nutritional status, known as hyperemesis gravidarum, may be an early symptom of hyperthyroidism. Beta-hCG has a thyroid-stimulating hormone–like effect on the maternal thyroid, and hyperthyroidism may be evident only by an increase in free T_4 instead of by both the TSH decrease and the free T_4 increase that are usually seen in women who are not pregnant (Turok & Schultz, 2008).

Contributing factors for pregnancy-related nausea and vomiting can include emotional factors and irregular eating habits. An increased incidence of *Helicobacter pylori* has recently been identified in pregnant women with intense nausea compared with those who had never experienced morning sickness (Reymunde, Santiago, & Perez, 2001). Conventional pregnancy-related nausea and vomiting commonly peak at about 10 to 15 weeks of gestation and resolve at approximately 20 weeks of gestation (Richter, 2007). Hyperemesis gravidarum occurs in only approximately 2% of pregnancies but is associated with nulliparity, increased body weight, history of migraines, multiple gestation, and molar pregnancies (Cashion, 2007; Harvey-Banchik, 2007). More than 50% of patients with hyperemesis gravidarum have elevated aminotransferase levels (Harvey-Banchik, 2007).

Pregnancy also increases the risk of developing gallstones owing to an increased progesterone level that reduces gallbladder emptying and therefore increases biliary stasis. Subsequent pregnancies exponentially increase the risk of cholelithiasis. Gallstones occur in approximately 7% of nulliparous women and 19% of multiparous women (Parangi & Pories, 2007). Upper endoscopy is a safe diagnostic procedure during pregnancy and does not carry an increased risk of preterm labor or other complications as compared to other diagnostic modalities such as diagnostic radiology studies (Ahmad & Frank, 2007). However, as a general rule, any procedures during pregnancy are usually postponed until after delivery or at least until after the first trimester unless the risk of the disease outweighs the risk of the procedure and definitive evaluation is needed.

If radiology studies are warranted, ultrasound is safe and effective in diagnosing intraabdominal conditions during pregnancy. Current knowledge indicates that magnetic resonance imaging (MRI) is safe during pregnancy, but computed tomography (CT) imaging exposes the fetus to doses of ionizing radiation (Sakornbut, 2008a).

Upper endoscopy may be indicated during pregnancy for significant GI bleeding, unresponsive nausea and vomiting, dysphagia, peptic ulcer disease, and severe abdominal pain. Bloody diarrhea, hematochezia, weight loss, and fatigue during pregnancy should initially be evaluated by stool samples for Gram stain and culture, ova and parasites, fecal leukocytes, and *Clostridium difficile* toxin. If these tests are negative, a flexible sigmoidoscopy or colonoscopy should be done. Sigmoidoscopy does not require conscious sedation and is not associated with any pregnancy complications (Ahmad & Frank, 2007).

NAUSEA AND VOMITING

Subjective

Initial questions regarding pregnancy-induced nausea and vomiting should include whether these symptoms occur more frequently during certain times of the day. Any pain should be assessed as to whether it has a gradual or rapid onset and whether eating either alleviates or exacerbates the condition. For example, nausea with pain that occurs with eating may indicate esophagitis, whereas symptoms that occur several hours postprandially suggests a duodenal ulcer. Hydration status can be assessed by asking about dark-colored urine and excessive thirst. Psychosocial distress also should be evaluated. Worrisome features in the history include fever, abdominal pain, abdominal cramping, diarrhea, jaundice, vaginal bleeding, headaches, neurological signs, projectile vomiting, hematemesis, and melena.

Objective

Vital signs should lie within normal limits and not be indicative of dehydration. There should not be any weight loss. The thyroid should be of normal size and shape. Uterine size should be appropriate for dates, and the presence of FHTs (after 12 weeks) is a reassuring sign. A complete blood count (CBC), complete metabolic panel containing liver enzymes and a calcium level, and a Hemoccult of the stool may eliminate other causes for the nausea and vomiting. Urine ketones and specific gravity should not be indicative of dehydration, and urine dipstick or urinalysis should be negative for infection or hematuria (to rule out renal calculus). Stool antigen for *H. pylori* can be attained to evaluate for current infection, since a serum titer will not differentiate between past and current infections.

Differential Diagnoses

Hyperemesis gravidarum, multiple gestation, hydatidiform gestation, molar pregnancy, intestinal obstruction, gastroenteritis, cholecystitis, pancreatitis, hepatitis, diabetes, thyroid dysfunction, migraine, food poisoning, emotional problems, eating disorders.

DYSPEPSIA

Subjective

Heartburn and epigastric/upper abdominal pain are the classic symptoms for dyspepsia, especially after heavy, fatty, fried, spicy, or gas-producing meals. Another symptom may include abdominal bloating or distention. Any psychosocial stressors or depression should be explored. Dyspepsia should be differentiated from dysphagia. Worrisome symptoms include associated chest pain, dyspnea, exercise intolerance, palpitations, diaphoresis, fatty stools, foul-smelling stools, melena, nausea, vomiting, diarrhea or constipation, or fever and chills.

Objective

Diagnosis for dyspepsia is usually made on history and physical examination. A CBC, complete metabolic panel, and a Hemoccult for blood in the stool may eliminate other causes for the dyspepsia. Presence of *H. pylori* can be addressed. Dyspepsia occurs at a higher incidence in people who are overweight or obese.

Differential Diagnoses

Dyspepsia related to pregnancy, cholecystitis, pancreatitis, cardiac etiology, ulcer, hiatal hernia.

ABDOMINAL PAIN

The uterine pressure increases as a result of the growing fetus and placenta and the increase in amniotic fluid volume. At 12 weeks, the fundus rises above the symphysis. When the pregnant woman is in an upright position, the broad and round ligaments anchor the uterus to the anterior abdominal wall in order to provide uterine stability (Baxley, 2008). The weight of the uterus may cause tension on these ligaments, creating inflammation and discomfort. This pain is often exacerbated with movement and is more often present on the right side. This ligament pain usually resolves when the woman assumes a supine position as the uterus descends backward.

Subjective

The woman should be asked whether the abdominal pain can be classified as acute, chronic, or recurrent; whether it has a gradual or rapid onset; and whether the pain has ever occurred before. The severity of the pain (on a scale of 1 to 10) and the progression or resolution of the pain should be noted. If there is sharp or dull pain on either or both sides of the abdomen, investigate whether the pain increases in intensity with movement. If there is tightening or pressure in the uterus, ask whether the pressure resolves with position change or with bladder emptying. Inquire about the timing and consistency of the last bowel movement. Worrisome symptoms include regular contractions that do not improve with position change or bladder emptying, nausea, vomiting, diarrhea, melena, hematochezia, hematemesis, fever, anorexia, periumbilical or right lower quadrant pain, one-sided abdominal pain that is constant and increases over time, urinary tract infection (UTI) symptoms, a tender lump in the groin that worsens with prolonged standing, vaginal bleeding or bloody show, or vaginal fluid leaking.

Objective

Vital signs and physical examination should be appropriate for the gestational age of the pregnancy. There should be no reproducible tenderness with palpation to the chest wall or pain with deep breathing. There should be no regular contractions felt; no cervical dilatation or effacement; no fluid leakage, possibly indicating rupture of membranes, or bleeding from the os; and no adnexal, abdominal, or pelvic masses or tenderness. Bowel sounds should be normal, and fetal activity should be present. Fetal heart sounds should be heard by Doppler if gestation is over 10 to 12 weeks. Ultrasonography should show a normal fetal heart motion and no worrisome signs, such as decreased fetal movement, abnormal placenta placement, or abnormal amniotic fluid levels. If the pregnancy is between weeks 4 and 8, the hCG levels should correspond with the gestational age of the fetus and should double every 2 to 3 days (Deutchman, 2008).

Differential Diagnoses

Normal fetal activity, ligament pain, Braxton Hicks contractions, preterm or true labor, ectopic pregnancy, abruptio placentae, placenta previa, threatened abortion, complete abortion, missed (incomplete) abortion, premature rupture of membranes, preeclampsia, vaginitis, pelvic inflammatory disease (PID), ovarian cyst rupture, constipation, intestinal obstruction, ulcer, diverticulitis, appendicitis, kidney stone, inguinal hernia, gastroenteritis, UTI, costochondritis.

■ Musculoskeletal Complaints

Low back pain is a common complaint during pregnancy. The pain may radiate to the legs and may increase at night. Back pain usually results from the exaggeration of the lumbar spine curvature that balances the woman's center of gravity over the lower extremities in response to the growing uterus. The release of the hormone relaxin causes ligaments in the pubic symphysis and sacroiliac joints to soften in preparation for vaginal delivery. An increased breast size may also result in upper back pain.

Carpal tunnel syndrome results from compression of the median nerve in the carpal tunnel, which results in paresthesias or weakness of the thumb, index, and middle fingers (Viera, 2003). Carpal tunnel syndrome occurs in 20% to 60% of pregnant women and often causes these women to awake with burning, numbness, and tingling in the median nerve distribution (Padua et al., 2001; Weimer et al., 2002). However, these symptoms usually tend to occur during the last trimester.

BACK PAIN
Subjective

Back pain is reported as a dull, aching pain in the upper or lower back that worsens as the day progresses. Standing or sitting for long periods may aggravate the back pain. The location of the pain is important, as is the information gathered via a PQRST report. This inquiry usually provides sufficient diagnostic information and comprises the *precipitating* (P) factors (what aggravates or alleviates the pain; the symptoms associated with the pain), the *quality* (Q) of the pain (achy, burning, cramping, shooting, etc.), the *radiation* (R) of the pain, the *severity* (S) of the pain (typically reported on a 1-to-10 scale and whether it interferes with the usual activities of daily living), and the *timing* (T) of the pain (sudden or gradual onset, duration). Worrisome symptoms include a history of back injuries, problems, or surgeries; UTI or vaginal infection symptoms; bowel changes; uterine contractions;

pain, numbness, or tingling that radiates either into the abdomen or down into the legs; and any neurological deficits.

Objective

The weight and body mass index of the woman should be noted. Lordosis, gait, paraspinal or costal vertebral angle (CVA) tenderness to palpation, straight leg raises, reflexes, and a neurologic examination should be assessed. A rectal examination should be done to assess for rectal tone and impaction. Urinary tract symptoms, vaginal discharge, or uterine contractions necessitate appropriate evaluation.

Differential Diagnoses

Backache related to pregnancy, muscle sprain or strain, sciatica, arthritis, herniated disk, uterine contractions, vaginal infection, UTI, kidney stone, pancreatitis, gallstones, ulcer.

MUSCLE CRAMPS

Subjective

The patient experiences calf, thigh, or buttocks cramps, occurring mostly at night or in the early morning. The woman may report excessive exercise or walking. Fluid and calcium intake should be checked through a diet recall. Worrisome symptoms include a history of deep vein thrombosis, a personal or family history of thrombophilic disorders (Table 19.4), recent trauma or surgery, lower back pain or arthritis, or neurologic complaints.

Table 19.4	
Thrombophilic States in Pregnancy	
Inherited Thrombophilias	**Acquired Thrombophilias**
Factor V Leiden	Pregnancy/postpartum
Prothrombin A20210	Immobilization
Antithrombin (AT) III	Trauma
Protein C	Postoperative state
Protein S	High estrogen levels
Homocysteine	Malignancy
	Nephrotic syndrome
	Heparin-induced thrombocytopenia
	Myeloproliferative disorders
	Paroxysmal nocturnal hematuria
	Congestive heart failure and atrial fibrillation
	Antiphospholipid antibody syndrome

Objective

Worrisome symptoms include a positive Homan's sign, unilateral swelling or tenderness, diminished pulses in the lower extremities, redness, abnormal warmth or coldness, numbness, or pale-appearing calf or leg. Orthostatic blood pressures and pulses should be taken if indicated. Electrolytes and serum calcium levels may need to be checked.

Differential Diagnoses

Muscle cramps, electrolyte imbalances, thromboembolic disease, varicosities, dehydration, arthritis, sciatica, nerve root compression.

NUMBNESS AND/OR TINGLING IN HAND(S)

Subjective

The patient reports a dull, achy pain in the wrist, forearm, or hand that may worsen at night. This pain may be associated with paresthesia or weakness in the hand. Edema in the hands or upper extremities may be noted. A history of repetitive activity of the upper extremity may be reported. Sitting, standing, and sleep posture (especially if the woman sleeps with the arm extended against the head) should be investigated.

Objective

Tinel's sign and Phalen's test should be performed. Upper extremity, grip, and finger strength should be assessed along with the ability to oppose the thumb to the fingers. An evaluation for thenar atrophy and dry skin on the thumb and index and middle fingers (median nerve distribution) should be completed. The size and shape of joints, skin color, pulses, and capillary refill should be noted.

Differential Diagnoses

Carpal tunnel syndrome, musculoskeletal pain, arthritis, infection, cervical neck injury or disease, nerve damage in the hand, cardiac problems, thoracic outlet syndrome, hyperventilation.

■ Respiratory Complaints

As the uterus enlarges, it presses against the abdominal organs and diaphragm, and this prevents the lungs from fully expanding and results in a decreased residual volume and functional residual capacity (Cline, 2008). Increased progesterone directly stimulates the central respiratory system to increase minute ventilation and tidal volume and to decrease blood P_{CO_2}. Oxygen consumption and basal metabolic rate also increases. These changes are the basis of an increased awareness of breathing or even dyspnea that is experienced during pregnancy. Nasal congestion or stuffiness may result from increased estrogen and progesterone levels, which increase perivascular edema and enlargement of the nasal turbinates (Baxley, 2008). These changes may also lead to episodes of epistaxis.

DYSPNEA (SHORTNESS OF BREATH)

Subjective

The pregnant woman may experience labored or heavy breathing, which may be associated with activity. Dizziness or lightheadedness may be reported. The woman's smoking history should be obtained. It is crucial to determine the onset (either acute or chronic), the progression, and any past history of dyspnea. Additional investigation should include whether the dyspnea occurred following an episode of eating, drinking, or potential allergen exposure, such as an insect bite. Severe dyspnea and significant oxygen deprivation requires an immediate assessment and referral. History should be negative for fever, cough, trauma, hemoptysis, night sweats, wheezing, chest pain, or GI symptoms. Past medical and family history should include assessment for deep vein thrombosis, recent immobilization or prolonged sitting, and thrombophilias such as factor V Leiden, protein C or S deficiency, and antiphospholipid syndrome.

Objective

Diagnostic tests are typically not necessary. Vital signs and physical examination, especially of the upper and lower respiratory tracts and cardiac system, should be within normal limits for gestational age. There should be no dependent edema. A CBC should not indicate anemia, and pulse oximetry should be 95% or above. A chest x-ray is not indicated unless absolutely necessary, especially until after 17 weeks of gestation. Ionizing radiation should not exceed a dose of more than 5 rads over the entire pregnancy (Wotring, 2004). A chest x-ray generally delivers 7 millirads (1 rad is equal to 1,000 millirads) to the ovary without shielding (Cline, 2008). A risk-versus-benefit assessment should be documented in the provider's note along with documentation that the abdomen had lead shielding and that the lowest exposure technique possible was used.

Differential Diagnoses

Pregnancy-related dyspnea, upper respiratory infection (URI), nasal congestion, asthma, bronchitis, pneumonia, pulmonary embolus, cardiac disease such as congestive heart failure (CHF), anemia, anxiety, hyperventilation, aspiration, anaphylaxis.

NASAL CONGESTION

Subjective

The woman may report nasal stuffiness, rhinorrhea, sneezing, postnasal drip, or cough. History may be positive for epistaxis. Worrisome symptoms include frontal headaches or sensation of fullness or pressure, teeth pain, or fever. Nasal spray and intranasal drug use should be investigated. Past medical history should include inquiries regarding allergic rhinitis, seasonal allergies, sinusitis, nasal or facial trauma, and hypertension.

Objective

Vital signs, particularly temperature and blood pressure, should be normal. Nasal turbinates may be pale to red, edematous, and may be either dry or have discharge. Clotted blood may be noted if epistaxis has occurred. Sinuses should be percussed and palpated. There should be no pain with forward head motion. No polyps should be noted, and the septum should be intact and not deviated.

Differential Diagnoses

Nasal congestion related to pregnancy, epistaxis, URI, sinusitis, allergic rhinitis, nasal polyps, cocaine or chronic nasal spray use, hypertension, facial trauma.

FATIGUE

Fatigue usually occurs during the first and third trimesters of pregnancy. First-trimester fatigue is often associated with the physical and psychosocial pregnancy changes. Fatigue may also be indicative of a more serious physical, emotional, or dietary problem.

Subjective

The woman may experience a higher than expected amount of fatigue despite a normal amount of energy expenditure and sleep. Worrisome symptoms include depression, anxiety, anorexia, exercise intolerance that is different from a prepregnancy state, chest pain or discomfort, dyspnea that is unrelated to pregnancy, pica, or other symptoms that may indicate an underlying cause.

Objective

Vital signs and physical examination, with attention to the thyroid and cardiac and pulmonary systems, should be normal. Weight gain during the pregnancy should be noted. A CBC and thyroid function tests (TSH and free T_4) are reasonable choices for screening. Other laboratory tests should be conducted as indicated by history or physical examination findings.

Differential Diagnoses

Fatigue due to pregnancy, anemia, thyroid disorder, or other pathological states.

■ Genitourinary Complaints

Urinary frequency is often at the top of the list of common pregnancy complaints. The kidneys change in size and shape as early as 10 weeks of gestation (Lowdermilk, 2007). Renal enlargement may originally be caused by increased tone and decreased smooth muscle motility, but after 20 weeks of gestation, it is caused by ureter compression caused by a growing uterus. Increases in circulating fluid volume and glomerular filtration rate may contribute to urinary frequency (Baxley, 2008). During the first trimester, the weight of the growing uterus begins to cause pressure on the bladder. Uterine displacement of the bladder by the end of the second trimester can result in urinary frequency and incontinence. Urinary infections and risk of trauma are greater owing to increased bladder tone relaxation, enlarged bladder capacity, increased bladder pressure, and increased edema of the bladder mucosa.

URINARY FREQUENCY

Subjective

The pregnant woman may complain of increased urination or nocturia. Worrisome symptoms include fever, back or flank pain, suprapubic pain, dysuria, urgency, hematuria, dark or cloudy urine, polyuria, polyphagia, or polydipsia.

Objective

Vital signs should be normal. An abdominal examination should rule out any uterine contractions or irritability. There should be no CVA or suprapubic tenderness. CBC and glucose levels should be within normal limits. Urine dipstick, urinalysis, and culture and sensitivity tests should be normal.

Differential Diagnoses

Pregnancy-related urinary frequency, UTI, pyelonephritis, kidney stone, diabetes.

URINARY INCONTINENCE

Subjective

The main complaint is an involuntary loss of urine possibly associated with coughing, sneezing, or laughing. The increased intra-abdominal pressure caused by these actions, along with the enlarging uterus, results in pressure on the bladder, leading to incontinence. Multigravidas may experience incontinence more often because of poor perineal muscle tone. Special attention should be given to fluid that does not smell like urine, that increases with lying down, or that gushes with initial standing. These patterns of fluid release may indicate rupture of membranes.

Objective

Abdominal examination should rule out any uterine contractions or irritability. Vaginal examination should not reveal any amniotic fluid pooling. Nitrazine and fern tests can differentiate between vaginal discharge and amniotic fluid. A sterile cotton-tipped applicator is used to place vaginal discharge on either nitrazine paper or on a clean microscope slide. If the nitrazine paper changes color and indicates a pH of 7, the discharge may be amniotic fluid. With a fern test, the discharge is allowed to dry on the slide and examined under a microscope. Amniotic fluid forms a fernlike pattern.

Differential Diagnoses

Stress urinary incontinence, rupture of membranes, leukorrhea, vaginitis.

■ Circulatory Complaints

A 30% to 50% increase in cardiac output occurs during pregnancy (Sakornbut, 2008b). This increase begins as early as 10 weeks of gestation and peaks at

20 to 24 weeks. A 40% to 50% increase in blood volume results in an increased venous pressure below the level of the uterus. This increased pressure can result in varicosities in the legs and perineum (hemorrhoids), especially when the pregnant woman is in an upright position, such as with prolonged sitting or standing. An enlarging uterus compresses the vena cava or pelvic and lower extremity veins, leading to venous pooling, which can result in edema, hypotension, dizziness, or even syncope. In order to lessen these complications, the pregnant woman should be instructed not to lie in a supine or recumbent position but rather in a left lateral tilt. Nasal capillaries may become engorged with blood, leading to nasal congestion or even epistaxis (see also the nasal congestion discussion in this chapter's subsection Respiratory Complaints).

DIZZINESS OR SYNCOPE

Subjective

Dizziness or faintness may be reported when the woman is standing, lying on her back, or changing positions. Information on caloric and fluid intake as well as substance abuse should be elicited. Disorientation to spatial relation (may report either that she feels like she is spinning or that the room is spinning) may be described. The practitioner should ask about precipitating and associated factors, such as micturition, defecation, hyperventilation, coughing, dyspnea, chest pain, palpitations, or exposure to a stressful event.

Objective

Vital signs with postural (orthostatic) blood pressures and physical examination, including hydration status and ear, nose, and throat examination, should be normal for gestational age. The CBC should be negative for anemia. Blood glucose, urine-specific gravity, and electrolytes should be normal.

Differential Diagnoses

Compression of the vena cava, orthostatic hypotension, dehydration, anemia, hypoglycemia, hyperventilation, psychosocial stress, inner ear or sinus disease, substance abuse, neurological disorders, cardiopulmonary disorders, situational dizziness.

EDEMA

Subjective

Swelling that worsens as the day progresses and gets better after rest and elevation is generally reported by pregnant women. Edema may be worse during warm weather or after prolonged sitting or standing. The woman should be questioned on the use of any type of constrictive clothing, such as pantyhose, girdles, or tight belts; nutrition, especially sodium and sugar intake; and medication use. There should be no numbness, strength or sensation loss, mental status changes, report of headaches, flashing lights, upper abdominal pain, nausea or vomiting, dyspnea, decreased fetal movement, or decreased urine output.

Objective

Vitals signs, especially blood pressure, should be normal for gestational age. Abnormal blood pressure readings that need to be evaluated include (1) 120/75 mm Hg or higher in midpregnancy, (2) 130/85 mm Hg in the last trimester, (3) a systolic rise of 30 mm Hg or diastolic rise of 15 mm Hg over baseline, or (4) a variation of 20 or more in postural (orthostatic) blood pressures (Lindheimer & Akbari, 2000). The woman's weight gain should be noted. An increase of more than 2 pounds per week should be investigated. Cardiac and pulmonary status should be evaluated. Deep tendon reflexes should be normal, and urine dipstick should be negative or no greater than a trace for protein. The location, amount, and extent of the edema should be documented. Worrisome symptoms include edema that does not respond to rest and leg elevation, rapidly progressing or generalized edema, hard or painful veins or legs, and temperature changes to the extremities.

Differential Diagnoses

Uncomplicated pregnancy-related lower extremity edema; preeclampsia; hemolysis, elevated liver enzymes, low platelets (HELLP) syndrome; superficial varicosities; phlebitis, renal, or liver disease; local trauma or infection in an extremity; CHF.

Pregnancy Complications

■ Anemia

Anemia is not a disease unto itself but a sign of an underlying disorder, which affects at least 20% of pregnant women (McAteer, 2007). Anemia can be defined either clinically as a decrease in the oxygen-carrying capacity of the blood or based on laboratory parameters as a decrease in the hemoglobin level or amount of red blood cells (RBCs). The normal hemoglobin for females is 12 to 16 g/dL. However, this may decrease to 11 g/dL during the first and third trimesters and to 10.5 g/dL in the second trimester (Julius & Kirchner, 2008; Pagana & Pagana, 2006). Anemia during pregnancy is associated with high-output CHF, premature delivery, low birth weight, and fetal demise.

The first step after evaluating the hemoglobin and identifying the presence of anemia is to evaluate the RBC indices. The mean corpuscular volume (MCV) classifies the average volume, or size, of a single RBC. The MCV is calculated by dividing the hematocrit by the RBC and multiplying by 10. The mean corpuscular hemoglobin concentration (MCHC) measures the average concentration or percentage of hemoglobin within a single RBC. If this value is not reported within the CBC, it can easily be determined by dividing the hemoglobin by the hematocrit and multiplying this number by 100. The RBC size distribution width (RDW) is an indirect measurement that indicates the degree of homogeneity of the RBC sample. Uniform RBCs will have a normal RDW, whereas a heterogeneous sample of RBCs (i.e., a sample containing some small and some normal RBCs) will have an increased RDW.

The etiology of the anemia can be classified according to the size and color of the RBCs (Table 19.5). The normal MCV is 80 to 100 fL and determines whether the anemia can be classified as normocytic, microcytic (below 80 fL), or macrocytic (above 100 fL). The normal MCHC is 32% to 36% but should be validated by a laboratory's normal range and determines whether the anemia can be categorized as normochromic, hypochromic (under 32%), or hyperchromic (above 36%). The primary purpose of the MCHC is to identify normochromic or hypochromic causes of anemia. Hyperchromic anemia is somewhat unusual (e.g., spherocytosis, cold agglutinin or intravascular hemolysis) and warrants a referral to a hematologist.

The anemias most often diagnosed during pregnancy are folic acid and iron-deficiency anemia (IDA). The principle etiologies for these anemias are inadequate nutrition, especially among women in lower socioeconomic groups, and the increased body requirements of pregnancy. The prevalence for IDA is 3.5% to 7.4% during the first trimester and may increase to 15% to 55% during the last trimester (Mandell, 2007). If IDA is suspected on the basis of a CBC (low hemoglobin and low RBC indices), iron studies should be attained. These iron studies will generally reveal a low serum iron level, decreased serum ferritin, increased total iron-binding capacity, and decreased transferrin saturation percentage. Anemia of chronic disease may be confused with IDA when the anemia is microcytic but will display low serum iron and total iron-binding capacity.

Table 19.5

Common Causes of Anemia

Normocytic (MCV 80–100 fL) Normochromic (MCHC 32%–36%)	Microcytic (MCV under 80 fL) Hypochromic (MCHC under 32%)	Microcytic (MCV under 80 fL) Normochromic (MCHC 32%–36%)	Macrocytic (MCV over 100 fL) Normochromic (MCHC 32%–36%)
• Iron deficiency (detected early) • Chronic disease • Acute blood loss • Dilutional • Aplastic anemia • Acquired hemolytic anemias (e.g., from prosthetic heart valves) • Dilutional (physiologic) anemia of pregnancy	• Iron deficiency (detected late) • Thalassemia • Lead poisoning • Neoplasms	• Renal disease	• Vitamin B_{12}/folate deficiency • Chemotherapy • Hypothyroidism • Chronic liver disease

MCHC = mean corpuscular hemoglobin concentration; MCV = mean corpuscular volume.

Folate is needed for normal DNA production, but the body stores of folate are limited to a 3-month reserve and may be depleted during high rates of cell turnover, such as during pregnancy. A folate and vitamin B_{12} level should be checked if the CBC suggests that a macrocytic anemia (low hemoglobin level and an MCV of greater than 100) is the cause.

Subjective

The woman may complain of fatigue and dyspnea on exertion.

Objective

Common findings include skin pallor, tachycardia, grade II/VI systolic heart murmur, and increased respiratory rate. The CBC will indicate potential causes (Table 19.5) and guide selection of additional diagnostic studies, such as iron panel, folate level, sickle cell screen or hemoglobin electrophoresis, and liver function tests.

Differential Diagnoses

The differential diagnosis includes iron deficiency, folate deficiency, vitamin B_{12} deficiency, sickle cell trait/anemia, thalassemia.

■ Gestational Diabetes

Diabetes is a group of metabolic disorders characterized by hyperglycemia resulting from defects in insulin secretion, insulin action, or both. Gestational diabetes mellitus (GDM) involves glucose intolerance that develops or is first discovered during pregnancy and hence may include women who have undiagnosed pregestational diabetes. GDM complicates 3% to 6% of all pregnancies with up to 50% of those women developing type 2 diabetes later in life (Beukema, Raiche, & Turok, 2008; Kim, Newton, & Knopp, 2002; Lobner et al., 2006). The greatest incidence of this conversion is within the first 5 to 10 years postdelivery, especially in women who are autoantibody positive, require insulin treatment during pregnancy, have a body mass index (BMI) greater than 30 kg/m², or have more than two prior pregnancies.

Screening for GDM remains controversial. Screening and treatment can reduce the rate of fetal macrosomia and fetal mortality but does not appear to reduce other adverse outcomes, such as cesarean delivery rate, birth injury, or the woman's perception of her health. Recommendations vary on whether and to what degree screenings are needed (Table 19.6).

Selective screening of women with risk factors for GDM has a high sensitivity but low specificity. In other words, it would identify 90% of all pregnant women at increased risk for GDM while falsely identifying others without the condition. Universal screening continues to be widely practiced within the United States between 24 and 28 weeks of gestation with a 50-g 1-hour Glucola test using a venous blood sample. An alternative to the Glucola is to have the woman eat

Table 19.6		

Gestational Diabetes Screening Recommendations

Universal Screening	Risk Factor–Based Screening	No Recommendation for Screening
• World Health Organization	• American Diabetes Association	• U.S. Preventive Services Task Force
• Third International Conference on Gestational Diabetes	• American College of Obstetricians and Gynecologists	• Canadian Task Force on the Periodic Examination
	• Society of Maternal–Fetal Medicine	

Note: This list is not all inclusive but a sampling of organizations that support each recommendation.

28 jelly beans within a 5-minute period (Beukema, Raiche & Turok, 2008). There are two thresholds for an abnormal test: (1) a venous plasma glucose cut-off of 130 mg/dL will identify over 90% of the women who will have a subsequent positive 100-g, 3-hour oral glucose tolerance test (OGTT), and (2) a cut-off of 140 mg/dL will detect 80% of women who will have a subsequent abnormal OGTT but will decrease the number of false positives (Beukema, Raiche & Turok, 2008). A 1-hour screening blood sugar of over 190 mg/dL may negate the need for a 3-hour OGTT. A fasting blood sugar (FBS) should be checked, and if it is elevated (above 95–105 mg/dL), the woman should be considered as having GDM. If the FBS is under 95 mg/dL, a 3-hour OGTT should still be done.

Unfortunately, there remains no universally accepted gold standard for diagnosing GDM, and North America and Europe are using different diagnostic test criteria. The measures used in the United States are based on a 100-g, 3-hour OGTT. These criteria were originally developed to identify mothers at risk for developing diabetes but not those whose newborns were at risk for complications, such as macrosomia. Whereas various expert groups in the United States have proposed different diagnostic values and all predict to some extent newborn complication risk, there is no evidence to date to support any one diagnostic standard (Table 19.7).

The 3-hour OGTT is usually administered after an overnight fast for at least 8, but not more than 14, hours. An FBS is obtained, and then a 100-g glucose load is given. Venous blood sugar samples are then obtained at 1, 2, and 3 hours after the glucose load. Either an elevated FBS or two elevated values on the 3-hour OGTT is diagnostic of GDM. If only one value on the OGTT is elevated, the test should be repeated between 32 and 34 weeks of gestation.

Subjective

The woman may be asymptomatic throughout the entire pregnancy or may report classic episodes of polyuria, polyphagia, or polydipsia. She may

Table 19.7			

Three-Hour OGTT in Pregnancy (Most Common Values Used)

	National Diabetes Data Group, 1979 (Venous Plasma)	Carpenter and Coustan, 1982 (Venous Plasma)	O'Sullivan and Mahan, 1964 (Venous Whole Blood)
Fasting (mg/dL)	105	95	90
1 hr (mg/dL)	190	180	165
2 hr (mg/dL)	165	155	145
3 hr (mg/dL)	145	140	125

Note: Using a standard 100-g glucose load. Fasting and 2-hr levels are most predictive, but diagnosis requires elevation in any two or more values.

experience more episodes of UTIs or vaginitis; therefore, recurrent infections should signal an earlier screening for diabetes or at least a random glucose level. Prior obstetric history should be investigated for unexplained stillbirths, spontaneous abortions, unexplained preterm birth, low-birth-weight infant (with undiagnosed preexisting diabetes), newborn weighing 4,000 g or more, or a previous incident of major congenital abnormality. Family history should be explored for diabetes, including GDM.

Objective

Maternal age and weight should be noted because major risk factors include an age over 35 years or a prepregnancy weight of more than 200 pounds. Excessive weight gain during pregnancy or a fundal height greater than expected is also worrisome. The blood pressure should be noted because women with diabetes are predisposed to hypertensive disorders, including preeclampsia. A retinal examination should be completed to assess for retinopathy. A urine dipstick should be evaluated for glycosuria and proteinuria.

Differential Diagnoses

GDM, undiagnosed type 1 DM or type 2 DM, hyperglycemia, macrosomia, recurrent UTI or vaginitis (not related to DM).

■ Hypertension

Hypertensive problems must be identified early and treated promptly during pregnancy to ensure good maternal and neonatal outcomes. Hypertensive disorders occur in 6% to 8% of all pregnancies and are the second leading cause of maternal deaths in the United States (NHBPEP, 2001). High blood pressure can occur in pregnancy in one of four ways (Table 19.8). The term "pregnancy-induced hypertension" is no longer used because it does not differentiate between gestational hypertension, which is relatively benign, and the more serious preeclampsia (NHBPEP, 2001). The appropriate clinical response to elevated

Table 19.8

Blood Pressure Classification in Pregnancy

NHBPEP Classification	Description
Chronic hypertension	• Hypertension preceding conception, or before the 20th week of gestation • Usually defined as blood pressure of 140/90 mm Hg or greater
Preeclampsia–eclampsia	• A pregnancy-specific systemic syndrome
Preeclampsia	• Systemic disease with hypertension accompanied by proteinuria after the 20th week of gestation • May also be diagnosed without proteinuria if there are other systemic symptoms (e.g., visual changes, headache, abdominal pain, abnormal laboratory values)
Eclampsia	• Convulsive stage of the disease; seizures cannot be attributed to other causes
Preeclampsia superimposed on chronic hypertension	• Women who are hypertensive before the 20th week of gestation who develop new-onset proteinuria • Women with both hypertension and proteinuria before 20 weeks of gestation • Sudden increase in blood pressure in women who previously had controlled hypertension • Women with thrombocytopenia (less than 100,000 cells/mm^3) and elevated liver enzymes (alanine aminotransferase [ALT] or aspartate aminotransferase [AST] • Most often associated with the most severe maternal–fetal complications • Prognosis is much worse than for either condition alone
Gestational hypertension	• High blood pressure detected for the first time after midpregnancy, without proteinuria • Diagnosis is made postpartum
Transient hypertension	• Elevated blood pressure that occurs without proteinuria late in pregnancy or in the early puerperium but returns to normal by 12 weeks postpartum
Chronic gestational hypertension	• Blood pressure remains elevated beyond 12 weeks postpartum but without evidence of preeclampsia

From National High Blood Pressure Education Program Working Group. Working group report on high blood pressure in pregnancy. (NHBPEP Publication No. 00-3029). Washington, DC: National Heart Lung and Blood Institute, 2000.

blood pressure during pregnancy is determined by the underlying pathology rather than the actual elevation in pressure (Peters & Flack, 2004).

The diastolic pressure usually drops by an average of 10 mm Hg below nonpregnant levels by midpregnancy and then slowly returns to nonpregnant levels in the third trimester (Poole, 2004). Determination of the woman's nonpregnant blood pressure is important in the evaluation of blood pressure during pregnancy.

If the systolic blood pressure increases by more than 30 mm Hg or the diastolic increases by more than 15 mm Hg over baseline, preeclampsia may still occur even if the blood pressure is still within the accepted "normal" range. A certain degree of caution should also be displayed for women with a blood pressure of 120/75 mm Hg or higher in midpregnancy or 130/85 mm Hg in later pregnancy (Lindheimer & Akbari, 2000).

Subjective

This condition may occur without the woman's awareness. Symptoms may include headache, visual disturbances, edema, heartburn, abdominal pain, and altered mental status.

Objective

Evaluation should include the presence of edema, blood pressure measurement, urine dip for proteinuria, reflex testing, retinal changes, hepatomegaly, or right upper quadrant tenderness.

Differential Diagnoses

Chronic hypertension (HTN), transient HTN, gestational HTN, preeclampsia, eclampsia, HELLP syndrome, disseminated intravascular coagulopathy.

■ Vaginal Bleeding

Approximately 20% of early pregnancies are complicated by vaginal bleeding, and about half of these will end in spontaneous abortion (Deutchman, 2008). Single or serial qualitative hCG levels can be helpful in evaluating vaginal bleeding during early pregnancy because the levels should double every 2 to 3 days during the fourth to eighth weeks of gestation. In about 30% of all cases, vaginal bleeding that occurs during the second and third trimesters is of unknown etiology. Episodes of bleeding are noted in 10% to 20% of all pregnancies and should always be considered serious and potentially life threatening (Poole, 2004).

Subjective

Assessment questions should be directed toward any precipitating factors of bleeding (e.g., after sexual intercourse), the amount of vaginal bleeding (saturation of sanitary napkins and frequency with which the napkins must be changed), the quality of the vaginal bleeding (clotted versus flowing), and whether the bleeding is actually coming from the vagina or from the urethral or rectal area. The presence of low back pain, abdominal cramping, foul odor, or any passage of products of conception also should be investigated. Any history of coagulation disorders, recent antiplatelet medication use, and Rh status need to be verified. A screening for intimate partner violence should also be done.

Objective

The vital signs should be normal for gestational age. Physical examination should concentrate on uterine size, fetal heart tones, a pelvic examination with cervix visualization, and a digital rectal examination. Other tests that may be useful include a transvaginal ultrasound, hCG level measurement, progesterone level, wet mount, urinalysis, and stool for occult blood. A CBC and coagulation studies should be considered.

Differential Diagnoses

Implantation bleeding, placenta previa, abruptio placentae, uterine rupture, threatened abortion, spontaneous abortion, ectopic pregnancy, gestational trophoblastic disease, vaginal infection, foreign body retention, abdominal or vaginal trauma, blood dyscrasias, intimate partner violence.

■ Vaginal Infections

Observational studies have demonstrated an association between bacterial vaginosis and certain adverse pregnancy outcomes, such as preterm labor, preterm delivery, premature rupture of membranes, and spontaneous abortions. Bacterial vaginosis can be treated with antibiotic therapy, but cure rates are erratic and recurrences are common. There is currently conflicting evidence on whether screening and treatment of asymptomatic bacterial vaginosis in high-risk pregnant women actually reduces the incidence of preterm delivery. The U.S. Preventive Services Task Force (PSTF) therefore neither recommends nor discourages routinely screening these women (U.S. PSTF, 2008). However, the U.S. PSTF does state that screening is not recommended in pregnant women at low risk for preterm delivery, but treatment is appropriate for symptomatic bacterial vaginosis infections (such as with patient complaints of vaginal discharge). Trichomoniasis is less common than other forms of infectious vaginitis during pregnancy, but vulvovaginal candidiasis occurs in 10% of women during the first trimester and in one-third to one-half of women during the third trimester (Rein & Liang, 1999).

Subjective

Inquire whether there have been multiple or new sexual partners, whether sexual activity has recently been resumed, whether there has been any recent douching or antibiotic use, or whether there is a history of abnormal Papanicolaou (Pap) smears. Further assessment should explore the presence of any vaginal discharge, perineal or vaginal sores or lesions, or UTI symptoms. Worrisome symptoms include excessive, malodorous, discolored, itchy, or irritating vaginal discharge; fever; abdominal pain; dysuria; or bleeding or pain after sexual intercourse.

Objective

The examination should begin with an inspection of the external genitalia. A pelvic examination should assess for vaginal discharge, signs of vaginal infections (including herpes), and any other vaginal or cervical abnormalities. A normal saline and potassium hydroxide test (wet mount) should be conducted from secretions of the vaginal pool to check for fungal organisms, trichomonas, clue cells, and bacteria. A gonorrhea and chlamydia specimen for culture should be obtained. A nitrazine or fern test should be done to evaluate for rupture of membranes. A Pap smear should be done if it has not been done previously in the initial obstetrical evaluation to assess for dysplasia, carcinoma, or human papillomavirus.

Differential Diagnoses

Leukorrhea, vaginitis, cervicitis, gonorrhea, chlamydia, UTI, rupture of membranes, condyloma acuminatum, genital herpes, or cervical dysplasia or neoplasia.

■ Urinary Tract Infections

Urinary tract infections consist of either cystitis, an infection in the bladder, or pyelonephritis, an infection in the kidneys. Cystitis occurs in about 1% to 2% of the pregnant population, and cultures usually grow out a single pathogen, typically *Escherichia coli* or a species from the genera *Staphylococcus, Proteus, Klebsiella,* or *Pseudomonas* (Moran, 2004). Untreated UTIs and pyelonephritis may result in preterm labor and delivery, maternal sepsis, or even septic shock and death.

Asymptomatic bacteriuria may be present in 2% to 10% of pregnancies and is diagnosed by the growth of 100,000 colonies per milliliter of a single pathogen that is cultured from a clean-voided urinary specimen (Cohen, 2008). This may be indicative of an underlying disorder, such as an anatomic urinary tract abnormality or chronic pyelonephritis. Asymptomatic bacteriuria may lead to pyelonephritis and is associated with an increased risk of preterm labor and low-birth-weight babies.

Subjective

Inquiries should be made about the presence of risk factors (frequent/recurrent UTIs, diabetes, urinary tract abnormalities, sexually transmitted diseases). Inquire also about any urgency, frequency, dysuria, suprapubic pain, abnormal urinary flow pattern, discolored or malodorous urine, fever, chills, flank pain, or GI complaints.

Objective

Evaluation includes documented fever, clean catch urine, pelvic examination/ wet mount (for vaginal infections), costovertebral angle or suprapubic tenderness, urine culture, CBC, and signs of shock (tachycardia, hypotension, and pallor).

Differential Diagnoses

Cystitis, pyelonephritis, asymptomatic bacteriuria, urethritis, vulvovaginitis, sexually transmitted diseases, preterm labor, renal stones.

■ Size Not Equal to Dates

A fetus may be found to be of a size that is not commensurate with normal growth rates (size not equal to dates) when the uterine size is measured and evaluated during routine prenatal visits. First-trimester uterine sizes are usually determined with bimanual examination, and size–date discrepancies are often not clinically relevant. After 20 weeks of gestation, fundal height measurements begin to correlate (within 2 cm) with gestational age. The fundus should be at the level of the umbilicus at 20 weeks of gestation, and it rises 1 cm per week until 32 weeks of gestation. False small-for-dates presentations may result from inaccurate last menstrual period dates, varying menstrual cycle lengths, improper fundal height measurement, or a fetus in a transverse lie. False large-for-dates presentations may likewise be produced by inaccurate last menstrual period dates and improper fundal height measurement as well as maternal obesity or short stature.

Small-For-Dates

Subjective

No subjective complaints are usually expressed by the pregnant woman; however, she may state that she does not appear as "big" as her gestational age. A 24-hour diet recall should be done.

Objective

Weight gain from prepregnancy weight should be noted. Fundal height measurements that are 3 to 4 cm smaller than the estimated gestational age during the 20- to 32-week gestational period require additional follow-up. Serial ultrasound examinations and measurements should be done for body ratios in order to plot growth velocity and to assess amniotic fluid volume.

Differential Diagnoses

Intrauterine growth restriction (either asymmetric or symmetric), which affects about 5% of the general population and as much as 10% of high-risk populations (Table 19.9), constitutionally small fetus, inaccurate pregnancy dating, improper fundal height measurement, transverse lie of the fetus, oligohydramnios.

Large-For-Dates

Subjective

Although no subjective complaints are usually expressed, the fundal height may appear to be increased, especially in pregnant women who are obese or short in stature. The woman may state that she appears "bigger" than her gestational age or that she is carrying multiple gestations. A 24-hour diet recall should be done.

Objective

Weight gain from prepregnancy weight should be noted. Fundal height measurements that are 3 to 4 cm larger than the estimated gestational age during the 20- to 32-week gestational period require additional evaluation. Serial ultrasound examinations and measurements for body ratios should be done in order to plot growth velocity and to assess amniotic fluid volume. A serum glucose and urine dip should be done to evaluate for GDM.

Table 19.9

High-Risk Populations for Intrauterine Growth Restriction

Associated Medical Conditions	Associated Obstetric Conditions
• Hypertension • Renal disease • Diabetes • Lupus • Sickle cell anemia • Tobacco use; substance abuse • Malnutrition • Maternal heart disorders, especially those with decreased cardiac output • Thrombophilias • Chronic lead poisoning	• Pregnancy-induced hypertension • Multiple gestation • Placental abnormalities • Intrauterine infections • Fetal/chromosomal abnormalities

Differential Diagnoses

Inaccurate pregnancy dating, improper fundal height measurement, fetal macrosomia, polyhydramnios, multiple gestation, uterine leiomyoma growth, molar pregnancy, gestational diabetes, maternal obesity.

■ Preterm Labor

Preterm labor is the onset of labor before 37 completed weeks of gestation. The accurate diagnosis of preterm labor is critical but often difficult. Fewer than half of the women who have four or more contractions per hour will deliver in 7 to 14 days of the preterm labor assessment. The diagnosis may be confirmed when there is a cervical dilatation of 3 cm or more in a woman without persistent contractions. Women who are having persistent contractions need a cervical change of at least 1 cm, a dilatation of 2 cm or more, or a positive fetal fibronectin assay for diagnosis (Bernhardt & Dorman, 2004). If the diagnosis is not confirmed, but the index of suspicion remains high, it is entirely reasonable to repeat the cervical examination at a later time. Transabdominal ultrasounds and home uterine activity monitoring have also been used in an effort to identify preterm labor but with mixed results.

Subjective

The most common complaint is contractions. The contractions should be evaluated for regularity, consistency, and location. Symptoms of preterm labor include pelvic pressure; a low, dull backache; menstrual-like cramps; a change or increase in vaginal discharge; uterine contractions that occur every 10 minutes or more frequently, with or without pain; intestinal cramping, with or without diarrhea; and contractions that do not resolve with rest and hydration. A history review should concentrate on any previous preterm labor/delivery and a determination of the gestational age. A complete review of systems should be accomplished to screen for precipitating conditions, such as cholecystitis or viral gastroenteritis.

Objective

Screening should be done for infection (urinalysis, gonorrhea, chlamydia, syphilis, group B streptococcus, bacterial vaginosis), urine specific gravity to assess for hydration status, nitrazine testing to assess for rupture of membranes, fetal fibronectin testing (should be done before a digital cervical examination), ultrasound cervical length examination, serial cervical examinations, and drug screening. Fetal fibronectin testing and cervical length evaluation both have a high negative predictive value and are therefore better at predicting when preterm delivery is unlikely to occur as opposed to when delivery will occur (Bernhardt & Dorman, 2004).

Differential Diagnoses

Preterm (true) labor, false labor, maternal dehydration, infectious etiologies (either urinary, vaginal, or sexually transmitted), incompetent cervix, premature rupture of membranes.

Summary

As stated at the beginning of this chapter, pregnancy should be considered a wellness condition and not a disease entity. Advanced practice nurses should tailor their education and interventions to the assessment of the pregnant woman and routinely reassess the clinical situation for any changes. Caring for pregnant women is well within the advanced practice nursing model, and advanced practice nurses should know what is needed, what they can provide, and when to refer.

REFERENCES

Ahmad, A., & Frank, B.B. (2007). Endoscopy in pregnancy. In American College of Gastroenterology (Eds.), *Pregnancy in Gastrointestinal Disorders*, 2nd ed. Bethesda, MD: American College of Gastroenterology, 10–16. www.acg.gi.org/physicians/pdfs/PregnancyMonograph. pdf (accessed March 16, 2011).

Baxley, E.G. (2008). Patient and family education. Section E. Physiologic changes and common discomforts of pregnancy. In Ratcliffe, S.D., Baxley, E.G., Cline, M.K., & Sakornbut, E.L. (Eds.), *Family Medicine Obstetrics*, 3rd ed. Philadelphia: Mosby Elsevier, 86–95.

Bernhardt, J., & Dorman, K. (2004). Pre-term birth risk assessment tools: Exploring fetal fibronectin and cervical length for validating risk. *Lifelines, 8*(1), 38–44.

Beukema, R., Raiche, M., & Turok, D. (2008). Complications of pregnancy. Section A. Gestational diabetes mellitus. In Ratcliffe et al. *Family Medicine Obstetrics*, 151–161.

Carpenter, M.W., & Coustan, D.R. (1982). Criteria for screening tests for gestational diabetes. *American Journal of Obstetrics and Gynecology, 144*, 768–773.

Cashion, K. (2007). Endocrine and metabolic disorders. In Lowdermilk, D.L., & Perry, S.E. (Eds.), *Maternity and Women's Health Care*, 9th ed. St. Louis: Mosby Elsevier, 826–848.

Choby, B. (2008). Content of prenatal care: Section C. Prenatal visits. In Ratcliffe et al., *Family Medicine Obstetrics*, 26–27.

Cline, M.K. (2008). Chronic medical conditions in pregnancy. Section A. Pulmonary problems in pregnancy. In Ratcliffe et al., *Family Medicine Obstetrics*, 202–213.

Cohen, D. (2008). Commonly encountered medical problems in pregnancy. XIV. Asymptomatic bacteriuria and urinary tract infection. In Ratcliffe et al., *Family Medicine Obstetrics*, 292–295.

Corbett, R.W. (2007). Nursing care during pregnancy. In Lowdermilk & Perry, *Maternity and Women's Health Care*, 380–427.

Dillon, P. (2007). *Nursing Health Assessment: A critical thinking, case studies approach.* Philadelphia: F.A. Davis.

Deutchman, M. (2008). Diagnosis and management of first-trimester complications. Section A. Diagnosis. In Ratcliffe et al., *Family Medicine Obstetrics*, 130–140.

Fowler, J.R., & Jack, B.W. (2008). Preconception care: Improving birth outcomes through care before pregnancy. In Ratcliffe et al., *Family Medicine Obstetrics*, 10–20.

Harvey-Banchik, L.P. (2007). Hyperemesis gravidarum and nutritional support. In American College of Gastroenterology, *Pregnancy in Gastrointestinal Disorders*, 26–31.

Julius, J.E., & Kirchner, J.T. (2008). Chronic medical conditions in pregnancy. Section E. Hematologic conditions in pregnancy. In Ratcliffe et al., *Family Medicine Obstetrics*, 227–232.

Kim, C., Newton, K.M., & Knopp, R.H. (2002). Gestational diabetes and the incidence of type 2 diabetes. *Diabetes Care, 25*(10), 1862–1868.

Lindheimer, M.D., & Akbari, A. (2000). Hypertension in pregnant. In Oparil, S., & Weber, M.A. (Eds.), *Hypertension: A Companion to Brenner and Rector's* The Kidney. Philadelphia: Saunders.

Lobner, K., Knoff, A., Baumgarten, A., Mollenhauer, U., Marienfeld, S., Garrido-Franco, et al. (2006). Predictors of postpartum diabetes in women with gestational diabetes mellitus. *Diabetes, 55,* 792–797.

Lowdermilk, D.L. (2007). Anatomy and physiology of pregnancy. In Lowdermilk & Perry, *Maternity and Women's Health Care*, 333–352.

Mandell, E. (2007). Anemias. In Buttaro, T.H., Trybulski, J., Bailey, P.P., & Sandberg-Cook, J. (Eds.), *Primary Care: A Collaborative Practice*, 3rd ed. St. Louis: Mosby, 922–940.

McAteer, J. (2007). Medical-surgical problems in pregnancy. In Lowdermilk & Perry, *Maternity and Women's Health Care*, 849–873.

Moore, M.C. (2007). Maternal and fetal nutrition. In Lowdermilk & Perry, *Maternity and Women's Health Care*, 353–379.

Moran, B.A. (2004). Maternal infections. In Mattson, S., & Smith, J.E. (Eds.), *Core Curriculum for Maternal-Newborn Nursing*, 3rd ed. St. Louis: Elsevier Saunders, 592–629.

National Diabetes Data Group. (1979). Classification and diagnosis of diabetes mellitus and other categories of glucose intolerance. *Diabetes, 28,* 1039–1057.

National High Blood Pressure Education Program (NHBPEP). (2001). Working group report on high blood pressure in pregnancy. (NHBPEP Publication No. 00–3029). Washington, DC: National Heart, Lung, and Blood Institute.

O'Sullivan, J.B., & Mahan, C.M. (1964). Criteria for the oral glucose tolerance test in pregnancy. *Diabetes, 13,* 278–285.

Padua, L., Aprile, I., Caliandro, P., Carboni, T., Meloni, A., Massi, S., et al. (2001). Symptoms and neurophysiological picture of carpal tunnel syndrome in pregnancy. *Clinical Neurophysiology, 112*(10), 1946–1951.

Pagana, K.D., & Pagana, T.J. (2006). *Mosby's Diagnostic and Laboratory Test Reference*, 8th ed. St. Louis: Mosby.

Pandolfino, J., & Vanagunas, A. (2000). Gastrointestinal complications of pregnancy. *Hospital Physician, 6*(4), 1–14.

Parangi, S., & Pories, S. (2007). Surgical problems in the pregnant patient. In American College of Gastroenterology, *Pregnancy in Gastrointestinal Disorders*, pp. 54–64.

Peters, R.M., & Flack, J.M. (2004). Hypertensive disorders of pregnancy. *Journal of Obstetric, Gynecologic, and Neonatal Nursing, 33*(2), 209–220.

Poole, J.D. (2004). Hemorrhagic disorders. In Mattson & Smith, *Core Curriculum for Maternal-Newborn Nursing*, 630–659.

Rein, M.F., & Liang, B.A. (1999). Diagnosis and treatment of infectious vaginitis. *Hospital Physician, 35*(10), 46–58.

Reymunde, A., Santiago, N., & Perez, L. (2001). *Helicobacter pylori* and severe morning sickness. *American Journal of Gastroenterology, 96*(7), 2279–2280.

Richter, J.E. (2007). Heartburn, nausea, vomiting during pregnancy. In American College of Gastroenterology, *Pregnancy in Gastrointestinal Disorders*, 18–25.

Sakornbut, E.L. (2008a). Abdominal pain and gastrointestinal illness. In Ratcliffe et al., *Family Medicine Obstetrics*, 306–311.

———. (2008b). Chronic medical conditions in pregnancy. Section B. Cardiovascular conditions. In Ratcliffe et al., *Family Medicine Obstetrics*, 213–219.

Turok, D., & Schultz, T. (2008). Chronic medical conditions in pregnancy. Section I. Endocrine problems. In Ratcliffe et al., *Family Medicine Obstetrics*, 243–254.

U.S. Preventive Services Task Force. (2008). Screening for bacterial vaginosis in pregnancy to prevent preterm delivery. *Annals of Internal Medicine, 148*(3), 214–219.

Viera, A.J. (2003). Management of carpal tunnel syndrome. *American Family Physician, 68*(7), 265–72, 279–280.

Weimer, L.H., Yin, J., Lovelace, R.E., & Gooch, C.L. (2002). Serial studies of carpal tunnel syndrome during and after pregnancy. *Muscle Nerve, 25*(6), 914–917.

Wotring, R. (2004). Environmental hazards. In Mattson & Smith, *Core Curriculum for Maternal-Newborn Nursing*, 201–224.

SUGGESTED READINGS

Adams, S.L. (1998). Urinary tract infections in pregnant women. In Collins-Bride, G.M., & Saxe, J.M. (Eds.), *Nurse Practitioner/Physician Collaborative Practice: Clinical Guidelines for Ambulatory Care*. San Francisco: UCSF Nursing Press.

Barron, W.M., & Lindheimer, M.D. (1995). Management of hypertension during pregnancy. In Largh, J.H., & Brenner, B.M. (Eds.), *Hypertension: Pathophysiology, Diagnosis, and Management*, 2nd ed. New York: Raven Press.

Corder-Mabe, J. (1998). Complications of pregnancy. In Youngkin, E.Q., & Davis, M.S. (Eds.), *Women's Health: A Primary Care Clinical Guide*, 2nd ed. Stamford, CN: Appleton & Lange.

Iams, J.D. (2003). Prediction and detection of early preterm labor. *Obstetrics and Gynecology, 101*, 402–412.

Mulley, Jr., A.G., & Goroll, A.H. (1995). Screening for anemia. In Goroll, A.H., May, L.A., & Mulley, Jr., A.G. (Eds.), *Primary Care Medicine: Office Evaluation and Management of the Adult Patient*, 3rd ed. Philadelphia: Lippincott-Raven.

Remich, M.C. (1998). Promoting a healthy pregnancy. In Youngkin & Davis, *Women's Health: A Primary Care Clinical Guide.*

Stanford, J.B., & Hobbins, D. (2001). Obstetric risk assessment. Section A. Preconception risk assessment. In Ratcliffe, S.D., Baxley, E.G., Byrd, J.E., & Sakornbut, E.L. (Eds.), *Family Practice Obstetrics*, 2nd ed. Philadelphia: Hanley & Belfus.

U.S. Preventive Services Task Force. (2001). Screening high-risk pregnant women for bacterial vaginosis. In *Guide to Clinical Preventive Services*, 2nd ed. Washington, DC: Office of Disease Prevention and Health Promotion.

Zinaman, M.J., Clegg, E., Brown, C.C., O'Connor, J., & Selevan, S.G. (1996). Estimates of human fertility and pregnancy loss. *Fertility & Sterility, 65,* 503–509.

Chapter 20

OLDER PATIENTS

Charon Pierson

The comprehensive assessment of elderly individuals requires an understanding of the physiologic changes of normal aging as well as the complex interplay among those changes, disease, and functional status. Performance of these assessments may need to be adapted to accommodate the frailty of the individual and the setting in which the assessment occurs. Finally, some well-recognized "syndromes" that either present in unusual ways or are rarely addressed in the typical clinical encounter require diligent investigation to prevent functional decline in the elderly. All of these factors contribute to the complexity of the comprehensive geriatric assessment and argue for a multidisciplinary approach in geriatrics.

This chapter addresses these issues by focusing on the concept of functional assessment, from its basic components to highly integrated aspects of role functioning, using the hierarchical model developed by the National Institute on Aging (2003). The model, illustrated in Figure 20.1, provides a holistic view of the individual and a guide to management options. Functional assessment is a performance-based approach that explores how disease affects the individual; it is a useful concept in many ways. For example, in the case of elders who have little disease but significant inability to function independently, the clinician is prompted to address management options that provide support to the individual and family in order to maintain as much independence as possible. Conversely, in elders who have significant comorbidities and who have adapted to their disease burden and remain independent, a functional assessment supports management options to allow for continued role functioning.

A functional assessment determines the degree to which an individual can perform those activities that enable him or her to live independently. The basic components are those that produce specific physical movements, such as the coordination and fine motor control required to grasp a fork or spoon. Specific movements are then required to take the grasping of the spoon to a goal-oriented activity, namely, eating a meal. A higher level of integration of the physical movements involved in eating with cognitive capability provides the basis for shopping for and preparing a meal or planning a holiday dinner for a larger family (Fig. 20-1). Degradation in the ability to perform these tasks

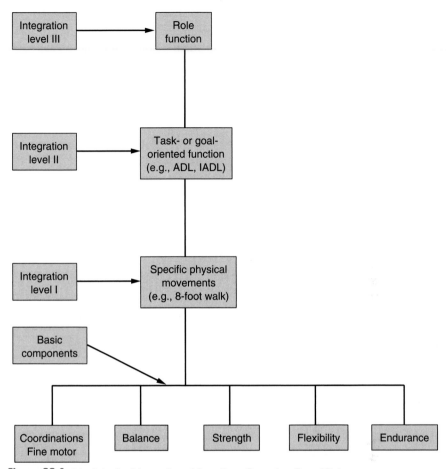

Figure 20.1 Model of a hierarchy of function. See also Box 20.1. National Institute on Aging, (2003).

results in greater dependence on others and often a change in living circumstances. Dependence among the elderly has implications for society as a whole owing to the demographic shift that has been occurring in most of the developed countries of the world.

The Demographics of Aging

According to U.S. census data, the elderly, aged 65 and older, amounted to 12.3% (35.6 million) of the population in 2002; it is estimated that number will double to about 70 million, or 20% of the population, by 2030. The fastest growing group among the elderly are those over 100 years of age. Most of these centenarians are considered to be among the most vulnerable to frailty and disability, which, coupled with the likelihood that they will live alone and therefore require support services, such as nursing home care, has caused dire predictions about the failure of the Medicare and Medicaid systems. Current data indicate that only 13% of the elderly population account for 90% of all nursing home expenditures; however, 44% of those who use nursing homes after age 65 start and end as private payers, and 14% spend down their assets to become eligible for Medicaid (www.elderweb.com/taxonomy/term/6391). This increase in the elderly population is occurring worldwide, and the projected socioeconomic impact on societies is of great concern to researchers, policymakers, and providers.

As the number of frail and dependent elderly increase, a concomitant rise in the proportion of those who are disabled will occur. The Administration on Aging, using the most optimistic ratios of disability to longevity, projects that the percentage of the population with limitations in performing the activities of daily living (ADL) will increase from the current 20% to at least 21.4%. Associated with these ADL limitations is the need for home- and community-based or institutional services. The level of services required will largely be determined by psychosocial and economic factors along with medical necessity, all of which should be determined through a comprehensive and perhaps multidisciplinary patient assessment. It is important to remember that aging is a life process that in and of itself does not inevitably produce functional decline.

Box 20.1

Functional Model Integration Levels

Basic Components The basic components of this model are viewed as functional units that form the building blocks of a series of increasingly complex functional tasks. The basic components include strength, balance, coordination, flexibility, and endurance.

Specific Physical Movements These are movement sequences that can be achieved by the integration of two or more basic components. Examples of specific physical movements include carry, reach, bend, stoop, transfer, chair rise, walk.

Task- or Goal-Oriented Activities This level requires all of the physical movements plus varying degrees of cognitive ability to conceptualize the task and follow through to achievement of the goal. Examples of these more complex tasks or activities include the activities of daily living and instrumental activities of daily living (bathing, grooming, dressing, toileting, shopping, managing money or medications, using the telephone, doing laundry).

Role Function This is the highest level of integration and the most difficult to assess because of its complexity. In the elderly, occupational activities might be replaced by volunteer activities; however, some elderly remain fully engaged in productive occupational activities until they die. This level of integration of functional abilities implies wide-ranging engagement in life, which can occur even in the presence of serious physical disability (e.g., amyotrophic lateral sclerosis, quadriplegia, multiple sclerosis) in the young as well as the old.

The Approach to the Assessment of Older Individuals

Older individuals are characterized by their heterogeneity; therefore, clinicians must adapt their approaches on the basis of the setting (outpatient, inpatient, or home), on the presenting complaint, and on the capabilities or limitations of the individual. In general, the elderly will have more physical complaints, more comorbidities, more medications, and longer medical and surgical histories than a younger person. Information about childhood immunizations may not be relevant, such as for those born before childhood immunizations were developed, and information about family history may not be complete. Certain components of the past history will be more relevant, such as occupational history; military service in wartime; environmental exposures; and functional changes in sensory, physical, or cognitive abilities over time. Lifestyle issues, such as habits, driving ability, nutrition, social support networks, and sleep and elimination patterns require particular attention. Advanced care planning, particularly advanced health-care directives and designation of durable power of attorney for health-care decisions, should be addressed with regular opportunities for discussion of changing priorities and status of significant members of the family (e.g., death of the spouse, who was the designated decision maker for health care). Losses, including loss of capability and independence as well as the loss of friends and family, become more frequent with aging. It is important to provide opportunities to discuss and grieve for such losses as frequently as possible during routine health-care encounters.

The approach to the physical examination of older adults will not differ greatly from standard examination techniques presented in this text. Some tests of functional ability are not routinely considered in the usual examination of the adult; those are presented in the various sections that follow. With older adults who are debilitated, it is important to focus the examination and reduce extraneous activities and distractions. Whenever possible, begin the examination with maneuvers that can be accomplished with the patient in his or her current position. For example, when the patient arrives to the examination seated in a wheelchair, check vital signs, heart rate, extremities, or anything else that can be done in the seated position first. If a patient's ability to transfer from the wheelchair is in question, observe the transfer before the patient becomes fatigued. The exertion of getting on the examination table could fatigue an individual enough to preclude optimal performance. Likewise, perform all supine or standing examinations together to preserve the patient's stamina. A reordering of the sequence of the examination should be done in a logical and thoughtful manner.

Attend to the safety of the elder person by removing obstructing objects, providing adequate lighting, and standing in close proximity to the individual to prevent falls. Turn off background music or television if possible, and speak clearly, facing the elder person, to facilitate good communication. Be aware that glare off windows and other shiny surfaces can cause discomfort as well as compromise vision during interviewing and testing.

The Physiology of Aging

A common adage indicates that aging changes consist of about one-third disease, one-third disuse, and one-third normal aging. The relationships among these three factors are important but often difficult to define. Although chronological aging does produce change in biochemical processes, actual function is remarkably well maintained in humans. Most of the impact of the changes relates to a decrease in physiologic reserve, and very little of the impairment seen among elderly populations is due to actual physiologic changes in the human organism. It is probably more helpful to view aging as a continuum upon which physiological and pathological processes seem to vary infinitely within a given population.

Table 20.1 lists the major physiological changes associated with aging and the known or postulated impacts those changes have on functional or disease states. Some of these changes are easily detected, such as the age-related attrition of oocytes in the ovaries that leads to the loss of female reproductive ability. Other changes are much less obvious, such as the loss of nephrons in the kidney that may affect the ability to excrete drug metabolites. The former, loss of female reproductive ability, is inevitable after a certain age, whereas the latter, loss of nephrons, is much more complex and variable. Although the loss of nephrons may be a given, the effect of that loss on an individual's function may vary considerably depending on other factors, such as disease states (e.g., hypertension) and other physiologic variables (e.g., intracellular fluid volume). Interactive effects from physiologic changes, such as the effect of declining levels of estrogen production following menopause on bone remodeling, complicate the picture. Thus, geriatric assessment is most effective when it is focused on functional impact rather than on disease states. Functional assessment allows the variability that occurs with the complex relationships among disease, disuse, and physiology to remain secondary to the development and implementation of a treatment plan.

Functional Assessment

Within the context of health assessment, functional assessment provides an alternative perspective on the health status of an individual. In the traditional model of health assessment taught in nurse practitioner programs, the focus is on the clinical diagnosis and the development of sound diagnostic reasoning. This medical model approach assumes that a reason for the client's presenting symptoms can be uncovered and an intervention can be instituted to cure the problem. Although some conditions are reversible in the elderly, many are not; thus, the focus of the assessment needs to be on maximizing the elderly client's function and maintaining or improving well-being.

In clinical trials, the effects of interventions on functional ability are frequently measured and reported as indicators of the quality of life. The domains of quality-of-life indicators encompass physical, emotional, spiritual, and

Table 20.1

Physiologic Changes of Aging and Their Impacts

Physiologic Change	Functional and Clinical Impact
Thinning of dermis and epidermis; decreased epidermal proliferation and collagen flexibility; changes in elastic fiber network	Increased skin fragility and cell irregularity; increased vulnerability to trauma and irritant dermatitis; susceptible to infection with break in epidermis; decreased elasticity; increased wrinkling and dryness; uneven pigmentation
Decreased amount of subcutaneous fat; decreased size of fat pads	Sagging of skin; decreased fat pads on soles of feet may change gait or ability to ambulate
Decreased sebaceous and eccrine gland activity; loss of hair pigment	Decreased rate of nail and hair growth; decreased sweating ability may lead to hyperthermia; thinning and graying of hair; increased susceptibility to infection
Increased threshold for pressure and touch; decreased vibratory sense in toes; decreased thermal sensitivity	Potential for injury and burns due to decreased sensation
Increased translucency and flattening of cornea; thickening and rigidity of choroid and iris; decreased production of aqueous humor; decreased mass of ciliary muscle; decreased number of rods, cones, and ganglion cells; increased yellowing and density and decreased elasticity of lens; liquefaction of vitreous body	Decreased accommodation to light intensity; impaired color discrimination; decreased night vision acuity; blurring and changes in visual acuity; pupils less reactive to light; floaters and light flashes increase; presbyopia; increased dryness; vulnerable to infection
Tympanic membrane thinner, less resilient; sclerotic changes to tympanic membrane; ossicles become calcified; pinna widens, elongates, and stiffens	Some degree of impaired auditory function; decreased sensitivity to high-frequency tones (presbycusis); ears may look larger
Decreased salivation, number of olfactory cells, and thirst	Decreased sensitivity to taste and smell; increased tendency to dehydration and undernutrition
Enlargement of alveolar duct; decreased elastic recoil; increased closing volume; loss of cilia; increased size and stiffening of trachea and bronchi; calcification of chest wall; decreased cough reflex, forced vital capacity, forced expiratory volume per second, and forced expiratory flow; increased residual volume, functional residual capacity, and residual volume/total lung capacity	Altered pulmonary function; decreased sensitivity to changes in levels of oxygen and carbon dioxide; loss of alveoli; decreased ability to clear infectious or environmental material

Continued

Table 20.1

Physiologic Changes of Aging and Their Impacts—cont'd

Physiologic Change	Functional and Clinical Impact
Increased weight of heart and vessels; left ventricular posterior wall and aortic thickness; decreased early diastolic closure rates of mitral valve; valves become more sclerotic; decreased response to beta-adrenergic stimulation	Decreased cardiac output and heart rate at rest and exercise, myocardial contractile efficiency, maximal oxygen uptake, and responsiveness to catecholamines; increased systolic pressure, left ventricular ejection time, and preejection period, stroke volume with progressive exercise, and ectopic activity; murmurs, S_4 heart sounds, and orthostatic blood pressure changes may occur
Decreased production of saliva, gastric juices (including intrinsic factor, peptic and hydrochloric acids); decreased gastric motility; mucosal and muscle atrophy; decreased size and activity of liver, hepatocytes, secretory acini and islets of Langerhans; decreased splenic blood flow	Decreased protection of teeth and tongue from bacteria, taste sensation, vitamins B_{12} and D, and carbohydrate absorption; protein, iron, and folic acid digestion; difficulty talking and chewing; delayed gastric emptying and maldigestion; impaired fat absorption; decreased drug metabolism and hepatic protein synthesis; decline in glucose tolerance
Decreased number of glomeruli, filtration of blood, and glomerular filtration rate as much as 30%–40%; thickened tubular membranes and fatty degeneration; stiffening and narrowing of renal vasculature; decreased expandability and compressibility of detrusor; decreased bladder sensation	Decreased clearance of medications and other waste products; decreased urine concentrating capacity; BUN and creatinine do not generally change; decreased creatinine clearance; decreased bladder capacity; increased urinary frequency and postvoid residual volume
Decreased secretion TSH and T_4, insulin, rennin, aldosterone, ACTH, growth hormone; decreased response to TRH, ACTH	Laboratory values may change and must be interpreted carefully; stress response is not as robust
Decreased bone mass, size and number of muscle fibers; lean body mass replaced by fat	Increased incidence of microfractures, decreased lean body mass and total body water; more vulnerable to fractures, balance, and gait problems
Decreased sleep efficiency; possible decreased total sleep time; increased sleep latency; more arousal during night; decreased REM latency and total REM sleep	Increased time to fall asleep; more time in bed waiting to fall asleep; earlier awakening; more daytime napping; no increase in daytime sleepiness

ACTH = adrenocorticotrophic hormone; BUN = blood urea nitrogen; REM = rapid eye movement; TRH = thyrotropin-releasing hormone; TSH = thyroid-stimulating hormone.
Data from Blair, 1990; Cotter & Strumpf, 2002; and Alessi, 2000.

psychosocial measures; many instruments have been developed for the purpose of measuring various indicators (Gerety, 2000). Many of these measures are self-reported; however, with elderly clients, caregiver reports and direct observations are commonly used. Moreover, measured domains frequently overlap, and it may be difficult to separate the effects that emotional or intellectual functions have on physical function. One way to overcome some of these measurement dilemmas is to use standardized performance-based measures that integrate basic components of a movement and provide the opportunity to observe a client perform a task or a goal-oriented function. This is the basis for the hierarchical model of function depicted in Figure 20.1.

■ Measures of Function

Two scales are commonly used to measure functional ability: the Physical Activities of Daily Living (Box 20.2) and the Instrumental Activities of Daily Living (IADL; Box 20.3). Although both scales are relatively crude, they have been largely accepted as adequate for determining the need for assistive services and for classifying the level of care required for institutional services. Both instruments are scored according to the level of independence in performance of the task, and they both provide snapshots of a person's ability to live independently. Most health professionals accept the goal-oriented activities depicted in Figure 20.1 as minimal criteria for independent functioning in the modern world.

For the well elderly, the 10-Minute Screener for Geriatric Conditions is recommended (American Geriatrics Society, 2003). This brief screening tool (Table 20.2) addresses vision, hearing, leg mobility, urinary incontinence, nutrition and weight loss, memory, depression, and physical disability. Using a combination of subjective and objective measures, the 10-Minute Screener covers all the basic ADL and IADL functions in a manner that fits well within the outpatient examination. A positive screen requires further evaluation, in some cases by a specialist or a geriatric specialist.

■ Measures of Cognitive Function

In primary care settings, assessment of cognitive function is often overlooked. Whether due to lack of time or lack of experience with appropriate screening measures, most clinicians in primary care fail to recognize early signs of cognitive impairment. Routine screening for dementia in adults in whom cognitive impairment is not suspected is not recommended at this time due to a lack of evidence to support the benefit (U.S. Preventive Services Task Force [USPSTF], 2003). In the primary care setting, two issues may be paramount: First, the time required for testing cognition may interfere with time requirements to attend to medical problems. Second, sensitivity and specificity of various instruments for testing cognition is an important consideration. Therefore, clinicians should be familiar with several possible instruments and decide which to use in their own settings. Harvan and Cotter (2006) provide a useful summary of the details of various dementia screening tools along with recommendations for their use in primary care (Table 20.3).

Box 20.2

Physical Self-Maintenance Scale (Activities of Daily Living [ADLs])

In each category, circle the item that most closely describes the person's highest level of functioning and record the score assigned to that level (either 1 or 0) in the blank at the beginning of the category.

A. Toilet

1. Care for self at toilet completely; no incontinence	1
2. Needs to be reminded, or needs help in cleaning self, or has rare (weekly at most) accidents	0
3. Soiling or wetting while asleep more than once a week	0
4. Soiling or wetting while awake more than once a week	0
5. No control of bowels or bladder	0

B. Feeding

1. Eats without assistance	1
2. Eats with minor assistance at meal times and/or with special preparation of food, or help in cleaning up after meals	0
3. Feeds self with moderate assistance and is untidy	0
4. Requires extensive assistance for all meals	0
5. Does not feed self at all and resists efforts of others to feed him or her	0

C. Dressing

1. Dresses, undresses, and selects clothes from own wardrobe	1
2. Dresses and undresses self, with minor assistance	0
3. Needs moderate assistance in dressing and selection of clothes	0
4. Needs major assistance in dressing, but cooperates with efforts of others to help	0
5. Completely unable to dress self and resists efforts of others to help	0

D. Grooming (neatness, hair, nails, hands, face, clothing)

1. Always neatly dressed, well-groomed, without assistance	1
2. Grooms self adequately with occasional minor assistance, eg, with shaving	0
3. Needs moderate and regular assistance or supervision with grooming	0
4. Needs total grooming care, but can remain well-groomed after help from others	0
5. Actively negates all efforts of others to maintain grooming	0

E. Physical Ambulation

1. Goes about grounds or city	1
2. Ambulates within residence on or about one block distant	0
3. Ambulates with assistance of (check one) a ( ) another person, b ( ) railing, c ( ) cane, d ( ) walker, e ( ) wheelchair 1.__Gets in and out without help. 2.__Needs help getting in and out	0
4. Sits unsupported in chair or wheelchair, but cannot propel self without help	0
5. Bedridden more than half the time	0

Box 20.2

Physical Self-Maintenance Scale (Activities of Daily Living [ADLs])—cont'd

F. Bathing

1. Bathes self (tub, shower, sponge bath) without help.	1
2. Bathes self with help getting in and out of tub.	0
3. Washes face and hands only, but cannot bathe rest of body.	0
4. Does not wash self, but is cooperative with those who bathe him or her.	0
5. Does not try to wash self and resists efforts to keep him or her clean.	0

For scoring interpretation and source, see note following the next instrument.

Scoring Interpretation: For ADLs, the total score ranges from 0 to 6, and for IADLs, from 0 to 8. In some categories, only the highest level of function receives a 1; in others, two or more levels have scores of 1 because each describes competence that represents some minimal level of function. These screens are useful for indicating specifically how a person is performing at the present time. When they are also used over time, they serve as documentation of a person's functional improvement or deterioration.

Box 20.3

Instrumental Activities of Daily Living (IADLs) Scale

In each category, circle the item that most closely describes the person's highest level of functioning and record the score assigned to that level (either 1 or 0) in the blank at the beginning of the category.

A. Ability to Use Telephone

1. Operates telephone on own initiative; looks up and dials numbers.	1
2. Dials a few well-known numbers.	1
3. Answers telephone, but does not dial.	1
4. Does not use telephone at all.	0

B. Shopping

1. Takes care of all shopping needs independently.	1
2. Shops independently for small purchases.	0
3. Needs to be accompanied on any shopping trip.	0
4. Completely unable to shop.	0

C. Food Preparation

1. Plans, prepares, and serves adequate meals independently.	1
2. Prepares adequate meals if supplied with ingredients.	0
3. Heats and serves prepared meals or prepares meals, but does not maintain adequate diet.	0
4. Needs to have meals prepared and served.	0

Continued

Box 20.3

Instrumental Activities of Daily Living (IADLs) Scale—cont'd

D. Housekeeping

1. Maintains house alone or with occasional assistance (e.g., heavy-work domestic help).	1
2. Performs light daily tasks such as dishwashing, bedmaking.	1
3. Performs light daily tasks, but cannot maintain acceptable level of cleanliness.	1
4. Needs help with all home maintenance tasks.	1
5. Does not participate in any housekeeping tasks.	0

E. Laundry

1. Does personal laundry completely.	1
2. Launders small items; rinses socks, stockings, etc.	1
3. All laundry must be done by others.	0

F. Mode of Transportation

1. Travels independently on public transportation or drives own car.	1
2. Arranges own travel via taxi, but does not otherwise use public transportation.	1
3. Travels on public transportation when assisted or accompanied by another.	1
4. Travel limited to taxi or automobile with assistance of another.	0
5. Does not travel at all.	0

G. Responsibility for Own Medications

1. Is responsible for taking medication in correct dosages at correct time.	1
2. Takes responsibility if medication is prepared in advance in separate dosages	0
3. Is not capable of dispensing own medication.	0

H. Ability to Handle Finances

1. Manages financial matters independently (budgets, writes checks, pays rent and bills, goes to bank); collects and keeps track of income.	1
2. Manages day-to-day purchases, but needs help with banking, major purchases, etc.	1
3. Incapable of handling money.	0

Scoring Interpretation: For ADLs, the total score ranges from 0 to 6, and for IADLs, from 0 to 8. In some categories, only the highest level of function receives a 1; in others, two or more levels have scores of 1 because each describes competence that represents some minimal level of function. These screens are useful for indicating specifically how a person is performing at the present time. When they are also used over time, they serve as documentation of a person's functional improvement or deterioration.

Table 20.2

10-Minute Screener for Geriatric Conditions

Problem	Screening Measure	Positive Screen
Vision	Two parts: Ask: "Do you have difficulty driving or watching television or reading or doing any of your daily activities because of your eyesight?" If yes, then: Test each eye with Snellen chart while patient wears corrective lenses (if applicable)	Yes to question and inability to read > 20/40 on Snellen chart
Hearing	Use audioscope set at 40 dB; test hearing using 1,000 and 2,000 Hz	Inability to hear 1,000 or 2,000 Hz in both ears, or inability to hear frequencies in either ear
Leg mobility	Time the patient after asking: "Rise from the chair. Walk 20 feet briskly, turn, walk back to the chair, and sit down."	Unable to complete task in 15 sec
Urinary incontinence	Two parts: Ask: "In the past year, have you ever lost your urine and gotten wet?" If yes, then ask: "Have you lost urine on at least 6 separate days?"	Yes to both questions
Nutrition, weight loss	Two parts: Ask: "Have you lost 10 lb over the past 6 months without trying to do so?" Weigh the patient	Yes to the question or weight < 100 lb
Memory	Three-item recall	Unable to recall all items after 1 min
Depression	Ask: "Do you often feel sad or depressed?"	Yes to the question
Physical disability	Six questions: "Are you able to . . ." ". . . do strenuous activities like fast walking or bicycling?" ". . . do heavy work around the house, like washing windows, walls, or floors?" ". . . go shopping for groceries or clothes?" ". . . get to places out of walking distance?" ". . . bathe, either a sponge bath, tub bath, or shower?" ". . . dress, like putting on a shirt, buttoning and zipping, or putting on shoes?"	No to any of the questions

Reprinted from Moore, A.A., et al. Screening for common problems in ambulatory elderly: clinical confirmation of a screen instrument, *American Journal of Medicine, 100,* 440. Copyright 1998, with permission from Excerpta Medica, Inc.

Table 20.3

Dementia Screening Tool Summary

Screening Tool	Method of Administration	Average Time of Administration	Scoring	Sensitivity (%)
Mini Mental State Exam (MMSE)	Verbal and written	5–12 min	11 items in five domains; score: 0–30; standard cutoff score for dementia: 23–24	86–92
Modified Mini Mental State Exam (3MS or mMMSE)	Verbal and written	12–15 min	15 items	87
Clock-drawing test (CDT)	Verbal	1–4 min	Varies: Manos (10 pt), Mendez (20 pt), Sunderland (10 pt), Rouleau (10 pt), Powlishta (5 pt)	59–74.7
General Practitioner Assessment of Cognition (GPCOG)	Verbal	4–5 min (patient <4 min; informant <2 min)	Patient maximum score = 9 on four items and informant maximum score = 6 on six items	82–85
7 Minute Screen (7MS)	Verbal	7 min	Four tests	89.4–92.9
Memory Impairment Screen (MIS)	Verbal	4 min	Four items	80–86
Mini-Cog	Verbal	2–4 min	Three-item recall + CDT; 1 pt per recalled word; 0 = positive screen for dementia; 1–2 with abnormal CDT = positive; 1–2 with normal CDT = negative; 3 = negative	76–99

pt = points.

From Harvan, J., & Cotter, V. (2006). Screening for dementia in primary care. *JAANP, 18,* 351–360, reproduced with permission of Blackwell Publishing, Ltd.

Specificity (%)	Reliability	Validity	Advantages	Disadvantages
92–99	Test–retest 0.887, internal consistency 0.86, interobserver 0.97	Content, predictive, construct with Wechsler 0.66–0.776	Strong predictor of dementia	Varying accuracy in patients of different ages, education levels, and ethnicities; cut points vary
89	Internal consistency 0.87–0.91, interrater 0.98, test–retest 0.78	Construct with MMSE 0.95	Marginally superior to MMSE in discriminating between severity of dementia and normals	May be susceptible to influences of age and education; too lengthy for primary care use
65.5–90	Test–retest 0.87–0.94, interrater 0.82–0.97	Construct with MMSE 0.73, construct with CAMCOG 0.80	Very short administration time; no equipment needed	May be affected by impairment in physical abilities (vision, handwriting)
83–86	*Patient:* interrater 0.75, test–retest 0.87, internal consistency 0.84; *informant:* interrater 0.56, test–retest 0.84, internal consistency 0.80	Construct with MMSE 0.683	Patient and informant data collected	Lack of informant at primary care visits
93.5	Test–retest 0.87–0.91	Construct	Better than MMSE to detect mild dementia	May be too lengthy for primary care use
96–97	Internal consistency 0.67	Construct with three-word memory test	Avoids effects of education (reading and writing)	
89–96	Interrater 0.93–0.95	Construct with MMSE	Not influenced by language or education; no special equipment needed	

One instrument that holds promise for rapid screening in primary care is the Mini-Cog (Box 20.4); it takes 2 to 4 minutes to administer and has good sensitivity (76%–99%) and specificity (89%–96%) and has been validated in primary care (Harvan & Cotter, 2006). A positive screen on the Mini-Cog requires a more thorough evaluation. The most commonly used and widely tested instrument (USPSTF, 2003) for the next step in the evaluation of cognitive function, which measures more than just short- and long-term memory, is the Mini-Mental State Examination (MMSE). Domains measured by the MMSE include orientation to time and place, registration, attention and calculation, recall, naming, repetition, comprehension, reading, writing, and drawing. Testing with the MMSE takes approximately 10 minutes, and it must be administered in a standard manner to

---

Box 20.4

Mini-Cog Assessment Instrument for Dementia

The Mini-Cog assessment instrument combines an uncued three-item recall test with a clock-drawing test (CDT). The Mini-Cog can be administered in about 3 minutes, requires no special equipment, and is relatively uninfluenced by level of education or language variations.

Administration

The test is administered as follows:
1. Instruct the patient to listen carefully to and remember 3 unrelated words and then to repeat the words.
2. Instruct the patient to draw the face of a clock, either on a blank sheet of paper, or on a sheet with the clock circle already drawn on the page. After the patient puts the numbers on the clock face, ask him or her to draw the hands of the clock to read a specific time, such as 11:20. These instructions can be repeated, but no additional instructions should be given. Give the patient as much time as needed to complete the task. The CDT serves as the recall distractor.
3. Ask the patient to repeat the 3 previously presented words.

Scoring

Give 1 point for each recalled word after the CDT distractor. Score 1–3.
- A score of 0 indicates positive screen for dementia.
- A score of 1 or 2 with an abnormal CDT indicates positive screen for dementia.
- A score of 1 or 2 with a normal CDT indicates negative screen for dementia.
- A score of 3 indicates negative screen for dementia.

The CDT is considered normal if all numbers are present in the correct sequence and position, and the hands readably display the requested time.

Source: Borson, S., Scanlan, J., Brush, M., Vitaliano, P., & Dokmak, A. (2000). The mini-cog: A cognitive "vital signs" measure for dementia screening in multi-lingual elderly. *International Journal of Geriatric Psychiatry, 15*(11), 1021–1027.

obtain valid results. The total possible score is 30 points; however, scores are highly correlated with age and educational level of the individual (Ashla, 2000; Harvan & Cotter, 2006). Scores on the MMSE will not differentiate between delirium and dementia, although both conditions will cause scores below the cutoff of 24 (Francis, 2000). Comprehensive information on the development, reliability and validity testing, and scoring of the MMSE can be found online (http://www4.parinc.com). The MMSE is available for purchase only to qualified health-care professionals through Psychological Assessment Resources (telephone 813-968-3003). A description of the qualifications for purchase can be found at www4.parinc.com.

Whenever there is a question of cognitive impairment, a screen for depression is warranted because depression and dementia commonly coexist. The most commonly used instrument is the Geriatric Depression Scale (GDS; Box 20.5). Originally, the GDS contained 30 items; a brief 15-item version is as reliable for

---

Box 20.5

Geriatric Depression Scale (GDS, Short Form)

Choose the best answer for how you felt over the past week.

1. Are you basically satisfied with your life?	yes/**no**
2. Have you dropped many of your activities and interests?	**yes**/no
3. Do you feel that your life is empty?	**yes**/no
4. Do you often get bored?	**yes**/no
5. Are you in good spirits most of the time?	yes/**no**
6. Are you afraid that something bad is going to happen to you?	**yes**/no
7. Do you feel happy most of the time?	yes/**no**
8. Do you often feel helpless?	**yes**/no
9. Do you prefer to stay at home, rather than going out and doing new things?	**yes**/no
10. Do you feel you have more problems with memory than most?	**yes**/no
11. Do you think it is wonderful to be alive now?	yes/**no**
12. Do you feel pretty worthless the way you are now?	**yes**/no
13. Do you feel full of energy?	yes/**no**
14. Do you feel that your situation is hopeless?	**yes**/no
15. Do you think that most people are better off than you are?	**yes**/no

Score 1 point for each bolded answer. Cut-off: normal (0–5), above 5 suggests depression.

Source: Courtesy of Jerome A. Yesavage, MD. For 30 translations of the GDS, see www.stanford.edu/?yesavage/GDS.html.

For additional information on administration and scoring refer to the following references:

1. Sheikh, J.I., & Yesavage, J.A. (1986). Geriatric Depression Scale: Recent evidence and development of a shorter version. *Clinical Gerontology, 5,* 165–172.
2. Feher, E.P., Larrabee, G.J., & Crook, T.H. 3rd. (1992). Factors attenuating the validity of the Geriatric Depression Scale in a dementia population. *Journal of the American Geriatric Society, 40,* 906–909.
3. Yesavage, J.A., Brink, T.L., Rose, T.L., et al. (1983). Development and validation of a geriatric depression rating scale: A preliminary report. *Journal of Psychiatric Research, 17,* 27.

screening. The presentation of depression in the elderly may be atypical, with fatigue and somatic symptoms predominating; therefore, traditional criteria (DSM-IV) for diagnosis of depression may not apply. Because depression is so difficult to detect and the suicide rate is so high in the elderly, routine screening has been suggested (Lesser & Banyas, 2000).

The Atypical Presentation of Common Conditions

The atypical presentation of common illnesses is a hallmark of geriatric care. Among the most common symptoms that may herald the onset of infection are cognitive changes, changes in the level of ADL or IADL abilities, decreased appetite, or sudden onset of urinary incontinence. Even those clients who are already debilitated may exhibit a measurable decline in function from baseline. The following two case studies compare the presentations of illness for a simple urinary tract infection in two females, one aged 23 years and the other 83 years. The cases contrast the clinical reasoning processes used to arrive at a diagnosis.

> CASE 1. Linda M. is a 23-year-old single female, gravida 0, who presents with a 24-hour history of severe dysuria, frequency, and urgency. Her symptoms began approximately 8 hours after sexual intercourse with her long-time male partner, with whom she has had a monogamous relationship for the past 2 years. She denies fever, flank pain, anorexia, or malaise. Last normal menstrual period began 2 weeks ago. She has been on a triphasic oral contraceptive for the past 4 years and has regular menstrual cycles every 28 days lasting 2 to 3 days without intermenstrual spotting or discharge. She denies vaginal discharge, odor, itching, or irritation. Although she has never had similar symptoms in the past, her sister has a long history of cystitis, so Linda attributes these symptoms to a urinary tract infection. She is

---

Box 20.6

Decision Support

When there is a suspicion of delirium as a cause of cognitive impairment, the Confusion Assessment Method (CAM) is the most widely used and accurate algorithm, with a sensitivity of 46% to 100% and specificity of 90% to 95% when applied by trained health-care professionals (Francis, 2000). Delirium is present if there is an acute onset and fluctuating course, plus inattention, plus either disorganized thinking or altered level of consciousness. The findings of inattention, disorganized thinking, and altered level of consciousness can be demonstrated by the MMSE plus a trained caregiver's or professional's observations.

---

otherwise in good health; does not smoke, drink alcohol, or take other drugs; and takes no medications other than her oral contraceptives and an occasional ibuprofen for headaches.

Physical signs include normal vital signs, mild suprapubic tenderness, and sensation of increased urgency with palpation over the bladder. There is no costovertebral angle tenderness. A clean-voided midstream urine sample reveals clear, straw-colored urine without obvious blood; dipstick analysis is positive for leukocyte esterase and nitrites.

CASE 2. Mrs. T. is an 83-year-old woman who has resided in a long-term care facility for the past 12 months. She has mild dementia of the Alzheimer's type; osteoporosis with a history of right femoral neck fracture status post–internal fixation and pinning 1 year ago; stage C congestive heart failure well controlled on a diuretic and a beta blocker; osteoarthritis of hands, knees, and low back; and a history of stage I breast cancer treated 10 years ago with lumpectomy and radiation. Functionally at baseline, Mrs. T. requires assistance with ADLs and IADLs and supervision for medications; she uses a walker and requires assistance to ambulate outside her room, but in her room she is able to get to the toilet or her chair by herself with her walker; she is normally continent of urine and stool with an occasional episode of enuresis; she requires assistance with bathing and grooming; her appetite is good, and she feeds herself and eats with others in the dining room; her mental status score on the Folstein mini-mental is 20/30, and she is alert, pleasant, and participates in many activities in the facility.

The nurse practitioner was called to the facility to see Mrs. T. for a sudden change in her condition, which began approximately 12 hours earlier. The nursing assistant on the evening shift reported that Mrs. T. did not eat any of her dinner and seemed more confused than usual. During the night, she was incontinent of urine three times, soaking the bed each time. When the charge nurse assessed her on rounds in the morning, Mrs. T. was very lethargic, did not know her name or where she was, could not respond appropriately to any questions, and became quite agitated when the nurse attempted to auscultate her heart and lungs. There had been no recent change in her medication regimen. Her vital signs were normal and she was afebrile. There had been no change in her weekly weights, and her bowel movements had been regular. By the time the nurse practitioner arrived to examine her, Mrs. T. was very agitated, shouting and crying out for her dead husband; she was trying to get out of her bed; she had been put in adult diapers, which were saturated with urine and stool. Her skin was warm and dry without any obvious lesions or erythema, her color was pale, and she was inconsolable and unable to respond coherently to any questions. Although the cardiac auscultation was less than ideal, the nurse practitioner did not appreciate any extra sounds or murmurs. Lung sounds were somewhat diminished at the bases bilaterally, although again, the examination was hampered by Mrs. T.'s agitation. The abdominal examination was also unremarkable.

■ Case Analysis

Nurse practitioners can feel comfortable treating a client such as Linda M. with a telephone consultation (University of Michigan Health System, 1999). Her symptoms do not suggest any complicating factors, and although the urine dipstick for leukocyte esterase is cost effective with good sensitivity (75%–96%) and specificity (94%–98%), treatment without an examination or urinalysis is an acceptable option (Gonzales & Kutner, 2003). In contrast, when faced with the situation of Mrs. T., the nurse practitioner must perform a more extensive examination, including at least a urinalysis and possibly a culture and sensitivity on a catheterized urine specimen, a complete blood count with differential, pulse oximetry if available, and possibly even a chest radiograph; blood cultures are rarely useful except in situations in which acute fulminant bacteremia is suspected (Bentley et al., 2001).

The differential diagnosis for an older client with a sudden change in condition includes infectious processes, most commonly involving the lungs, skin, and gastrointestinal or urinary tracts; cardiac decompensation; drug toxicity; fecal impaction; and occult trauma from an undocumented fall or injury. With such a varied differential, a comprehensive examination is essential, and a thorough knowledge of the client and the environment is more likely to guide the process of clinical reasoning. In the case of Mrs. T., the nurse practitioner examined the skin for obvious cellulitis; reviewed the record for changes in medication, weight, and stool pattern; and examined the heart, lungs, and abdomen for obvious signs of cardiac decompensation and pain. Armed with knowledge of the client's previous level of function and the meager clinical findings, the nurse practitioner will prioritize the differential diagnoses with the following considerations.

Although Mrs. T. has Alzheimer's disease, a sudden worsening of cognitive status or level of consciousness is not characteristic of the progression of dementia and usually indicates what is commonly called delirium. Delirium is a reversible condition frequently caused by infection (Table 20.4). According to the nurse practitioner's chart review, Mrs. T. is not on any new medications or any medications likely to cause toxicity; there is a fairly stable record of normal bowel movements, so impaction or gastroenteritis are not the likely culprits; there was no recent weight gain, which is common in worsening congestive heart failure, although another weight should be obtained to compare with the most recent one. When a client resides in an institution, the environment is a strong consideration in the analysis of the problem. In this case, there had been no recent outbreak of upper respiratory infection or influenza in the facility, so pneumonia is unlikely to be the cause. Tachypnea of greater than 25 breaths per minute, not seen in the case of Mrs. T., is one of the few physical findings with a positive predictive value (90%) for pneumonia, although pulse oximetry is helpful in absolutely ruling out pneumonia as a source of infection (Bentley et al., 2001). The physical examination did not reveal any other possible sources of sepsis, such as skin infections. The sudden onset of complete incontinence in a client who has been mostly continent could be due to either the cognitive

Table 20.4

Differentiating Dementia, Depression, and Delirium in the Elderly

Characteristic	Dementia	Depression	Delirium
Onset	Insidious	Insidious or precipitated by an event	Acute
Duration	Months–years	Months–years	Hours–days
Fluctuations	No or occasional due to stress	Some, may feel worse in the morning	Prominent with abnormal day/night cycles
Affect	Labile	Flat	Variable
Alertness	Normal or lethargic	Normal or lethargic	Highly variable from lethargy to agitation
Attention	Normal to progressively abnormal inattention	Normal to mildly distracted	Prominently abnormal, fluctuates
Orientation	Impaired but may be close to correct	Normal	Usually abnormal, may fluctuate
Memory	Abnormal	Normal	Normal when registers
Speech/language	Anomic or worse	Normal to slightly slowed	Dysarthric/misnaming
Speech content	Empty or sparse	Normal	Confused or incoherent
Perceptual	Normal to moderately abnormal	Normal	Hallucinations common

changes attendant to delirium or an infection in the urinary tract. Several urinary pathogens, most notably some of the strains of *Escherichia coli*, have a direct irritative effect on bladder mucosa and can cause incontinence.

Clinical and laboratory findings that support a diagnosis of urinary tract infection include an elevated white blood cell (WBC) count higher than $14,000/mm^3$ and/or a left shift; pyuria on the microscopic urinalysis of greater than 10 WBCs per high-power field; and/or a positive leukocyte esterase test. The absence of pyuria is equally significant in that it provides a negative predictive value approaching 100% and is therefore more useful in excluding the diagnosis of urinary tract infection (Bentley et al., 2001). Additionally, clinical practice guidelines suggest that in 77% of episodes of functional decline in long-term care residents, infection is the cause, and the most frequent site of such infection is the urinary tract (55%). Taking all of this into consideration, urinary tract infection is the most likely diagnosis for Mrs. T. at this point.

It is clear from this case analysis that a simple urinary tract infection can cause widespread and rapid physical decline in frail elders, particularly those who are institutionalized. The assessment process is much more involved and less focused when there is an atypical presentation, which is common among the elderly regardless of whether they reside in long-term care or present to the emergency room from home. Adequate treatment of the underlying infection should resolve the delirium, and the patient should return to baseline functioning.

Geriatric Syndromes

There is no commonly accepted definition or list of "geriatric syndromes." There is, however, some agreement about their common characteristics. Geriatric syndromes tend to be multifactorial in nature, have vague or atypical presentations, progress and result in frailty, and are often interrelated and display some degree of iatrogenesis or medical error. In short, they are often precipitated by a convergence of events that causes a cascade of further problems and ends in a serious change of health status. Case 2 in the preceding section is an example of the geriatric syndrome of delirium, which is precipitated by a urinary tract infection and also leads to urinary incontinence. It is not unusual for such a situation to progress rapidly to additional adverse events: a fall as the patient attempts to climb out of bed, malnutrition and dehydration owing to the loss of appetite and the presence of infection, and skin breakdown resulting from the constant presence of urine on the perineal and coccygeal areas. Many of the geriatric syndromes are adverse events that occur as a result of immobility and hospitalization or inappropriate prescribing of medications; such syndromes require systems interventions to improve or change outcomes. Among these syndromes are four—falls, delirium, pressure ulcers, and underfeeding—that have been labeled as "medical errors" because they are largely preventable in hospitalized elders (Tsilimingras, Rosen, & Berlowitz, 2003).

It is important that nurse practitioners have a basic understanding of the risk factors, causes, and clinical presentations of geriatric syndromes and routinely assess for factors that may be amenable to intervention beyond the medical issues. Prevention is particularly important in managing geriatric syndromes both in the hospitalized and in the community-residing elder. For example, falls in the home can be prevented with a thorough evaluation of any senior who reports a single fall or who demonstrates an unsteady gait; an appropriate intervention should be instituted for any problems detected.

Details of the fall provide direction for further investigation. Not only are the date, time, and location of the fall important, but also detail about what the patient was experiencing before the fall can provide important clues. Ask about the presence of dizziness, blurred vision, weakness, palpitations, and a sensation of faintness preceding the fall and an awareness or lack thereof of the sensation of falling in an effort to uncover possible medical reasons for the fall. The get up and go test is a simple screening measure that takes only minutes and can be conducted by trained staff. Instruct the patient to stand up from a seated position without using his or her arms or the chair arms for support, walk a few feet away, turn around and return to the chair, and sit down again without using any support. If the examiner observes any instability or difficulty with this test, further evaluation of gait and balance is required.

Using the example of falls again, a home safety evaluation that includes questions about lighting, clutter on floors, footwear, bathroom configuration, stairways, sidewalks, and the availability of help in the case of a fall can focus attention on areas where safety can be improved to prevent falls. A useful tool that can be completed by patients or their families is available online at the Practicing Physicians Education Project in its Falls Toolkit (http://www .gericareonline.net/tools/eng/falls). In the case of patients who have fallen frequently, a home visit by a nurse or physical therapist is very helpful to determine what risk factors are modifiable. When patients fall in hospitals or long-term care facilities, similar attention to environmental and other system factors that increase risk has been shown to reduce falls by as much as 30% (Tsilimingras, Rosen, & Berlowitz, 2003). Owing to the multifactorial nature of the risk of falling, interventions are most successful when they go beyond a simple plan to treat medical risk factors. A multidisciplinary approach that includes patient and family education, training in gait and balance, strengthening exercises, nutrition counseling, behavior modification, and elimination of environmental hazards has been found to be most successful.

Pressure ulcers are another common condition that is preventable both in the home and in institutional settings. Tissue trauma occurs when soft tissue is compressed between a bony prominence and a hard or rough surface or when shearing of the skin occurs with movement. The trauma produces visible change of the skin, ranging from a mild erythema or discoloration to deep ulceration down to bone. The important point to remember when assessing individuals who are immobile and dependent in ADLs and being cared for at home is to include the caregivers in the process. Ask about caregivers' knowledge of the importance of keeping skin clean and dry and their ability to move, transfer, and position the patient. Support for caregivers is a crucial part of geriatric care and one that is often forgotten in clinical practice. Provide links to aging services, such as respite care, caregiver support groups, and educational classes to help families cope with the burden of caregiving.

The Assessment of Physical Activity Readiness

Older adults are increasingly turning to exercise for socialization and fitness, and this trend should be supported. The question always arises: How much screening and assessment should be conducted prior to initiating an exercise program? The Canadian Society for Exercise Physiology (www.csep.ca; 2002) has developed a useful evidence-based, seven-question screening tool, the Physical Activity Readiness Questionnaire (PAR-Q) for screening adults up to age 69. The recommendation for those over age 69 who are not accustomed to being active is to consult with a health-care provider prior to initiating a formal exercise program. The questions on the PAR-Q require a yes or no response; any response of yes requires further screening by a health-care provider. There is a companion form, the PARmed-X, for the clinician to complete prior to the individual beginning a formal exercise program. The PARmed-X includes a clearance as well as suggestions for special prescriptions for conditions such as chronic obstructive pulmonary disease. There are relatively few absolute contraindications to exercise listed on the PARmed-X; they include acute infectious processes, dissecting aortic aneurysm, severe aortic stenosis, active or recent myocarditis, acute myocardial infarction or heart failure, and acute thrombotic or embolic processes. Once any acute illness is resolved, the adult should be rescreened and allowed to exercise to tolerance. These guidelines could serve as a screening tool in primary care for older adults who are just beginning an exercise program; however, it is important to remove barriers to exercise whenever possible for those who wish to begin exercising at any age.

The Assessment of Driving Safety

Most people rely on the automobile as the most convenient and efficient mode of transportation for obtaining medical services, groceries, and other necessities of life, as well as for maintaining social contacts with friends, families, and organizations, such as a church or place of employment. The need to drive might be related to a lack of public transportation as well as a sense of independence that seniors are reluctant to relinquish. The ability of an older individual to drive safely is dependent on a number of factors, which need to be considered in a comprehensive assessment of that individual. Drivers 65 years and older will account for at least 16% of all motor vehicle crashes and 25% of all fatal crashes, making unsafe driving among the elderly a significant and growing public health problem (American Medical Association [AMA], 2003).

■ General History

At least one or two questions about driving should be included in the comprehensive history of any older adult. Questions might be as simple as "Do you drive an automobile?" "Have you changed your driving patterns recently?" "Are there any situations in which you feel uncomfortable driving?" Many seniors voluntarily restrict their driving when they recognize a feeling of discomfort with, for example, driving after dark or driving on high-speed highways. In addition, families might express concerns about the ability of a senior to drive safely with such comments as "He's had a couple of 'near misses' with the car recently" or "No one will ride with her anymore because it's too scary." Comments from family members should always be addressed both with the family and the client. It is important to remember that increasing chronological age is not an indicator of an inability to drive safely.

■ Focused History

Another option is to give all older clients the questionnaire *Am I a Safe Driver?* (available at www.ama-assn.org/ama1/pub/upload/mm/433/appendixb.pdf). Positive responses can provide a starting point for a more comprehensive evaluation of driving safety. The American Medical Association (AMA) resource on safe driving contains other useful resources for practice to ensure that this issue is addressed.

Certain medical conditions or medications should be red flags to the nurse practitioner as areas for exploration of medically impaired driving. Obvious acute events include myocardial infarction, stroke, brain injury, syncope, vertigo, seizures, delirium, or recent surgery. Other chronic conditions include those that affect vision, cognition, strength, mobility, and uncontrolled diabetes mellitus. The most common offending medications are listed in Box 20.7. Any new medication has the potential to affect driving ability temporarily; thus, clients should be cautioned to restrict driving at least temporarily until the response to the new medication is known.

■ Habits

Alcohol consumption is known to impair driving ability in any driver and may be an even greater concern among the elderly. Ask specifically about the

---

Box 20.7

Medications That Might Affect Driving Ability

1. Alcohol
2. Anticholinergics
3. Anticonvulsants
4. Antidepressants
   a. Bupropion
   b. Mirtazapine
   c. Monoamine oxidase (MAO) inhibitors
   d. Selective serotonin reuptake inhibitors (SSRIs)
   e. Tricyclic antidepressants (TCAs)
5. Antiemetics
6. Antihistamines
7. Antihypertensives
8. Antiparkinsonians
9. Antipsychotics
10. Benzodiazepines and other sedatives/anxiolytics
11. Muscle relaxants
12. Narcotic analgesics
13. NSAIDs
14. Stimulants

type, quantity, and timing of drinking behavior, and verify with an independent observer if possible.

■ Physical Examination

The AMA guidelines provide useful information on appropriate physical examination techniques to validate medical recommendations about driving ability; however, the report cautions that there are currently no tests that predict crash risk. These tests focus on vision, cognition, and motor function and can be integrated into the routine examination. Begin with a general observation of the client, including appearance, gait, interactive ability, looking specifically for signs of depression, dementia, delirium, motor instability, or generalized weakness. Vision is responsible for 95% of driving-related inputs (AMA, 2003), and vision testing should at least include tests for acuity and visual fields. Although contrast sensitivity is an important factor in the ability to distinguish objects against a background, currently there are no validated clinical measures for this dimension of vision. Decreased accommodation also contributes to comfort with driving at night and is easily tested but not easily quantified.

Cognition is the most complex variable to test in the driving safety assessment. The ability to drive the car and navigate from one point to another requires many complex cognitive skills: crystallized and working memory, selective and divided attention, visual perception and processing as well as visuospatial skills, and executive skills (AMA, 2003). These skills are not adequately tested on the MMSE; therefore, supplemental tests specific to the higher executive functions are suggested, such as the clock-drawing test and the trail-making test (available at http://www.ama-assn.org/resources/doc/public-health/older-drivers-chapter3.pdf). There are specific criteria for scoring each of these additional tests as well as clear directions for their administration. Research has demonstrated that the trail-making test, part B, is a reasonable predictor of "at-fault" crashes in older drivers (Staplin et al., 2003). It is possible that a client with mild dementia on the MMSE could still score well enough on these supplemental tests to continue driving. The problem arises when the dementia progresses and those afflicted fail to recognize that they have become unsafe drivers. This usually results in family members being forced to take away the driving privilege and request the assistance of the nurse practitioner or other professionals.

Motor ability testing involves testing range of motion in the neck, motor strength in both upper limbs and the right lower limb, and trunk stability and balance. Adequate range of motion of the neck without excessive pain or hesitation is essential for checking behind and to the sides of the car. Often a client with a lack of central vision owing to macular degeneration can still drive safely if the peripheral vision is intact and the ability to turn the head quickly allows adequate scanning of the street and traffic situations. Although adequate range of motion is difficult to quantify, it is rarely the sole reason for restriction of driving. Upper limb strength is essential for steering, and the lower right limb is usually the one used for acceleration and braking. Strength should be graded on a scale of 0 to 5, with 4 to 5 signifying adequate strength against at least some resistance. Adaptive technologies in some automobiles may compensate for less than adequate strength in one or more areas. The rapid pace walk is specifically suggested (AMA, 2003) as a good predictor of driving safety. The client is timed walking as swiftly as possible along a 10-foot path marked on the floor both away from and toward the examiner. A cane can be used, but this should be noted on the chart. A completion time of greater than 9 seconds indicates a possible need for intervention.

■ Resources

Many states now have safe-driving programs for at-risk drivers that provide further testing and driver rehabilitation. Testing might include on-road tests or computerized simulations of driving situations. Some vision problems can be corrected with lenses or other medical interventions, although a referral might be needed to an ophthalmologist or low-vision specialist. Automobiles that are easier to drive, have controls in more convenient locations, have better visibility, and are fully automatic rather than manual may compensate for restricted movement and strength, allowing an elder to continue driving. Restricting driving to familiar locations, daylight hours, low-traffic situations, and good weather may also suffice in some situations. The AMA (2003) strongly recommends against the use of a "copilot" to allow unsafe drivers to continue driving, although this practice has been accepted by some state driver-licensing agencies. Even the best and most observant copilots might not have time to alert the driver to a potential hazard, and the driver might not respond quickly enough to avoid a crash.

Addressing client and family concerns about safe driving for an elderly person is one of the most common issues in clinical practice. It is incumbent on nurse practitioners to know the laws in the state where they practice regarding reporting medically unsafe drivers; reporting guidelines vary across the country. Besides reporting or referring questionably safe drivers for further evaluation, it is important to help clients and their families plan for a transition to a nondriving status because everyone who drives will stop driving one day. Make available resources, both local and national, for clients facing this dilemma (Box 20.8). Open the dialogue at every opportunity with clients and their families to monitor changes and the need for further interventions. Incorporate an awareness of the need for and an ability to accomplish an evaluation of an older person for safe driving.

Head, Eyes, Ears, Nose, and Mouth

Specific attention should be directed toward those organs that affect functional ability: the eyes, ears, and mouth directly affect one's ability to see, hear,

Box 20.8

Resources for Safe Driving

AARP 55 ALIVE Driver Safety Program
1 888 227–7669
American Automobile Association (AAA) Foundation for Traffic Safety
1 800 993–7222   *www.aaafoundation.org*
AAA Safe Driving for Mature Operators Program
Call your local AAA club to find a class near you.
National Safety Council Defensive Driving Course
1 800 621–7619
Driving School Association of the Americas, Inc.
1 800 270–3722

and eat. There are some particular points to remember when assessing these systems.

- An examination of the eyes should always include measuring ocular pressure to rule out glaucoma, which is a serious cause of blindness and is more common with aging; screening for close and distance vision, particularly when there are questions related to driving or medication-taking ability; dilating the pupil to examine the retina for macular degeneration, a common cause of blindness in the elderly; and screening for cataracts, also increasingly common with age. Referral to an optometrist or an ophthalmologist is ideal and may be covered by Medicare and other insurance depending on the diagnosis.
- Examination of the ears should include carefully inspecting and removing cerumen impactions, which are a common cause of hearing loss. In addition to the whisper test, screening with an audioscope at 40 dB and testing both ears using 1,000 and 2,000 Hz provides reasonable sensitivity (94%) and specificity (72%) in community-dwelling populations (American Geriatric Society, 2003). Referral to an audiologist is ideal; however, many seniors do not have the ability to pay for hearing aids, and in some cases hearing aids do not help with speech discrimination.
- Examination of the mouth should include a through inspection of the teeth. Ill-fitting or missing dentures and loose teeth can severely affect the ability to chew and eat sufficient food to maintain nutrition. Referral to a dentist is ideal; however, many seniors without dental insurance do not have the ability to pay for dental services or replacement dentures.

Neuromuscular System

Specific attention should be directed toward gait and mobility, which greatly affect functional ability and predict risk of falling. Beyond the usual examination of range of motion and strength, there are several specific tests to measure performance that can be incorporated into an examination.

- The timed get up and go test should be administered to all clients who have experienced a fall or who report difficulty with strenuous activities, such as fast walking, heavy housework, shopping, or climbing stairs. It is easy to perform and takes very little additional time during the examination. Place a chair in an unobstructed location and instruct client to rise from the seated position, walk 20 feet, turn, walk back to the chair, and sit down. Time this activity with a stopwatch. In populations that cannot complete the task in 15 seconds or less, research has shown a strong correlation (0.6–0.8) with other measures of gait and balance (Gerety, 2000).

- Contributors to pathologic gait include foot or joint pain, weakness, sensory impairment, bone and joint abnormalities, and an impaired neurological system. The Tinetti Performance-Oriented Mobility Assessment (POMA) scale is a more sensitive and specific test of gait, balance, and mobility (Box 20.9). The gait and mobility components of the POMA include opportunities to evaluate the initiation of gait, adequacy of step length and height, step and path symmetry and continuity, and ability to turn and pick up speed. Balance is tested by observing immediate standing balance; balance during tandem, one-leg, heel, and toe standing; and a nudge to the sternum or tug from behind. The POMA is sensitive and reproducible and can be used to measure improvement over time; thus, it is often used in clinical trials of exercise interventions.

- The functional reach test is another useful test for upper extremity function that correlates well with an increased risk for falls and dependence (Behrman et al., 2002). Give the client the following instructions: stand with your feet hip-width apart and your right (dominant) side next to but not touching a wall. Extend your right arm (or whichever is closest to the wall) parallel to the floor at shoulder height with your fingers extended. Now reach forward as far as you can, bending at the waist, but do not lift your heels off the floor. The examiner measures the distance in centimeters from the back of the shoulder to the tip of the middle finger in the "normal reach" position and again in the "forward reach" position. Differences greater than 25 cm are a significant predictor of falls and increased dependence in ADLs and IADLs.

Nutritional Assessment

Nutritional deficiencies are a prevalent problem among the elderly, ranging from 15% among community-dwelling elderly to as much as 65% among hospitalized patients. Undernourishment among institutionalized elders increases mortality rates as well as places discharged individuals at risk for serious

Box 20.9

Tinetti Balance and Gait Evaluation

Balance

Instructions: Seat the subject in a hard armless chair. Test the following maneuvers. Select one number that best describes the subject's performance in each text, and add up the scores at the end.

1. Sitting balance
   Leans or slides in chair =0
   Steady, safe =1_____
2. Arising
   Unstable without help =0
   Able but uses arms to help =1
   Able without use of arms =2_____
3. Attempt to arise
   Unable without help =0
   Able but requires more than one attempt =1
   Able to arise with one attempt =2_____
4. Immediate standing balance (first 5 seconds)
   Unsteady (staggers, moves feet, marked trunk sway) =0
   Steady but uses walker or cane or grabs other objects for support =1
   Steady without walker, cane, or other support =2_____
5. Standing balance
   Unsteady =0
   Steady but wide stance (medial heels more than 4 inches apart) =1
   or uses cane, walker, or other support
   Narrow stance without support =2_____
6. Nudging (with subject's feet as close together as possible, push
   lightly on the sternum with palm of hand three times)
   Begins to fall =0
   Staggers and grabs, but catches self =1
   Steady =2_____
7 Eyes closed (at same position in No. 6)
   Unsteady =0
   Steady =1_____
8. Turning 360 degrees
   Discontinuous steps =0
   Continuous steps =1_____
   Unsteady (grabs and staggers) =0
   Steady =1_____
9. Sitting down
   Unsafe (misjudges distance, falls into chair) =0
   Uses arms or lacks smooth motion =1
   Safe, smooth motion =2_____

GAIT

Instructions: The subject stands with the examiner, and then walks down the hallway or across the room, first at the usual pace and then back at a rapid but safe pace, using a cane or walker if accustomed to one.

10. Initiation of gait (immediately after being told to go)
    Any hesitancy or several attempts to start =0
    No hesitancy =1_____

Box 20.9

Tinetti Balance and Gait Evaluation—cont'd

11. Step length and height
    Right swing foot:
    Fails to pass left stance foot with step   =0
    Passes left stance foot   =1_____
    Fails to clear floor completely with step   =0
    Completely clears floor   =1_____
    Left swing foot:
    Fails to pass right stance foot with step   =0
    Passes right stance foot   =1_____
    Fails to clear floor completely with step   =0
    Completely clears floor   =1_____
12. Step symmetry
    Right and left step length unequal   =0
    Right and left step equal   =1_____
13. Step continuity
    Stopping or discontinuity between steps   =0
    Steps appear continuous   =1_____
14. Path (observe excursion of either left or right foot over about
    10 feet of the course)
    Marked deviation   =0
    Mild to moderate deviation or uses walking aid   =1
    Walks straight without aid   =2_____
15. Trunk
    Marked sway or uses walking aid   =0
    No sway but flexion of knees or back or spreads arms out while walking =1
    No sway, flexion, use of arms, or use of walking aid   =2_____
16. Walking stance
    Heels apart   =0
    Heels almost touching while walking   =1_____
    Balance score _____ 16   Gait score:
                                                                            _____ 12

Total score: _____ 28

Modified from Tinetti, M. (1986). Performance-oriented assessment of mobility problems in elderly patients. *Journal of the American Geriatric Society, 34,* 119–126.

malnutrition; malnutrition then predisposes the elder to frailty, dependence, and long-term care placement.

One of the key factors in tracking malnutrition is measuring and recording clients' heights and weights. Most adults overestimate their height and underestimate their weight on self-report; height is a particular problem because adults tend to lose 1 inch of height every 20 years after age 35 to 40. Measurement of standing height is difficult if there is any degree of kyphosis (underestimates the actual height). The following are some tips to ensure accurate height and weight measures in difficult situations.

• Ask the client to stand with his or her head flat against the wall; the lower border of the eye should be aligned with the upper opening of the auditory canal (the Frankfurt plane). If the head does not touch wall, measure and record that distance to estimate the degree of kyphosis.

- Estimates of actual adult height can be made with either a wingspan or knee-to-heel measurement. For the wingspan method, measure from the center of the sternum to the tip of the middle finger with the arm extended straight and supported at a 90-degree angle from the body. Take two measurements and use the average if there is a difference. To measure knee height, have the client seated on a straight chair, with hips, knees, and ankles at a 90-degree angle, which you can check with a goniometer if necessary. Measure (in centimeters) from the top of the knee to the bottom of the heel with a rigid tape measure or large wooden calipers, if available. Trunk-to-limb proportion varies by gender, ethnicity, and race; however, the following formulas for whites have been validated with larger northern Europeans as well as smaller southern Europeans.

$$\text{Males} = (2.02 \times \text{knee ht.}) - (0.04 \times \text{age}) + 64.19$$
$$\text{Females} = (1.83 \times \text{knee ht.}) - (0.24 \times \text{age}) + 84.88$$

- Obtain an accurate weight, and make sure the scale is calibrated. For residents of long-term care facilities, always use the same scale for the same patient and, if there is a change in scale, make sure to note that beside the weight. Document what the patient is wearing, and always weigh in that same state. Significant weight loss is a quality indicator measure, and a pattern of weight loss in any facility will trigger an investigation by state and federal regulatory agencies. Ask the patient's usual body weight if possible. Calculate ideal body weight using the same formula as for any other population.
- Once you have obtained an accurate height and weight, calculate the body mass index (BMI). For amputees, add the following percentages of the weight obtained on the scale prior to calculating the BMI: below knee 6%, at knee 9%, above knee 15%, arm 6.5%, arm below elbow 3.6%. The formula for calculating BMI is the same for the elderly as for any other population. A BMI of less than 21 or a total body weight of less than 100 pounds is an indicator of a high risk for protein–energy malnutrition.
- Useful laboratory measures that indicate protein–energy malnutrition or potentially poor outcomes in hospitalized elders include a serum albumin level below 3.4 g/dL and total cholesterol below 160 mg/dL.
- Nutrition screening can be accomplished by asking clients to complete diet records or food frequency questionnaires or by screening for other risk factors, such as those in the Nutrition Screening Initiative (Box 20.10). The Nutrition Screening Initiative (2005) is appropriately used with well elderly and provides a screening tool with support documentation online (http://www .ncbi.nlm.nih.gov/pmc/articles/PMC1694757/pdf/amjph00531-0046.pdf). For residents in long-term care facilities, the Mini Nutritional Assessment is the best validated instrument for screening; it is available at http://mna-elderly.com/ along with supporting documentation.
- Although a lot of attention is devoted to undernutrition, obesity, defined as a BMI of greater than 30, or 20% greater than ideal body weight, is also an independent risk factor for functional decline in the elderly. Women have a

Box 20.10

Nutritional Screening Tool

The Warning Signs of poor nutritional health are often overlooked. Use this Checklist to find out if you or someone you know is at nutritional risk.

Read the statements below. Circle the number in the Yes column for those that apply to you or someone you know. For each "yes" answer, score the number in the box. Total your nutritional score.

DETERMINE YOUR NUTRITIONAL HEALTH

	YES
I have an illness or condition that made me change the kind and/or amount of food I eat.	2
I eat fewer than 2 meals per day.	3
I eat few fruits or vegetables or milk products.	2
I have 3 or more drinks of beer, liquor, or wine almost every day.	2
I have tooth or mouth problems that make it hard for me to eat.	2
I don't always have enough money to buy the food I need.	4
I eat alone most of the time.	1
I take three or more different prescribed or over-the-counter drugs a day.	1
Without wanting to, I have lost or gained 10 pounds in the last 6 months.	2
I am not always physically able to shop, cook, and/or feed myself.	2
TOTAL	

Total your nutritional score. If it's

0–2   **Good! Recheck** your nutritional score in 6 months.

3–5   **You are at moderate nutritional risk.** See what can be done to improve your eating habits and lifestyle. Your office on aging, senior nutrition program, senior citizens center or health department can help. Recheck your nutritional score in 3 months.

6 or more   **You are at high nutritional risk.** Bring this Checklist the next time you see your doctor, dietitian, or other qualified health or social service professional. Talk with them about any problems you may have. Ask for help to improve your nutritional health.

Remember that warning signs suggest risk, but do not represent a diagnosis of any condition. Turn the page to learn more about the Warnings Signs of poor nutritional health.

These materials are developed and distributed by the Nutrition Screening Initiative, a project of:

■ AMERICAN ACADEMY OF FAMILY PHYSICIANS

■ THE AMERICAN DIETETIC ASSOCIATION

■ THE NATIONAL COUNCIL ON THE AGING, INC.

The Nutrition Screening Initiative • 1010 Wisconsin Avenue, NW • Suite 800 • Washington, DC 20007
The Nutrition Screening Initiative is funded in part by a grant from Ross Products Division of Abbott Laboratories. Inc.

higher prevalence of functional decline than men at the upper end of the BMI categories (three times greater risk at a BMI of greater than 35), independent of the usual factors, such as depression and polypharmacy (Jensen & Friedmann, 2002).

- Dehydration is common in the elderly and has serious consequences. The average fluid intake for community-dwelling elderly persons is less than 1,000 mL per day. Thirst is not a reliable indicator of the need for fluids, and most elderly individuals need reminders to drink fluids. The best method for monitoring hydration status is with the BUN/creatinine ratio; anything greater than 20:1 is highly suggestive of dehydration.
- The prevalence of constipation is about 30% among the elderly regardless of their state of health. The type and amount of food and fluids strongly influences the occurrence of constipation among the elderly. Additionally, the elderly are very likely to take laxatives; routine laxative use occurs with more than 50% of residents of long-term care facilities. With a decrease in gastrointestinal motility and fluid intake, a tendency to eat easily digestible foods (i.e., less fibrous), and the common use of medications that are constipating, special attention should be directed toward the prevention of constipation. Besides causing great discomfort, constipation can lead to fecal impaction, which can be life threatening.

Advance Care Planning

Discussions about clients' preferences for limits on medical intervention should be initiated long before clients become incapable of making their wishes known; such discussions should also be a routine part of primary care practice (Agency for Healthcare Research and Quality, 2003). All states recognize and provide guidelines for some type of official document that outlines an individual's care preferences. Nurse practitioners should become familiar with these documents and make them available to their clients or provide referrals to a service that can facilitate this process. Most of the time, clients make these decisions with their family members; however, it is not uncommon for families to disagree over the details of a plan. For nurse practitioners who care for residents of long-term care facilities, family discussions and case conferences are a useful way to resolve issues of disagreement.

In order to make good decisions, clients need to feel comfortable asking questions about death, dying, and medical interventions. They also need to be assured that having an advance care directive does not mean they will be abandoned by the health-care team. Decisions reached at any point are never irreversible; in fact, advance care decisions should be revisited at least annually and whenever a significant change in the client's or the family's condition has occurred. Nurse practitioners can play a significant role in educating clients and their families about the realities of cardiopulmonary resuscitation, tube feedings, artificial ventilation, and other invasive procedures by giving factual and unhurried explanations. Most people have only seen optimal outcomes after

Box 20.11	

Decision Support Box

Murphy and colleagues (1994) interviewed 287 elderly patients (mean age, 77 years) in a geriatrics practice about their wishes to undergo CPR following a cardiac arrest during an acute illness. Before learning the facts about the probability of survival to discharge for elderly patients, 41% opted for CPR. After learning the probability of survival (10%–17%), only 22% opted for CPR; of that number, only 6% over age 85 would choose to undergo CPR in the same conditions. Using a scenario of having a chronic illness and choosing CPR when there was a life expectancy of 1 year or less, only 11% opted for CPR before learning the probability of survival to discharge after CPR declines to 0% to 5%; after the discussion, the number decreased to 5%. Prognostic information, when given during a discussion of decisions related to end-of-life choices, has a significant influence on elders' decisions.

heroic efforts at resuscitation portrayed in the media; the realities of likely or average outcomes need to be addressed in order for individuals to make decisions consonant with their own values and wishes.

Conclusion

The assessment of older individuals requires a thorough understanding of physiology, awareness of the client's environment, good communication skills, avoidance of ageist thinking, and good critical thinking ability—plus time and patience. It is often the lack of time that leads to problems. Sufficient time to perform some of the additional tests of functional ability, as well as time to talk with family and caregivers, is optimal. Ideally, home assessments can be made in cases of a concern about safety and the ability to function independently. A multidisciplinary team approach facilitates management of complex situations and affords families and their elders the best opportunities for maximizing health and quality of life.

REFERENCES

Agency for Healthcare Research and Quality. (2003). "Advance Care Planning: Preferences for Care at the End of Life." *Research in Action*, Issue 12. AHRQ Publication Number 03–0018. www.ahrq.gov/research/endliferia/endria.htm (accessed March 21, 2011).

Alessi, C. (2000). Sleep. In Osterweil, D., Brummel-Smith, K., & Beck, J. (Eds.), *Comprehensive Geriatric Assessment*. New York: McGraw-Hill.

American Geriatrics Society. (2003). "Geriatrics at Your Fingertips." www.geriatricsatyourfingertips. org (accessed March 21, 2011).

American Medical Association. (2003). "Physician's Guide to Assessing and Counseling Older Drivers." http://www.ama-assn.org/ama/pub/physician-resources/public-health/ promoting-healthy-lifestyles/geriatric-health/older-driver-safety/assessing-counseling-older-drivers.page (accessed March 21, 2011).

Ashla, M. (2000). Cognitive function, mood, and behavior assessments. In Osterweil, Brummel-Smith, & Beck, *Comprehensive Geriatric Assessment.*

Behrman, A., Light, K., Flynn, S., & Thigpen, M. (2002). Is the functional reach test useful for identifying falls risk among individuals with Parkinson's disease? *Archives of Physical Medicine and Rehabilitation, 83*(4), 538–542.

Bentley, D., Bradley, S., High, K., Schoenbaum, S., Taler, G., & Yoshikawa, T. (2001). Practice guideline for evaluation of fever and infection in long-term care facilities. *Journal of the American Medical Directors Association, 2*(5), 246–258.

Blair, K. (1990). Aging: Physiological aspects and clinical implications. *Nurse Practitioner, 15*(2), 14–16, 18, 23, 26–28.

Canadian Society for Exercise Physiology (2002). Physical activity readiness questionnaire (PAR-Q). www.csep.ca (accessed March 16, 2011).

Cotter, V., & Strumpf, N. (2002). *Advanced Practice Nursing with Older Adults: Clinical Guidelines.* New York: McGraw-Hill.

Francis, J. (2000). Delirium. In Osterweil, Brummel-Smith, & Beck, *Comprehensive Geriatric Assessment.*

Gerety, M. (2000). Health status and physical capacity. In Osterweil, Brummel-Smith, & Beck, *Comprehensive Geriatric Assessment.*

Gonzales, R., & Kutner, J. (2003). *Current Practice Guidelines in Primary Care.* New York: Lange Medical Books.

Harvan, J., & Cotter, V. (2006) An evaluation of dementia screening in the primary care setting. *Journal of the American Academy of Nurse Practitioners, 18*(8), 351–360.

Jensen, G., & Friedmann, J. (2002). Obesity is associated with functional decline in community-dwelling rural older persons. *Journal of the American Geriatrics Society, 50,* 918–923.

Lesser, I., & Banyas, C. (2000). Depression. In Osterweil, Brummel-Smith, & Beck, *Comprehensive Geriatric Assessment.*

Manos, P. (1994). The ten point clock test: A quick screen and grading method for cognitive impairment in medical and surgical patients. *International Journal of Psychiatry in Medicine, 24*(3), 229–244.

Mendez, M., Ala, T., & Underwood, K. (1992). Development of scoring criteria for the clock drawing task in Alzheimer's disease. *Journal of the American Geriatrics Society, 40*(11), 1095–1099.

Murphy, D., Burrows, D., Santilli, S., Kemp, A., Tenner, S., Kreling, B., et al. (1994). The influence of the probability of survival on patients' preferences regarding cardiopulmonary resuscitation. *New England Journal of Medicine, 330*(8), 545–549.

National Institute on Aging (2003). The measurement of physical functioning in older adult populations. Report of meeting held on December 12, 2003.

Nutrition Screening Initiative. (n.d.). http://www.ncbi.nlm.nih.gov/pmc/articles/PMC1694757/pdf/amjph00531-0046.pdf (accessed March 21, 2011).

Powlishta, K., Von Dras, D., Stanford, A., Carr, D., Tsering, C., Miller, J., & Morris,, J. (2002). The clock drawing test is a poor screen for very mild dementia. *Neurology, 59,* 898–903.

Practicing Physicians Education in Geriatrics (2003). Toolkits. http://www.gericareonline.net/tools/index.html (accessed March 21, 2011).

Rouleau, I., Salmon, D., & Butters, N. (1996). Longitudinal analysis clock drawing in Alzheimer's disease patients. *Brain and Cognition, 31*(1), 17–34.

Staplin, L., Lococo, K., Gish, K., & Decina, L. (2003). *Model Driver Screening and Evaluation Program: Final Technical Report Volume II: Maryland Pilot Older Driver Study.* Department of Transportation and Highway Safety, Document # 809 583. www.nhtsa.dot.gov/people/injury/olddrive/modeldriver/2_chap_4a.htm (accessed March 21, 2011).

Sunderland, T., Hill, J., Mellow, A., Lawlor, B., Gundershelmer, J., Newhouse, P., & Grafman, J. (1989). Clock drawing in Alzheimer's disease: A novel measure of dementia severity. *Journal of the American Geriatrics Society, 37*(8), 725–729.

Tsilimingras, D., Rosen, A., & Berlowitz, D. (2003). Patient safety in geriatrics: A call for action. *Journals of Gerontology: Medical Sciences, 58A*(9), 813–819.

University of Michigan Health System. (1999). "UTI in Adult Women: Diagnosis and Management." http://cme.med.umich.edu/pdf/guideline/UTI.pdf (accessed March 21, 2011).

U.S. Preventive Services Task Force. (2003). "Screening for Dementia: Recommendation and Rationale." Retrieved from National Guidelines Clearinghouse. http://www.uspreventiveservicestaskforce.org/3rduspstf/dementia/dementrr.htm (accessed March 21, 2011).

Index

A

α₁-antitrypsin deficiency, 34
Abdomen
  abnormalities, 246–248
  differential diagnosis of chief complaints, 249–295
  history of patient, 243–244
  laboratory values for, 251
  pediatric patients, assessment of, 538–539
  physical examination, 244–249
  red flags, 539
  regions, 244, 245
Abdominal pain, 249–250
  differentiating types of, 252
  epigastric, 259–261
  history of patient, 251–252, 260, 263–264
  laboratory studies, 254–255, 266
  left upper quadrant, 258–259
  pelvic, 270–271
  physical examination for, 252, 258, 260–261, 264
  in pregnancy, 575–576
  red flags, 250
  right and left lower quadrant, 263–270
  right upper quadrant, 250–258
  suprapubic, 270–271
Abducens nerve, 546
Abortions, 568, 589
Abscesses
  brain, 463–464
  peritonsillar, 156–157
Abstract thoughts, 452
Acanthosis nigracans, 61
Accessory nerve, 546
Accutane, 511
Ace inhibitor-induced cough, 217
Achalasia, 85, 88
Achilles tendonitis, 447
Achondroplasia, 32
Acne vulgaris, 55
Acoustic nerve, 135–136, 546
Acoustic neuroma, 135–136, 475
Actinic keratoses, 56
Activities of daily living (ADLs), 600, 605, 606–608
Acute bronchitis, 215
Acute closed-angle glaucoma, 93, 94, 103
Acute otitis media (AOM), 127, 533
  with perforation, 131
Acute rheumatic fever, 423
Addiction, 517
Addison's disease, 49, 479, 484–485
Adenovirus, 274, 279
ADHD. See Attention deficit-hyperactivity disorder (ADHD)
Adhesive capsulitis, 435
Adnexa, 376
Adolescents
  anticipatory guidance and safety, 565
  bipolar disorder in, 513
  communication with, 531
  development milestones in, 554, 556
  eating disorders in, 518–519
  nutrition, assessment of, 560–561
Adrenal dysfunction, 401, 484–485
Adrenocorticosteroids, 45

Adrenocorticotropic hormone (ACTH), 45, 308
Advance care planning, 601, 630–631
Affect, 503
Affected, 13
Afterload, 197
Aging. See also Older patients
  demographics of, 599–600
  eyes and, 114
  physiology of, 602, 603–604
Airway obstruction, 221
Alanine aminotransferase (ALT), 254
Albinism, 49
Albumin, 255
Albuterol, 506
Alcohol abuse, 180, 518
Alcohol dependence, 518
Alcohol use, 70, 71, 81
  breast disorders and, 227
  driving ability and, 621–622
  pancreatitis and, 180
Aldosterone, 484
Alertness, 503
Algorithms, 7
Alignment, eye, 95
Alkaline phosphatase, 255
Allergic reactions
  conjunctivitis, 106–107
  facial swelling and, 77, 78
  fever and, 494–495
Allergies, 144
Allopurinol, 47
Alpha-thalassemia, 25
ALT. See Alanine aminotransferase (ALT)
Altered mental status, 467–472
Alzheimer's disease, 35, 471, 472
Amaurosis fugax, 93, 103–104
Amebic dysentery, parasitic, 280
Amenorrhea, 376–377, 399, 400–403
Amylase, 178, 255
Amyotrophic lateral sclerosis, 490–491
Anabolic steroid use, 369
Analgesic rebound headache, 466
Anatomic abnormality, in genitourinary system, 326
Androgens, 484
Andropause, 367
Anemia, 49, 221, 479
  fatigue and, 481–482
  hemolytic, 291
  in pregnancy, 583–585
Aneuploidy, 28–29
Aneurysms
  aortic, 179, 248
  thoracic, 179
Angina, 74, 178
Angioedema, 78
Angiomas, 63
Ankle pain, 446–448
Ankle-brachial index (ABI), 203–204
Ankylosing spondylitis, 431
Anorexia nervosa, 518, 519–520
Anovulation, 399
Anterior chamber, of eye, 95
Anterior cruciate ligament (ACL), 442

R